OXFORD MEDICAL PUBLICATIONS

Oxford Handbook of Practical Drug Therapy

Oxford Handbooks

Oxford Handbook of Clinical Medicine 6/e
Oxford Handbook of Clinical Specialties 6/e
Oxford Handbook of Accident and Emergency Medicine 2/e
Oxford Handbook of Acute Medicine 2/e
Oxford Handbook of Anaesthesia
Oxford Handbook of Applied Dental Sciences
Oxford Handbook of Clinical and Laboratory Investigation
Oxford Handbook of Clinical Dentistry 3/e
Oxford Handbook of Clinical Genetics
Oxford Handbook of Clinical Haematology 2/e
Oxford Handbook of Clinical Immunology
Oxford Handbook of Clinical Surgery 2/e
Oxford Handbook of Critical Care
Oxford Handbook of Dental Patient Care
Oxford Handbook of Dialysis 2/e
Oxford Handbook of Endocrinology and Diabetes
Oxford Handbook of General Practice
Oxford Handbook of Obstetrics and Gynaecology
Oxford Handbook of Oncology
Oxford Handbook of Operative Surgery
Oxford Handbook of Palliative Care
Oxford Handbook of Patients' Welfare
Oxford Handbook of Practical Drug Therapy
Oxford Handbook of Psychiatry
Oxford Handbook of Public Health Practice
Oxford Handbook of Rehabilitation Medicine
Oxford Handbook of Rheumatology
Oxford Handbook of Tropical Medicine 2/e

Oxford Handbook of Practical Drug Therapy

Duncan Richards

Clinical Lecturer in Clinical Pharmacology,
Department of Clinical Pharmacology,
University of Oxford,
UK

Jeffrey Aronson

Clinical Reader in Clinical Pharmacology,
Department of Clinical Pharmacology,
University of Oxford,
UK

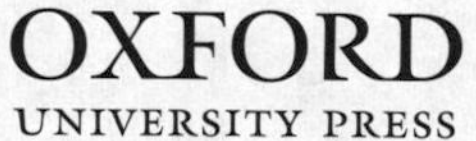

OXFORD
UNIVERSITY PRESS

Great Clarendon Street, Oxford OX2 6DP

Oxford University Press is a department of the University of Oxford. It furthers the University's objective of excellence in research, scholarship, and education by publishing worldwide in

Oxford New York

Auckland Cape Town Dar es Salaam Hong Kong Karachi Kuala Lumpur Madrid Melbourne Mexico City Nairobi New Delhi Shanghai Taipei Toronto

With offices in

Argentina Austria Brazil Chile Czech Republic France Greece Guatemala Hungary Italy Japan South Korea Poland Portugal Singapore Switzerland Thailand Turkey Ukraine Vietnam

Oxford is a registered trade mark of Oxford University Press in the UK and in certain other countries

Published in the United States
by Oxford University Press Inc., New York

First published 2005

Reprinted 2005 (with corrections), 2006

A catalogue record for this title is available from the British Library

ISBN 0-19-853007-2 ISBN-13 978-0-19-853007-7

10 9 8 7 6 5 4 3

Typeset by Cepha Imaging Pvt Ltd

Printed in China
on acid-free paper by
Phoenix Offset

Contents

Detailed contents

Abbreviations

Not all these abbreviations are internationally recognized and recommended, but they have been included because they are used commonly.

Ab	Antibody
ABC	Airways, breathing, circulation (resuscitation)
ABG	Arterial blood gas(es)
ACE	Angiotensin converting enzyme
ACh	Acetylcholine
AChE	Acetylcholinesterase
ACTH	Adrenocorticotrophic hormone
ADH	Antidiuretic hormone (vasopressin)
ADP	Adenosine diphosphate
AF	Atrial fibrillation
AIDS	Acquired immunodeficiency syndrome (due to infection with HIV)
ALP	Alkaline phosphatase
AlT	Alanine transaminase (aminotransferase)
ANA	Antinuclear antibody
ANF	Antinuclear factor
APTT	Activated partial thromboplastin time
ARB	Angiotensin receptor antagonist (blocker)
AsT	Aspartate transaminase (aminotransferase)
BCG	Bacille Calmette–Guérin (see vaccines)
bd (bid)	Twice daily (bis [in] die)
BMI	Body mass index
BNF	British National Formulary
BP	Blood pressure
BPH	Benign prostatic hyperplasia
CA	Carbonic anhydrase
CD4	Cell surface marker for T-helper lymphocytes
CK	Creatine kinase
CMV	Cytomegalovirus
CNS	Central nervous system
COMT	Catechol-o-methyl transferase
COPD/COAD	Chronic obstructive pulmonary (airways) disease
COX	Cyclo-oxygenase
CPAP	Continuous positive airways pressure
CRP	C-reactive protein
CSF	Cerebrospinal fluid
CSM	Committee on Safety of Medicines
CT	Computed tomography

CVP	Central venous pressure
CVS	Cardiovascular system
CXR	Chest X-ray (radiograph)
CYP	Cytochrome P450 isoenzyme
DC	Direct current
DKA	Diabetic ketoacidosis
DMARD	Disease-modifying antirheumatic drug
DNA	Deoxyribonucleic acid
DVLA	Driver and Vehicle Licensing Agency (UK)
DVT	Deep vein thrombosis
EBV	Epstein–Barr virus
ECG/EKG	Electrocardiogram
ED	Erectile dysfunction
EEG	Electroencephalogram
EMEA	European Medicines Evaluation Agency (Regulatory Authority)
ESR	Erythrocyte sedimentation rate
FDA	Food and Drugs Administration (USA)
FEV	Forced expiratory volume
FSH	Follicle stimulating hormone
FVC	Forced vital capacity
G6PD	Glucose 6-phosphate dehydrogenase
GABA	Gamma aminobutyric acid
GnRH	Gonadorelin releasing hormone
GP	General practitioner (UK)
HAART	Highly active antiretroviral treatment
Hb	Haemoglobin
HDL	High-density lipoprotein
HIV	Human immunodeficiency virus
HONK	Hyperosmolar non-ketotic coma (non-ketotic hyperglycaemia)
HPA	Hypothalamic/pituitary/adrenal
HRT	Hormone replacement therapy
HSV	Herpesvirus
HT	Hypertension
ICP	Intracranial pressure
Ig	Immunoglobulin
INR	International normalized ratio (see warfarin)
IR	Immediate-release (formulation of a drug)
ITU/ICU	Intensive therapy (care) unit
LDL	Low-density lipoprotein
LEMS	Lambert–Eaton myasthenic syndrome
LH	Luteinizing hormone
LMWH	Low molecular weight heparins
LOC	Loss of consciousness
MAB	Monoclonal antibody

MAOI	Monoamine oxidase inhibitor
MDI	Metered-dose inhaler
MHRA	Medicines and Healthcare Products Regulatory Agency (UK)
MR	Modified-release (formulation of a drug)
MRI	Magnetic resonance imaging
NHS	National Health Service (UK)
NICE	National Institute of Clinical Excellence (UK)
NNRTI	Non-nucleoside reverse transcriptase inhibitor (used to treat HIV)
NRTI	Nucleoside reverse transcriptase inhibitor (used to treat HIV)
NSAID	Non-steroidal anti-inflammatory drug
NYHA	New York Heart Association (heart failure rating scale)
od	Once daily (omni die)
PCA	Patient-controlled analgesia
PE	Pulmonary embolus/embolism
PEFR	Peak expiratory flow rate
PG	Prostaglandin
PI	Protease inhibitor (used to treat HIV)
pINN	Proposed International Non-proprietary Name
$PPAR_{\gamma}$	Peroxisome proliferator activated receptor
PPI	Proton pump inhibitor
prn	When required (pro re nata)
PT	Prothrombin time
PTCA	Percutaneous transluminal coronary angioplasty
qds	Four times daily (quater die sumendus)
RA	Rheumatoid arthritis
rINN	Recommended International Non-proprietary Name
RNA	Ribonucleic acid
R_x	Prescription sign (derived from the sign of the 'Eye of Horus')
SA	Sinoatrial
SIADH	Syndrome of inappropriate ADH secretion
SSRI	Selective serotonin reuptake inhibitor
stat	Immediately
SVT	Supraventricular tachycardia
TB	Tuberculosis
TCA	Tricyclic antidepressant drug
tds	Three times daily (ter die sumendus)
TIA	Transient ischaemic attack
TNF	Tumour necrosis factor
TPA	Tissue plasminogen activator
TSH	Thyroid stimulating hormone
UC	Ulcerative colitis
VF	Ventricular fibrillation
VT	Ventricular tachycardia

VTE	Venous thromboembolism
VZIG	*Varicella zoster* immunoglobulin
VZV	*Varicella zoster* virus
WHO	World Health Organization
ZIG	Zoster-immune globulin

How to use this book

The overall structure of this handbook is similar to that of the *British National Formulary*; it is arranged broadly by therapeutic category. When a drug has several different uses, these are brought together in a single article (e.g. lidocaine is used as an antiarrhythmic drug and as a local anaesthetic); this will allow the reader to appreciate its full range of actions, whether therapeutic or adverse.

This is not a textbook of pharmacology, but the safe and effective use of medicines requires a sound knowledge of pharmacology. When a drug illustrates a particular pharmacological principle, this is expanded on in the 'teaching point' section at the end of an article. As readers use the book, they will increase their basic knowledge in this practical way.

A 'cookbook' approach to drug therapy is inappropriate, since each prescription constitutes an individual experiment in that patient. However, the text includes boxes giving guidance on the approach to therapy of specific diseases and clinical problems (e.g. the treatment of gout and the symptomatic treatment of vomiting). In some cases, algorithms for the treatment of clinical emergencies are also given (e.g. hypoglycaemia, cardiac arrest).

- A box at the start of each article gives a graphical representation of the pharmacological actions of the drug.
- This section gives a list of the potential uses of the drug. When these are specialized or unlicensed, this is indicated. If NICE or other national bodies have issued guidance on the use of that drug, this is included (see *www.nice.org.uk*).
- The contraindications and cautions section is intended to be read before the drug is prescribed. It gives guidance on patients for whom the drug may not be suitable or in whom the dosage may need to be adjusted.
- The how to use section gives practical advice on the use of the drug for its major indications. Unusual or specialized uses may not be covered in detail.
- In contrast to many other sources, in which adverse effects of drugs are often given as a long, exhaustive list, this section gives the most common and most serious adverse effects. Whenever possible, this will include incidence information and the mechanism of the effect. Advice is also given on ways of avoiding or mitigating adverse effects.
- Drug interactions are important; for each drug, the major drug–drug interactions are listed. Metabolism interactions are the most common, but other types are also included.
- Monitoring for the therapeutic and adverse effects of drug therapy is essential for successful treatment. The monitoring section gives practical advice on measures of efficacy for the drug and how to detect adverse effects.
- The patient information section provides advice of particular importance to the patient (e.g. the effect of the drug on ability to drive).

  The prescribing section gives limited prescribing information for the most commonly used drugs and formulations. Specialized uses are not usually covered.

Introductory sections

Contents

Writing a prescription

Before writing a prescription, review the patient's drug therapy, even if you are rewriting a drug chart in hospital. Ask yourself the following questions:

- How will the new drug fit in with the existing therapy for this disease?
  - Will it add to symptom relief?
  - Will it modify the pathophysiology of the disease?
  - Will it prevent the disease or its progression?
- Will the drug have an effect on any other diseases?
  - Diuretics given for heart failure can worsen gout; beta-blockers can precipitate and worsen asthma.
- Will the drug interact with any other drugs that the patient is taking? Remember:
  - Drugs prescribed by others (doctors, nurses, pharmacists)
  - Over-the-counter drugs including herbal remedies and other non-prescribed drugs

Practical prescription writing

Prescribers are encouraged to use recommended International Non-proprietary Names (rINN); proprietary names can cause confusion. See p. 179 for more information on drug names. Do not use abbreviations or acronyms (e.g. GTN for glyceryl trinitrate)

- **State the dose**
  - mg and mL can be used
  - Write 'micrograms' out in full (µg is not acceptable, it can be confused with mg)
  - Use the word 'units' (do not use U or Θ, these can be confused with a zero)
  - Whenever possible, avoid decimal points — if they are unclear the dose can be misinterpreted (e.g. .5 mL looks like 5 mL). When a decimal is required, put in a zero (e.g. 0.5 mL).
- **State the route**

The following abbreviations are generally recognized:

po	by mouth
im	intramuscularly
iv	intravenously
sc	subcutaneously

- **State the frequency of administration (dosage interval)**

The following abbreviations are commonly used; some are from Latin:

od	once daily
bd	twice daily
tds	three times daily
qds	four times daily
prn	when required (state a maximum daily dose)
stat	immediately

- **Give special instructions if necessary**
  - Dietary instructions (e.g. take with food)
  - When to take the drug (e.g. at night)
- **Sign and date the prescription**

N.B. prescriptions for controlled drugs—see opioids article (p. 672) for information.

Repeat prescriptions

- Many drug treatments need to be taken long-term and will therefore require a repeat prescription.
- About 75% of all prescriptions issued by GPs are repeat prescriptions. Computer systems have made the practicalities of issuing a repeat prescription easier, but before doing so consider the following:
  - Is long-term treatment required or justified (e.g. corticosteroids, antidepressants, benzodiazepines)? Each of these should be given for a defined period with a clinical review at the end. See individual articles for more information.
  - The duration of each repeat prescription should be no longer than 3 months. All long-term therapy should be reviewed with the patient in person at least once a year.
  - Take the opportunity to review all the patient's medication. Computer systems can alert you to possible drug–drug interactions, but consider drug–disease interactions as well.
  - Ask whether you have clear targets for the patient's treatment, and whether the drug regimen is optimal.
- If you are discharging a patient from hospital, make clear which drugs should be continued long-term and whether any further dose titration is required.

'Off-licence' drugs

- Drugs are commonly prescribed outside the terms of their product licence (e.g. in children or for an unlicenced indication). An unlicensed drug does not have a licence for human use for any indication or age group (in that country). An unlicensed drug should only be used under certain circumstances:
    - As part of a clinical trial.
    - When it has been imported from a country where it does have a licence.
    - When it has been prepared extemporaneously (e.g. a specialist dermatological mixed formulation for topical use; a mixture of a corticosteroid and local anaesthetic for injection into a joint).
    - When it is prepared under a special licence (e.g. a liquid formulation for patients with difficulty in swallowing; a reduced-dose formulation for children).
    - When the licence has been suspended, revoked, or not renewed, but the product is made available for named patients under specific circumstances (e.g. thalidomide is used for the treatment of multiple myeloma, leprosy, HIV infection).
    - If the drug is not considered a medicine but is used to treat a rare condition (e.g. a rare metabolic disease).

Practical advice

- Tell the patient that the drug is being used off-licence and why you think that it is appropriate to use the drug. This is important both from the medico-legal point of view and because the patient information leaflet may not make sense to the patient if the drug is used off-licence.
- Off-licence prescribing should usually be limited to consultant-level specialists familiar with all the alternatives and prevailing expert opinion. In some circumstances it may be appropriate to continue this prescribing in primary care, but this should always be by mutual agreement.

Cautionary and advisory labels

- Most medicines are dispensed by pharmacists. They will always label a medicine with essential details (the name of the medicine, the dose, and the frequency of administration), and in some cases will add cautionary and advisory labels.
- Standard labels offer advice but are not exhaustive. Remember that labels are not a substitute for adequate counselling by prescribers and dispensers but are intended to reinforce essential information.
- Recommended label wording can offer advice about:
  - Timing of doses in relation to food.
  - Completing the course of treatment.
  - What to do if a dose is missed.
  - The correct storage of a medicine.
  - Dissolution of the medicine in water before taking it.
  - Limits to the number of tablets that should be taken in a given time.
- Recommended label wording can offer warnings about:
  - Effects of the medicine on driving or work (e.g. through drowsiness).
  - Foods or medicines that should be avoided.
  - Avoidance of exposure of the skin to sunlight or sun lamps.
  - Medicines that can discolour the urine.
  - Medicines that can stain clothes or skin.

The World Health Organization (WHO) essential medicines list

- The original 1977 WHO definition of essential medicines was that they were 'of utmost importance, basic, indispensable, and necessary for the healthcare needs of the population'. The difficulty of putting this into practice is reflected in the rather longer and more categorical 2002 definition: 'Essential medicines are those that satisfy the priority healthcare needs of the population. They are selected with due regard to public health relevance, evidence on safety and efficacy, and comparative cost-effectiveness. Essential medicines are intended to be available within the context of functioning healthcare systems, at all times, in adequate amounts, in the appropriate dosage forms, with assured quality and adequate information, and at a price the individual and the community can afford. The implementation of the concept of essential medicines is intended to be flexible and adaptable to many different situations; exactly which medicines are regarded as essential remains a national responsibility.'
- The constituents of the list remain controversial. The list is divided into two sections:
  - Core medicines that are efficacious, safe, and cost-effective medicines for priority conditions.
  - Medicines that are efficacious, safe, and cost effective, but that are not necessarily affordable, or for which specialized healthcare services are required.
- Cost effectiveness is difficult to define and is the subject of fierce debate between producers and purchasers of drugs.
- The number of drugs on the list has nearly doubled, from 186 in 1977 to 320 in 2002. The range has increased substantially over the years and now includes antimigraine drugs, antidotes, and antineoplastic drugs. The list is important because it forms the basis of national drug policies in many countries, both developed and developing (e.g. South Africa, Eritrea).
- For more information: see http://www.who.int/medicines/

Compliance, adherence, and concordance

- It has been estimated that about half of those for whom medicines are prescribed do not take them in the recommended way. Until recently this was termed non-compliance, which was sometimes regarded as a manifestation of irrational behaviour or wilful failure to observe instructions, although forgetfulness is probably a more common reason. We prefer to talk about adherence to a regimen rather than compliance. There are many reasons why patients do not take medicines in the ways that health professionals expect them to, for example:
  - Lack of agreement that a prescription medicine is the best treatment for an illness
  - Concern about the effectiveness of a treatment or about possible adverse effects
  - Failure to appreciate the reasons for therapy
  - Forgetfulness
- In this book we highlight issues that may be of particular concern to patients in the 'patient information' sections.
- There have been many studies of the effects of different strategies in improving adherence to therapy. These include reducing the frequency of administration during the day and reducing the numbers of medicines the patient has to take. However, evidence that such measures are effective is lacking. Nevertheless, it seems likely that adherence can be improved by taking care to explain the benefits and adverse effects of a drug; in a busy clinic it is all too easy to issue a prescription with little or no explanation. Reducing the frequency of administration to once or, at most, twice a day also makes sense, despite lack of convincing evidence that this is effective.
- Concordance is a term that has been coined to reflect the changing nature of the relationship between patients and prescribers. It encapsulates the notion that there should be an explicit agreement between the patient and the prescriber; an impression that agreement has been reached is not enough. It recognizes that patients should have the casting vote and may decide not to take a medicine, even when it appears to be in their best interests. The corollary of this is that patients should take greater responsibility for their treatment and the consequences of their actions.

Guidelines

Clinical guidelines are intended to improve the quality of healthcare by implementing the best available information. They are not a substitute for thought; prescribers should always consider the extent to which the guidelines apply to their clinical problem. Clinical guidelines vary in quality — some are based on a careful review of all the available data, others represent little more than the opinion of a small group. Do not forget that political and economic considerations can influence the ways in which guidelines are written and their contents. The scope of guidelines varies — some consider clinical effectiveness only, while others consider cost as well. This can lead to contradictory recommendations.

UK common law considers that minimum acceptable standards of clinical care derive from responsible customary practice, not from guidelines. Thus, thoughtless implementation of guidelines does not provide immunity from rebuke or prosecution.

Guidelines issued by the National Institute for Clinical Excellence (NICE) are expected to be binding on professionals working in the NHS. However, NICE guidance does not override the individual's responsibility to make decisions appropriate to the circumstances of the individual patient, in consultation with the patient and/or their guardian or carer. For example, if an individual patient is allergic to a drug recommended in a guideline, it would be appropriate for them to be given an alternative.

This book refers to NICE guidance, when it has been issued, and to guidance from other bodies that we feel is helpful. Whenever possible, we have given information to guide rational implementation of the guideline.

Guidelines are produced by many different bodies, and there is no single repository of the best. The following list is a guide to sites that might be helpful.

- National Institute for Clinical Excellence (www.nice.org.uk)
  - NICE is part of the UK NHS; its role is to provide patients, health professionals, and the public with authoritative, robust, and reliable guidance on current 'best practice'.
- National Electronic Library for Health (*http://www.nelh.nhs.uk/guidelinesfinder/*)
  - A library of over 600 clinical guidelines
- Further guidelines at *www.prodigy.nhs.uk* (e.g. treatment of epilepsy)

Other UK Government/NHS resources

- Antibiotic guidelines — Health Protection Agency (*www.hpa.org.uk/infections/topics_az/antimicrobial_resistance/guidance.htm*)
- Immunization against infection (*http://www.dh.gov.uk/PublicationsAndStatistics/Publications/PublicationsPolicyAndGuidance/PublicationsPolicyAndGuidanceArticle/fs/en?CONTENT_ID=4072977&chk=87uz6M*)
- Blood transfusion — 'Handbook of Transfusion Medicine' (*www.transfusionguidelines.org.uk*)
- Investigation and treatment of suspected poisoning — National Poisons Information Service (*www.spib.axl.co.uk*)
- Information on the law regarding driving — Driver Vehicle Licensing Agency (*www.dvla.gov.uk*)

Guidelines produced by expert groups

- Guidelines on many aspects of the treatment of HIV — British HIV Association (*http://www.bhiva.org*)

- Investigation and treatment of asthma — British Thoracic Society/ Scottish Intercollegiate Guidelines Network guidelines (*http://www.brit-thoracic.org.uk/sign/index.htm*)
- Guidelines for the monitoring of second-line drugs for rheumatoid arthritis — British Society for Rheumatology (*http://www.msecportal.org/portal/editorial/PublicPages/bsr/536883013/3.doc*)
- Guidelines on many aspects of haematology including antithrombotic treatment — British Society for Haematology (*www.bcshguidelines.com*)
- Treatment of hypertension (*BMJ* 2004; **328**:634–40)
- Treatment of osteoporosis — Royal College of Physicians UK (*http://www.rcplondon.ac.uk/pubs/wp_osteo_update.htm*)

Other resources

- Evidence-based medicine (*http://www.cebm.utoronto.ca/*)
- 'Clinical evidence' (*http://www.clinicalevidence.com*)
  - Summaries of the available evidence on a wide range of topics. Produced by the British Medical Journal Publishing Group, and made available by the National Electronic Library for Health.

Efficacy of drugs

The therapeutic effect of a drug depends on the translation of its actions, through a series of steps, from its initial molecular action into the final outcome, as illustrated below. Anything that interferes with one of these steps can alter the action of the drug.

The therapeutic process	A clinical example: digoxin for atrial fibrillation	Interfering factors
Molecular pharmacology	Inhibits the sodium/pottasium pump (Na/K ATPase)	Altered binding to the Na/K ATPase (e.g. enhanced binding in hypokalaemia)
Cell pharmacology	Altered intracellular sodium and calcium concentrations	
Cell physiology	Altered electrophysiology	
Tissue physiology	Slowed conduction through AV node	Anomalous conduction pathways (unaffected by digoxin)
Organ physiology	Reduced ventricular rate	Paroxysmal atrial fibrillation (worsened by digoxin)
Clinical effect	Sensation of fast heart rate and breathlessness improved	

Adverse drug reactions

Relation to dose

Relation to time-course

Adverse drug reactions

- It is a truism that any drug that can produce therapeutic benefit can also cause unexpected effects, which are usually (but not always) adverse. For each drug covered in this book, we list important adverse effects and, when possible, indicate their frequencies. However, for several reasons this information is sometimes hard to come by:
  - Clinical trials are primarily designed to study beneficial outcomes, rather than adverse effects (*BMJ* 2004, 3 July).
  - Beneficial effects of drugs are well identified in advance of a trial, whilst adverse effects are generally not.
  - Drugs usually have single beneficial effects (e.g. the reduction of blood pressure by an ACE inhibitor in a patient with hypertension), but can have several adverse effects (e.g. hypotension, cough, hyperkalaemia, angio-oedema), each with a lower individual incidence than the beneficial effect.
  - The beneficial effects of drugs can be quantified by systematic reviews of many trials if the individual trials are too small, but this is much more difficult for adverse effects, because much larger numbers of subjects are needed and data on adverse effects are often poorly reported.
- All this implies that during drug therapy it is important to monitor individual patients not only for the beneficial effects of the drug but also for its adverse effects. Understanding how to classify adverse reactions will help in doing this. Adverse reactions can be classified according to the important features of the three aspects of the reaction. We call this system DoTS (Dose, Time-course, and Susceptibility) (*BMJ* 2003, **327**:1222–5).

Relation to dose

- Adverse reactions that occur at doses *above the usual therapeutic dosage range* are called *toxic* reactions or effects (e.g. bleeding due to too high a dose of warfarin). They can be avoided by using minimally effective doses and treated by reducing the dose when they occur. If a reaction is truly toxic it is often not necessary to withdraw the drug altogether or at least not permanently.
- Adverse reactions that occur *in the usual therapeutic dosage range* are called *collateral* reactions or effects (e.g. the anticholinergic effects of tricyclic antidepressants). (Here we avoid the term 'side effects', which is often loosely used to mean all adverse effects.) They generally cannot be avoided and may not be amenable to dosage reduction, since that will also result in loss of the therapeutic effect.
- Adverse reactions that occur at doses *below the usual therapeutic range* are called *hypersusceptibility* reactions or effects (e.g. penicillin allergy). They can only be avoided by foreknowledge of the patient's susceptibility to them and they imply permanent avoidance of the drug.

Relation to time-course

- Some adverse effects are independent of the duration of therapy (e.g. bleeding due to too high a dose of warfarin can occur at any time during therapy); these are usually toxic effects. The implications are the same as those for toxic effects (above).
- *Rapid reactions* occur when a drug is infused too rapidly (e.g. the massive histamine release ('red man' syndrome) that occurs when intravenous vancomycin is given too quickly). Such reactions can be avoided by infusing the drug slowly.

- *First-dose reactions* occur after the first dose of a course of treatment and not necessarily thereafter (e.g. hypotension after the first dose of an ACE inhibitor). They can be minimized by taking special precautions before the first dose is given, but do not need monitoring thereafter.
- *Early reactions* occur early in treatment then abate with continuing treatment. These are reactions to which patients develop tolerance (e.g. nitrate-induced headache). The patient can be told that the effect will wear off.
- *Intermediate reactions* occur after some delay; but during longer-term therapy the risk falls (e.g. neutropenia due to carbimazole). If after a certain time there is no reaction, there is little or no risk that it will occur later. Early monitoring is important, but if the reaction does not occur after a certain time vigilance can be relaxed.
- *Late reactions* occur rarely or not at all at first, but the risk increases with continued or repeated exposure (e.g. many of the adverse effects of corticosteroids). This type of reaction implies a need for long-term monitoring and perhaps preventive measures (e.g. the use of bisphosphonates to prevent corticosteroid-induced osteoporosis).
- *Withdrawal reactions* are late reactions that occur when, after prolonged treatment, a drug is withdrawn or its effective dose is reduced (e.g. the opiate withdrawal syndrome). They imply the need for slow withdrawal after long-term therapy.
- *Delayed reactions* are observed some time after exposure, even if the drug is withdrawn before the reaction appears. Examples are carcinogenesis (e.g. vaginal adenocarcinoma in women whose mothers took diethylstilbestrol during pregnancy) and teratogenesis (e.g. phocomelia due to thalidomide). Theoretically these effects can be avoided by avoiding the drug in a patient with known susceptibility; however, often that is not known.

Relation to patient susceptibility

- Genetic susceptibility (e.g. succinylcholine apnoea can be predicted if there is a family history). The drug should be avoided or used in a low dose.
- Age. Lower doses are usually required in older people.
- Sex. Women are sometimes more susceptible to adverse effects (e.g. they are more likely to develop cardiac arrhythmias with drugs that prolong the QT interval).
- Physiological changes, such as occur in pregnancy, can modify drug actions. Doses may need to be changed.
- Endogenous factors, such as drug interactions (p. 14) can modify drug actions. Doses may need to be changed or certain combinations avoided.
- Diseases. Renal or hepatic insufficiency can alter dosage requirements.

If you can use the DoTS system to classify an adverse drug reaction, you will be able to plan how to manage it (either to avoid it or to treat it when it occurs).

Drug interactions

- A drug interaction occurs when an effect of one drug alters the effects of another. The result is usually adverse, although it can sometimes be beneficial. Knowing the mechanism of an interaction will help you to predict whether it is likely to be important and how to manage it (avoid it, detect it when it occurs, and treat it). There are three broad mechanisms of drug interactions:
  - Pharmaceutical
  - Pharmacokinetic
  - Pharmacodynamic
- Pharmaceutical interactions occur when two drugs interact physicochemically in solution. For example, the addition, during a cardiac arrest, of calcium gluconate to an infusion of sodium bicarbonate causes precipitation of insoluble calcium carbonate. There are too many of these to remember. Avoid them by following some simple principles:
  - Never add drugs to any infusion solution other than saline or 5% dextrose.
  - Never mix two or more drugs in an infusion solution, unless you know the mixture to be safe (e.g. insulin plus potassium chloride).
- Pharmacokinetic interactions occur when one drug alters the disposition (absorption, distribution, or elimination) of another drug. This can result in drug toxicity or loss of effect.
  - Absorption interactions are uncommon and are easily avoided by giving the two drugs at different times; for example, divalent and trivalent cations (calcium, magnesium, aluminium, iron) are chelated by tetracyclines, and the absorption of both is impaired. Pharmacists put a warning label on bottles or packets containing tetracyclines telling patients to avoid co-administration by 2–3 hours.
  - Distribution interactions usually involve altered protein binding of one drug by another. They are rarely important. However, for a discussion of the interpretation of the plasma phenytoin concentration when phenytoin protein binding is altered see p. 253.
  - Inhibition of metabolism of one drug by another is often important. Many drugs are eliminated by hepatic metabolism involving enzymes of the cytochrome P450 series, such as CYP2D6 and CYP3A4. For lists of drugs that inhibit these see pp. 91 and 347. Interactions of this kind occur soon after introduction of the inhibitor; they should be avoided by avoiding co-administration. A few other interactions are due to inhibition of enzymes other than the P450 series (e.g. monoamine oxidase and xanthine oxidase).
  - Stimulation (induction) of metabolism of one drug by another is often important. Drugs that induce P450 enzymes include carbamazepine, phenobarbital, phenytoin, rifampicin, and St John's wort. For example, if oestrogen metabolism is induced in a woman taking an oral contraceptive she may become pregnant. Avoid co-administration; if co-administration is unavoidable increase the dose of oestrogen and warn her to look out for mid-cycle spotting. Induction interactions take a week or two to occur and lead to increased dosage requirements; then, when the inducer is withdrawn, rebound toxicity can occur if the dose is not again reduced.

- Inhibition of renal excretion of one drug by another is often important (e.g. thiazide diuretics inhibit the renal excretion of lithium). Avoid such combinations or reduce the dose of the affected drug.

- Pharmacodynamic interactions occur when one drug alters the action of another drug. This can result in drug toxicity or loss of effect.
  - Direct potentiating interactions. When two drugs act in the same way at the same site of action their effects can be potentiated (e.g. alcohol potentiates the effects of all drugs that act on the brain). It is generally best to avoid such combinations.
  - Direct inhibitory interactions. When two drugs act in opposing ways at the same site of action the effects of one can be inhibited by the other. Usually such effects are beneficial, since they are used to reverse the adverse effects of a drug (e.g. naloxone reverses opiate toxicity and vitamin K reverses warfarin toxicity).
  - Indirect physiological interactions. These occur when one drug produces a physiological change that alters the action of another drug. For example, diuretics can cause potassium depletion, which can potentiate the actions of digoxin without a change in digoxin dose. Avoid such combinations or take steps to avoid the physiological change that precipitates the interaction (e.g. by giving a potassium-sparing diuretic).
  - Indirect pathological interactions. These occur when one drug produces a pathological change that alters the action of another drug. For example, aspirin causes gastric erosions; if gastric bleeding occurs and the patient is also taking warfarin the bleeding will be worse or more prolonged; impaired platelet aggregation by aspirin worsens the problem. In general, avoid such combinations.

Placebos

- A placebo is a formulation that does not contain any active drug ingredients. However, that does not mean that it cannot have a therapeutic effect.
- Placebo effects are well known and reflect several of the components of the therapeutic process. They can arise from:
  - The therapeutic relationship between healthcare provider and patient.
  - The transience of some symptoms (e.g. those resulting from musculoskeletal injury).
  - The fact that some disease processes improve with time (e.g. most peptic ulcers will heal without drugs, but treatment with a proton pump inhibitor increases the 6-week healing rate to over 90%).
- The most common appropriate use of placebos is as dummy comparators in clinical trials. Their purpose is to reduce subjective bias in the assessment of the results of treatment. When there is no effective alternative treatment the use of an inert placebo may be appropriate, but there is increasing pressure for drug developers to compare new treatments with existing ones.
- Some uses of placebos are not appropriate:
  - To 'test' the patient (e.g. saline injections given for pain that is thought to be factitious).
  - To terminate a consultation early because the patient has difficult symptoms.
  - Do not give drugs that you believe are unlikely to have any therapeutic effect. This can act as a distraction, delay diagnosis, and undermine the therapeutic relationship.

Changing the doses of drugs

- It is good practice to start drug treatment with a low dose and then to titrate to the maximum tolerated or most effective dose. This reduces the incidence of adverse effects and allows treatment to be tailored to individual requirements.
- When increasing the total dose the choice is often between increasing the amount of each dose and reducing the time between doses; in some cases you may want to do both. Each of these has different effects on the pharmacokinetics of the drug and you should choose that which is most appropriate (see Fig. 2).
- Some drugs, for example those with unusual kinetic properties (e.g. bisphosphonates) or those with very long half-lives (e.g. amiodarone), may not behave in this way. See relevant pages for more information.

Intervention	Pharmacokinetic effects	Possible consequences
Increase the amount of the dose	Higher peak plasma concentration	Greater pharmacological effect but adverse effects are more common. The therapeutic effect will depend on whether the action is related to the peak plasma concentration or not. See vancomycin and gentamicin monographs for an example.
	Greater fluctuation in plasma concentration	Adverse effects may be more common. The ratio between the trough and peak concentration can be important for the therapeutic action of some drugs. See angiotensin receptor blockers monograph for more information on trough-to-peak ratios.
Increase frequency of administration	Less fluctuation in plasma concentration	The average plasma concentration will be the same as if the dose were increased but the variation around the mean will be less. This can be an advantage if the drug has a narrow therapeutic range. Very frequent administration can be inconvenient and can lead to missed doses. This will reduce the therapeutic effect.

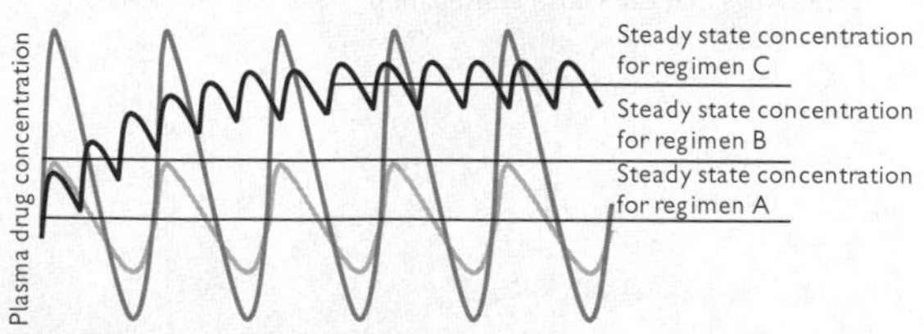

The figure shows two ways of increasing the steady state concentration of a drug. The original dosing regimen (A) is shown in light blue type. Increasing the dose and frequency will increase the steady state concentration (B); the inter-dose fluctuation in concentration will be greater (intermediate blue type). If the dose is kept the same but the frequency of administration increased (C), the drug will accumulate until a new higher steady state is reached (dark blue type).

Renal insufficiency

- See p. 462.

Hepatic insufficiency

- The majority of drugs are metabolized by the liver and under normal circumstances there is considerable reserve. If, however, the metabolic capacity of the liver is markedly reduced (e.g. in cirrhosis), the metabolism of drugs will be reduced.
- Creatinine clearance provides a measure of renal function and can be used to classify renal insufficiency (see p. 462). Unfortunately, no equivalent measure of hepatic function exists. Hepatic enzyme concentrations in plasma provide a poor marker, as they reflect liver damage rather than liver metabolic function. The prothrombin time reflects the synthesis of clotting factors and is a useful measure of hepatic synthetic capacity, but does not reflect metabolic capacity.
- In the majority of patients, it is not possible to predict the extent to which hepatic insufficiency will affect drug metabolism. The following clinical features are suggestive of severe disease; take care if any of these are present:
    - Jaundice
    - Ascites
    - Encephalopathy
- Hepatic insufficiency also affects the action of drugs through other mechanisms, for example:
    - Biliary obstruction will prevent the excretion of some drugs (e.g. rifampicin) and prevent the action of others (e.g. colestyramine).
    - Hypoalbuminaemia caused by hepatic insufficiency will complicate the interpretation of plasma phenytoin concentrations (see phenytoin p. 253).
    - Reduced hepatic synthetic function will increase a patient's sensitivity to drugs such as warfarin.
    - Hepatic insufficiency is associated with fluid overload; avoid the use of drugs that could exacerbate this (e.g. NSAIDs, corticosteroids).
    - Drugs can precipitate hepatic encephalopathy; avoid the following in hepatic insufficiency:
        - Sedative drugs
        - Diuretics (can cause hypokalaemia)
        - Drugs that can cause constipation

An approach to rational prescribing

Prescribing should follow a rational algorithm. All too often, however, it is a reflex decision taken at the end of a consultation.

Principles

When planning therapy consider your interventions in the following categories:

- Treatments that relieve symptoms of the disease.
- Treatments that modify the pathophysiology of the disease.
- Treatments that are aimed at secondary (and primary) prevention.

These treatments can be both pharmacological and non-pharmacological.

Drug selection

- Do I need a drug at all?

If I need a drug —

- What sort of drug do I need?

Consider —

- What is the target? (receptor, enzyme, transport protein, etc.)
- Where is the target found?
  - Does the drug reach its site of action? (e.g. vancomycin is not absorbed when given by mouth)
- Can I focus my treatment on one subtype or location?
  - Pharmacodynamic targeting (receptor subtypes) (e.g. a relatively β_1-selective beta-blocker)
  - Pharmacokinetic targeting (routes of delivery) (e.g. β_2 agonists given by inhalation)
- Is the onset of action of this drug appropriate for the indication?
  - Some drugs take days to act, is this fast enough? (e.g. antidepressant drugs take at least 2 weeks to act)
- How will I deliver this drug?
  - Route (e.g. by inhalation)
  - Formulation (e.g. modified-release)
- Have I taken into account any important kinetic factors?
  - Renal or hepatic insufficiency (see 'cautions' sections in this book)
- Have I considered any interactions:
  - With the disease/physiology (e.g. a sulphonylurea will not work in most cases of type I diabetes — the islet cells have been destroyed)
  - With drugs
    - Metabolic interactions (enzyme induction)
    - Pharmacological interactions (e.g. beta-blockers and verapamil)

Monitoring therapy

- Having selected a drug, it is essential to set targets for your therapy. Make a note of the effect you expect the drug to have (e.g. by how much you want the blood pressure to fall). The 'monitoring' sections in this book give guidance on the sorts of targets to set.
- Warn the patient about any predictable adverse effects and other points to note (see 'patient information' sections).
- Arrange appropriate follow-up.
- At follow-up, assess the success of your intervention. This should include assessment of both the therapeutic and adverse effects.
- Set a new target for your therapy and repeat the process. Do not give patients drugs without a clear idea of what you are hoping to achieve.

Drug therapy and breastfeeding

- Drugs taken by a mother can cause (adverse) pharmacological effects in the breastfeeding infant.
- Some drugs are excreted in breast milk in sufficient quantities to cause dose-related pharmacological effects in the child (e.g. antithyroid drugs).
- The drug need not enter the breast milk in large quantities to cause adverse effects if the child is hypersensitive to it (e.g. penicillin) or if the child is more susceptible to adverse effects owing to altered pharmacokinetics (e.g. sulfonamides can cause kernicterus).
- When considering drug therapy in a woman who wishes to breastfeed:
  - Decide whether drug therapy is essential.
  - If possible select a drug that is considered safe (see below and consult the BNF).
  - If drug therapy is essential and the drug required is not safe (e.g. high dosages of corticosteroids), advise the mother that she should not breastfeed.

The following drugs appear to be safe in breastfeeding:

- ACE inhibitors
- ACTH
- Adrenaline
- Antihistamines
- Baclofen
- Beta-blockers (can cause neonatal bradycardia and hypoglycaemia)
- Carbamazepine
- Chloroquine
- Clomethiazole
- Codeine
- Digoxin
- Disopyramide
- Ethambutol
- Furosemide
- Heparin
- Inhaled $beta_2$ adrenoceptor agonists
- Inhaled corticosteroids in moderate dosages
- Insulin
- Methyldopa
- Neuroleptic drugs in moderate dosages (e.g. chlorpromazine, haloperidol)
- Nifedipine
- Nortriptyline
- NSAIDS
- Rifampicin
- Thyroid hormones
- Tricyclic antidepressants (except doxepin)
- Valproate
- Verapamil
- Warfarin

Chapter 1

Gastrointestinal system

Contents

Histamine H_2 receptor antagonists

Antagonists at the histamine H_2 receptor

The principal effect of these drugs is inhibition of histamine-driven production of stomach acid. Gastric acid is produced through three major pathways (see teaching point below). One of these is stimulated by histamine. These drugs are effective antacid drugs but, because they act on only one of the pathways, they are not able to suppress gastric acid secretion completely, even at high dosages.

Drugs in this class

- Cimetidine
- Famotidine
- Nizatidine
- Ranitidine
- Ranitidine bismuth citrate

- When suppression of gastric acid is required.
  - Healing of gastric and duodenal ulcers.
  - Reflux oesophagitis.
  - May be used in prophylaxis against gastric ulceration in an ICU (see prescribing information).
  - Also available over the counter for short-term relief of dyspeptic symptoms.
- Use famotidine, nizatidine, or ranitidine in preference to cimetidine, because of drug interactions with cimetidine.

- Bear in mind that dyspeptic symptoms may be the result of gastric malignancy, especially in older patients. H_2 receptor antagonists can mask these symptoms and delay the diagnosis.
- H_2 receptor antagonists are effective in the treatment of reflux oesophagitis, but less so than proton pump inhibitors.
- Intravenous H_2 receptor antagonists are not effective in acute haematemesis; they do not improve outcome.
- Of these drugs, only ranitidine bismuth citrate is recommended as part of a *Helicobacter pylori* eradication regimen (see proton pump inhibitors, p. 28).
- Halve the dose in severe renal or hepatic insufficiency.
- There is no information on the safety of these drugs in pregnancy. Avoid using them.

- These drugs are best taken in divided doses to give adequate 24-hour cover. Some patients do not require full 24-hour cover, in which case a single dose taken at night may be sufficient.
- Usual treatment periods:
  - Duodenal ulcer, 4–6 weeks
  - Gastric ulcer, 6 weeks
  - NSAID-associated ulceration, 8 weeks
- If the ulcer is the result of *Helicobacter pylori* infection, and this has been eradicated, the patient does not usually need maintenance treatment.
- If the cause of the ulcer is a NSAID drug, it should be withdrawn. If the NSAID is essential, the patient should be given maintenance treatment with a proton pump inhibitor at half the normal treatment dose (NICE guidance).

- These drugs have a good adverse effects profile, and are generally well tolerated.
- The most common adverse effects are diarrhoea, altered liver function, rash, headache, and dizziness.

- Cimetidine inhibits oxidative hepatic metabolism by P450 enzymes. It can therefore increase the plasma concentrations of several drugs, in particular warfarin, theophylline, and phenytoin. Nizatidine, famotidine, and ranitidine do not do this.

Safety

- Beware of prolonged treatment with these drugs without a diagnosis; they can mask the symptoms of gastric malignancy.

Efficacy

- Efficacy is usually judged by symptom relief.
  - If ineffective reconsider the diagnosis.
  - If the diagnosis is reflux oesophagitis, a proton pump inhibitor may be preferable.

- Obesity and smoking are important risk factors for reflux oesophagitis (and peptic ulcer). Address these issues as well as providing drug treatment.

Prescribing information: **Histamine H_2 receptor antagonists**

Famotidine

- Ulcer healing, by mouth: 40 mg at night.
- Maintenance dose, by mouth: 20 mg at night.
- Reflux oesophagitis, by mouth: 20–40 mg bd.

Nizatidine

- Ulcer healing, by mouth: 150 mg bd or 300 mg at night.
- Maintenance dose, by mouth: 150 mg at night.
- Reflux oesophagitis, by mouth: 150–300 mg bd.
- Also available in parenteral formulations (see note below).

Ranitidine

- Ulcer healing, by mouth: 150 mg bd or 300 mg at night.
- Maintenance dose, by mouth: 150 mg at night.
- Reflux oesophagitis: 150–300 mg bd.
- Also available in parenteral formulations (see note below).
- Parenteral use of these drugs is usually limited to prophylaxis against stress ulceration on the ICU.
- The usual dose of ranitidine for this indication is 50 mg tds; this should be reduced to 25 mg tds in severe renal insufficiency.

TEACHING POINT Pathways of stomach acid secretion

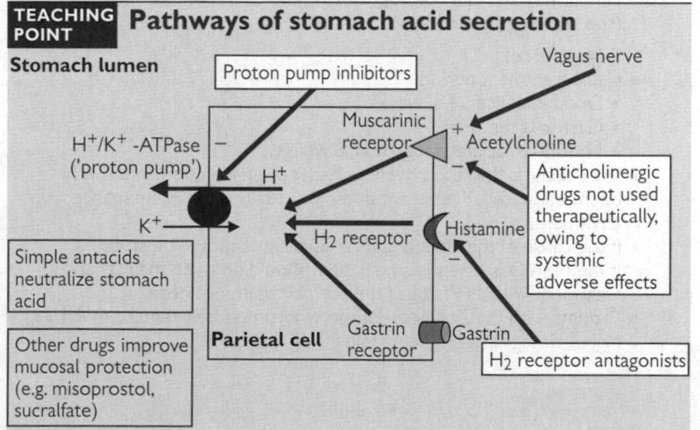

Proton pump inhibitors (PPIs)

Irreversible inhibitors of the H^+/K^+-ATPase ('proton pump')

These drugs bind irreversibly to the H^+/K^+-ATPase, located in the secretory cannaliculae of parietal cells. The drug must be absorbed into the body to do this; it does not act directly from the stomach lumen. It also requires an acid environment to be activated; this provides a negative feedback mechanism—inhibition of acid production reduces the activation of the PPI. The H^+/K^+-ATPase is the final common pathway of gastric acid secretion, so these drugs are powerful antacids. See H_2 antagonists section (p. 24) for details of acid secretion.

Drugs in this class
- Omeprazole
- Esomeprazole
- Rabeprazole
- Pantoprazole
- Lansoprazole

- When suppression of gastric acid is required.
  - Healing of gastric and duodenal ulcers.
  - Reflux oesophagitis.
  - Eradication of *Helicobacter pylori* infection, in combination with antibacterial drugs (see teaching point below).
  - Treatment of Zollinger–Ellison syndrome.
  - High-dose intravenous omeprazole has been used as adjunctive treatment in patients with high-risk bleeding duodenal ulcer (unlicensed indication).

- Bear in mind that dyspeptic symptoms can result from gastric malignancy, especially in older patients. PPIs can mask these symptoms and delay the diagnosis.
- PPIs are not suitable for acute haematemesis.
- PPIs are metabolized by the liver; dosage adjustment is not usually required, but take care in severe hepatic insufficiency.
- There is no information on the safety of these drugs in pregnancy. Avoid using them.

- Note that omeprazole and lansoprazole capsules can be opened and the contents suspended in fruit juice or yoghurt for patients with difficulty swallowing. Lansoprazole is also available as a suspension (see teaching point below).

Peptic ulcer
- Usual treatment periods:
  - Duodenal ulcer, 4–6 weeks
  - Gastric ulcer, 6 weeks
  - NSAID-associated ulceration, 8 weeks
- If the ulcer is the result of *Helicobacter pylori* infection, and this has been eradicated, the patient does not usually need maintenance treatment.
- If the cause of the ulcer is an NSAID drug, it should be stopped. If the NSAID is essential, the patient should be given maintenance treatment with a PPI at half the normal treatment dose.
- Patients with the Zollinger–Ellison syndrome often require much higher dosages (e.g. omeprazole 80 mg daily).

Reflux oesophagitis

- Treatment of reflux oesophagitis often requires higher dosages and treatment for longer (8 weeks) than for peptic ulcer.
- Most patients with reflux symptoms will relapse after a period of treatment. If this is frequent and severe consider maintenance treatment with half the treatment dose.
  - NICE has recommended that patients with a history of oesophageal stricture, ulcer, or haemorrhage should receive maintenance treatment at the full dose.
- Many patients use these drugs in an on-demand manner; they take the PPI for a period of a few days or weeks whenever symptoms recur.
  - Only esomeprazole is licensed for use in this way.
- Standard doses of these drugs are sufficient for most patients. Esomeprazole has the most powerful acid suppressant action and may be useful in patients with resistant symptoms.

Bleeding peptic ulcer

- The process of haemostasis is inhibited by a low pH (acid). Omeprazole, given at very high dosages (200 mg/day) iv, has been shown in one study to reduce the re-bleeding rate in patients with high-risk peptic ulcer after endoscopic treatment.
  - This indication is unlicensed and should only be considered in consultation with a specialist. Use your local protocol.
  - This treatment should not be used instead of, or to delay, endoscopic treatment.

- These drugs have a good adverse effects profile, and are generally well-tolerated.
- The most common adverse effect is diarrhoea, particularly with long-term use.
- Other rare adverse effects include rash, liver enzyme abnormalities, and interstitial nephritis.
- Long-term treatment with these drugs causes carcinoid tumours in the stomachs of laboratory animals, but has not been observed in clinical practice. Always consider whether maintenance treatment is required.

- The potential for drug interactions with these drugs is low.
- Lansoprazole, omeprazole, and esomeprazole inhibit hepatic cytochrome P450 enzymes to some degree. This effect is not great, but may enhance the actions of warfarin and phenytoin (see erythromycin, p. 347, for more information).

Safety

- Beware of prolonged treatment with these drugs without a diagnosis; they can mask the symptoms of gastric malignancy.
- Patients with Barrett's oesophagus require regular endoscopic follow-up.

Efficacy

- Efficacy is usually judged by symptom relief. If ineffective, reconsider the diagnosis.

- Ensure that patients who require follow-up (e.g. for Barrett's oesophagus) understand why they need to be seen again.
- Obesity and smoking are important risk factors for reflux oesophagitis (and peptic ulcer). Address these issues as well as providing drug treatment.
- If the capsules are opened, tell the patient not to chew the granules.

Prescribing information: **Proton pump inhibitors**

Omeprazole

- Ulcer healing, by mouth: 20 mg daily.
- Maintenance dose, by mouth: 10–20 mg daily (see notes above).
- Reflux oesophagitis, by mouth: 20–40 mg daily.
- Also available in an intravenous formulation.

Esomeprazole

- Reflux oesophagitis, by mouth: 40 mg daily.

Lansoprazole

- Ulcer healing, by mouth: 30 mg daily.
- Maintenance dose, by mouth: 15–30 mg daily (see notes above).
- Reflux oesophagitis, by mouth: 30 mg daily.

Pantoprazole

- Ulcer healing, by mouth: 40 mg daily.
- Maintenance dose, by mouth: 20–40 mg daily (see notes above).
- Reflux oesophagitis, by mouth: 20–40 mg daily.

Rabeprazole

- Ulcer healing, by mouth: 20 mg daily.
- Maintenance dose, by mouth: 10–20 mg daily (see notes above).
- Reflux oesophagitis, by mouth: 10–20 mg daily.

Helicobacter pylori **eradication regimens** BNF Reference 1.3

- *Helicobacter pylori* infection is thought to be responsible for almost all duodenal ulcers and a high proportion of gastric ones. The prevalence of infection varies; for example, it once affected 50% of adults in Western Europe, but this has now fallen dramatically.
- Suppressing acid secretion will heal ulcers, but long-term cure requires eradication of *Helicobacter pylori*, if that is the cause of the ulcer.
- The following 7-day regimens eradicate *Helicobacter pylori* in over 90% of cases.
    - PPI at the ulcer-healing dose given **twice daily** (or ranitidine bismuth citrate 400 mg bd)
    - + amoxicillin 1 g bd
    - + clarithromycin 500 mg bd
- If eradication is unsuccessful, repeat the course, substituting metronidazole 400 mg bd for the clarithromycin.
- If this is unsuccessful, seek a specialist opinion.
- If the patient has an ulcer they should continue the PPI (**once daily**) or H_2 antagonist alone for the 6-week healing period.
- If the patient does not have an ulcer, no continuing treatment is usually required.

TEACHING POINT Patients who have difficulty swallowing tablets

- Some patients report that they cannot swallow tablets because they do not wish to take the drug, or because they are worried about adverse effects of the drug.
- Identify whether difficulty swallowing tablets is in fact a symptom of a more general swallowing problem. Causes include:
  - Oesophageal strictures (benign and malignant)
  - Stroke
  - Muscle weakness (e.g. myasthenia gravis)
- Some patients may have problems because they do not take tablets with water; this is potentially hazardous. Tablets can stick to the oesophageal muscoa and cause ulceration; this has been a particular problem with bisphosphonate drugs, which should be taken with a full glass of water.
- Some patients find gelatin capsules more difficult to swallow than tablets; a change of formulation may solve the problem.
- A modified-release formulation may mean that the drug needs to be given less often.
  - Some drugs (e.g. alendronate) are available in a formulation that can be given once weekly.
- There are several options for patients with persistent problems in swallowing tablets:
  - Prescribe an elixir or melt formulation.
  - Some capsules can be opened and the contents suspended in yoghurt or fruit juice (e.g. Lansoprazole, Zomorph®). Warn the patient not to chew the granules.
  - Discuss with a pharmacist whether a specially prepared suspension or elixir can be produced.
  - Parenteral administration is an option but is rarely ideal, although subcutaneous administration may be suitable.

Misoprostol

Synthetic prostaglandin analogue

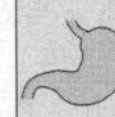

- Reduces the volume and proteolytic action of gastric juice.
- Also increases bicarbonate and mucus secretion.
- See prostaglandins section (p. 450) for more information.

Risk factors for NSAID-induced gastric ulceration

- Linear increase in risk with increasing age (especially over 65 years).
- History of peptic ulceration.
- Debilitated patients.
- Long-term treatment with maximal doses of NSAIDs.
- Concomitant treatment with drugs that can cause bleeding.

- Treatment and prevention of benign gastric and duodenal ulcers.
  - Its most common use is as prophylaxis against gastric ulceration in those at risk who need to continue taking NSAIDs.
- Unlicensed use to induce a medical abortion and to induce labour.

- Misoprostol increases uterine tone and can induce abortion. It is contraindicated in women who are pregnant or planning pregnancy.
  - The manufacturers advise against use in all women of childbearing age, unless they are fully aware of the risks.
- Misoprostol has the potential to cause hypotension, although this is not commonly seen in practice. Consider alternatives for those in whom hypotension can precipitate severe complications (e.g. cerebrovascular and cardiovascular disease).
- No dosage reduction is usually required in renal or hepatic insufficiency.

Gastric ulceration

- Consider misoprostol for those who are at high risk of gastric ulceration but who require NSAIDs for other reasons. See box above for risk factors.
- The risk of bleeding from NSAIDs is relatively constant over time. The longer the patient takes an NSAID, the greater the risk.
  - Not all NSAIDs carry the same risk of bleeding (see NSAIDs, p. 658).
  - Consider these factors when prescribing misoprostol for prophylaxis against gastric ulceration.
- Always think — can I stop or change the NSAID, rather than adding misoprostol to the prescription chart?
- Misoprostol is available in combination with naproxen and diclofenac as single tablets.
  - Note that co-administration of a PPI with an NSAID is an alternative to a combination of misoprostol with a NSAID.

Obstetric uses

- Misoprostol is used systemically, and topically to induce and augment labour (it can also be used to induce abortion). This is a specialized use.

- Misoprostol can cause diarrhoea; in some cases this can be severe and necessitate withdrawal of the drug.
- Non-specific gastrointestinal disturbance is also seen.
- Less common effects include rash, dizziness, and abnormal vaginal bleeding (includes intermenstrual bleeding, menorrhagia, postmenopausal bleeding).

- Misoprostol is subject to few drug interactions.

- In patients taking a prostaglandin to prevent NSAID-induced blood loss, blood loss can nevertheless occur and can be occult and chronic. Have a low threshold for measuring a full blood count. Chronic diseases are often associated with anaemia, but ensure that it is not due to iron deficiency through blood loss.

- Advise patients that this drug can reduce the risk of bleeding from the gut, but that they should seek immediate medical attention if they have blood in the stool, or dark, tarry stools.
- Warn women that they should not take misoprostol if they are planning a pregnancy.

Prescribing information: **Misoprostol**

Benign gastric and duodenal ulceration and NSAID-associated ulceration

- By mouth, 800 micrograms daily (in 2–4 divided doses) with breakfast (or main meals) and at bedtime; treatment should be continued for at least 4 weeks and can be continued for up to 8 weeks if required.

Prophylaxis of NSAID-induced gastric and duodenal ulceration

- By mouth, 200 micrograms 2–4 times daily (depending on the perceived risk of bleeding in that patient), taken with the NSAID.

TEACHING POINT **Combination formulations: Advantages and disadvantages**

A combination formulation contains two or, rarely, three drugs of different types. Many combination products are available, but they are only acceptable or even preferable when the following minimum criteria are met:

- When the frequency of administration of the two drugs is the same
- When the fixed doses in the combination product are therapeutically and optimally effective in most cases (i.e. when it is not necessary to alter the dose of one drug independently of the other)
  - It is the second criterion that is the most difficult to achieve in clinical practice. For example, patients may require different dosages of an NSAID over time, but the dose of misoprostol does not need to change. A new prescription of the combination product will be required each time the dose of NSAID is changed; this is expensive and may be confusing for the patient.

Nevertheless, combination products do have a number of potential advantages:

Potential Advantages	Examples
Antituberculosis drugs (rifampicin + isoniazid) Ferrous sulfate and folic acid (pregnancy)	Improved compliance
Triple vaccine (diphtheria, tetanus, pertussis) Combined insulins (e.g. Mixtard®)	Ease of administration
Amoxicillin + clavulanic acid (co-amoxiclav)* Combined oral contraceptive (oestrogen + progestogen)	Synergistic or additive effects
Levodopa + decarboxylase inhibitors (Parkinson's disease)	Reduced adverse effects

*Even so, co-amoxiclav is often given as combination tablets plus extra amoxicillin in separate tablets.

Constipation

- The word constipation is used to describe many disorders of bowel motility. Take a careful history to determine the specific symptoms that are causing the problem (e.g. a hard stool, a feeling of incomplete evacuation, straining).
- Constipation may be secondary to another disease:
  - Diseases of the colon (e.g. cancer, anal fissure, proctitis).
  - Metabolic disturbances (e.g. hypercalcaemia, hypothyroidism, diabetes mellitus).
  - Neurological disorders (e.g. spinal cord lesion, Parkinsonism).
  - Drug treatments (e.g. opioids, iron).
- If one of these is the cause and can be corrected, then correct it. In many cases, however, treatment is symptomatic. Constipation develops as a result of two principal disorders of colorectal motility: slow-transit constipation and pelvic floor dysfunction. If the cause is pelvic floor dysfunction, pelvic floor exercises and biofeedback training are of some benefit. If the principal problem is slow transit, a gradual increase in dietary fibre intake will usually suffice.
- If drug treatment is required consider:
  - Bulk-forming laxatives for those with small, hard stools. Increasing the amount of dietary fibre and fluid intake is preferable to long-term treatment.
  - **Bran:** by mouth, 1 sachet 2–3 times daily.
  - **Ispagula husk** (Fybogel®, Regulan®): by mouth, 1 sachet twice daily.
  - **Methylcellulose:** by mouth, 3–6 tablets twice daily.
  - All of these should be taken with plenty of water.
- As an alterative to bulk-forming laxatives use osmotic laxatives. These act by retaining fluid in the bowel, so an adequate fluid intake is essential.
  - **Lactulose:** by mouth, initially 15 mL bd. Adjust the dose according to the patient's needs. Given in hepatic encephalopathy because it discourages the growth of ammonia-producing organisms in the gut.
  - **Magnesium hydroxide:** by mouth, 25–50 mL when required. Avoid in renal failure; magnesium can accumulate.
  - **Polyethylene glycols:** doses vary; refer to manufacturers' material.
- Stimulant laxatives are most useful when reduced colonic transit is the cause of constipation. However, prolonged use can cause an atonic non-functioning colon and hypokalaemia. Therefore, these drugs should only be used for short periods. Dantron (co-danthramer, co-danthusate) is only licensed for use in palliative care because of potential carcinogenicity.
  - **Senna**: doses vary; refer to manufacturers' material.
  - **Bisacodyl:** by mouth, 5–10 mg at night.
  - **Glycerol:** suppositories, 2 g when required.
  - Stimulant laxatives are also used when there is faecal impaction and for bowel cleansing before clinical investigations and surgery.

Treatment of faecal impaction

- Docusate is given first, because it is a faecal softener as well as a stimulant laxative. By mouth, up to 500 mg daily in divided doses. Also available as an enema.

- An alterative faecal softener is arachis (peanut) oil. This is given as an enema. Do not give this if the patient has history of nut allergy.
- Once the stool has been softened, evacuation can be encouraged with a phosphate enema (an osmotic laxative).

Bowel cleansing for clinical investigations and surgery

- Bowel cleansing solutions are given to clear the bowel of any solid matter before investigations or surgery; they are not suitable treatment for constipation.
- Warn the patient that these solutions will cause profuse watery diarrhoea and that they should drink plenty of fluid. Take care if the patient is at risk from the large fluid shifts these solutions can cause (e.g. renal insufficiency, heart failure, elderly patients). Do not give these solutions if the patient has any form of gastrointestinal obstruction.
- **Sodium picosulfate** (Picolax®): by mouth, 1 sachet at 08.00 and 1 sachet at 14.00 on the day before the procedure.
- **Polyethylene glycol** (Klean-prep®): by mouth, 250 mL every 10–15 minutes until 4 litres consumed.
- **Magnesium carbonate and citric acid** (Citramag®): by mouth, 1 sachet at 08.00 and 1 sachet at 14.00 on the day before the procedure.

Co-phenotrope (Lomotil®)

Mixture of the opioid diphenoxylate hydrochloride and the anticholinergic drug atropine sulfate in a ratio of 100 : 1

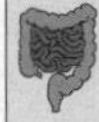

- Diphenoxylate hydrochloride is an opioid. For actions of opioids, see p. 668.
- Atropine is an antagonist at muscarinic cholinergic receptors. It causes relaxation of smooth muscle of bowel, increased heart rate, pupillary dilatation, and reduced bronchial secretions.

Alternative anti-motility drugs

- Codeine
- Morphine
- Loperamide
- Bile salt sequestrants (e.g. colestyramine, aluminium hydroxide) for patients who have had an ileal resection or who have ileal disease.

- As an adjunct to rehydration in the treatment of acute diarrhoea.
- Chronic mild ulcerative colitis.

- Do not use instead of rehydration. Avoid when there is a suspicion of acute infective diarrhoea.
- Contraindicated in active ulcerative colitis and antibiotic-associated colitis.
- May induce hepatic coma in those with advanced liver disease.
- Licensed for use in the young, but not recommended.

- See codeine (p. 664) for advice on treatment of diarrhoea.
- Acute diarrhoea is usually a symptom of another disease. Do not use antimotility drugs when there is any suspicion that the cause may be an infection.
- Do not use instead of rehydration.

- Excessive use can cause intestinal obstruction (both mechanical and paralytic). Warn the patient to stop if bloating or distension develop.
- In overdose, other opioid effects occur: drowsiness, respiratory depression, etc. (see p. 668). These can be treated with naloxone.
- Atropine effects: flushing, dry mouth, tachycardia, urinary retention (anticholinergic effects).
    - Note that patients with Down's syndrome are more susceptible to these effects.

Safety

- Tolerance and dependence can develop with prolonged use.

Efficacy

- Review patients with acute diarrhoea after a few days to ensure that the episode has resolved; if it has not, review the diagnosis.

- Warn the patient to stop the drug if bloating or abdominal distension occur.

Prescribing information: **Co-phenotrope**

- **By mouth**, co-phenotrope 2.5/0.25 (diphenoxylate hydrochloride 2.5 mg, atropine sulfate 25 micrograms).
    - Initially 4 tablets, followed by 2 tablets every 6 hours until diarrhoea is controlled.

TEACHING POINT Drugs with names beginning co-

Drugs that have names beginning with co- are mixtures of two different drugs. The theoretical advantage of this is that two synergistic drugs are combined in a single tablet to aid compliance. However, this advantage is often outweighed by the disadvantage of giving two drugs with different actions when one would be sufficient. See misoprostol article (p. 31) for more information on combination formulations. The Table below shows a few examples.

Formulation	Component drugs	Potential advantages	Potential disadvantages
Co-codamol	Paracetamol Codeine	Opioid/ paracetamol synergy.	Opioid can cause confusion.
Co-amilofruse	Furosemide Amiloride	Potassium-sparing actions of amiloride.	Amiloride not always required, especially in those also taking ACE inhibitors.
Co-fluampicil	Ampicillin Flucloxacillin	Broader antibacterial spectrum.	Wider spectrum rarely required. May encourage bacterial resistance if used inappropriately.
Co-tenidone	Atenolol Chlorthalidone	Single tablet for the treatment of hypertension.	Two drugs are not always required. Not suitable for dose titration.
Co-careldopa	Carbidopa L-dopa	Peripheral dopa decarboxylase inhibitor (carbidopa) reduces adverse effects from the peripheral conversion of L-dopa to dopamine.	

Loperamide (Immodium®)

Opioid receptor agonist

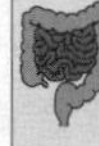

- Binds to opioid receptors in the gut wall, reducing peristalsis.
- Also increases anal tone.
- See opioids section (p. 668) for more information.

Alternative antimotility drugs

- Codeine
- Morphine
- Co-phenotrope
- Bile salt sequestrants (e.g. colestyramine, aluminium hydroxide) for patients who have had an ileal resection or who have ileal disease.

- As an adjunct to rehydration in acute diarrhoea.
- Symptomatic treatment of chronic diarrhoea (adults only).

- This drug is an opioid, but it is not an analgesic because it does not penetrate the central nervous system well (see opioids, p. 668).
- Do not use instead of rehydration.
- Avoid when there is a suspicion of acute infective diarrhoea.
- Contraindicated in active ulcerative colitis and antibiotic-associated colitis, in which it can cause toxic dilatation of the bowel.
- There is no information about the safety of loperamide in pregnancy. Avoid using it.

- See codeine (p. 664) for advice on treatment of diarrhoea.
- Acute diarrhoea is usually a symptom of another disease. Do not use antimotility drugs when there is any suspicion that the cause may be an infection.
- Do not use instead of rehydration.
- Loperamide should be taken immediately after a bowel movement.

- Excessive use can lead to bowel obstruction (both mechanical and paralytic).
- Skin reactions, including urticaria, are reported.
- In overdose, loperamide can cause opioid effects: drowsiness, respiratory depression, nausea and vomiting. These can be treated with naloxone (see p. 626).

- Loperamide antagonizes the gastric emptying actions of domperidone and metoclopramide.

Efficacy

- Review patients with acute diarrhoea after a few days, to ensure that the episode has resolved. If it hasn't resolved, review the diagnosis and the use of loperamide.

- Discuss the dosage regimen, so that the patient feels empowered to adjust the dose to optimize symptom control.
- Warn the patient to stop the drug if bloating or abdominal distension develop.

Prescribing information: **Loperamide**

Acute diarrhoea

- 4 mg initially, followed by 2 mg after each loose stool for up to 5 days; usual dose 6–8 mg daily.
- Maximum dose 16 mg daily.

Chronic diarrhoea in adults

- Initially 4–8 mg daily in divided doses, subsequently adjusted according to response and given in two divided doses for maintenance.
- Maximum dose 16 mg daily.

Mesalazine and related compounds (aminosalicylates)

Mesalazine is the recommended International Non-proprietary Name (rINN) for 5-aminosalicylic acid

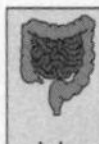

The active ingredient of all of these drugs is 5-aminosalicylic acid. The mechanism of its action in inflammatory bowel disease is not fully understood, although it may act by altering cytokine function. However, what is important is that the drug is delivered to the site of action, usually the large bowel or distal ileum. Each of the drugs in this class does this in a different way after oral administration.

Mesalazine formulations. Modified-release formulations provide delivery of 5-aminosalicylic acid to the large bowel.

Olsalazine is a dimer of 5-aminosalicylic acid; it is cleaved in the lower bowel to release 5-aminosalicylic acid.

Balsalazide is mesalazine attached by an diazo bond to a carrier molecule. This bond is cleaved in the colon to release active mesalazine.

Sulfasalazine is 5-aminosalicylate coupled to a carrier sulfapyridine molecule. This drug has different properties from the others in the class and is the subject of a separate article.

Aminosalicylates

- Sulfasalazine
- Mesalazine
- Balsalazide
- Olsalazine

- Treatment of mild to moderate ulcerative colitis, and maintenance of remission.
- Maintenance of remission in Crohn's ileo-colitis (balsalazide).

- Mesalazine is excreted via the kidneys. It is contraindicated in moderate or severe renal impairment and in severe hepatic impairment.
- Hypersensitivity to salicylates is relatively common (see aspirin, p. 116).
- Mesalazine is not contraindicated in pregnancy; negligible quantities of drug cross the placenta.

- Mesalazine is available as tablets for colitis, enemas for distal colitis, and suppositories for proctitis. Mesalazine is absorbed systemically from each of these, and so its effects may not be limited to the site of delivery. The precise choice of formulation will depend on the nature and extent of the individual patient's disease. The dose of mesalazine in each of the manufacturers' formulations varies (see prescribing information).
- Balsalazide is only available in oral formulations; consider alternatives for distal disease when topical treatment may be more appropriate.

- Risk of blood dyscrasias (agranulocytosis, aplastic anaemia, leukopenia, neutropenia, thrombocytopenia) with all aminosalicylates. Be alert to this possibility and check a full blood count if suspicious. Warn the patient (see patient information).
- Hypersensitivity phenomena: rash, urticaria, interstitial nephritis, lupus-like syndrome.
- Diarrhoea, nausea, vomiting, abdominal pain, cholelithiasis.
  - Watery diarrhoea seems to be more common with olsalazine than some of the other aminosalicylates; it may be reduced by taking the drug after meals.
- Can occasionally exacerbate the symptoms of colitis.

- Do not co-prescribe lactulose or other drugs that will alkalinize the gut contents, as this will prevent the formation of 5-aminosalicylic acid from mesalazine.
- Mesalazine is subject to few drug interactions, but take care when giving it with other drugs that can suppress the bone marrow (e.g. azathioprine).

Safety

- Check the full blood count if you suspect a blood dyscrasia.
- Mesalazine is renally excreted; be aware of accumulation in people with renal impairment (especially the elderly).

Efficacy

- Measure markers of inflammation (ESR, CRP) and ask the patient to keep a diary of stool frequency.

- Advise patients to report immediately any unexplained purpura, bruising, bleeding, fever, sore throat, or malaise, as these may be indicative of a blood dyscrasia.

Prescribing information: **Mesalazine**

Asacol®

- Tablets contain mesalazine 400 mg. Dose is 6 tablets daily in divided doses for an acute attack. Titrate to between 3 and 6 tablets daily for maintenance of remission.
- Foam enema. Delivers mesalazine 1 g. Used for acute attacks. One dose per day for rectosigmoid disease, increased to two doses for disease affecting the descending colon.
- Suppositories. Available as 250 mg and 500 mg doses. Dose is 750–1500 mg daily in divided doses, last dose taken at bedtime.

Pentasa®

- Modified-release tablets contain mesalazine 500 mg. Dose is up to 4 g in divided doses to control an acute attack. Maintenance dose is usually 1.5 g daily, in divided doses.
  - Do not chew the tablets; doing so will destroy the modified-release system.
- Modified-release granules contain mesalazine 1 g per sachet. Dose is 4 g in divided doses to control an acute attack. Maintenance dose is usually 2 g daily, in divided doses.
  - Do not chew the granules; doing so will destroy the modified-release system.
- Retention enema contains mesalazine 1 g. Dose is 1 g at bedtime.
- Suppositories contain mesalazine 1 g. Dose is one suppository at bedtime for an acute attack. Maintenance dose is usually one suppository daily.

Salofalk®

- Tablets contain mesalazine 250 mg. Dose is 6 tablets daily in 3 divided doses. Maintenance titrated to between 3 and 6 tablets in divided doses.
- Suppositories contain mesalazine 500 mg. Dose for an acute attack is 1–2 suppositories given 2–3 times per day according to response.
- Enemas contain mesalazine 2 g. Dose is 1 enema at bedtime for control of acute attack or for maintenance.

Prescribing information: **Balsalazide**

- Capsules contain balsalazide 750 mg. Dose for an acute attack is 2.25 g 3 times daily until remission occurs or for up to maximum of 12 weeks.
- Maintenance dose is 1.5 g twice daily, adjusted according to response (maximum 6 g daily).

Prescribing information: **Olsalazine**

- Dose for an acute attack, 1 g daily in divided doses after meals, increased if necessary over 1 week to a maximum of 3 g daily (maximum single dose 1 g).
- Maintenance dose, 500 mg twice daily after meals.

Sulfasalazine

Sulfasalazine is a derivative of 5-aminosalicylic acid (see mesalazine, p. 38)

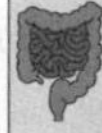

- Sulfasalazine is 5-aminosalicylate coupled to a carrier sulfapyridine molecule.
- Sulfasalazine itself is poorly absorbed from the gut.
- In inflammatory bowel disease, hydrolysis of sulfasalazine by colonic bacteria releases the active moiety mesalazine (5-aminosalicylate) in the large bowel. The precise mechanism by which 5-aminosalicylate acts in inflammatory bowel disease is not known, but it may alter cytokine function.
- By contrast, the sulfapyridine moiety causes many of the adverse effects of sulfasalazine and is thought to be the active ingredient in rheumatoid arthritis. Again the mechanism of action is unknown.

Aminosalicylates (also see p. 38)

- Sulfasalazine
- Mesalazine
- Balsalazide
- Olsalazine

- Treatment of mild, moderate, and severe ulcerative colitis, and maintenance of remission.
- Active Crohn's disease.
- Sulfasalazine is also used as a disease-modifying agent in rheumatoid arthritis.

- Contraindicated in moderate or severe renal impairment, and in severe hepatic impairment.
- Hypersensitivity to salicylates is relatively common (see aspirin, p. 116).
- G6PD deficiency (see p. 387).
- Sulfasalzine is not contraindicated in pregnancy, There is a potential risk of haemolysis in the neonate in the third trimester, owing to folate deficiency; give folate supplements.

Ulcerative colitis

- Sulfasalazine is given by mouth, by suppository, or by enema for the treatment of acute ulcerative colitis. It is given by mouth as maintenance therapy to prevent recurrence.

Rheumatoid arthritis

- Introduce gradually to avoid gastrointestinal adverse effects. Suggested dosage 500 mg daily in the first week, rising to 1 g twice daily in the fourth and subsequent weeks.

- 75% of adverse events are reported in the first 3 months, hence the close monitoring suggested during this period (see below).
- The adverse effects are those associated with the other aminosalicylates and with sulphur-containing drugs (see sulfonamides, p. 351, for a list).
- Risk of blood dyscrasias with all aminosalicylates: agranulocytosis (1 in 700 patients), aplastic anaemia and leukopenia (1.5% of patients), neutropenia, thrombocytopenia, megaloblastic anaemia, haemolytic anaemia. Be alert to this possibility and check a full blood count if suspicious. Warn the patient (see patient information).
- Hypersensitivity reactions are common, usually an urticarial rash, but sometimes Stevens–Johnson syndrome, interstitial nephritis, or a lupus-like syndrome. (See sulfonamides, p. 351, for more information on sulphur allergy.)

- Diarrhoea, nausea, vomiting, abdominal pain, cholelithiasis.
- Lung complications: fibrosing alveolitis, eosinophilia.
- CNS: aseptic meningitis, vertigo, tinnitus, peripheral neuropathy, depression, hallucinations.
- Renal: proteinuria, crystalluria, haematuria, nephrotic syndrome.
- Can exacerbate the symptoms of colitis.

Safety

- The following monitoring regimen is suggested: measure a full blood count (looking for myelosuppression) fortnightly, and liver function tests monthly for the first 12 weeks of treatment, and 3-monthly thereafter. Suspend treatment if any of the following occur:
  - White blood cell count below 4.0×10^9 /l or neutrophil count below 2.09×10^9 /l.
  - Platelet count below 150×10^9 /l or if there are clinical signs of thrombocytopenia.
  - A greater than two-fold rise in AsT, AlT, or alkaline phosphatase.
  - Ask about rash or oral ulceration.
- Some manufacturers recommend regular renal function testing, but the practical predictive value of this has not been demonstrated.

- Sulfasalazine is subject to few drug interactions, but take care when giving it with other drugs that can suppress the bone marrow (e.g. azathioprine).

- Advise patients to report immediately any unexplained purpura, bruising, bleeding, fever, sore throat, or malaise, as these may be indicative of a blood dyscrasia.
- Can turn tears and urine orange, and can stain soft contact lenses.

Prescribing information: **Sulfasalazine**

- Tablets and enteric-coated tablets, 500 mg per tablet.
- For an acute attack the usual dose is 1–2 g 4 times daily until control is achieved; this may require concomitant corticosteroids. The maintenance dose is usually 500 mg 4 times daily.
- Suppositories for rectal treatment. Usual dose 0.5–1 g morning and night.
- Enema for distal colonic disease. Usual dose 3 g at night, retained for at least 1 hour.

Salazopyrin®

- Tablets and enteric-coated tablets. Contain 500 mg per tablet.
- Suspension. Contains 250 mg sulfasalazine per 5 mL.
- Suppository. Contains 500 mg sulfasalazine per suppository.
- Retention enema. Contains 3 g sulfasalazine per enema.

Cholic acids

Bile acids

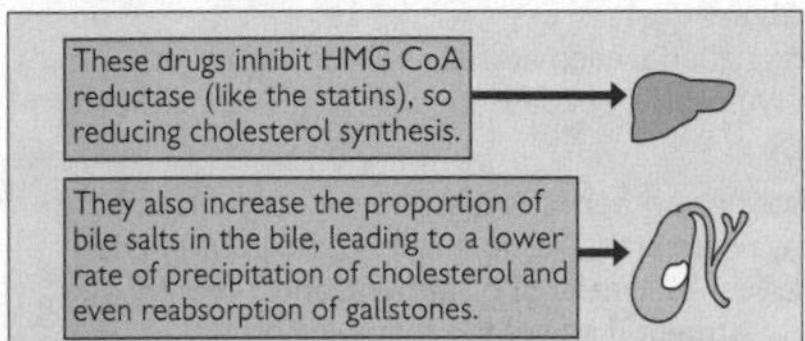

Drugs in this class
- Ursodeoxycholic acid
- Chenodeoxycholic acid

- Treatment of cholesterol gallstones (not other types of gallstone).
- Ursodeoxycholic acid is used in the treatment of primary biliary cirrhosis and primary sclerosing cholangitis. These are unlicensed, specialist uses.

- Cholic acids can worsen liver impairment in those with existing disease.
- Cholic acids can worsen peptic ulcer and symptoms from ileal disease; avoid in these patients.
- The manufacturer advises that these drugs should not be used in pregnancy, although there is no evidence of harm.

Gallstones

- These drugs will act only on cholesterol gallstones (which are radiotranslucent).
- Laparoscopic cholecystectomy is the treatment of choice for symptomatic gallstone disease.
- If the patient is unsuitable for surgery, consider treatment with the cholic acids.
  - Treatment can be for up to 2 years.
  - Stop the treatment 3 months after the stone has disappeared.
  - A repeat ultrasound examination should be performed 4–12 weeks after the stone has disappeared to confirm this.
  - The recurrence rate is high once treatment has stopped; it is estimated to be 25% after 1 year and 50% by 5 years.

- Diarrhoea is common, owing to disturbance of water and electrolyte reabsorption. Tolerance develops with time.
- Nausea and vomiting can occur.
- Treatment with these drugs can cause gallstones to calcify.

- Oestrogens and clofibrate oppose the action of these drugs.
  - Use a progestogen-only oral contraceptive, or preferably a non-hormonal method of contraception.

Safety and efficacy
- Regular ultrasound examination is required to monitor the progress of treatment.
- The manufacturers advise regular measurement of liver function tests, but the value of this has not been established.

- Warn the patient about the possibility of diarrhoea and advise that it may improve with time.

Prescribing information: **Cholic acids**

- Ursodeoxycholic acid is given as an example.
  - Dissolution of gallstones, 8–12 mg/kg daily as a single dose at bedtime *or* in 2 divided doses. Treat for up to 2 years, and continue for 3–4 months after stones dissolve.
  - Primary biliary cirrhosis, 10–15 mg/kg daily in 2–4 divided doses.

Colestyramine and colestipol

Exchange resins

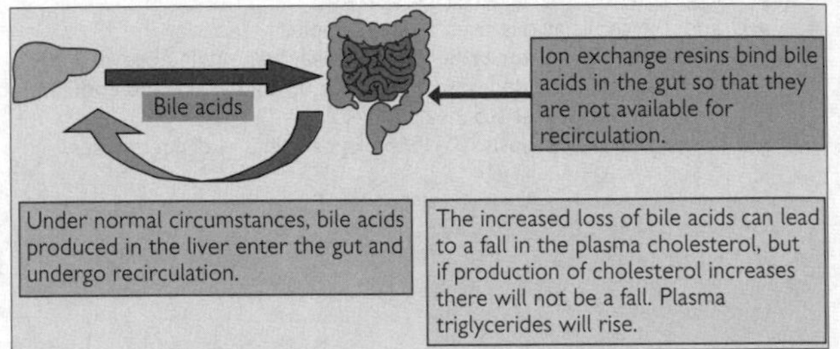

- Treatment of type IIa familial hypercholesterolaemia.
- Treatment of pruritus due to bile acids in the skin in partial obstructive jaundice (but note caution below).
- Diarrhoea caused by excess bile acids in the gut in ileal disease.

- These drugs can aggravate hypertriglyceridaemia.
- Owing to their mechanism of action, these drugs will not work if biliary obstruction is complete.
- The manufacturer advises caution in pregnancy; these drugs are not absorbed so should not cause harm, but the reduction in absorption of certain vitamins (see below) carries the potential for harm.
- These drugs are not absorbed systemically; no dosage reduction is usually required in renal or hepatic insufficiency.

Hypercholesterolaemia

- Exchange resins are not first-line treatments for hypercholesterolaemia. Use a statin instead.

Pruritus due to biliary obstruction

- Exchange resins can provide symptomatic relief for this distressing symptom, but only if obstruction is incomplete.
- Note that these drugs will not have any effect on the underlying cause of the obstruction.

Diarrhoea

- Exchange resins can be very effective for the diarrhoea caused by excess bile acids in the lower bowel in patients with ileal disease.
- Diarrhoea of this type is a symptom not a diagnosis; arrange for further investigation.

- These drugs cause constipation in 50% of patients.
- Nausea and heartburn are common.
- These drugs will reduce absorption of the vitamins A, D, E, and K; prolonged treatment can cause deficiency. Give vitamin A, D, and K supplements to those taking long-term treatment.
- These drugs rarely cause a hypochloraemic acidosis.

- The absorption of warfarin, levothyroxine, tri-iodothyronine (T3), digitoxin, and leflunomide can be reduced.

Safety and efficacy

- Measure the total cholesterol, cholesterol fractions, and plasma triglycerides before and during treatment.

- Advise the patient not to take any other drugs either 1 hour before or 4–6 hours after taking these drugs.

Prescribing information: **Colestyramine and Colestipol**

Colestyramine

- For lipid reduction or diarrhoea: introduce gradually over 3–4 weeks. Maintenance dosage usually 12–24 g daily in water (or another suitable liquid) in single or up to 4 divided doses.
    - Up to 36 g daily can be used if necessary
- For pruritus: 4–8 g daily in water (or other suitable liquid).

Colestipol

- For lipid reduction: 5 g 1–2 times daily in liquid, increased if necessary at intervals of 1–2 months to a maximum of 30 g daily (in single or 2 divided doses).

HMG CoA reductase inhibitors ('statins')

Drugs affecting lipid metabolism

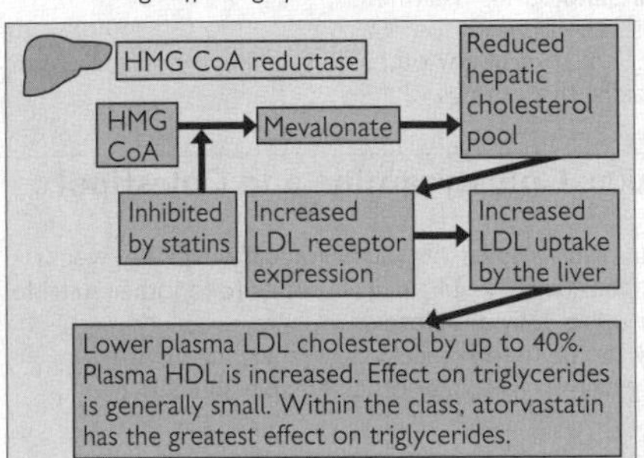

Drugs that lower plasma cholesterol

First-line
- HMG CoA reductase inhibitors ('statins')

Second-line
- Fibrates (used occasionally)
- Nicotinic acid (in high doses it inhibits cholesterol synthesis)
- Resins (colestyramine and colestipol)
- Omega 3 fish oils

Drugs in this class

Substrates for CYP 3A4
- Atorvastatin
- Lovastatin
- Simvastatin
- (Cerivastatin withdrawn)

Substrate for CYP 2C9
- Fluvastatin

Not metabolized by P450 enzymes
- Pravastatin

- Treatment of hyperlipoproteinaemia, especially types IIa and IIb.
- Primary and secondary prevention of coronary artery disease.

- Statins are contraindicated during pregnancy; in addition, women should avoid becoming pregnant during treatment and for 1 month after stopping these drugs. The reduction in cholesterol may affect embryonic development. Toxicity has been observed in animals.
- Patients with renal insufficiency may be at an increased risk of myositis.
- Do not give these drugs to patients with hepatic insufficiency or to patients with persistently raised transaminases.

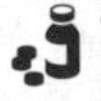

- The statins are considerably more effective at reducing plasma cholesterol than plasma triglycerides. The relative contribution of each to the development of coronary artery disease is still debated but the results of large-scale clinical trials suggest that lowering cholesterol is most important.

Secondary prevention of coronary artery disease
- All patients who have had an event (stroke, angina, or myocardial infarction) should be treated with a statin.
- There is evidence that all patients over 55 years of age benefit from treatment with a statin, even if their initial total cholesterol is <5 mmol/L.

Primary prevention of coronary artery disease
- Use a cardiac risk assessor (tables or computer program) to determine whether your patient requires treatment for primary prevention.
  - Current UK guidelines suggest that patients with a 10-year risk of coronary artery disease greater then 30% should be treated, although there is evidence that patients at lower risk will also benefit.
  - NICE has recommended that patients with type II diabetes mellitus should be given a statin if their total cholesterol is >5 mmol/L (or LDL cholesterol >3 mmol/L) and/or tyriglyceride concentration >2.3 mmol/L, if they fail to respond to a 3-month trial of diet and exercise.

- The most important adverse effect of these drugs is a myopathy; although uncommon, it can be fatal.
  - It is characterized by muscle pain and stiffness and can progress to rhabdomyolysis.
  - A transient asymptomatic rise in creatine kinase (CK) is more common.
  - It is difficult to define an incidence rate but one estimate is less than 0.05%.
  - The following factors increase the risk substantially:
    - — The risk is dose-related.
    - — Concomitant treatment with fibrates. The combination of cerivastatin with a fibrate drug seems to carry the highest risk and cerivastatin has been withdrawn as a result.
    - — Concomitant treatment with ciclosporin.
    - — Renal insufficiency.
- These drugs are usually well tolerated. The most common adverse effects are headache, nausea, and abdominal cramps.

- The risk of myopathy is increased when these drugs are given with fibrates or ciclosporin. Avoid these combinations unless the benefit outweighs the risk (e.g. some forms of familial hyperlipidaemia).

Safety and efficacy

- Measure plasma triglycerides, total cholesterol, and HDL cholesterol before starting treatment in order to select the most appropriate drug (statin or fibrate). If a lipid-lowering drug is required for secondary prevention, a statin is recommended.
  - Measure these again once maintenance treatment has been established and adjust the dose according to your targets. Many prescribers give the maximum tolerated dose.
  - Targets change, and will depend on the patient's risk. NICE has recommended that for patients with type II diabetes mellitus, treatment should reduce total cholesterol to below 5 mmol/L, or by 25–30%, whichever is the greater. If LDL is used, it should be below 3 mmol/L or be reduced by 30%.
  - Some advocate the use of the highest dose in all patients as the risk reduction is linear.
- Measure liver function tests (transaminases) before treatment, after 1–3 months' treatment, and at 6 and 12 months.
  - An increase in transaminases is reported in 1–2% of patients and usually occurs in the first 3 months.
  - Stop the drug if this rise is greater than three times normal or baseline.
- Measure CK activity urgently if the patient reports muscle pain. Stop the drug.

- Advise the patient to report any generalized muscle weakness or pain immediately.
- Advise the patient to take the tablet at night-time, when the drug is supposed to have a slightly greater effect. The reasons for this are not known, but hepatic cholesterol synthesis is greater at night.

Prescribing information: **Statins**

Atorvastatin

- By mouth, usual dose 10 mg daily.
- Can be increased up to 40 mg daily.

- In the treatment of heterozygous familial hypercholesterolaemia the maximum dose is increased to 80 mg daily (specialist use only).

Fluvastatin
- By mouth, usual dose 20–40 mg daily.
- Can be increased up to 40 mg twice daily.

Pravastatin
- By mouth, usual dose 10–40 mg daily.

Simvastatin
- By mouth, usual dose 10–40 mg daily. Note that the 10 mg dose is often inadequate; many clinicians begin with a dose of 20 mg.
- Can be increased up to 80 mg daily if required (e.g. treatment of primary hypercholesterolaemia, heterozygous familial hypercholesterolaemia, or combined hyperlipidaemia).

Fibrates

Drugs affecting lipid metabolism

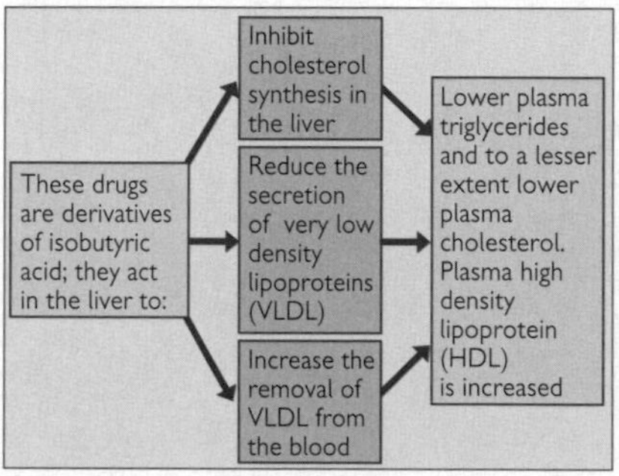

Drugs that lower plasma cholesterol

First-line
- HMG CoA reductase inhibitors ('statins')

Second-line
- Fibrates (used occasionally)
- Nicotinic acid (in high doses it inhibits cholesterol synthesis)
- Resins (colestyramine and colestipol)
- Omega 3 fish oils

Drugs in this class
- Bezafibrate
- Ciprofibrate
- Fenofibrate
- Gemfibrozil

- Treatment of hyperlipoproteinaemia, especially types IIa, IIb, III, IV, V.
- Primary prevention of coronary artery disease (licence is for men only).

- Fibrates are contraindicated during pregnancy; they are embryotoxic in animals.
- Do not use these drugs in patients with primary biliary cirrhosis or gall bladder disease.
- Patients with renal insufficiency are at an increased risk of myositis from these drugs. Consider alternatives.
- Do not give fibrates to patients with severe hepatic insufficiency.

- Fibrates are considerably more effective at reducing plasma triglycerides than plasma cholesterol.
  - Hypercholesterolaemia is much more common than hypertrigyceridaemia.
- Gemfibrozil has a licence for the primary prevention of coronary artery disease in middle-aged men. Note that the evidence base for the use of statins in primary prevention is considerably larger and covers a much wider group of patients.
- Use a cardiac risk assessor (tables or computer program) to determine whether your patient requires treatment for primary prevention.
  - Current UK guidelines suggest that patients with hypertriglyceridaemia and a 10-year risk of coronary artery disease greater than 30% should be treated, although there is evidence that patients at lower risk will also benefit.
  - NICE has recommended that patients with type II diabetes should be given a fibrate if their plasma triglycerides exceed 10 mmol/L, whether or not they are taking a statin. Consider adding a fibrate if the plasma triglycerides remain above 2.3 mmol/L despite treatment with a statin, although the evidence base for this is less strong.

- The most important adverse effect of these drugs is myositis; although uncommon, it can be fatal.
  - Characterized by muscle pain and stiffness and can progress to rhabdomyolysis.
  - It is difficult to define an incidence rate but the following factors increase the risk substantially:
    - — Concomitant treatment with HMG CoA reductase inhibitors ('statins').
    - — Concomitant treatment with ciclosporin.
    - — Renal insufficiency.
- Hypersensitivity to these drugs manifests as urticaria, pruritus, and a photosensitive rash.
- Gastrointestinal adverse effects, such as nausea and vomiting, are common.

- The risk of myositis is increased when these drugs are given with statins and ciclosporin. Avoid these combinations unless the benefit outweighs the risk (e.g. some familial hyperlipidaemias).
- Fibrates enhance the anticoagulant action of warfarin.

Safety and efficacy

- Measure plasma triglycerides, total cholesterol, and HDL cholesterol before starting treatment in order to select the most appropriate drug.
  - Measure the triglycerides again once maintenance treatment has been established, and adjust the dose according to your target (usually <2.3 mmol/L).
- Measure renal function (creatinine) and stop the drug if this is deteriorating.
- Measure CK activity urgently if the patient reports muscle pain. Stop the drug.

- Advise the patient to report any generalized muscle weakness or pain immediately.

Prescribing information: **Fibrates**

Bezafibrate and gemfibrozil are given as examples.

Bezafibrate

- By mouth, 200 mg 3 times daily, after food.

Genfibrozil

- By mouth, dosage range is from 900 mg to 1500 mg daily, usually 600 mg twice daily.

Orlistat

Inhibitor of pancreatic lipase

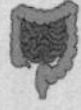

- Orlistat inhibits the action of pancreatic lipase within the gut lumen; orlistat is barely absorbed. Because less fat is digested, less is absorbed.
- The increased fat content of the faeces can cause adverse effects (see below).

Body Mass Index (BMI)

$$\text{BMI} = \frac{\text{Mass (kg)}}{\text{Height (m)}^2}$$

For example:
weight = 70 kg,
height =180 cm,
BMI = 21.6 kg/m²

	BMI (kg/m²)
Underweight	<18.5
Ideal weight	18.6–24.9
Overweight	25–29.9
Obese	30–39.9
Morbidly obese	>40

- As an adjunct to diet and exercise in the treatment of morbid obesity.
  - If the patient has a BMI >30 kg/m² or if the BMI is > 28 kg/m² and the patient has other risk factors for cardiovascular disease (e.g. type II diabetes, hypertension, hypercholesterolaemia).

- Pregnant women need about 100–200 additional kilocalories daily. Advise women to avoid excessive weight gain during pregnancy, but drug treatment is inappropriate.
- Orlistat can reduce the absorption of fat-soluble vitamins; it should not be given to patients with malabsorption or cholestasis.
- No dosage adjuustment is usually required in hepatic or renal insufficiency.

- NICE has recommended that orlistat should only be given if the patient has lost 2.5 kg over 1 month by diet and exercise alone.
  - Counselling and support are an essential part of a weight loss programme.
  - See sibutramine (p. 59) for general advice on the treatment of obesity.
- Review the success of the regimen regularly; see below for advice on target weight loss.

- Orlistat is barely absorbed so the risk of systemic adverse effects is low.
  - Hypersensitivity and hepatitis have been observed, but are very rare.
- Inhibition of fat absorption commonly causes oily stools, abdominal pain, and faecal incontinence.

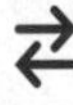

- The absorption of fat-soluble vitamins (A, D, E, K) is reduced by treatment with orlistat. Consider giving supplements to patients who are at risk of deficiency. Take the supplement at least 2 hours after a dose of orlistat. Most patients are not at risk of vitamin deficiency.

Efficacy

- Treatment with orlistat should only continue beyond 3 months if the patient has lost more then 5% of their body weight, and beyond 6 months only if they have lost 10%.
- Treatment should not usually continue beyond 2 years.

- Warn the patient about the risk of oily stools and faecal soiling. Many patients find these adverse effects intolerable.
- Warn the patient that the effects of drug treatments are modest; continued weight loss depends on the programme of diet and exercise.
- Warn the patient of the risk of weight gain on stopping the drug treatment. A sensible diet and appropriate programme of exercise should be lifelong.
- Advise the patient to omit the dose of orlistat if they miss a meal or if the meal contains no fat.

Prescribing information: **Orlistat**

- Adjunct to diet and exercise in the treatment of morbid obesity.
  - 120 mg taken immediately before, during, or up to 1 hour after each main meal.

  Maximum dose 360 mg daily.

Sibutramine

Inhibitor of the reuptake of serotonin and noradrenaline

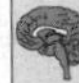
Sibutramine is a centrally acting appetite suppressant. Pharmacologically it an inhibitor of the reuptake of serotonin and noradrenaline.

Body Mass Index (BMI)

$$BMI = \frac{\text{Mass (kg)}}{\text{Height (m)}^2}$$

For example:
weight = 70 kg,
height =180 cm,
BMI = 21.6 kg/m^2

	BMI (kg/m^2)
Underweight	<18.5
Ideal weight	18.6–24.9
Overweight	25–29.9
Obese	30–39.9
Morbidly obese	>40

- As an adjunct to diet and exercise in the treatment of morbid obesity.
  - If the patient has a BMI >30 kg/m^2 or if the BMI is >28 kg/m^2 and the patient has other risk factors for cardiovascular disease (e.g. type II diabetes, hypertension, hypercholesterolaemia).

- Sibutramine can cause hypertension.
- Avoid it if the patient has a blood pressure greater than 145/90 mmHg.
- Patients who have sleep apnoea commonly have hypertension; avoid sibutramine.
- Sibutramine should not be given to patients who have coronary artery disease, heart failure, or a history of cardiac arrhythmias.
- Avoid sibutramine if the patient has closed angle glaucoma or prostatic hyperplasia.
- Avoid sibutramine if the patient has severe renal or hepatic insufficiency; metabolites can accumulate.
- Sibutramine is a stimulant of the central nervous system; avoid it if there is a history of a psychiatric disorder, an eating disorder, or substance abuse.
- Pregnant women need about 100–200 additional kilocalories daily. Advise women to avoid excessive weight gain during pregnancy, but drug treatment is inappropriate.

- NICE has recommended that sibutramine should only be given if the patient has lost 2.5 kg over 1 month by diet and exercise alone.
  - Counselling and support are an essential part of a weight loss programme.
  - See below for general advice on the treatment of obesity.
- Review the success of the regimen regularly; see below for advice on target weight loss.

- Stimulant cardiovascular effects are common: tachycardia, palpitation, and hypertension. See monitoring section below.
- Other common adverse effects include constipation, dry mouth, insomnia, and sweating.

- Sibutramine increases concentrations of serotonin in the brain; avoid any drugs that also do this, especially monoamine oxidase inhibitors and SSRIs.

Safety

- Measure the pulse and blood pressure every 2 weeks for the first 4 months of treatment, and monthly thereafter.

- Stop sibutramine if the resting heart rate increases by more then 10 beats per minute or the blood pressure rises by more than 10 mmHg.

Efficacy

- If the patient has lost less than 2 kg after 4 weeks' treatment and they are complying with the dietary and exercise regimen, consider increasing the daily dose of sibutramine to 15 mg. If the patient loses less than 2 kg over the following 4 weeks, withdraw the drug.
- Treatment with sibutramine should only continue beyond 3 months if the patient has lost more than 5% of body weight, and beyond 6 months only if they have lost 10%.
- Treatment should not usually continue beyond 1 year.

- Warn the patient that the effects of drug treatments are modest; continued weight loss depends on a programme of diet and exercise.
- Warn the patient of the risk of weight gain on stopping the drug treatment. A sensible diet and appropriate programme of exercise should be lifelong.

Prescribing information: **Sibutramine**

- Adjunct to diet and exercise in the treatment of morbid obesity.
  - By mouth, initially 10 mg daily in the morning.
  - This can be increased to 15 mg daily if weight loss is less than 2 kg after 4 weeks.
  - Discontinue drug treatment if weight loss less than 2 kg after 4 weeks at the higher dose.

TEACHING POINT Treatment of obesity

- Obesity is increasingly common. For example, 17% of adults in the UK are classed as obese (BMI >30). The changes in metabolism associated with obesity are central to the pathophysiology of insulin resistance and type II diabetes; obesity is also an important risk factor for hypertension and coronary artery disease; and there is an increased incidence of osteoarthritis of weight-bearing joints.
- Medical causes of obesity (e.g. Cushing's syndrome, hypothyroidism) are rare, but should be excluded before starting treatment.
- Weight gain results from an imbalance between energy intake and expenditure. The only long-term solution is to reduce intake and increase energy expenditure through exercise. Diets should be low in calories, but not very low. Aim for a total daily intake of around 1000 kCal. In patients who are motivated to lose weight, drug treatments can increase the amount of weight lost as part of a diet and exercise programme. Drug treatments are ineffective if given alone, and should not be continued for long periods (see individual articles for details).
- Ideally, obesity should be managed by a multidisciplinary team, but in many countries such expertise and resources are scarce.
- NICE has advised that patients with a (e.g. BMI >30 kg/m^2 should receive treatment. Patients with complications arising from obesity (obstructive apnoea, hypertension, type II diabetes) have most to gain from weight reduction and represent a priority group for treatment. Consider treatment in this group if they have a BMI >28 kg/m^2.
- Treatment of obesity should form part of a wider assessment of a patient's lifestyle and risk factors for cardiovascular disease. Help with stopping smoking can be particularly beneficial (see p. 236).
- Many patients are desperate to lose weight but find it difficult to modify their lifestyle; these patients are particularly vulnerable to those offering 'miracle treatments'. Many of these contain amphetamines, diuretics, and thyroid hormones. They have no place in the treatment of obesity and can cause significant harm.
- Fenfluramine, dexfenfluramine, and phenteramine are centrally-acting appetite suppressants structurally related to amphetamines. They have been withdrawn because they can cause pulmonary hypertension.
- Bulk-forming supplements (e.g. methylcellulose) are unlikely to cause harm, but there is little evidence that they are effective.

Metoclopramide

Antiemetic drug

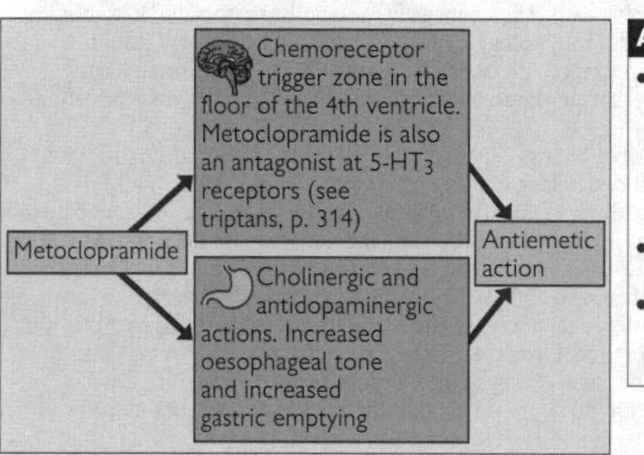

Antiemetic drugs

- Dopamine receptor antagonists
  - Phenothiazines
  - Domperidone
  - Metoclopramide
- 5-HT_3 receptor antagonists
- Antihistamines
  - motion sickness only

- Treatment and prevention of nausea and vomiting, especially:
  - Drug-induced
  - Postoperatively
  - Associated with migraine
- To stimulate gastric emptying:
  - During radiological investigations
  - In patients with gastroparesis due to diabetic neuropathy (specialized use)

- Metoclopramide is metabolized by the liver. Reduce the dose in hepatic insufficiency.
- Antiemetic drugs are rarely needed for vomiting associated with pregnancy. If severe seek specialist advice. Metoclopramide is an option in such cases.
- Do not use metoclopramide in patients with gastrointestinal obstruction or haemorrhage; the actions on the stomach may be dangerous.
- Do not use metoclopramide in patients with Parkinsonian symptoms; the antidopaminergic actions can worsen these.
- Do not give metoclopramide to patients with phaeochromocytoma; it can precipitate a hypertensive crisis.
- The use of metoclopramide in patients under 20 years old is specialized; seek expert advice (see below).

- Nausea and vomiting are symptoms, not diagnoses. Always consider the underlying cause. Long-term treatment should be of the cause, rather than with antiemetic drugs.
- Like the treatment of pain, the treatment of nausea and vomiting should be based on avoidance and prophylaxis, rather than waiting for symptoms to occur before tackling them.
- Metoclopramide is used widely but is especially useful:
  - For nausea owing to gastrointestinal, biliary, and liver disease; however, it should not be used if there is gastrointestinal obstruction.
  - In high dosages for emesis associated with chemotherapy, but it has largely been replaced by the $5HT_3$ receptor antagonists for this indication.

- Consider the following factors:
  - Identify patients who are at high risk of postoperative nausea and vomiting and give them treatment early. A dose of 10 mg alone is often inadequate for postoperative nausea and vomiting.
  - Treat pain, as this is often a contributory factor.
  - Refer to the teaching point in $5HT_3$ receptor antagonists (p. 73) for information on the treatment of nausea and vomiting due to chemotherapy.
  - Metoclopramide is unlikely to be effective for motion sickness; this is mediated through the vestibular system.

- Extrapyramidal (antidopaminergic) adverse effects affect 1% of patients.
  - These can range from dystonia to an oculogyric crisis.
  - Young people (<20 years) are at greatest risk.
  - Treat this adverse effect with diazepam or procyclidine.
- The antidopaminergic action of metoclopramide can also cause:
  - Parkisonian symptoms and signs.
  - Prolactin release, leading to galactorrhoea, gynaecomastia, and menstrual disturbances.
- Other CNS adverse effects include dizziness and drowsiness.

- Metoclopramide enhances the action of other antidopaminergic drugs.
- Anticholinergic and opioid drugs antagonize the actions of metoclopramide on the gut, reducing its efficacy.
- Increased gastric emptying due to metoclopramide can increase the speed of absorption of other drugs.
  - This effect will not usually be apparent, as the extent of absorption of drugs will remain the same.
  - Analgesics, such as aspirin and paracetamol, may act a little more quickly; this has been used in the treatment of migraine.

Efficacy

- If a patient has had postoperative nausea and vomiting in the past, discuss strategies to prevent this with the anaesthetist.

- Warn the patient that metoclopramide can cause dizziness that may interfere with skilled motor tasks (e.g. driving). Patients who are given metoclopramide should not drive (e.g. after day surgery).

Prescribing information: **Metoclopramide**

- By mouth, intramuscular injection, or intravenous injection (over 1–2 minutes), 10 mg tds.
- High-dose metoclopramide can be used with cytotoxic chemotherapy; seek specialist advice.

Prochlorperazine (Stemetil®)

Antiemetic phenothiazine

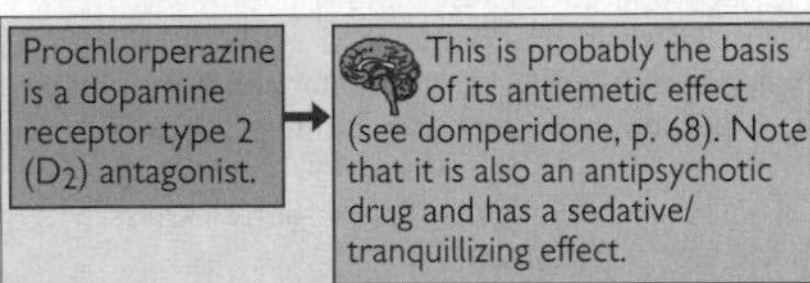

Prochlorperazine also has anticholinergic, antihistamine, and anti-α-adrenergic actions. The contribution of these to its antipsychotic effect is not known, but they do cause adverse effects.

Phenothiazine drugs

- Chlorpromazine
- Fluphenazine
- Prochlorperazine
- Thioridazine
- Trifluoperazine

Note

- Other antipsychotic drugs are not routinely used for their antiemetic actions, as they are very sedative.
- The sedative action can be useful when used for nausea and vomiting in palliative care, see box below.

- Treatment and prevention of nausea and vomiting, especially:
  - Due to cytotoxic chemotherapy
  - Due to diffuse neoplastic disease
  - Opioid-induced
  - Postoperatively

- Antiemetic drugs are rarely needed for vomiting associated with pregnancy. If severe seek specialist advice. Prochlorperazine is an option in such cases.

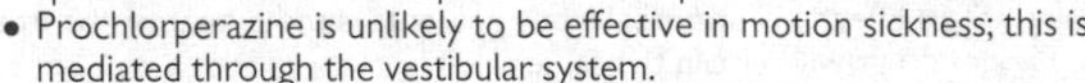

- Prochlorperazine is unlikely to be effective in motion sickness; this is mediated through the vestibular system.
- Do not give prochlorperazine to patients with hepatic insufficiency; it can induce hepatic coma.
- Use smaller initial doses if the patient has renal insufficiency; they are more susceptible to the sedative effects.
- Do not give prochlorperazine to patients with Parkinsonian symptoms; the antidopaminergic actions can worsen these.
- Prochlorperazine has anticholinergic actions; avoid it in patients with closed angle glaucoma or urinary retention.
- Prochlorperazine lowers the seizure threshold; avoid using it in patients with epilepsy.
- Do not give prochlorperazine to patients with phaeochromocytoma; it can precipitate a hypertensive crisis.

- Nausea and vomiting are symptoms, not diagnoses. Always consider the underlying cause. Long-term treatment should be of the cause, rather than with antiemetic drugs.
- Like the treatment of pain, the treatment of nausea and vomiting should be based on avoidance and prophylaxis rather than waiting for symptoms to occur before tackling them.
- Prochlorperazine is especially useful for postoperative nausea and vomiting.
  - Prochlorperazine is less sedative than chlorpromazine but still has a sedative effect.
- Note that the dose is different for each route of administration.
- See teaching point below for more guidance on the treatment of acute vertigo.

- Prochlorperazine can cause the neuroleptic malignant syndrome (see antipsychotic drugs, p. 290).
    - This is characterized by fever, anorexia, rigidity, lowered level of consciousness, and autonomic disturbance (tachycardia, hyperthermia), and can be fatal (see SSRIs, p. 283).
    - Stop the drug immediately. There are no established effective treatments, but cooling, bromocriptine, and dantrolene can be helpful.
    - The syndrome usually lasts 5–7 days.
- Extrapyramidal (antidopaminergic) adverse effects are common.
    - These can range from dystonia and akathisia to an oculogyric crisis.
    - The young, elderly, and the debilitated are at greatest risk.
    - Treat this adverse effect with diazepam or procyclidine.
- The antidopaminergic actions can also cause prolactin release, leading to galactorrhoea, gynaecomastia, and menstrual disturbances.
- The anticholinergic actions can cause dry mouth, blurred vision, and urinary retention.
- Hypersensitivity phenomena, such as a photosensitive rash, are common.
- Prochlorperazine can cause cardiac arrhythmias by prolonging the QT interval.
- Prochlorperazine can cause hypotension, especially in hypovolaemic patients. Take care in postoperative patients.
- Prochlorperazine can lower the body temperature. This has been used therapeutically.
- Rare adverse effects include blood dyscrasias and liver toxicity (cholestatic jaundice).

- Prochlorperazine potentiates the actions of other sedative drugs (e.g. alcohol).
- Prochlorperazine potentiates the actions of other drugs that lower the blood pressure.
- Avoid giving prochlorperazine to patients taking other drugs that can prolong the QT interval (this includes tricyclic antidepressant drugs).
- The risk of neurotoxicity from lithium is increased by prochlorperazine.

- If a patient has had postoperative nausea and vomiting in the past, discuss strategies to prevent this with the anaesthetist.

- Warn the patient that prochlorperazine can cause dizziness, which may interfere with skilled motor tasks (e.g. driving).
- Prochlorperazine is available over the counter for patients who have nausea and vomiting associated with previously diagnosed migraine. Ensure that a formal diagnosis has been made if the patient is taking the drug for this indication.

Prescribing information: **Prochlorperazine**

- By mouth
    - Acute treatment 20 mg initially, followed by 10 mg after 2 hours.
    - Prevention 5–10 mg bd or tds.
- By deep intramuscular injection
    - 12.5 mg, followed after 6 hours by an oral dose.
- By rectum, in suppositories
    - 25 mg, followed if necessary after 6 hours by an oral dose.

TEACHING POINT Routes of administration of drugs

- The choice of route of administration will depend on the nature of the effect desired and whether the drug can act when given by that route. An intravenous bolus dose can achieve a high plasma concentration quickly, but it is likely to have a limited duration of action owing to distribution and metabolism of the drug. A prolonged action can be achieved by following a bolus dose with an infusion. Although a rapid onset of effect is sometimes needed, it is rarely necessary during long-term therapy.
- Administration by mouth is often favoured for long-term therapy because it is convenient. Other kinetic factors are important, but this route can produce a long duration of action because of continued delivery of the drug, especially when given in a modified-release formulation. A more rapid onset of effect can be achieved by giving a loading dose, but modified-release formulations are not suitable for this purpose.
- It is often convenient to deliver drug treatments directly to the site of disease (e.g. topical corticosteroids for eczema). This can reduce systemic exposure to the drug, but remember that systemic exposure can still occur and cause adverse effects.
- Not all drugs can be given by every route; for example, a drug must be relatively lipid soluble in order to be absorbed through the skin.
- The table below summarizes the advantages and disadvantages of the major routes of administration.

Advantages and disadvantages of the major routes of administration

Route of administration	Advantages	Disadvantages
By mouth	Convenient. Sustained delivery possible (e.g. modified-release formulations).	Slow onset of action. Cannot give peptides by this route. Absorption can be inadequate or unpredictable.
Intramuscular	Rapid onset of action. Useful if the patient is vomiting (e.g. metoclopramide).	Invasive. Can cause haematoma or sterile abscess. Some drugs are painful when given by this route. Some drugs are erratically absorbed by this route (e.g. phenytoin).
Depot formulations	Prolonged duration of action (e.g. depot contraceptives).	Once the dose has been given it cannot be withdrawn if adverse effects occur (e.g. phenothiazines).
Intravenous	Very rapid onset of action. Allows precise dose titration. Dose delivered is the dose received.	Very invasive. Complex administration. Risk of systemic infection. Not generally suitable for long-term administration.

(continued)

Advantages and disadvantages of the major routes of administration—cont'd

Route of administration	Advantages	Disadvantages
Subcutaneous	Simple administration. Suitable for long-term administration. An alternative to intravenous administration of large volumes of saline.	Absorption can be unpredictable (e.g. adrenaline). Can cause lipodystophy (e.g. insulin).
Inhalations (dry powders, aerosols, and solutions for nebulization)	Direct delivery to the lungs for respiratory diseases.	Systemic absorption of drugs is significant (e.g. corticosteroids).
Rectal	Rapid systemic delivery. Suitable if the patient is vomiting (e.g. domperidone). Direct delivery for some bowel diseases (e.g. steroids for ulcerative colitis).	Limited social acceptance.
Vaginal	Local treatment.	Not appropriate for delivery of many drugs.
Nasal	Local treatment (e.g. allergic rhinitis). Can give peptides by this route (e.g. calcitonin).	Systemic absorption is unpredictable.
Buccal, sublingual, and 'melt' formulations	Rapid onset of action.	Short duration of action.
Eye drops	Direct delivery to the eye.	Systemic absorption can occur (e.g. beta-blockers).
Topical (skin)	Direct treatment of isolated skin diseases.	Some drugs are absorbed through the skin, and can cause systemic adverse effects (e.g. corticosteroids)
Creams/ointments	Limited systemic exposure (e.g. corticosteroids). Convenient.	
Transdermal patches	Sustained delivery.	Limited systemic delivery. Potential for tolerance (e.g. nitrates).
Intrathecal	Direct delivery to the CNS (e.g. treatment of leukaemia).	Potential for severe adverse effects (e.g. vinca alkaloids).
Epidural	Allows regional anaesthesia.	Invasive. Risk of sepsis.
Intraperitoneal	Direct treatment of peritoneal infection. Good systemic delivery.	Only available in a limited number of patients. Risk of introduction of infection.

TEACHING POINT Drugs and dizziness

Drug toxicity

- Drugs can cause dizziness through toxic effects on the vestibular apparatus.
  - For example, high trough concentrations of aminoglycoside antibiotics (see p. 340 for advice on safe use of these drugs).
  - Excessively rapid infusion of large doses of furosemide can cause ototoxicity.
- Adverse effects occurring in the therapeutic range.
  - For example, phenothiazines.
- Drugs that can cause hypotension (especially postural hypotension).
  - For example, nitrates.

Drugs used to treat symptoms of dizziness

It is important to make a diagnosis; if the underlying cause can be treated, that is preferable; and none of the symptomatic treatments is very effective.

Acute severe vertigo with nausea and vomiting

- A phenothiazine by intramuscular injection (e.g. prochlorperazine 12.5 mg).
- If the extrapyramidal adverse effects of phenothiazines are likely to cause problems consider giving a benzodiazepine instead.

Moderate vertigo with nausea

- An antihistamine by mouth (e.g. cinnarizine 30 mg tds).

Ménière's disease

- A diuretic alone or combined with salt restriction may provide symptomatic relief for vertigo associated with Ménière's disease.
- Betahistine is an analogue of histamine that is licensed for symptomatic relief of Ménière's disease; it may act by reducing endolymphatic pressure.
  - By mouth, initially 16 mg tds, with food.
  - Usual maintenance dose 24–48 mg daily, in divided doses.

Motion sickness

- Antiemetics should be given prophylactically for the prevention of motion sickness rather than after nausea or vomiting develop. The most effective drug for the prevention of motion sickness is hyoscine.
- Sedative antihistamines are slightly less effective against motion sickness, but are generally better tolerated than hyoscine.
- Promethazine is useful but very sedating; slightly less sedating antihistamines such as cyclizine or cinnarizine are usually preferred.
  - The $5HT_3$ antagonists, domperidone, metoclopramide, and the phenothiazines (except the antihistamine phenothiazine promethazine) are ineffective in motion sickness.

Domperidone

Antiemetic drug

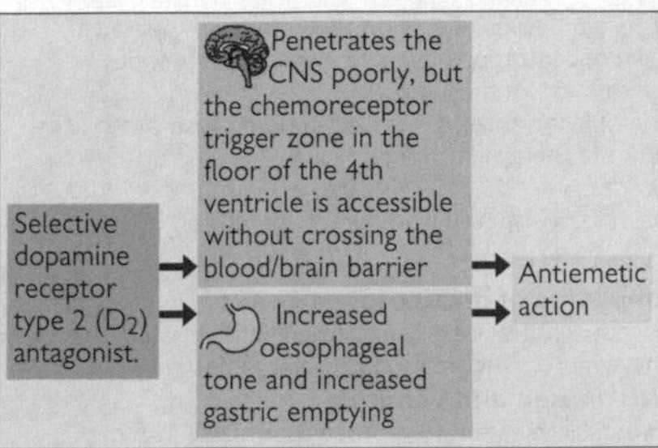

Antiemetic drugs

- Dopamine receptor antagonists
  - Phenothiazines
  - Domperidone
  - Metoclopramide
- 5-HT_3 receptor antagonists
- Antihistamines
  - Motion sickness only

- Treatment and prevention of nausea and vomiting, especially:
  - Due to cytotoxic chemotherapy
  - Due to dopamine receptor agonists and levodopa

- Domperidone is not recommended in pregnancy.
- Domperidone is unlikely to be effective in motion sickness, which is mediated through the vestibular system.
- Do not use domperidone in patients with gastrointestinal obstruction or haemorrhage; the actions on the stomach may be dangerous.
- Domperidone is not recommended for routine prevention and treatment of postoperative nausea and vomiting.
- No dosage adjustment is usually required in hepatic or renal insufficiency.

- Nausea and vomiting are symptoms, not diagnoses. Always consider the underlying cause. Long-term treatment should be of the cause, rather than with antiemetic drugs.
- Like the treatment of pain, the treatment of nausea and vomiting should be based on avoidance and prophylaxis, rather than waiting for symptoms to occur before tackling them.
- Domperidone is especially useful for nausea and vomiting due to dopamine receptor agonists and levodopa. Because it penetrates the CNS poorly it will not antagonize their CNS actions. For the same reason, domperidone does not usually cause Parkinsonian adverse effects, although they can occur.
- Domperidone is a first-line drug for the treatment of nausea and vomiting due to cytotoxic chemotherapy. See teaching point for 5-HT_3 receptor antagonists (p. 73) for further details.

- The antidopaminergic action of domperidone can cause prolactin release, leading to galactorrhoea, gynaecomastia, and menstrual disturbances.
- Extrapyramidal (antidopaminergic) adverse effects are uncommon.
- Domperidone can cause a rash.

- The absorption of domperidone is reduced by histamine H_2 receptor antagonists (e.g. ranitidine), food, and antacids.
- Anticholinergic and opioid drugs antagonize the actions of domperidone on the gut, reducing its efficacy.

- Continuous treatment (for nausea due to drugs) should be for a maximum of 12 weeks.

- Domperidone is available over the counter for short-term relief of postprandial fullness and bloating. Consider investigation if symptoms are severe or prolonged. Regular treatment should not exceed 12 weeks.

Prescribing information: **Domperidone**

- By mouth, 10–20 mg every 4–8 hours.

Serotonin 5-HT$_3$ receptor antagonists

Antiemetic drugs

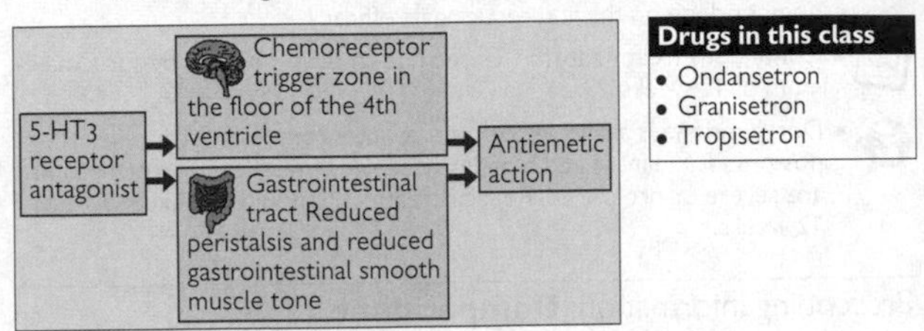

Drugs in this class

- Ondansetron
- Granisetron
- Tropisetron

- Treatment and prevention of nausea and vomiting, especially:
  - During radiotherapy or chemotherapy
  - Postoperatively

- These drugs are metabolized by the liver. Limit the maximum dose (e.g. ondansetron 8 mg daily) in hepatic insufficiency.
- There is little information about the safety of these drugs in pregnancy.
  - Antiemetic drugs are rarely needed for vomiting associated with pregnancy. If severe seek specialist advice.

- Nausea and vomiting are symptoms, not diagnoses. Always consider the underlying cause. Long-term treatment should be of the cause, rather than with antiemetic drugs.
- Like the treatment of pain, the treatment of nausea and vomiting should be based on avoidance and prophylaxis rather than waiting for symptoms to occur before tackling them.
  - Identify patients who are at high risk of postoperative nausea and vomiting and give them treatment early.
  - Treat pain, as this is often a contributory factor.
  - Refer to teaching point below for information on the treatment of nausea and vomiting due to chemotherapy.
  - These drugs are not very effective for delayed vomiting.
- Although these drugs can be given by mouth, they are usually given by injection for the majority of indications for which they are most useful.

- These drugs are usually well tolerated.
- They can cause headache, especially with repeated administration. This can be severe and require withdrawal of the drug.
- There are 5-HT$_3$ receptors in the gut and these drugs can cause constipation.
- Rapid intravenous injection can cause flushing.
- Hypersensitivity reactions are rare.

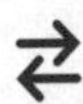

- The antiemetic action of these drugs is enhanced by co-administration with steroids (see below).

Efficacy

- Review the patient at the end of a cycle of chemotherapy and assess how effective the antiemetic treatment was. Increase the treatment by giving it more frequently if the response is unsatisfactory. Anticipatory symptoms are very difficult to treat once they have developed.
- If a patient has had postoperative nausea and vomiting in the past, discuss strategies to prevent this with the anaesthetist.

- Warn the patient that these drugs can cause dizziness, which can interfere with skilled motor tasks (e.g. driving). Patients who are given these drugs should not drive home (e.g. after day surgery).

Prescribing information: **5-HT$_3$ receptor antagonists**

There are many regimens. Ondansetron is given as an example.

Postoperative nausea and vomiting

Prevention

Several regimens are available. Discuss with the anaesthetist which is the most appropriate for the proposed surgery.

- By mouth, 16 mg 1 hour before anaesthesia.
- By mouth, 8 mg 1 hour before anaesthesia, followed by 8 mg for 2 further doses at intervals of 8 hours.
- By intramuscular or slow intravenous injection, 4 mg at induction of anaesthesia.

Treatment

- By intramuscular or slow intravenous injection, 4 mg.

Severely emetogenic chemotherapy (first 24 hours)

- By intramuscular or slow intravenous injection, 8 mg immediately before treatment.
- Followed by:
  - Either intramuscular or slow intravenous injection, 8 mg for further 2 doses at intervals of 2–4 hours.
  - Or intravenous infusion 1 mg hourly for 24 hours.

Severely emetogenic chemotherapy (for next 5 days maximum)

- By mouth, 8 mg every 12 hours.

TEACHING POINT

Treatment of emesis associated with chemotherapy

Prevention and pre-treatment are important, as anticipatory symptoms (symptoms that occur in advance of a course of treatment) are difficult to treat once they have developed.

	Risk of nausea		
	Low	**Medium**	**High**
Example drugs	Fluorouracil, etoposide, vinca alkaloids, methotrexate, abdominal radiotherapy.	Doxorubicin, cyclophos-phamide, high-dose methotrexate, mitoxantrone	Cisplatin, dacarbazine, high-dose cyclophos-phamide
Pre-treatment	Metoclopramide or domperidone	Add dexamethasone 6–10 mg orally and lorazepam 1–2 mg orally	Use a 5-HT_3 receptor antagonist plus dexamethasone
Duration of treatment	24 hours after chemotherapy	24 hours after chemotherapy	Usually 5 days, but may last a week

Delayed symptoms Dexamethasone plus either metoclopramide or prochlorperazine; 5-HT_3 receptor antagonists are less effective

Anticipatory symptoms Difficult to treat. Consider lorazepam 1–2 mg orally.

Chapter 2

Cardiovascular system

Contents

A pharmacological approach to the treatment of arrhythmias

The treatment of arrhythmias is controversial. The following is intended as a general guide to their acute treatment. See relevant pages for guidance on the use of the drugs suggested. Seek expert advice on the long-term treatment of arrhythmias.

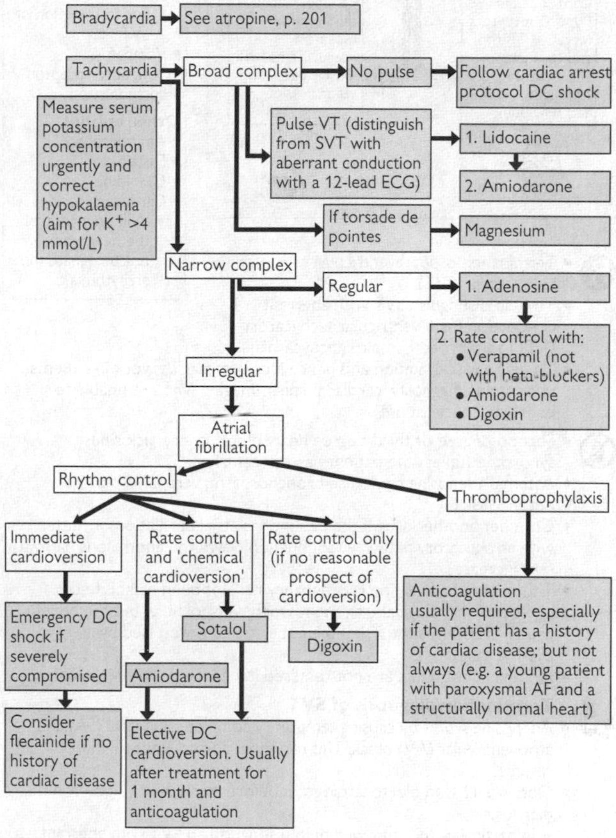

Adenosine

Antagonist at purine A_2 receptors

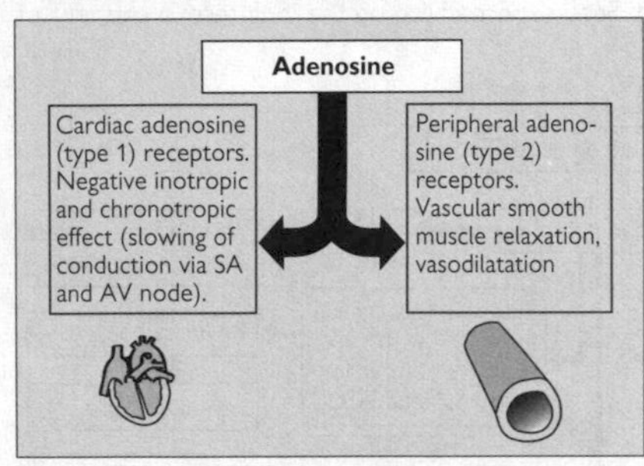

Drugs used for SVT

First-line
- Adenosine
  - For termination of SVT
- Verapamil
- Beta-adrenoceptor antagonists

Other options
- Amiodarone
- Flecainide
- Quinidine
- Cardiac glycosides
  - Will only control the heart rate; will not terminate the arrhythmia

- Termination of supraventricular tachycardia (SVT).
- To help distinguish SVT with aberrant conduction from ventricular tachycardia (VT) (both broad-complex tachycardias).
- To cause vasodilatation and hence increase cardiac work in patients undergoing diagnostic cardiac nuclear imaging who are unable to exercise (specialist use).

- Second-degree or third-degree heart block, or the sick sinus syndrome (unless the patient has a pacemaker).
- Asthma: adenosine can cause bronchospasm; verapamil may be a better choice.
- Consider another drug if the patient has atrial fibrillation or flutter with an accessory pathway (conduction down the anomalous pathway may increase).
- The safety of adenosine in pregnancy has not been established; avoid pharmacological treatment whenever possible, but the benefit usually outweighs the risk if the patient is compromised by a dysrhythmia.
- Dosage adjustments are not required in hepatic or renal insufficiency.

Termination/diagnosis of SVT

- Adenosine works by causing temporary complete sinoatrial (SA) and atrioventricular (AV) block. This can allow normal sinus rhythm to resume.
- Obtain a 12-lead electocardiogram before treatment, to confirm the diagnosis.
  - In particular, this may well help distinguish an SVT with aberrant conduction from VT.
  - If the patient is compromised and you suspect VT, do not delay treatment by using adenosine for diagnostic purposes.
- Ensure that there are adequate facilities for resuscitation, and that the patient has continuous cardiac monitoring.
- Adenosine is given by intravenous bolus only. See below for a suggested regimen.

- The pharmacological action of adenosine on the heart is associated with a sensation often described as a 'thump' within the chest. A few patients even feel as if they are 'about to die'. The duration of action of adenosine is very short (10–20 seconds), and so this feeling is short-lived. Warn the patient that they may experience unpleasant sensations but that they will not last.
- Other reported effects include flushing and headache, owing to vasodilatation.
- Adenosine can cause bronchospasm.
- Transplanted hearts are especially sensitive to the actions of adenosine; reduce the initial dose to 0.5–1 mg.

- Dipyridamole (an antiplatelet drug) inhibits the uptake of adenosine into cells. This is the main route by which adenosine is cleared from the plasma. Co-administration of dipyridamole will therefore greatly increase the effect of adenosine. Reduce the initial dose of adenosine to 0.5–1 mg.
- The effect of adenosine will be enhanced if the patient is already taking another antiarrhythmic drug; start treatment at a lower dose.
- Treatment with theophylline increases the dose of adenosine required to convert a SVT.

Safety and efficacy

- Ensure that adequate resuscitation facilities are immediately available.
- The patient should have continuous cardiac monitoring during administration of adenosine.
- Obtain a 12-lead electrocardiogram before and after treatment.

- The action of adenosine on the heart causes a sensation like a thump within the chest. This is transient, and may be mild, but can be very frightening for patients. Warn patients that they may experience this sensation, and assure them that it will not last long. Warn them also that they will experience flushing and increased respiration.

Prescribing information: **Adenosine**

Termination/diagnosis of SVT

- *By rapid intravenous injection* into a central or large peripheral vein.
  - The recommended initial dose is 3 mg, but many patients do not respond to this, so some doctors begin with 6 mg.
  - If the first dose is ineffective, repeat after 1–2 minutes with 6 mg and then 12 mg.
  - Follow each dose with a large (10–20 mL) saline flush to ensure rapid delivery to the heart.
  - Do not increase the dose if high-degree AV block develops at any dose.
  - If adenosine is ineffective after 12 mg, stop and consider another drug (see box above) or direct current (DC) cardioversion.

Myocardial nuclear imaging (specialized use)

- By continuous intravenous infusion. Suggested dosage 140 micrograms/kg/min for 6 minutes.

Safety and efficacy

TEACHING POINT Loss of consciousness and fitness to drive

- The legal basis of fitness to drive lies in the EC directives on driver licensing, the Road Traffic Act 1988, and subsequent regulations, including in particular the Motor Vehicles (Driving Licences) Regulations 1999.
- Because this is the subject of legislation, prescribers should take care to limit themselves to advising the patient of the rules, and not to try to interpret them. The DVLA rules apply to anyone who is at risk of losing consciousness whatever the cause. Cardiac causes are responsible for 50% of cases of loss of consciousness.
- See lamotrigine (p. 261) for information on epilepsy and driving.
- It is the responsibility of the patient to inform the DVLA about their medical condition. Respect for patient confidentiality usually prohibits healthcare professionals from disclosing information about a patient to a third party such as the DVLA. Recent changes in the case law in the UK, however, allow this confidence to be broken if you have reason to suspect that a patient is driving when they should not. The need to protect the public overrides the individual's rights in this case.
- The rules below apply to Group 1 drivers; the rules for Group 2 drivers (e.g. heavy goods vehicles, passenger service vehicles) are much more strict; seek advice from the DVLA.
- Remind patients that they should contact their insurance company as well as the DVLA; failure to do so could invalidate their insurance.

Assessment of loss of consciousness

Presumed diagnosis	Investigations	Likelihood of recurrence	Duration of driving ban
Simple faint	Normal	Low	None
'Unexplained syncope'	Normal ECG, neurological and cardiovascular examination	Low	4 weeks
Syncope	Can be normal or abnormal	High	If the cause is identified, can drive 4 weeks after treatment. If no cause is identified, driving banned for 6 months.
Possible epileptic seizure	History includes any of the following features: amnesia, injury, tongue biting, incontinence, confusion, or headache	Unknown	1 year
Loss of consciouness with no clinical pointers	Normal	Unknown	6 months

For more information see *www.dvla.gov.uk*

Procainamide

Antiarrhythmic drug

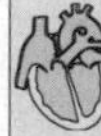

- In the Vaughan–Williams classification, procainamide is a class Ia antiarrhythmic drug. All of these drugs have complex actions on the electrophysiology of cardiac tissues.
- At the simplest level procainamide inhibits the fast depolarizing sodium channels.
- The effect is to reduce automaticity, decrease the rate of depolarization and conduction velocity, and increase the refractory period.
- Procainamide has an active metabolite (N-acetyl-procainamide, acecainide) that has class III antiarrhythmic actions.
- As with all antiarrhythmic drugs, it can be difficult to correlate the electrophysiological actions with the clinical effects.

Class I antiarrhythmic drugs

- Ia Drugs that prolong the action potential (*quinidine, procainamide, disopyramide, propafenone*)
- Ib Drugs that shorten the action potential (*lidocaine, mexiletine, tocainide*)
- Ic Drugs that leave the action potential duration unchanged (*flecainide*)

- Can be used for the treatment of acute and chronic ventricular arrhythmias, but its principal use is intravenously for the acute termination of VT.
  - Not a treatment for ventricular fibrillation or torsade de pointes.
  - Lidocaine is the first-line drug treatment for VT.

- The kinetics of procainamide are altered in patients with heart failure; reduce the dose.
- Reduce the dose in patients with renal insufficiency; both procainamide and its active metabolite, acecainide, are renally excreted.
- Reduce the dose in patients with hepatic insufficiency, as the metabolism of procainamide to its active metabolite will be reduced.
- Hypokalaemia (a common adverse effect of diuretics) will reduce the efficacy of procainamide and predispose to cardiac arrhythmias. Correct hypokalaemia as a matter of urgency in patients at risk of arrhythmias.
- Avoid using procainamide in patients with 2nd or 3rd degree heart block or sinus node disease.
- Avoid procainamide in pregnancy; there is no evidence that it is safe.

- Procainamide is available as an intravenous injection, and as immediate-release and modified-release tablets. It is most commonly given by intravenous injection (followed by infusion when necessary) for the treatment of ventricular arrhythmias.
- Procainamide can be given as a series of 100 mg boluses (up to 600 mg), or as an infusion of 500–600 mg over 30 minutes. Do not inject or infuse at a rate exceeding 50 mg /min.
- Stop once the arrhythmia has been terminated.
  - Wait 3–4 hours before the next (oral) dose is given.
  - The decision to use procainamide for long-term prophylaxis should only be made by a specialist; its use is not recommended.
- The metabolism of procainamide depends on the acetylator status of the patient. See teaching point below.

- Procainamide causes dose-related falls in blood pressure, heart block, and ventricular arrhythmias.
- Procainamide can cause a drug-induced lupus-like syndrome.
  - See teaching point below.
  - The antinuclear factor (ANF) antibody is usually positive if the patient develops the syndrome, but 60–70% of patients given procainamide will be ANF positive and only 20–30% of these will develop lupus.
- Procainamide can cause hypersensitivity, characterized by fever and agranulocytosis.
  - There is a suggestion that this is more common (although rare) with modified-release oral formulations.
- Giddiness and psychosis have been reported rarely.
- Anorexia, nausea, and vomiting are also reported.

- Procainamide prolongs the QT interval; avoid giving it with other drugs that prolong the QT interval (see teaching point in antihistamines, p. 610, for a list).
- Take care in patients taking diuretics; hypokalaemia reduces the efficacy of procainamide and increases the risk of cardiac arrhythmias.

Safety and efficacy
- Only give intravenous procainamide with continuous cardiac monitoring.
- Measure the plasma potassium concentration and correct it urgently if low.

- If procainamide is to be used long-term, tell the patient to report symptoms of arthritis (which can indicate the development of lupus).

Prescribing information: **Procainamide**

Treatment of ventricular arrhythmias after myocardial infarction
- *Either slow intravenous injection*, 100 mg, repeated at 5-minute intervals until the arrhythmia is controlled (at a rate not exceeding 50 mg/minute).
- *Or intravenous infusion*, 500–600 mg over 25–30 minutes.

TEACHING POINT Acetylator status and drug metabolism

- Liver drug metabolism is of two types:
  - Oxidative reactions (see flecainide and erythromycin, pp. 91 and 347).
  - Conjugation reactions.
- Important conjugation reactions are acetylation, sulphation, glucuronidation, and methylation.
- Procainamide is an example of a drug that is acetylated as part of its metabolism; see list below for other examples.
- Acetylation is polymorphic. Slow acetylation is autosomal recessive.
- Patients who are slow acetylators are more likely to suffer adverse effects from these drugs. They are at particular risk of developing a drug-induced lupus-like syndrome (see box below).

Drugs metabolized by acetylation

Isoniazid	Hydralazine
Procainamide	Phenelzine
Dapsone	Some sulfonamides

TEACHING POINT Drug-induced lupus-like syndrome

- Several drugs can cause a syndrome mimicking systemic lupus erythematosus.
  - The syndrome is dose-dependent.
  - In the cases due to procainamide and hydralazine it is more common among slow acetylators.
- The syndrome is characterized by arthralgia, arthritis, fever, pleurisy, rash, pulmonary involvement, and pericarditis; renal involvement is rare.
- The syndrome usually resolves after withdrawal of the drug but it may take months to do so.
- Features that may help distinguish drug-induced from idiopathic lupus erythematosus are:

Feature	Idiopathic lupus erythematosus	Drug-induced lupus-like syndrome
Age and sex	Usually young women	Any
Renal involvement	Common	Rare
Serum complement	Often low	Usually normal
Antinuclear antibodies	Anti double-stranded DNA antibodies common	Anti single-stranded DNA antibodies common Antihistone antibodies common

Drugs that can cause a lupus-like syndrome

Alpha-methyldopa	Fluphenazine	Minocycline	Procainamide
Atenolol (rare)	Griseofulvin	Oestrogens (rare)	Propafenone
Co-trimoxazole	Hydralazine	Oxcarbazepine	Propylthiouracil
Ethosuximide	Isoniazid	Penicillamine	Sulfasalazine
Flutamide		Phenytoin	

Quinidine

Antiarrhythmic drug

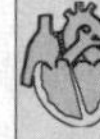

- In the Vaughan–Williams classification, quinidine is a class Ia antiarrhythmic drug. All of these drugs have complex actions on the electrophysiology of cardiac tissues.
- At the simplest level, quinidine inhibits the fast depolarizing sodium channels.
- The effect is to reduce automaticity, decrease the rate of depolarization and conduction velocity, and increase the refractory period.
- In addition, quinidine has anticholinergic effects and has α-adrenoceptor antagonist actions.
- As with all antiarrhythmic drugs, it can be difficult to correlate the electrophysiological actions with the clinical effects.
- Quinidine is the dextrorotatory diastereoisomer of quinine.

Class I antiarrhythmic drugs

- Ia Drugs that prolong the action potential (*quinidine, procainamide, disopyramide, propafenone*)
- Ib Drugs that shorten the action potential (*lidocaine, mexiletine, tocainide*)
- Ic Drugs that leave the action potential duration unchanged (*flecainide*)

- Quinidine can be used for the treatment of SVT and VT, but it has largely been superceded by other, safer drugs.
  - Not a treatment for ventricular fibrillation or torsade de pointes.
  - See adenosine (p. 78) for more information on treatment of SVT.
- Quinidine is effective for the treatment of falciparum malaria, but quinine is preferred. This indication is not considered further here.

- Quinidine is negatively inotropic; avoid using it in patients with, or at risk of developing, heart failure.
- Quinidine has anticholinergic effects; avoid it in patients with prostatic enlargement or closed angle glaucoma.
- Hypokalaemia (a common adverse effect of diuretics) will reduce the efficacy of quinidine and predisposes to arrhythmias. Correct hypokalaemia as a matter of urgency in patients at risk of arrhythmias.
- Avoid using quinidine in patients with 2nd or 3rd degree heart block or sinus node disease.
- Avoid quinidine in pregnancy; the related compound quinine is teratogenic.
- Reduce the dose by 25% in hepatic insufficiency.

- The decision to use quinidine should only be made by a specialist.
- Use a modified-release formulation as this reduces fluctuations in plasma concentrations.
- Give a test dose of 200 mg of immediate-release quinidine before starting long-term treatment. Some patients are hypersensitive to quinidine.

- Adverse effects of quinidine are common, even at therapeutic dosages. The most common are nausea, vomiting, and diarrhoea.
- As well as suppressing arrhythmias, quinidine can cause them, by prolonging the QT interval and reducing sinus node function.
- The anticholinergic adverse effects of quinidine include dry mouth, blurred vision, exacerbation of glaucoma, constipation, and urinary retention.
- The α-adrenoceptor antagonist action of quinidine can cause postural hypotension.

- Hypersensivity can manifest as a rash, thrombocytopenia, and haemolytic anaemia (rare).
- Overdose is associated with the syndrome called cinchonism. This is characterized by tinnitus, deafness, blurred vision, nausea, headache, and, in more serious cases, delirium and psychosis.
- At high doses quinidine can cause hypoglycaemia.

- Quinidine prolongs the QT interval; avoid giving it with other drugs that prolong the QT interval (see teaching point in antihistamines, p. 610, for a list).
- Avoid giving quinidine with other drugs with anticholinergic actions (e.g. tricyclic antidepressants).
- Take care in patients taking diuretics; hypokalaemia reduces the efficacy of quinidine.
- Avoid giving quinidine with other negatively inotropic drugs (e.g. beta-blockers and some calcium channel blockers).
- Quinidine doubles the steady-state plasma concentration of digoxin. Avoid this combination. Quinidine also opposes the positive inotropic action of digoxin.
- Inducers of hepatic enzymes will increase the rate of metabolism of quinidine; the dose may need to be increased.
- Quinidine can potentiate the actions of warfarin; the mechanism of this is not clear.

Safety and efficacy

- The target plasma concentration of quinidine is 3–6 micrograms/L, measured after 1 week. However, routine measurement of plasma quinidine concentrations has not been shown to be useful.
- Measure the plasma potassium concentration and correct it urgently if low.

- If quinidine is to be used long-term, warn the patient about anticholinergic adverse effects.

Prescribing information: **Quinidine**

Long-term prophylaxis of supraventricular and ventricular arrhythmias (specialist use only)

- *Immediate-release tablets:* quinidine sulfate 200–400 mg 3–4 times daily.
  - Quinidine sulfate 200 mg = quinidine bisulfate 250 mg.
- Modified-release tablets: quinidine bisulfate 500 mg bd.

Flecainide

Antiarrhythmic drug

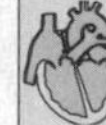

- In the Vaughan–Williams classification, flecainide is a class Ic antiarrhythmic drug. All of these drugs have complex actions on the electrophysiology of cardiac tissues.
- At the simplest level, flecainide inhibits the fast depolarizing sodium channels.
- The effect is to broaden the QRS complex, but there is no effect on the action potential duration.
- As with all these drugs, it can be difficult to correlate the electrophysiological actions with the clinical effects.

Class I antiarrhythmic drugs

- Ia Drugs that prolong the action potential (*quinidine, procainamide, disopyramide, propafenone*)
- Ib Drugs that shorten the action potential (*lidocaine, mexiletine, tocainide*)
- Ic Drugs that leave the action potential duration unchanged (*flecainide*)

- Flecainide can be used for the treatment of SVT and VT, but its principal use is for the termination of acute atrial fibrillation.
  - It can be used in patients with Wolff–Parkinson–White syndrome.
  - See adenosine (p. 78) for more information on treatment of SVT.

- Avoid using flecainide after myocardial infarction and in patients with heart failure or structural cardiac abnormalities; it may precipitate VT by prolonging the QT interval.
- Flecainide should not be used for the conversion of long-standing atrial fibrillation; it is unlikely to be successful.
- Hypokalaemia (a common adverse effect of diuretics) will reduce the efficacy of flecainide and predispose to cardiac arrhythmias. Correct hypokalaemia as a matter of urgency in patients at risk of arrhythmias.
- Avoid using flecainide in patients with 2nd or 3rd degree heart block or sinus node disease.
- Avoid flecainide in pregnancy; toxicity has been observed in animal studies.
- Reduce the dose or avoid in severe hepatic insufficiency. The manufacturer advises that the initial dose should be 100 mg in patients with renal insufficiency, and that the plasma concentration should be measured, but that is not usually available.

- Flecainide is most useful for the termination of atrial fibrillation in patients without ischaemic or structural heart disease. Many of these patients have paroxysmal atrial fibrillation.
  - For this indication flecainide is given by intravenous injection, with continuous cardiac monitoring.
- Flecainide can be given by mouth for long-term prophylaxis against paroxysmal atrial fibrillation, but see notes on the CAST trial opposite. The treatment of paroxysmal atrial fibrillation is complex, especially in the absence of ischaemic heart disease. An assessment of cardiac structure and function is required. Pharmacological treatment is not always the most appropriate choice; seek a specialist opinion for your patient.

Flecainide and the CAST trial

Ventricular extra beats in patients with ischaemic heart disease are a risk factor for the development of sustained ventricular arrhythmias. Class Ic antiarrhythmics suppress this abnormal electrical activity. The Cardiac Arrhythmia Suppression Trial (CAST) was designed to ascertain whether treatment with these drugs (encainide, flecainide, moricizine) improved outcome in patients with ectopic activity following myocardial infarction (with left ventricular impairment). However, the study showed that those taking Ic antiarrhythmic drugs had a 3.6 fold *greater* chance of arrhythmia-related death than those taking placebo.

It is always difficult, and potentially hazardous, to extrapolate findings from a clinical trial to everyday clinical practice, but most doctors would not recommend the use of flecainide in patients with ischaemic heart disease, whatever the indication.

CAST trial investigators, *New Engl J Med* 1989, **321:** 406–12.

- All drugs that block fast sodium channels can interfere with neuronal conduction in the CNS. This can cause toxicity.
  - This is characterized by lightheadedness initially, followed by sedation and twitching. If severe it can progress to seizures and coma.
- As well as suppressing arrhythmias, flecainide can cause them, by prolonging the QT interval.
- Rare adverse effects of flecainide include reduced haemopoiesis, corneal deposits, and a photosensitive rash.
- Flecainide is metabolized in the liver by the cytochrome P450 isoenzyme CYP2D6; see teaching point below.

- Flecainide prolongs the QT interval; avoid giving it with other drugs that prolong the QT interval (see teaching point in antihistamines, p. 610, for a list).
- Flecainide is subject to pharmacokinetic interactions with several drugs. Avoid using it in patients taking amiodarone, fluoxetine, quinidine, ritonavir; the plasma concentration will be increased.
- Take care in patients taking diuretics; hypokalaemia reduces the efficacy of flecainide and increases the risk of cardiac arrhythmias.
- Avoid giving flecainide with other negatively inotropic drugs (e.g. beta-blockers and some calcium channel blockers).

Safety and efficacy

- The manufacturer advises that the target plasma concentration of flecainide is 0.2–1 mg/l. This is of limited use, as the assay is not available in most hospitals.
- Measure the plasma potassium concentration and correct it urgently if low.

- If the patient has paroxysmal atrial fibrillation, try to identify and avoid any precipitating factors (e.g. coffee, alcohol).

Prescribing information: **Flecainide**

Long-term prophylaxis of supraventricular and ventricular arrhythmias (specialist use only)

- *By mouth*, for ventricular arrhythmias, initially 100 mg twice daily. Maximum dose 400 mg daily in exceptional cases.
- By mouth, for supraventricular arrhythmias, 50 mg twice daily, increased if required to a maximum of 300 mg daily

Termination of acute supraventricular arrhythmias, especially atrial fibrillation

- *By slow intravenous injection*, 2 mg/kg over 10–30 minutes. Maximum dose 150 mg.
- Can be followed by *infusion* at a rate of 1.5 mg/kg/hour for 1 hour, subsequently reduced to 100–250 micrograms/kg/hour for up to 24 hours, if required.
  - Maximum cumulative dose in first 24 hours, 600 mg.

TEACHING POINT Cytochrome P450 isoenzyme 2D6 (CYP 2D6)

- Liver drug metabolism is of two types:
  - Oxidative reactions.
  - Conjugation reactions (see procainamide, p. 85).
- Oxidations are of several types, catalzed by a group of enzymes called cytochrome P450.
- The important isozymes of cytochrome P450 are CYP 3A4 and CYP 2D6
- Most drugs that are metabolized by the liver are metabolized by several pathways, usually including the cytochrome P450 isoenzyme 3A4 (see erythromycin, p. 347).
- If a drug is metabolized by several pathways it is less likely to be subject to drug interactions, as effects on one pathway may be compensated for by another pathway.
- A small number of drugs (listed below) are almost exclusively metabolized by CYP 2D6.
- CYP 2D6 is polymorphic; reduced activity of this isoenzyme is inherited in a homozygous recessive manner. It affects 9% of patients in Caucasian populations. They metabolize the listed drugs much more slowly and are at considerably increased risk of adverse effects. It has been suggested that identification of these patients by genomic technologies could be a means of tailoring treatment to the individual and of reducing the incidence of serious adverse effects.

Drugs metabolized by CYP 2D6

Debrisoquine	Captopril
Nortriptyline	Perhexiline
Codeine	Phenacetin
Flecainide	Phenformin
Metoprolol	Propafenone
Sparteine	Timolol

Cardiac glycosides (digitalis)

Inhibitors of Na^+/K^+-ATPase (the Na^+/K^+ pump)

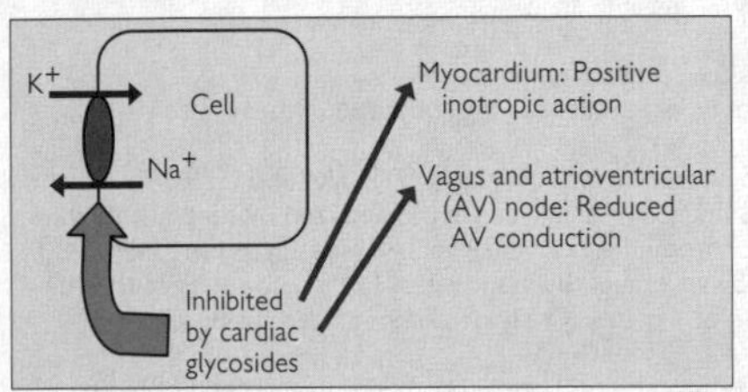

Choice of cardiac glycoside

- We prefer digoxin to other cardiac glycosides, such as digitoxin.
- Digitoxin has a very long half-life which can make it difficult to use.
- Digitoxin also differs from digoxin in that it is metabolized by the liver and is highly protein bound.

- Rate control for supraventricular arrhythmias, especially atrial fibrillation.
- Symptom relief in some patients with heart failure; digoxin also reduces the number of hospital admissions in these patients.

- Digoxin slows conduction via the AV node. It should therefore be avoided in:
    - Intermittent complete heart block.
    - Second-degree AV block.
- Digoxin does not slow conduction via accessory pathways. It should therefore be avoided in:
    - SVT associated with the Wolff–Parkinson–White syndrome and related syndromes. Block of the AV node allows the alternative pathway to conduct at the atrial rate, with catastrophic consequences.
- The risk of arrhythmias is greatly increased by hypokalaemia.
    - Always check the plasma potassium concentration before starting digoxin.
    - If there is hypokalaemia give potassium supplements before starting digoxin; during treatment for heart failure the potassium-sparing effects of an ACE inhibitor and spironolactone will usually suffice.
- Digoxin is not contraindicated in pregnancy, but should only be used under specialist supervision.
- Digoxin is excreted by the kidneys; see below for dosage adjustments according to renal function.

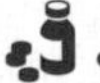

Atrial fibrillation (AF)

- Digoxin will only provide rate control in AF; it will not cause reversion to sinus rhythm. If there is reversion to sinus rhythm the diagnosis is paroxysmal AF and the digoxin should be withheld.
- Digoxin is not effective in paroxysmal AF and may prolong bouts when they occur.
- Always consider alternative measures, such as cardioversion by DC shock or pharmacological cardioversion (e.g. amiodarone, flecainide), especially in AF of recent onset.
- When starting digoxin, and if a rapid effect is required, a loading dose should be given (see below).
- Digoxin is excreted from the body via the kidneys.
    - Renal function is therefore the major determinant of the maintenance dose (usual range 62.5–500 micrograms daily).

- Use the plasma digoxin concentration to determine the optimal dose.
- Once the patient is established on a dose, regular monitoring is not usually required, unless circumstances change (see monitoring below).

Heart failure

- Digoxin is used for its small positive inotropic effect.
- This treatment should be in addition to diuretics and an ACE inhibitor, not instead of.
- Patients treated with digoxin sometimes feel better, but treatment does not prolong life.
- A loading dose is not usually required.
- The doses used are usually lower than those used for AF.
  - Usual range 62.5–250 micrograms per day.

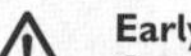

Early

- Over-rapid infusion of digoxin can cause cardiac arrhythmias, heart block, and hypertension.
  - Follow the regimen given below.
- Beware hypokalaemia in patients taking digoxin; the risk of arrhythmias is greatly increased.
  - Be especially careful in those taking diuretics.
  - Check the plasma potassium concentration and give potassium supplements or a potassium-sparing diuretic when required; in heart failure the potassium-sparing effects of an ACE inhibitor and spironolactone will usually suffice.
  - Aim to keep the plasma potassium concentration above 4 mmol/L.
- Digoxin is renally excreted, so expect to use a lower maintenance dose in renal insufficiency.
- Elderly people are especially susceptible to digoxin toxicity, partly because of renal impairment and partly because their tissues are more sensitive to its actions.
  - The features of acute toxicity are non-cardiac (nausea and vomiting, diarrhoea and abdominal pain, visual disturbances, confusion, and delirium, especially in elderly people) and cardiac (arrhythmias, heart block, and often a combination, for example, SVT with block).
  - For patients with severe digoxin toxicity consider treatment with antidigoxin antibody Fab fragments (Digibind®). If the plasma potassium rises above 5 mmol/L Fab fragments should be used. The dose of antibody should be calculated as shown in the box below. It should be infused over 20 minutes, and in some cases an extra dose may have to be given if the first dose is not completely effective. It starts to act from before the end of the infusion to about 30 minutes after.

Calculating the appropriate dose of antidigoxin antibody fragments to treat digoxin overdose

When the dose of digoxin is known:

(a) Tablets	Dose in mg × 40
(b) Elixir	Dose in mg × 48
(c) Capsules	Dose in mg × 55
(d) Intravenous	Dose in mg × 60

When the plasma (or serum) digoxin concentration is known:

microgram/L × lean body weight × 0.34
or nmol/L × lean body weight × 0.26

- The introduction of drugs that impair renal function can affect the plasma digoxin concentration (e.g. ACE inhibitors, NSAIDs).
- Diuretics can cause hypokalaemia, resulting in digoxin toxicity without a change in plasma concentration.
- Digoxin may need to be combined with another antiarrhythmic drug for optimal rate control of ventricular rate in AF, but be aware that the effect of the combination is often much greater than either alone. Be prepared to reduce the dose as required.
  - Drugs that are used in these circumstances include beta-blockers, amiodarone, verapamil, and diltiazem.
- Drugs that reduce digoxin renal clearance include amiodarone, quinidine, spironolactone, and verapamil.

Efficacy

- In AF, count the ventricular rate at the apex; it should ideally be 80–90 beats per minute, to ensure a good average stroke volume, and should not be below 60.
- Once the desired clinical effect has been achieved, confirm that the plasma digoxin concentration is in the target range — usually 0.8–2.0 microgram/L (1.0–2.6 nmol/L).

Safety

- Measure the plasma digoxin concentration:
  - Whenever the dose of digoxin is changed.
  - After a drug that may affect digoxin elimination is introduced or stopped.
  - Whenever toxicity is suspected.
- The risk of toxicity increases greatly at plasma digoxin concentrations over 2.0 microgram/L (2.6 nmol/L).
- Digoxin has a long half-life.
  - 40 hours when renal function is normal.
  - Nearly 5 days when there is no renal function.
  - Wait 4 days after changing the dose before checking the plasma concentration; times to steady state are given in prescribing information below.

ECG lead II rhythm strips from two different patients suffering from digitalis toxicity. Both show a junctional rhythm, but differing ventricular rates. Digitalis treatment often causes sagging ST segment depression (seen in both examples here); this is an effect of digitalis but it does not necessarily indicate digitalis toxicity.

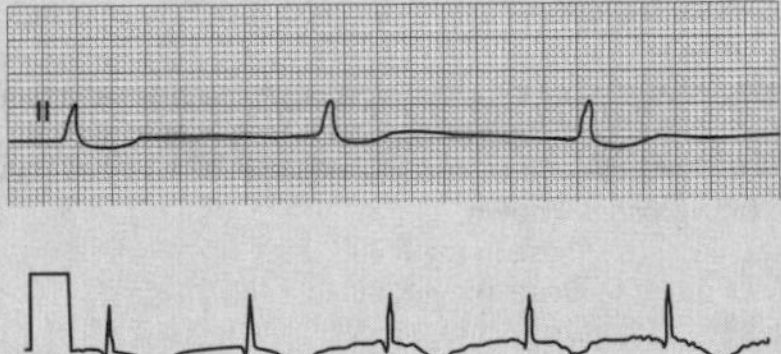

Digitalis toxicity can cause almost any type of dysrhythmia or conduction disturbance. Common digitalis toxic rhythms include:

- Ventricular extra beats
- Paroxysmal atrial tachycardia with block
- AF with a regular ventricular response
- Junctional tachycardia
- Complete heart block

- Collect the sample for plasma digoxin concentration at least 6 hours and preferably 12 hours after the last dose was taken.
  - Tell the patient to take the dose in the evening; a blood sample taken the next day will then be suitable.
- Toxicity is more likely in elderly people and in the presence of hypokalaemia.

- Warn the patient that loss of appetite, nausea, or vomiting may be early signs of toxicity and that they should seek medical attention.

Prescribing information: **Digoxin**

Loading dose

- Rapid digitalization by mouth: 15 micrograms/kg lean body weight in 3 divided doses over 12 hours.
  - For example, a 60-kg man would be given 1 mg (as 0.5 mg, 0.25 mg, and 0.25 mg at 6-hourly intervals), monitoring before the 2nd and 3rd doses for clinical evidence of acute toxicity.
  - If a therapeutic effect has not occurred and there is no evidence of toxicity, give another 5 micrograms/kg lean body weight as a 4th dose.
  - See azathioprine (p. 515) for more information on calculating drug dosages by body weight.

Maintenance dose

- 62.5–500 micrograms/day (usually in 1 dose, but higher doses may be divided). Adjust the dose according to renal function (see below) and, in AF, according to ventricular rate response; usual range 125–250 micrograms daily (a lower dose is usually appropriate in elderly people).
- The box below shows an example of maintenance dose alteration according to renal function in a patient whose usual maintenance dose with normal renal function would be 250 micrograms/day.

Creatinine clearance (mL/min)	Ratio of usual dose to renal impairment dose	Exact maintenance dose (micrograms/day)	No. of tablets (to nearest tablet size)	Half-life (hrs)	Approximate time to new steady state (days)
100	1	250	1 × 250 micrograms	40	6
50	3:4	187	3 × 62.5 micrograms	60	9
10	3:6	125	1 × 125 micrograms	90	13
0	3:8	94	1 × 62.5 micrograms	110	15

- Note: these doses are a first approximation; always check the plasma digoxin concentration for further adjustments.

- Remember that an elderly patient with a serum creatinine concentration in the reference range (up to 150 micromol/L) probably has no more than 50% of normal renal function.

Intravenous administration

- If the patient cannot swallow give digoxin elixir by nasogastric tube if possible.
- Use intravenous digoxin only if there is no alternative; it does not act significantly quicker than oral digoxin.
- Do not use intravenous digoxin in the hope of producing a more rapid response than by oral administration.
- Suggested regimen: 5 micrograms/kg lean body weight in 50 mL of 0.9% saline or 5% glucose, over at least 2 hours; repeat after 6 hours; if this is ineffective another 3 micrograms/kg can be given 6 hours later.
- Intravenous ouabain offers no major advantages over digoxin.

Do not give digoxin intramuscularly

- It is painful.
- It causes muscle damage.
- It is slowly and unreliably absorbed.

Disopyramide

Antiarrhythmic drug acting mainly on ventricular tissues

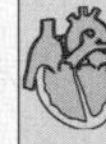

- In the Vaughan–Williams classification, disopyramide is a class Ia antiarrhythmic drug. All of these drugs have complex actions on the electrophysiology of cardiac tissues.
- At the simplest level disopyramide inhibits the fast depolarizing sodium channels.
- The effect is to reduce automaticity, decrease the rate of depolarization and conduction velocity, and increase the refractory period.
- In addition, disopyramide has potent anticholinergic effects and is negatively inotropic.
- As with all antiarrhythmic drugs, it can be difficult to correlate the electrophysiological actions with the clinical effects.

Class I antiarrhythmic drugs

- Ia Drugs that prolong the action potential (*quinidine, procainamide, disopyramide, propafenone*)
- Ib Drugs that shorten the action potential (*lidocaine, mexiletine, tocainide*)
- Ic Drugs that leave the action potential duration unchanged (*flecainide*)

Disopyramide is an example of a drug that is highly protein bound. See teaching point below for more information

- Major use is for the treatment of VT following myocardial infarction.
  - Not a treatment for ventricular fibrillation or torsade de pointes.
  - Lidocaine is the first-line treatment for VT.
- Can be used for the treatment of SVT, but consider other drugs first (see adenosine, p. 78, for more information).
- Disopyramide has a specialist use in patients with hypertrophic cardiomyopathy.

- Disopyramide is negatively inotropic; avoid using it in patients with, or who are at risk of developing, heart failure.
- Disopyramide has anticholinergic effects; avoid in patients with prostatic enlargement or closed angle glaucoma.
- Hypokalaemia (a common adverse effect of diuretics) will reduce the efficacy of disopyramide and predispose to arrhythmias. Correct hypokalaemia as a matter of urgency in patients at risk of arrhythmias.
- Avoid using disopyramide in patients with 2nd or 3rd degree heart block or sinus node disease.
- Avoid disopyramide in pregnancy; it can induce labour.
- Halve the dose of disopyramide in renal insufficiency. Reduce the dose in hepatic insufficiency.

- Disopyramide is given by intravenous injection (followed by infusion when necessary) for the treatment of ventricular arrhythmias.
- Avoid over-rapid infusion, as this can precipitate or worsen heart failure.
- Disopyramide should only be given with continuous cardiac monitoring, and when resuscitation facilities are immediately available.
- The decision to use disopyramide for long-term prophylaxis should only be made by a specialist.

- The anticholinergic adverse effects of disopyramide include dry mouth, blurred vision, exacerbation of glaucoma, constipation, and urinary retention.
- Less common adverse effects include nausea, vomiting, and diarrhoea.
- Hypoglycaemia has been reported rarely.

- Disopyramide prolongs the QT interval; avoid giving it with other drugs that prolong the QT interval (e.g. amiodarone); see also teaching point in antihistamines (p. 610) for a list.
- Avoid giving disopyramide with other negatively inotropic drugs (e.g. beta-blockers and some calcium channel blockers).
- Avoid giving disopyramide with other drugs with anticholinergic actions (e.g. tricyclic antidepressants).
- Take care in patients taking diuretics; hypokalaemia reduces the efficacy of disopyramide and increases the risk of arrhythmias.

Safety and efficacy

- Only give intravenous disopyramide with continuous cardiac monitoring.
- Measure the plasma potassium concentration and correct it urgently if low.

- If disopyramide is to be used long-term warn the patient about anticholinergic adverse effects.

Prescribing information: **Disopyramide**

Treatment of ventricular arrhythmias after myocardial infarction

- *By slow intravenous injection*, 2 mg/kg over at least 5 minutes to a maximum of 150 mg.
  - See azathioprine (p. 515) for more information on giving drug dosages by body weight.
- Followed immediately *by:*
  - Either 200 mg *by mouth*, then 200 mg every 8 hours for 24 hours.
  - *Or* 400 micrograms/kg/hour *by intravenous infusion*.
- Maximum dosages are 300 mg in first hour and 800 mg daily.

Long-term prophylaxis (specialist use only)

- *By mouth*, 300–800 mg daily in divided doses.

TEACHING POINT **Plasma protein binding of drugs**

- Many drugs are bound to circulating proteins. Acid drugs bind to albumin and basic ones to acid glycoproteins. Only the fraction of drug that is not bound to proteins is available to produce its pharmacological action.
- Changes in protein binding can be important, but only if:
  - The proportion of drug that is bound to protein is high. If only 10% of a drug is protein-bound, a halving of the bound fraction to 5% will only increase the unbound (free) fraction from 90% to 95%. But if 95% of the drug is usually highly protein-bound (say 95%), a fall to 85% increases the unbound fraction from 5% to 15% (a three-fold increase).
  - The drug is not widely distributed to the tissues (i.e. has a small volume of distribution). If a drug is widely distributed, any increase in unbound drug in the plasma will rapidly be 'mopped up' by the tissues.
- Examples of drugs that are highly protein-bound and have a low volume of distribution: phenytoin, tolbutamide, warfarin.
- Note: the protein binding of disopyramide is saturable at therapeutic doses; the fraction of disopyramide bound varies between 35% at high therapeutic doses and 95% at low therapeutic doses. This means that small increases in the dose of disopyramide can produce disproportionately large changes in effect.

Amiodarone

Antiarrhythmic drug acting on atrial and ventricular tissues

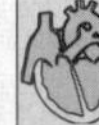

- Amiodarone has a complex mechanism of action that is incompletely understood, but is probably mediated through effects on cardiac potassium channels.
- Amiodarone prolongs the action potential and refractory period homogeneously throughout the heart.
- The principal ECG change is a prolongation of the QT interval.
- Amiodarone is a class III antiarrhythmic drug in the Vaughan–Williams classification.

- Amiodarone should be introduced under hospital or specialist supervision.
- Used for the treatment of:
  - Paroxsysmal supraventricular, nodal, and ventricular tachycardias.
  - AF and flutter.
- Emergency treatment of ventricular fibrillation (VF) or pulseless VT.

- Amiodarone slows the heart rate and AV conduction. It is contraindicated in sinus bradycardia, sino-atrial disease, and heart block.
- Avoid bolus intravenous administration in severe heart failure and cardiomyopathy, as this may lead to a precipitous drop in blood pressure.
- Amiodarone is contraindicated in those who are sensitive to iodine or have thyroid disease (see box below).
- Contraindicated in pregnancy; it may affect the fetal thyroid gland.
- Contraindicated in breast feeding.
- Amiodarone interacts with many other drugs (see below).
- Dosage adjustments are not usually required in hepatic or renal insufficiency.

- Amiodarone is an effective antiarrhythmic drug and has the advantage of causing relatively little cardiac depression. It is, however, associated with a significant risk of adverse effects, especially in the long term. It is reserved for those patients in whom other antiarrhythmic therapy has been either ineffective or poorly tolerated.
- An implantable cardioverter defibrillator is more effective than amiodarone for the treatment of ventricular arrhythmias. NICE has issued guidance about those patients who are most likely to benefit from an implantable cardioverter defibrillator.
- Amiodarone has a very long half-life (50 days; see teaching point below). When taken by mouth it takes weeks to have its full effect. If a rapid effect is required, amiodarone can be given by intravenous infusion.
  - Intravenous amiodarone is very irritant to veins and should be given via a central line. In an emergency it can be given via a large-bore peripheral cannula, but ensure that this is fully patent and flushed through well.
  - If it is anticipated that amiodarone therapy is to continue long-term following intravenous administration, it is recommended that the patient should also receive amiodarone in a loading dose by mouth concomitantly with the intravenous treatment.
- Amiodarone is widely distributed throughout the body and a loading dose is usually given when initiating treatment.
  - This is usually 200 mg tds for 1 week, then 200 mg bd for 1 week, then 200 mg daily.

    - This regimen may be altered depending on the clinical circumstances, and especially if amiodarone is being used in combination with another antiarrhythmic drug. Seek expert advice in each case.
    - The maintenance dose should be the lowest effective dose, usually 100–200 mg daily.
    - Review the need for amiodarone every 6 months.
- Emergency use in cardiopulmonary resuscitation.
    - Amiodarone 300 mg (pre-filled syringe) should be considered after adrenaline to treat VF or pulseless VT that is refractory to defibrillation.

- Adverse effects from amiodarone are much more common if the maintenance dose is 400 mg or more daily.
- Most patients taking amiodarone will develop corneal lipofuscin microdeposits.
    - In most cases these are not a problem and are reversible on stopping the drug. They cause a visual flare effect, especially when driving at night, in about 2% of patients.
- Treatment with amiodarone makes many patients sensitive to sunlight.
    - Advise patients to use a high SPF sun cream with UVA and UVB protection.
    - Amiodarone can cause a persistent slate-grey skin discolouration.
- Amiodarone can cause a pneumonitis (in about 2% of patients). This is a steroid-responsive pulmonary lipofuscin alveolitis and it can be severe. Have a high index of suspicion if the patient develops breathlessness.
- Amiodarone can cause a reversible peripheral neuropathy; this is thought to be demyelinating in origin.
- Amiodarone contains a great deal of iodine (37.5 mg iodine per 100 mg of amiodarone). It can have complex effects on thyroid function. This affects about 4% of patients. See box below.
- Rare but important adverse effects include:
    - Hepatotoxicity characterized by raised transaminases; may be severe. Raised liver transaminases occur in about 1% of patients; frank toxicity is much rarer.
    - Hypersensitivity phenomena and vasculitis.
    - Haemolytic or aplastic anaemia.

Amiodarone interacts with many drugs

- Warfarin. Amiodarone inhibits the metabolism of warfarin. Measure the INR and be prepared to reduce the dose of warfarin.
- Digoxin. Amiodarone inhibits renal P-glycoprotein. This reduces the excretion of digoxin. Measure the plasma digoxin concentration and be prepared to reduce the dose of digoxin. A dosage reduction of about one third is often required. Measure the plasma digoxin concentration again once a steady state has been achieved (3–4 months later).
- Any drug that prolongs the QT interval. Avoid using these drugs with amiodarone.
    - Antiarrhythmic drugs: quinidine, disopyramide, procainamide, sotalol.
    - Antibiotics: co-trimoxazole, intravenous erythromycin.
    - Antipsychotic drugs.
    - Antidepressants: lithium and tricyclic antidepressants.
    - Antiepileptic drugs: phenytoin.
- Any drug that also reduces the heart rate. Avoid combining amiodarone with these drugs.
    - Calcium channel blockers: diltiazem and verapamil.

Safety

- Before starting treatment, assess baseline thyroid function (TSH, T4, and T3), liver transaminases, and an ECG. Obtain a chest X-ray to allow comparison if the patient should develop evidence of pneumonitis.
- Measure thyroid function and liver function every 6 months.
- Ensure that the patient has continuous cardiac monitoring if administering amiodarone intravenously.
- Perform an ECG if the patient's symptoms worsen; measure the QT interval.
- Regular eye examinations are not usually recommended, but they should be performed if the patient has visual symptoms.

Efficacy

- The measures of efficacy will depend on the arrhythmia being treated, but review should include a consideration of whether the benefits of continued treatment outweigh the risks of adverse effects.

- Advise the patient that they may become more sensitive to the sun, and that they should use a high SPF sun cream.
- Warn the patient about the possibility of persistent slate-grey skin discolouration.
- Advise the patient to seek immediate medical advice if they become breathless (pneumonitis).

Amiodarone and thyroid function

- Thyroid dysfunction related to treatment with amiodarone affects about 4% of patients.
- Amiodarone contains a great deal of iodine (37.5 mg iodine per 100 mg of amiodarone).
- Amiodarone can cause symptoms of hyperthyroidism or hypothyroidism.
- Amiodarone reduces the peripheral conversion of T4 to T3. T4 may therefore be raised without symptoms of hyperthroidism; measure TSH and T3 as well.
- Amiodarone can cause hyperthyroidism by two mechanisms.
  - Type 1 — iodine-induced excessive synthesis of thyroid hormone (occurs particularly in patients with underlying thyroid disease). If amiodarone is essential, consider treatment with antithyroid drugs.
  - Type 2 — amiodarone-induced destructive thyroiditis. If amiodarone is essential, consider treatment with corticosteroids.
  - It can be refractory to conventional antithyroid drugs.
- If hypothyroidism develops, replacement therapy can be given; the amiodarone can be continued if it is essential.

Prescribing information: **Amiodarone**

- Treatment by mouth
  - 200 mg 3 times daily for 1 week reduced to 200 mg twice daily for a further week.
  - Maintenance dose, usually 200 mg daily or the minimum required to control the arrhythmia.
- Treatment by intravenous infusion
  - Via a central line, 5 mg/kg over 20–120 minutes with ECG monitoring; maximum 1.2 g in 24 hours.
- Emergency treatment during cardiopulmonary resuscitation
  - VF or pulseless VT, 300 mg *by intravenous injection* over at least 3 minutes (pre-filled syringe).

TEACHING POINT Drugs with a long half-life. Onset and offset of action.

- Amiodarone is an example of a drug with a very long half-life (about 50 days). The half-life of a drug is the time taken for the plasma concentration of the drug to fall by half, and is a measure of how quickly a drug is eliminated from the body.
- When a second dose of a drug is taken, its pharmacokinetic profile is superimposed on that of the first dose, and so on for subsequent doses. For a given dose, the pattern of plasma concentrations that results will depend upon two factors: the dosage interval and the half-life of the drug. A consequence of first-order pharmacokinetics (essentially exponential decay) is that during repeated administration, drug accumulation occurs. This is because the higher the plasma concentration is, the faster it falls. Eventually, during a dosage interval, the plasma concentration falls as fast as it rises. At this point a steady state is reached, after about four half-lives of administration, provided that the dosage interval is not excessively long. Before such a steady state has been reached one cannot say that the drug has reached its maximum effect.
- The practical consequence of this is that the maximum effect of amiodarone is not reached until about 4 half-lives have elapsed, about 200 days, unless a loading dose is given.
- It is unwise to declare that a drug is not effective until a steady state has been reached. Prematurely increasing the dose may lead to excessive accumulation and toxicity.
- In the same way as it takes a very long time for amiodarone to have its maximum effect, it takes a very long time for amiodarone to be eliminated from the body once it has been stopped. Adverse effects and drug interactions can occur weeks after amiodarone has been stopped.

Drugs with long half-lives

• Bisphosphonates	Years (in bone)
• Amiodarone	50 days
• Choloroquine	48 days
• Hydroxychloroquine	18 days
• Gold salts	
◆ Auranofin	21 days
◆ Sodium aurothiomalate	6 days
• Alfacalcidol	14 days
• Levothyroxine	7 days
• Digitoxin	5 days
• Phenytoin	Variable, up to 60 hours or more
• Fluoxetine	48 hours
• Digoxin	40 hours
• Warfarin	24 hours

Heparins (unfractionated and low molecular weight)

Anticoagulants

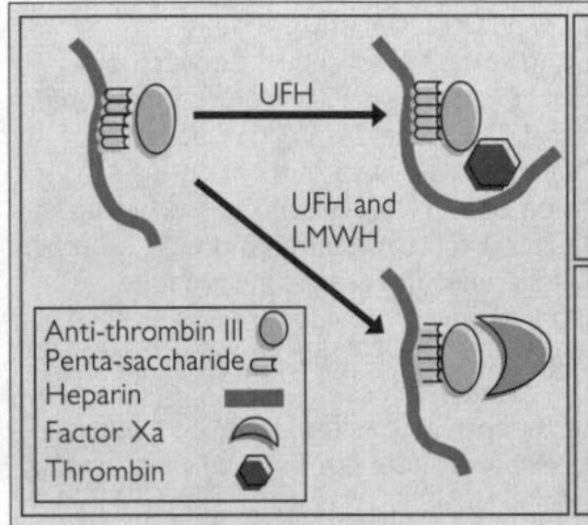

Unfractionated heparin (UFH) has penta-saccharides along its length. These bind to antithrombin III and increase its activity. This then forms a ternary complex with thrombin (upper arrow) deactivating it. In addition, heparin binds factor X (lower arrow) and deactivates it.

Low molecular weight heparins (LMWH) cannot form the ternary complex (upper arrow), because they are shorter. They can only deactivate factor X (lower arrow). LMWH are often more effective anticoagulants because they have more predictable kinetic properties.

Drugs in this class

- UFH
- LMWH
  - Certoparin
  - Dalteparin
  - Enoxaparin
  - Reviparin
  - Tinzaparin

Note on heparinoids

Danaparoid is a factor X antagonist. It can be used in patients who require anticoagulation but have developed immune-mediated thrombocytopenia with conventional heparins.

- Parenteral anticoagulant drugs.
- Used in full anticoagulant doses whenever rapid anticoagulation is required, for example:
  - Thromboembolic disease.
  - Acute coronary syndromes.
- Used in lower doses as prophylaxis against thromboembolic disease, especially during the peri-surgical period.
- Used to prevent blood clotting in extracorporeal circuits (dialysis membranes, cardiopulmonary bypass) and intravenous lines (e.g. Hickman lines).
  - Sodium chloride is as effective as heparinized saline for maintaining the patency of peripheral venous catheters.

- These drugs can only be given parenterally; they are therefore not suitable for long-term treatment, unless there is no alternative (e.g. pregnancy, see below).
- The decision to anticoagulate a patient should always involve assessment of risk and benefit. There are certain situations in which anticoagulation would not be recommended, as the risks are considered very great:
  - Haemophilia and inherited disorders of coagulation.
  - Patients with thrombocytopenia have a very high risk of bleeding. Note that heparins can cause thrombocytopenia (see below).
  - Patients with severe hepatic disease have disordered coagulation, but are also at increased risk of thrombosis. These patients may have oesophageal varices. See expert advice before giving heparin.

  - Elderly and debilitated patients are at greater risk of bleeding.
  - Recent severe trauma or surgery. This will depend on the site and nature of the injury. For example, anticoagulation would not be recommended after trauma to the eye or brain.
    — Avoid in patients with recent cerebral haemorrhage (subarachnoid or stroke).
  - Severe renal insufficiency increases the risk of bleeding.
  - Avoid in patients with active peptic ulcer unless the indication is overwhelming. The decision is more difficult in patients with a history of peptic ulcer; assess the potential benefits carefully.
  - Severe or uncontrolled hypertension increases the risk of bleeding.
- Pregnant women.
  - Avoid these drugs whenever possible; there is a risk of bleeding.
  - Oral anticoagulants (e.g. warfarin) are contraindicated in the first trimester of pregnancy and the last few weeks, so heparins have to be used if anticoagulation is indicated.
- Do not give these drugs by intramuscular injection because of the risk of haematoma.

- Heparins are most effective for venous thrombosis and that associated with sluggish blood flow (so called 'red clot'). Antiplatelet drugs are more effective for arterial clots that are composed mainly of platelets ('white clot').
- Unfractionated heparin (UFH) shows a great deal of variation in its pharmacokinetic and pharmacodynamic properties. This is true whether given it is by intravenous infusion or by subcutaneous injection, making it a difficult drug to use. Low molecular weight heparins (LMWH) have much more predictable actions, and when given by subcutaneous injection they provide reliable anticoagulation based upon body weight, without the need for routine measurement of clotting parameters. They have largely replaced UFH for the major indications. UFH, given intravenously, is still used when anticoagulation is required but needs to be stopped for a period (e.g. during a surgical procedure; see teaching point in warfarin, p. 115).
  - Both LMWH and UFH are given in low doses for prophylaxis against thromboembolic disease.
- If parenteral anticoagulation is to be followed by oral anticoagulation (e.g. warfarin) the heparin should be continued for 5 days, or until the INR has been in the target range (usually 2.5 +/– 0.5) for 2 days, whichever is the longer.

Low molecular weight heparins (LMWH)

- These drugs are given by subcutaneous injection only.
- The dose is calculated according to body weight (see below). It may be given either once or twice daily. If the patient is perceived to be at risk of bleeding, give the drug twice daily.
- The dose given for thromboembolic disease is slightly different from that given in acute coronary syndromes. This is a quirk of the doses used in clinical trials. Refer to your local protocol, but the difference is not likely to be important clinically.
- Because these drugs have a predictable action, routine measurement of clotting parameters is not required. See monitoring section for special arrangements if monitoring is required.

Unfractionated heparin (UFH)

- To anticoagulate a patient using intravenous infusion, give an initial bolus followed by a continuous infusion (see below for doses). The only advantage of this method is that the effect of the drug will disappear quickly once it has been stopped (e.g. during surgery or interventional radiological procedures).
  - Many of the thrombolytic protocols call for anticoagulation with UFH following thrombolysis. Follow your local policy.
  - Find out the local policy regarding the use of LMWH in patients who may need cardiac catheterization.
  - UFH is still widely used to prevent clotting in extracorporeal circuits. Remember that in most cases the patient will be exposed to at least a proportion of this heparin.
- UFH may be used to anticoagulate a patient by subcutaneous injection. The degree of anticoagulation is unpredictable; consider using LMWH instead.
  - UFH is still widely used in low doses for prophylaxis against thromboembolic disease; this is because it is considerably less expensive than LMWH.

- The greatest risk from these drugs is haemorrhage (LMWH, major bleeding risk 0–3% during clinical trials).
  - Consider the patient factors listed above.
  - See the box below for treatment of bleeding . See warfarin (p. 115) for assessment of excessive anticoagulation and anticoagulation during surgery.
  - Remember, heparins do not usually cause bleeding but make what would ordinarily be trivial bleeding worse. Always investigate the cause of the bleeding.
- These drugs can cause thrombocytopenia in about 5% of patients.
  - This is usually immune-mediated. The risk is greater if treatment is for longer than 5 days.
  - Stop the drug if the platelet count falls by more than 50%.
  - Seek expert haematological guidance.
  - Consider treatment with a heparinoid (see box above).
- These are large molecules and can cause hypersensitivity, characterized by urticaria, angio-oedema, and anaphylaxis.
- These drugs inhibit aldosterone secretion. This can cause hyperkalaemia. Those at greatest risk include:
  - Patients with renal insufficiency.
  - Patients given heparin for more than 7 days.
  - Patients with diabetes mellitus.
  - Patients also taking potassium-sparing diuretics.
- These drugs can cause osteoporosis with long-term use. This is an issue in women who are pregnant and require long-term treatment with heparin, because warfarin is contraindicated. These patients should be managed by a specialist.

- Take care when giving heparin to patients taking other drugs that also increase the risk of bleeding: NSAIDs, antiplatelet drugs (e.g. aspirin), and corticosteroids.
  - In some cases this increased risk will be justified, but ensure that you have considered it before prescribing the drug.
  - Consider giving a PPI or misoprostol.

Efficacy

- When given in a low dose for prophylaxis against thromboembolic disease, neither UFH nor LMWH affects the APTT.
  - Look for evidence of venous thrombosis even if prophylaxis has been given.
- LMWH. Routine monitoring is not usually required. LMWH only affects the APTT to a moderate degree; this cannot be used to measure the adequacy of anticoagulation. If there is a need to measure the degree of anticoagulation (e.g. in very obese patients), measure the antifactor Xa activity. This is a special assay, and you will need to arrange it with the laboratory.
- UFH. Measure the APTT 6 hours after starting an infusion and every 12 hours thereafter. Aim for the APTT to be 2–3 times normal (control).

Safety

- Measure the platelet count and clotting parameters before starting treatment. Measure the platelet count if treatment is likely to continue for more than 5 days or if bruising appears.
- Measure the plasma potassium if the patient is at risk of hyperkalaemia (see above).

- Explain that these drugs can cause bleeding; this risk has to be balanced against the potential benefits.
- Advise the patient that these drugs can cause bruising around injection sites but that they should report any large or unexpected bruises immediately (measure the clotting parameters and platelet count).
- Advise the patient to avoid over-the-counter formulations containing aspirin or NSAIDs (e.g. ibuprofen).

Prescribing information: **Heparins**

Unfractionated heparin

Full anticoagulation

- By intravenous infusion, initial bolus of 5000 units (10 000 units in severe pulmonary embolism), followed by an infusion of 15–25 units/kg/hour. Adjust the rate according to the APTT.
- By subcutaneous injection, initially 15 000 units every 12 hours. Adjust the dose according to the APTT.

Thromboprophylaxis

- By subcutaneous injection, 5000 units 2 hours before surgery, followed by 5000 units every 8–12 hours for 7 days, or until the patient is ambulant. Monitoring is not usually required (see section above).

Dalteparin

Several types of LMWH are available (see list above); dalteparin is given as an example.

Full anticoagulation

- By subcutaneous injection once daily for treatment of venous thromboembolism, 200 units/kg (see box below).

Body weight (kg)	Daily dose (may be divided)
<46	7500 units
46–56	10 000 units
57–68	12 500 units
69–82	15 000 units
83 and over	18 000 units
	Maximum daily dose 18 000 units

- By subcutaneous injection 12-hourly for treatment of unstable angina, 120 units/kg.
  - Maximum dose is 10 000 units/12 hours.
  - Treatment may continue for 8 days if considered of benefit by the physician.

Thromboprophylaxis

- By subcutaneous injection.
  - *Moderate risk*: 2500 units 2 hours before surgery, followed by 2500 units every 24 hours for 7 days, or until the patient is ambulant.
  - *High risk*: 2500 units 2 hours before surgery, followed by 5000 units every 24 hours for 7 days, or until the patient is ambulant.

TEACHING POINT Treatment of bleeding in patients given anticoagulant drugs

- Patients may bleed because:
  - They are at high risk (see notes above). Consider the risk carefully before starting anticoagulant treatment.
  - The degree of anticoagulation is excessive. The risk of bleeding increases greatly once the APPT is >3 times normal or if the INR is >3.
  - They have been given a drug that may cause them to bleed (e.g. an antiplatelet drug (such as aspirin) or NSAID). Anticoagulation makes this bleeding worse.
- Resuscitate the patient if required.
- Treat the bleeding locally, if possible. For example, apply local pressure to a cannula site or arrange endoscopic intervention for a bleeding peptic ulcer.
- Reverse the anticoagulation if required. Assess which is the greater danger, bleeding or thrombosis. For example, it would be inappropriate to reverse anticoagulation fully in a patient with severe pulmonary embolism on account of minor cannula site bleeding.

The reversal treatment depends on the anticoagulant drug.

- UFH. Use protamine; 1 mg of protamine reverses the effect of 100 units of heparin. The maximum dose of protamine is 50 mg. Protamine is given by slow iv injection over 10 minutes.
- LMWH. Protamine is less effective for these drugs (about 50%). However, the dose is the same.
- Warfarin. Use vitamin K. Full reversal 5 mg iv. Use lower doses (0.5–2.0 mg iv) if complete reversal is not desired. Adjust the dose according to response. Note that it may be very difficult to re-anticoagulate the patient after giving vitamin K.

- If bleeding is severe or reversal is inadequate, consider giving prothrombin complex concentrate (contains clotting factors) 50 units/kg or, if this is not available, fresh frozen plasma 15 mL/kg.
- In the most severe cases, consider cryoprecipitate, pooled platelets, and whole blood. Seek specialist haematological guidance.

Warfarin

Coumarin anticoagulant

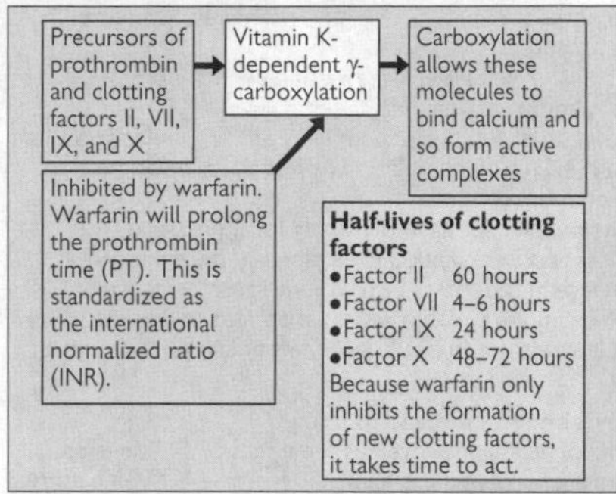

Other oral anticoagulants

- Acenocoumarol (nicoumalone)
- Phenprocoumon
- Phenindione

Risk factors for venous thromboembolism

- Malignancy (may be occult)
- Prolonged immobilization (car and aeroplane journeys)
- Surgery and trauma, especially of the pelvis and lower limb
- Oral contraceptive use
- Smoking
- Obesity
- Severe heart failure
- Pregnancy
- Polycythaemia/severe dehydration
- Previous thrombosis

Patients taking anticoagulants who require surgery

See teaching point below

- Oral anticoagulant drug.
- Used whenever long-term anticoagulation is required, for example:
  - Prophylaxis and treatment of thromboembolic disease (e.g. AF, prosthetic heart valves, ventricular clot).

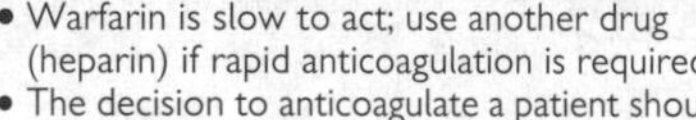

- Warfarin is slow to act; use another drug (heparin) if rapid anticoagulation is required.
- The decision to anticoagulate a patient should always involve an assessment of risk and benefit. There are certain circumstances in which anticoagulation would not be recommended, as the risks are considered very great:
  - Haemophilia and inherited disorders of coagulation.
  - Patients with thrombocytopenia, who are at very high risk of bleeding.
  - Patients with severe hepatic disease, who have disordered coagulation but are also at increased risk of thrombosis. These patients may have oesophageal varices. Seek expert advice before giving warfarin.
  - Elderly and debilitated patients, who are at greater risk of bleeding.
  - Recent severe trauma or surgery. This will depend on the site and nature of the injury.
    - — For example, anticoagulation would not be recommended after trauma to the eye or brain.
    - — For example, avoid in patients with recent cerebral haemorrhage.
  - Severe renal insufficiency increases the risk of bleeding.
  - Avoid in patients with active peptic ulcer. The decision is more difficult in patients with a history of peptic ulcer; assess the potential benefits carefully.
  - Severe or uncontrolled hypertension, in which the risk of bleeding is increased.
- Pregnant women.
  - Warfarin is teratogenic; do not use it during the first trimester of pregnancy and in the last few weeks before term (see heparin, p. 104).

- Advise women taking long-term anticoagulation to seek medical advice before they become pregnant, so that appropriate arrangements can be made.

- Warfarin is most effective for venous thrombosis and that associated with sluggish blood flow (so-called 'red clot'). Antiplatelet drugs are more effective for arterial clots that are composed mainly of platelets ('white clot').
- Treatment with warfarin can be started de novo (e.g. in patients with AF to reduce their risk of stroke), but it is most commonly given after initial treatment with heparin for medium- to long-term treatment of thromboembolic disease (see below for suggested durations of treatment).
- Treatment with warfarin is often started at the same time as heparin, in order to shorten the length of time a patient has to stay in hospital. Remember that heparin needs to be given for a minimum of 5 days, even if the INR has risen into the target range. Also remember that treatment with warfarin takes time to stabilize; do not stop treatment with heparin until the INR has been above 2.0 for 1 or 2 days.
- Warfarin is subject to a large number of drug interactions; these are most likely to occur whenever interacting drugs are started or stopped.

Starting warfarin

- There are several regimens; the following is offered as an example of a simple practical method.
  - Measure the INR before starting treatment.
  - Give 10 mg daily*; measure the INR (see below) daily from the second day onwards. Once the INR has reached 2, count the number of days since treatment started. This number, converted into milligrams is the approximate maintenance dose. (For example, the INR is 2.1 after 3 days at 10 mg daily. The estimated maintenance dose is 3 mg.)
  - Fine tuning of the dosage thereafter is usually required to maintain the INR at the usual target value (2.5).

(*If the patient is at high risk, is taking interacting drugs, or has hepatic or cardiac disease, consider reducing this to 5 mg daily. In this case the maintenance dose calculation is halved as well.)

- If anticoagulation is not urgent, initiation with a low dose (2 mg daily), gradually adjusted as required, is an alternative.

Target INR and duration of treatment

(Based on British Society for Haematology guidelines: *www.bcshguidelines.com*)

- Always set a target for the duration of anticoagulation. Arrange to review the patient after this period. Consider whether any risk factors persist (see box above), and whether anticoagulation treatment should continue beyond the initial period.
- **Venous thromboembolism**
  - First event pulmonary embolism or proximal vein thrombosis: INR 2.5 for 6 months.
  - Calf vein thrombosis in a non-surgical patient with no persistent risk factors: INR 2.5 for 3 months.
  - Postoperative calf vein thrombosis without persistent risk factors: INR 2.5 for 6 weeks.
  - Recurrence while taking warfarin: increase INR to 3.5.
  - First recurrence after stopping warfarin: treat again as above; look for persistent risk factors.
  - Second recurrence on or off warfarin: consider long-term treatment and seek expert advice.

- **Inherited thrombophilia**
  - No clinical episodes. Long-term anticoagulation is not recommended. Remember prophylaxis for risk periods.
  - First clinical episode: treat as above. Consider long-term treatment; seek expert advice.
- **Atrial fibrillation**
  - INR 2.5.
  - Cardioversion: INR 2.5 for 3 weeks before and 4 weeks after cardioversion.
  - Paroxysmal AF: seek expert advice; depends on the risk of embolism.
- **Prosthetic heart valves**
  - Mechanical valve: INR 3.5.
  - Bioprosthetic valves: anticoagulation not usually required in the absence of AF.

- The greatest risk from warfarin is haemorrhage. Other adverse effects are uncommon.
  - Consider the patient factors listed above.
  - See the box below for treatment of excessive anticoagulation. See heparin (p. 109) for treatment of bleeding.
  - Remember that warfarin does not usually cause bleeding but makes what would ordinarily be trivial bleeding worse. Always investigate the cause of the bleeding.
- Warfarin can rarely cause hypersensitivity, characterized by a maculopapular rash.
- Other adverse effects include alopecia, diarrhoea, hepatic dysfunction, and pancreatitis.

- Warfarin is affected by a large number of other drugs (see below).
- Also remember that the risk of bleeding is increased when given with drugs that can cause gastrointestinal ulceration.
  - NSAIDs, antiplatelet drugs (e.g. aspirin), and corticosteroids.
  - In some cases this increased risk will be justified, but ensure that you have considered it before prescribing the drug.
  - Consider giving a PPI or misoprostol.
- Foods vary in their contents of vitamin K. Some enteral feeds contain vitamin K. Measure the INR more frequently if the patient changes their diet significantly.

Drugs that enhance the anticoagulant effect	Drugs that reduce the anticoagulant effect
Alcohol, anabolic steroids	Anti-infective drugs: rifampicin, griseofulvin
Antiarrhythmic drugs: amiodarone, propafenone, and quinidine	St John's wort
Anti-infective drugs: macrolides (e.g. erythomycin, clarithromycin), some quinolones (e.g. ciprofloxacin), sulphonamides	Antiepileptics: phenytoin, carbamazepine, phenobarbital, primidone
Antifungals: drugs ending with '–conazole'	
Disulfiram	
Hormone antagonists: danazol, flutamide, tamoxifen	
Lipid-regulating drugs: statins and fibrates	
Testosterone	
Thyroid hormones	
Ulcer-healing drugs: omeprazole, cimetidine	

Efficacy and safety

- Measure the prothrombin time and other clotting parameters before starting anticoagulation treatment. If these are abnormal at baseline, reconsider treatment or reduce the initial dose.
- Warfarin prolongs the prothrombin time; this is compared with an internationally agreed standard to produce the INR. An INR of 2.0 means that the prothrombin time is twice the control value.
- Measure the INR daily when initiating treatment. Once the patient is stabilized, the time between INR measurements can be increased. The maximum recommended time between measurements during stable therapy is 12 weeks.
- Aim for smooth control of the INR. Do not make frequent, large changes to the dose; this will lead to great variations in the INR. Many anticoagulation clinics use computer programs that examine the pattern of a patient's INR in relation to daily dose and recommend dosage adjustments accordingly.
- Remember that the INR will vary with time of day and from day to day. For this reason, a target INR is given; if the actual INR is within +/– 0.5 units of the target, that is acceptable.
- Remember that the INR is a continuous variable. An INR of 1.9 does not confer zero protection, and an INR of 2.1 does not confer complete protection. Once the INR rises above 3.0 the risk of bleeding increases exponentially. For this reason, the target INR is usually around 2.5 (see above). This seems to provide the best ratio between benefit and risk; however, in some cases that balance is altered (e.g. recurrent thrombosis).

- Explain that warfarin can cause bleeding, and that the risk has to be balanced against the potential benefits.
- Advise the patient that warfarin can cause bruising but that they should report any large or unexpected bruises immediately (measure the clotting parameters).
- Advise the patient to avoid over-the-counter formulations containing aspirin or NSAIDs (e.g. ibuprofen).
- Advise the patient to take the warfarin tablets at the same time of day; this will improve the smoothness of control.
- Warfarin is supplied as tablets of differing strengths and colours. Ensure that the patient knows which is which, so that they can safely adjust their dose when advised to (see below).
- Give the patient an anticoagulant card.

Prescribing information: **Warfarin**

See above for treatment targets and advice on starting warfarin.

- By mouth, usual daily dose in the range of 2–9 mg.
  - 0.5 mg tablets are white
  - 1 mg tablets are brown
  - 3 mg tablets are blue
  - 5 mg tablets are pink

TEACHING POINT Treatment of excessive anticoagulation with warfarin

- See 'treatment of bleeding' in heparin (p. 109) for management of severe bleeding.
- Remember, warfarin does not usually cause bleeding but makes what would ordinarily be trivial bleeding worse. If there is bleeding, investigate the cause.
- Excessive anticoagulation is usually the result of a failure to take account of a factor that will enhance the anticoagulant effect of warfarin:
  - The patient has a severe intercurrent illness and the dose of warfarin is not reduced.
  - A drug that enhances the action of warfarin is started.
  - A drug that reduces the effect of warfarin is stopped.
  - The maintenance dose is incorrect, but the INR has not been measured.
- INR >8.0
  - No bleeding. Stop warfarin and restart at a lower dose once the INR is <5.0.
  - If the patient is at high risk of bleeding consider giving 0.5 mg vitamin K_1 iv or 5 mg by mouth.
- INR 5.0–8.0
  - No bleeding. Stop warfarin and restart at a lower dose once the INR is <5.0.
- INR >0.5 units above target but <5.0
  - No bleeding. Continue warfarin at a lower dose.

TEACHING POINT Anticoagulation and surgery

- If you can delay surgery until the patient is no longer taking an anticoagulant, do so. Make sure that the patient's risk factors have been thoroughly investigated and modified before surgery is planned.
- In most cases, the risk of bleeding from anticoagulation is greater than the risk of thrombosis, even for patients at moderately high risk.
- Anticoagulation should therefore be stopped 3 or 4 days before major surgery. It may be restarted 48–72 hours after the operation. If the patient is unable to take medications by mouth, initial treatment with heparin will be required.
- Make sure that the patient receives adequate thromboprophylaxis (compression stockings, low-dose heparin, early mobilization).
- Guidelines suggest that it is safe to operate if the INR is <2.5, but this will depend on the procedure (e.g. neurosurgical procedures often require a lower INR). Make sure that you know the target INR before the day of operation.
- Use vitamin K very cautiously if the INR needs to be brought down (dosages of 0.5 mg iv); large doses will make it very difficult to re-anticoagulate the patient after the operation.
- A few patients are at very high risk of thromboembolism; these patients may require interim treatment with heparin once the INR falls below 3.0.
  - For example, patients with ball-and-cage prosthetic heart valves and patients with adenocarcinoma who have previously suffered a thrombotic event.

Acetylsalicylic acid (aspirin)

Irreversible inhibitor of cyclo-oxygenase

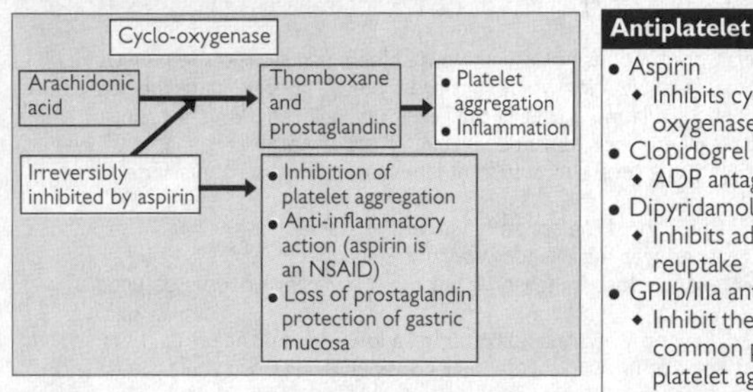

Antiplatelet drugs

- Aspirin
  - Inhibits cyclo-oxygenase
- Clopidogrel
  - ADP antagonist
- Dipyridamole
  - Inhibits adenosine reuptake
- GPIIb/IIIa antagonists
  - Inhibit the final common pathway of platelet aggregation

- Primary and secondary prevention of complications of atherosclerotic disease.
  - Angina.
  - Myocardial infarction.
  - Stroke.
  - Peripheral vascular disease.
- Analgesia.
- Anti-inflammatory drug for rheumatoid arthritis (high doses only; specialist use).

- Aspirin can cause bleeding; avoid using it in patients who are at a high risk of bleeding or in whom the consequences of bleeding could be catastrophic:
  - Active peptic ulceration.
  - Uncontrolled/accelerated phase hypertension.
  - Severe renal or hepatic insufficiency.
  - Haemophilia.
  - Pregnant women. Risk of intrauterine bleeding and closure of ductus arteriosus in utero.
- Aspirin can cause asthma and worsen the control of intrinsic asthma.
- Aspirin's active metabolite, salicylate, is renally excreted. Avoid large (anti-inflammatory doses) in renal insufficiency.
- Avoid if the patient has G6PD deficiency.
- Aspirin can cause Reye's syndrome. Avoid using it in children under the age of 16.

- Antiplatelet drugs are most effective for arterial clots that are composed mainly of platelets ('white clot'). Anticoagulant drugs are more effective for venous thrombosis and that associated with sluggish blood flow, so called ('red clot').

As an antiplatelet drug

- The antiplatelet action of aspirin is achieved by small daily dosages (75 mg daily or less). Increasing the dose does not increase protection. If aspirin prophylaxis proves to be ineffective, consider adding another drug rather than increasing the dose.
- Aspirin is effective in the secondary treatment of atherosclerotic disease. It is also effective for primary prevention, particularly for those aged over 55. Do not use antiplatelet drugs indiscriminately. If the risk is low, the risk of bleeding (gastrointestinal and intracranial) will outweigh the potential benefit.

- Once started appropriately, treatment with aspirin should be lifelong.
- Uncontrolled hypertension increases the risk of bleeding on aspirin. Ensure that the blood pressure is controlled before starting an antiplatelet drug.
- Aspirin is considerably less effective than anticoagulation (with warfarin) for the prevention of stroke in patients with AF (see box below).
- Early aspirin treatment saves lives in acute ischaemic stroke. Most strokes are ischaemic rather than haemorrhagic. There is some debate whether it is always necessary to confirm this before starting treatment, but most doctors wait until the brain has been imaged (see box below).
- Early treatment with aspirin in patients with myocardial infarction saves as many lives as thrombolysis.

Analgesia
- Aspirin is an effective simple analgesic and is a component of many proprietary compound formulations.
- Dispersible (soluble) formulations act more quickly.

Anti-inflammatory
- Aspirin has little anti-inflammatory action at daily dosages below 3 g.
- Aspirin used to be the treatment of choice for symptom relief in rheumatoid arthritis, but other NSAIDs are now preferred.

- Aspirin treatment will cause 4 major extracranial bleeds and 2 intracranial bleeds per 1000 patients treated per year. This risk needs to be set against any potential benefits of treatment (see above).
  - The risk of bleeding with aspirin is constant; it does not diminish with time.
  - Enteric-coated formulations do not reduce the risk.
- Gastrointestinal disturbance (other than bleeding) and tinnitus are common at high dosages.
- Hypersensitivity is variously reported as occurring in between 1% and 50% of patients. It is characterized by rash, urticaria, and angio-oedema.
- Aspirin can cause bronchospasm, and aspirin and NSAIDs can precipitate asthma; patients in whom this happens sometimes also have nasal polyps.
- Aspirin causes thrombocytopenia rarely.

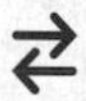

- Take care when giving aspirin to patients taking drugs that increase their risk of bleeding: warfarin, other antiplatelet drugs, corticosteroids.
  - In some cases this increased risk will be justified, but ensure that you have considered it before prescribing the drug.
- Aspirin can antagonize the action of diuretics and cause fluid retention (especially at higher dosages).
- Some NSAIDs (e.g. ibuprofen, but not diclofenac) inhibit the antiplatelet action of aspirin. It is wise to avoid these drugs, especially if the patient has unstable cardiac disease.
- Aspirin reduces the excretion of methotrexate, increasing the risk of toxicity.

Safety and efficacy
- Routine monitoring is not required for low dosages.
- If high dosages are used (for rheumatoid arthritis) measurement of plasma concentrations is recommended to individualize the dose.

- Advise patients to seek immediate medical attention if they have blood in the stool or dark, tarry stools.
- See teaching point below.

Prescribing information: **Acetylsalicylic acid**

Antiplatelet action

- Aspirin has an antiplatelet action at low dosages (75 mg daily or less), but many of the clinical trials used higher dosages (150–300 mg daily). Most clinicians use 75 mg daily for long-term treatment, but check local protocols.
- A one-off dose of 300 mg is recommended (dispersible or chewed) for patients who present with suspected acute myocardial infarction.

Analgesia

- By mouth, 300–900 mg every 4–6 hours. Maximum of 4 g daily.

Anti-inflammatory (specialized use)

- By mouth, 0.3–1 g every 4 hours after food.

TEACHING POINT Concepts of benefit and harm

- Treatment with aspirin for its antiplatelet action illustrates one of the major challenges of modern medicine — explaining the concept of a benefit/harm balance.
- Giving a patient penicillin for pneumococcal pneumonia is a fairly straightforward decision. Untreated, the condition may well be fatal, but treated the prognosis is good. There is a risk that the patient may be allergic to the drug, but set against the almost certain benefit this is a reasonable risk to take.
- Early treatment with aspirin after an acute ischaemic stroke will save 9 vascular events per 1000 patients treated. The 9 events are made up of 4 non-fatal strokes and 5 deaths from a vascular cause. This needs to be set against the risk: aspirin treatment will cause 4 major extracranial and 2 intracranial bleeds per 1000 patients treated per year.
- There are many difficulties in interpreting this for the patient, not least that these figures are derived from different clinical trials and so may not apply to the patient sitting in front of you. Even if the figures do apply, you do not know if the patient before you will be one to have an event saved, suffer a serious adverse event, or neither. Communicating this uncertainty to patients can be very difficult.
- Most prescribers will not see a thousand patients with acute ischaemic stroke in a year, so the concept of events saved per 1000 treated is difficult to comprehend. Figures like 'number needed to treat (or harm)' or 'percentage risk' are a little more user-friendly, but still require the prescriber and patient to take a wider view.
- Faced with the individual patient, it is all too easy to default to giving the drug in the hope that the patient will derive benefit and not harm. When the benefits are measured in numbers of events per 1000 treated, this will not always be so.
- There are no easy answers, but it is especially important to assess the risk and benefit as accurately as you can. Calculators such as the 10-year cardiovascular risk tables go some way to providing more objective evidence to inform your decision. The benefits of drugs are often well defined by clinical trials, but information on the associated risks is much more difficult to find.

TEACHING POINT Treatment of stroke

Prevention

Stroke can be fatal, but in terms of healthcare and social resources it is a better recognized major cause of severe morbidity. Because the resultant disability can be severe and none of the treatments is particularly effective, prevention of stroke is more important than treatment.

Risk factors for stroke

- *Hypertension* is the single most important risk factor and most of the long-term benefits of antihypertensive therapy are in reducing the risk of stroke. See p. 158 for guidance on the treatment of hypertension.
- *Atrial fibrillation* is associated with an annual risk of stroke of 7%; this can be reduced to about 2% with anticoagulation with warfarin. Anticoagulation can cause severe haemorrhage; in most cases this risk is justified by the reduction in risk of stroke, but make sure that you have assessed your patient's risk and taken any action required to minimize this. See warfarin (p. 110) for more information. Treatment with aspirin is less effective than anticoagulation but should be considered if the patient cannot take warfarin or is at very high risk of haemorrhage.
- *Hypercholesterolaemia* Treatment with a statin reduces the risk of stroke.
- *Carotid stenosis* Carotid endartectomy may be indicated in some patients; those most likely to benefit are those with a stenosis of 60–99%, a low surgical risk (less than 3% risk of death), and a life expectancy greater than 5 years. Seek expert advice.

Primary and secondary prevention

- Patients at high risk and those who have already had an event (stroke or TIA) should be given antiplatelet therapy with aspirin. Adding dipyridamole confers additional protection for those patients who have a further event while taking aspirin. See aspirin and dipyridamole (pp. 116 and 124) for more information.
- Clopidogrel can be considered as an alternative to aspirin.

Treatment

- Confirm the diagnosis (haemorrhage or infarction) using a CT scan of the brain.

Specific treatments for acute stroke

- *Thrombolytic therapy*. Some patients benefit from thrombolysis with alteplase if they present within 3 hours; the diagnosis must be confirmed with a CT scan. Very few patients present and can be investigated within this period, and alteplase can cause major haemorrhage. For these reasons, this treatment is currently restricted to a few specialist centres; see fibrinolytic drugs (p. 128) for more information.
- *Antiplatelet therapy*. Aspirin, given within 48 hours of cerebral infarction, reduces mortality and the risk of recurrent stroke. This is a small but statistically significant effect.
- *Anticoagulation*. Early anticoagulation following stroke should not be given routinely. The risks outweigh the benefits, except in some circumstances:
  - Stroke due to cardiac emboli with a high risk of recurrence (e.g. AF, endocarditis).
  - Established thrombophilia.
  - Symptomatic dissection of extracranial and intracranial arteries.
  - Symptomatic internal carotid stenosis before operation.
  - Crescendo TIAs.
  - Venous sinus thrombosis.

Supportive treatments

- Protect the airway and provide adequate oxygenation.
- Do not treat hypertension in the initial phase after a stroke unless the systolic blood pressure is more than 220 mmHg or the diastolic pressure is above 140 mmHg on repeated measures. The blood pressure is often labile and hypotension can cause more cerebral damage. If drug treatment is required, seek expert advice. See also beta-blockers (p. 147) for more information on the emergency treatment of hypertension.
- Electrolyte and blood glucose disturbances are common; correct them.
- If the patient is immobile, consider thromboprophylaxis with low-dose heparin. Early full anticoagulation with heparin or warfarin after an acute stroke is not recommended (see above).

Rehabilitation

- Rehabilitation after a stroke requires a multidisciplinary approach. Nursing the patient on a dedicated stroke unit improves survival and rehabilitation.
- Ensure that the patient has a pressure-relieving mattress and chair.
- Attend to the patient's nutritional needs; some patients require feeding through a nasogastric tube.

Clopidogrel

Adenosine diphosphate (ADP) receptor antagonist

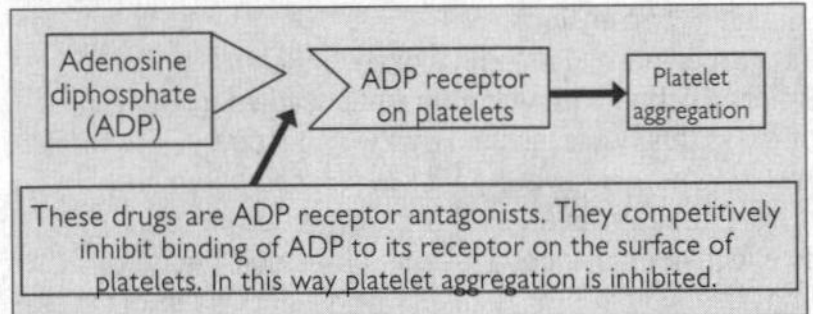

Antiplatelet drugs

- Aspirin
  - Inhibits cyclo-oxygenase
- Clopidogrel
  - ADP antagonist
- Dipyridamole
  - Inhibits ADP reuptake
- GPIIb/IIIa antagonists
  - Inhibit the final common pathway of platelet aggregation

- Secondary prevention of the complications of atherosclerotic disease.
  - Angina.
  - Myocardial infarction.
  - Stroke.
  - Peripheral vascular disease.
- Acute coronary syndromes and following percutaneous transluminal coronary angioplasty (PTCA).

Note on ticlopidine

Ticlopidine is another ADP antagonist that has been used following PTCA. It can cause agranulocytosis and so its use is not recommended.

- Clopidogrel can cause bleeding; avoid using it in patients who are at a high risk of bleeding, or in whom the consequences of bleeding could be catastrophic:
  - Active peptic ulceration.
  - Uncontrolled/accelerated phase hypertension.
  - Severe renal or hepatic insufficiency.
  - Haemophilia.
  - Pregnant women; risk of intrauterine bleeding.

- Antiplatelet drugs are most effective for arterial clots that are composed mainly of platelets ('white clot'). Anticoagulant drugs are most effective for venous thrombosis and that associated with sluggish blood flow ('red clot').

As an antiplatelet drug

- Clopidogrel is an effective antiplatelet drug and in one large trial was slightly more effective than aspirin. However, this effect is very small (relative risk reduction of 8%, see teaching point below) and so is very costly.
  - Clopidogrel is sometimes used in combination with aspirin (see below).
- Consider clopidogrel for patients who are:
  - Hypersensitive to aspirin.
  - Unable to tolerate aspirin.
- Clopidogrel does cause gastrointestinal bleeding, but less often than aspirin. If a patient has had a bleed from aspirin, and antiplatelet treatment is still required, options include:
  - Adding a PPI.
  - Adding misoprostol.
  - Switching to clopidogrel.
- Uncontrolled hypertension increases the risk of bleeding on clopidogrel. Ensure that the blood pressure is controlled before starting an antiplatelet drug.

Acute coronary syndromes

- Clopidogrel improves outcome when added to existing aspirin treatment in patients with acute coronary syndromes.
- It is also used in addition to aspirin for the first 28 days following PTCA, whether elective or emergency. It is unclear whether continued treatment after 28 days confers any significant further benefit.

- Clopidogrel can cause bleeding. The relative risk reduction for gastrointestinal bleeding compared with aspirin is 25% (there is probably no difference in the number of intracranial bleeds). This translates into a very small number of actual events saved. (See teaching point below.)
  - This risk needs to be set against any potential benefits of treatment.
- Clopidogrel can cause abdominal pain and nausea.
- Rare adverse effects include dizziness, vertigo, paraesthesia, and hepatic and biliary damage.

- Adding clopidogrel to existing aspirin treatment increases the antiplatelet effect but also markedly increases the risk of bleeding. The combination should only be used when this risk is outweighed by the potential benefit (e.g. acute coronary syndromes).
- Take care when giving clopidogrel to patients taking drugs that increase their risk of bleeding: warfarin, other antiplatelet drugs, corticosteroids.
  - In some cases this increased risk will be justified, but ensure that you have considered it before prescribing the drug.

Safety and efficacy

- Routine monitoring is not usually required. The key to successful treatment with clopidogrel is ensuring appropriate patient selection in the first place.

- See teaching point below.

Prescribing information: **Clopidogrel**

- By mouth, 75 mg once daily.

TEACHING POINT Relative and absolute risk reductions

- Promotional material and reports of clinical trials commonly quote the relative risk reduction associated with a particular treatment. For example, patients who take treatment A only had half as many events as those in the control group. This is a relative risk reduction of 50%. This sounds very impressive, and in terms of efficacy for many drugs would be very impressive. The piece of information that is missing is the background incidence of these events. If the event affects 50 out of 100 patients, then a relative risk reduction of 50% will mean that a further 25 events per 100 patients are avoided. This is an absolute risk reduction of 25% — a very effective intervention. If, however, the incidence of the event is only 2 in 100, a 50% relative risk reduction will only reduce the incidence to 1 in 100, an absolute risk reduction of 1%.
- Clopidogrel is an effective antiplatelet drug. Treatment with clopidogrel in the CAPRIE trial resulted in a relative risk reduction of 8.7% for the primary endpoint (ischaemic stroke, myocardial infarction, or vascular death), compared with aspirin. The annual event rate was 5.83% in the aspirin group and 5.32% in the clopidogrel group. This is an absolute risk reduction of 0.5%. You would have to treat 200 patients with clopidogrel rather than aspirin to save one additional event. Clopidogrel is not very expensive (about £30 per month), but aspirin is very cheap. This means that the incremental cost to save those additional events is very high.
- When faced with information about relative risk reduction, put it in context by considering:
  - What is the background incidence of this event — is it common or rare?
  - What is the absolute risk reduction?
  - How many patients would need to be treated to save an additional event (the number needed to treat)
  - Is there a significant difference in cost between the two interventions?
  - Do the interventions carry different risks of adverse events?

CAPRIE trial, *Lancet* 1996, **348**: 1329–39.

Dipyridamole

Antiplatelet drug

The mechanism of action of dipyridamole is not fully understood. It probably acts by inhibiting the reuptake of adenosine into platelets and so reduces ADP-induced aggregation.

Antiplatelet drugs

- Aspirin
  - Inhibits cyclo-oxygenase
- Clopidogrel
  - ADP antagonist
- Dipyridamole
  - Inhibits adenosine reuptake
- GPIIb/IIIa antagonists
  - Inhibit the final common pathway of platelet aggregation

- Secondary prevention of stroke following a stroke or transient ischaemic attack (TIA).
- Adjunct to oral anticoagulation for prophylaxis of thromboembolism associated with prosthetic heart valves.

- Dipyridamole can cause bleeding, but this is less common than with other antiplatelet drugs. Avoid using it in patients who are at a high risk of bleeding, or in whom the consequences of bleeding could be catastrophic:
  - Active peptic ulceration.
  - Uncontrolled/accelerated phase hypertension.
  - Severe renal or hepatic insufficiency.
  - Haemophilia.
- Although there is no formal evidence of its safety, dipyridamole has been used in pregnancy without adverse effects.

- Antiplatelet drugs are most effective for arterial clots that are composed mainly of platelets ('white clot'). Anticoagulant drugs are most effective for venous thrombosis and that associated with sluggish blood flow ('red clot').

As an antiplatelet drug

- Used alone, diypridamole is a weak antiplatelet drug and its use is not generally recommended.
- If the patient is at a high risk of bleeding and antiplatelet treatment is required consider:
  - Aspirin with either a PPI or misoprostol.
  - Clopidogrel.
- Dipyridamole provides additional protection when given with aspirin to patients who have had either a stroke or TIA.
  - These trials used the 200 mg modified-release formulation.

⚠

- Dipyridamole can cause bleeding, but this is less common than with other antiplatelet drugs.
- Gastrointestinal disturbance is probably the most common adverse effect.
- Dipyridamole can cause vasodilatation; this in turn causes hot flushes, headache, and tachycardia.
- Hypersensitivity reactions are rare.

- Dipyridamole will greatly enhance the effect of adenosine. Avoid giving adenosine to patient taking dipyridamole.
- Take care when giving dipyridamole to patients taking drugs that increase their risk of bleeding: warfarin, other antiplatelet drugs, corticosteroids.
  - In some cases this increased risk will be justified, but ensure that you have considered it before prescribing the drug.

Safety and efficacy

- Routine monitoring is not usually required. The key to successful treatment with dipyridamole is appropriate patient selection in the first place.

- Warn the patient to report any unusual bleeding or bruising immediately.

Prescribing information: **Dipyridamole**

Secondary prevention of stroke

- By mouth, 200 mg modified-release bd; in combination with aspirin.

Adjunct to oral anticoagulation for prophylaxis of thromboembolism associated with prosthetic heart valves

- By mouth, 300–600 mg daily in 3 or 4 divided doses before food.

Glycoprotein IIb/IIIa antagonists

Antagonists at the platelet GPIIb/IIIa receptor

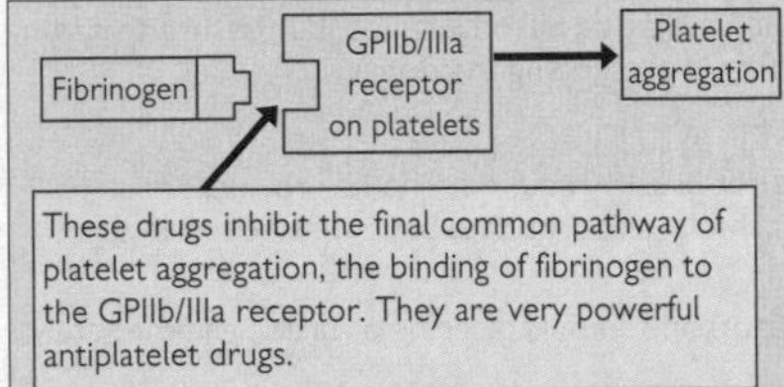

Antiplatelet drugs

- Aspirin
  - Inhibits cyclo-oxygenase
- Clopidogrel
  - ADP antagonist
- Dipyridamole
  - Inhibits adenosine reuptake
- GPIIb/IIIa antagonists
  - Inhibit the final common pathway of platelet aggregation

Abciximab is a monoclonal antibody raised against the GPIIb/IIIa receptor.
Eptifibatide and **tirofiban** are non-peptide antagonists at the GPIIb/IIIa receptor.

- Adjunctive treatment of unstable angina and non-Q-wave myocardial infarction (specialist use only).
- Adjunctive treatment to PTCA (specialist use only).

- These drugs can cause severe bleeding; avoid using them in patients who are at a high risk of bleeding, or in whom the consequences of bleeding could be catastrophic. Different manufacturers vary in their recommendations for exclusion. The following is not an exhaustive list; assess each patient individually.
  - Active peptic ulceration.
  - Uncontrolled/accelerated phase hypertension.
  - Severe renal or hepatic insufficiency.
  - Haemophilia.
  - Pregnant women; risk of intrauterine bleeding.
  - Intracranial neoplasm or other neoplasm at risk of causing severe bleeding.
  - Major or cranial surgery within 2 months.
  - Recent trauma.
  - Recent stroke (recommendations vary between 30 days and 2 years).
  - Arterio-venous malformations.
  - Aortic dissection.
  - Thrombocytopenia.
  - Vasculitis.
  - Retinopathy (hypertensive or diabetic).

- These drugs should only be given under specialist supervision.
- Remember that they are adjunctive, and are intended to be given with aspirin and an anticoagulant (heparin).
- All are given by intravenous infusion; the regimens vary considerably. Consult your local protocol for details.
- NICE has recommended that these drugs should be given to:
  - Patients with high-risk unstable angina or non-Q-wave myocardial infarction.

- As an adjunct to PTCA if:
  - The procedure is indicated, but delayed.
  - The patient has diabetes mellitus.
  - The procedure is complex.
- Patients receiving these drugs should be monitored closely (e.g. in a coronary care unit).
- Stop the infusion if emergency surgery or arterial balloon pump insertion is required.
- It can take 12 hours or more for platelet function to be restored after stopping the infusion.
- Remember that these patients should also be receiving anticoagulants.

- GPIIb/IIIa antagonists can cause severe bleeding. This is most common at the site of femoral puncture for PTCA, and can be severe. Estimates of the incidence vary depending on the definition of severe bleeding, but overall it is probably twice as common in patients given GPIIb/IIIa antagonists.
  - Take care to make a clear assessment of the risks and potential benefits before starting treatment with a GPIIb/IIIa antagonist. Only those at a high risk of infarction are likely to benefit.
- These drugs can cause thrombocytopenia.
- Other adverse effects include hypotension, headache, fever, and hypersensitivity reactions.
- Abciximab is a monoclonal antibody; it should only be used once, as neutralizing antibodies form.

- These drugs should be used with anticoagulants and antiplatelet drugs, but remember that these combinations increase the risk of bleeding.

Safety
- Measure the PT, APTT, haemoglobin concentration, platelet count, and haematocrit at baseline. Do not give the drug if these are abnormal.
- Measure the haemoglobin concentration and haematocrit at 12 and 24 hours.
- Measure the platelet count at 4 and 24 hours.

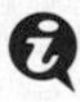

- Many of the drugs used for acute coronary syndromes increase the risk of bleeding. Warn the patient about this. A small amount of bleeding around cannula sites may seem trivial but can be very frightening for patients.

Prescribing information: **Glycoprotein IIb/IIIa antagonists**
- These drugs should only be given under specialist supervision.
- Regimens vary according to the drug used and the indication. Use your local protocols.

Fibrinolytic drugs

Activators of plasmin

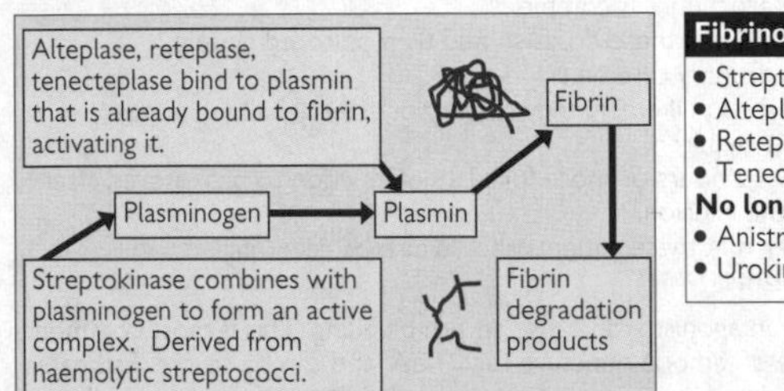

Fibrinolytic drugs

- Streptokinase
- Alteplase (tPA)
- Reteplase
- Tenecteplase

No longer available

- Anistreplase
- Urokinase

- These drugs are used when there is an urgent need to break down fibrin clot, for example:
  - Acute myocardial infarction.
  - Acute stroke.
  - Life-threatening venous thrombosis and pulmonary embolism.
- These drugs are also used less acutely when fibrin deposition is a clinical problem, for example:
  - Used to break down fibrin walls in loculated pleural effusions and empyemas.
  - Used to unblock venous catheters (e.g. Hickman lines).
  - Used to unblock thrombosed arteriovenous shunts.
  - Streptokinase can be applied topically to deslough wounds.

- These drugs can cause bleeding; avoid using them in patients who are at a high risk of bleeding or in whom the consequences of bleeding could be catastrophic. The following list of contraindications is offered as a guide. In some cases the benefits may outweigh the risk; treat each patient as an individual.
  - Active peptic ulceration.
  - Uncontrolled/accelerated phase hypertension (systolic BP >180 mmHg or diastolic BP >100 mmHg).
  - Severe renal or hepatic insufficiency (oesophageal varices).
  - Haemophilia.
  - Pregnancy, postpartum, and menstruation.
  - Previous haemorrhagic stroke or any stroke within the last 6 months.
  - Surgery or trauma within last 2 weeks.
  - Laser therapy for retinopathy within the last week (proliferative diabetic retinopathy).
  - Pericarditis, infective endocarditis.
  - Pulmonary disease with cavitation.
  - Acute pancreatitis.
- Anticoagulant and antiplatelet drugs are important components of the treatment of diseases such as acute myocardial infarction, but they increase the risk of bleeding from fibrinolytic drugs.
- Patients who have been given streptokinase in the past may form neutralizing antibodies. If they require fibrinolytic therapy again, they should be given an alternative drug, such as alteplase.

Acute myocardial infarction

- Fibrinolytic drugs reduce mortality in acute myocardial infarction by about 2–3%.
- They act on fibrin; however, early arterial clots are composed mainly of platelets ('white clot'). Early treatment with antiplatelet drugs (aspirin) saves as many lives as thrombolysis in myocardial infarction.
- They are more effective the earlier they are given. There is little benefit from thrombolysis if it is begun more than 12 hours after the start of the event.
- The UK National Service Framework demands a call-to-needle time of less than 60 minutes. This requires a streamlined admission and assessment procedure for patients at risk of myocardial infarction.
- Although it is important to give these drugs early, this should not be at the expense of proper assessment of the patient and the risks. See above for a list of contraindications.
  - It is especially important to try to distinguish myocardial infarction from acute dissection of the aorta. Giving a fibrinolytic drug in the latter case could be catastrophic.
- There are differences between these drugs (see adverse effects), but NICE has advised that careful assessment of the patient is more important than the choice of fibrinolytic drug.
- Hypertension increases the risk of bleeding from these drugs. The blood pressure should be reduced to below 180/100 mmHg using a nitrate infusion before thrombolysis starts.
- Treatment with alteplase, tenecteplase, and reteplase, but not streptokinase, should be followed by heparin.
- Cardiac arrhythmias are common as the myocardium reperfuses. Ensure that resuscitation facilities, including defibrillation equipment, are immediately available. These patients should ideally be nursed in a coronary care unit or high-dependency area.
- There is increasing evidence that immediate percutaneous intervention is more effective than thrombolysis. The availability of angiographic intervention varies widely; seek advice from a cardiologist.

Acute stroke (see also teaching point in aspirin, p. 118)

- There is evidence that alteplase is effective in acute stroke, but only in specific circumstances.
  - Thrombolytic treatment with tissue plasminogen activator (tPA) should only be given within 3 hours of the onset of stroke symptoms if haemorrhage has been definitively excluded and if the patient is in a specialist centre with appropriate experience and expertise.
- Thrombolytic therapy significantly increases symptomatic and fatal intracranial haemorrhage. These risks are offset by a reduction in disability in survivors, so that there is, overall, a significant net reduction in the proportion of patients dead or dependent in activities of daily living.
  - Wardlaw JM, del Zoppo G, Yamaguchi T. (2003) Thrombolysis for acute ischaemic stroke (Cochrane Review). In: *The Cochrane Library*, Issue 1. Oxford, Update Software.
- Alteplase is currently licensed for this indication in the UK under the guidance of a specialist neurologist.

Life-threatening venous thromboembolism or pulmonary embolism

- The use of thrombolytic therapy for venous thromboembolism remains controversial.
- Patients who are cardiovascularly unstable may be considered for this treatment.
    - An alternative is surgical thrombectomy.
- Patients with massive ileofemoral clot seem to be those with the most to gain from this treatment, but only if it is given within 1 week of the incident.
- Seek expert guidance before staring this treatment.

Thrombolysis for loculated pleural effusions and empyemas

- There is currently insufficient evidence to support the routine use of intrapleural fibrinolytic therapy in the treatment of parapneumonic effusion and empyema. This is the subject of a large-scale clinical trial.

Topical streptokinase

- Streptokinase can be used topically on ulcers to remove slough and clot. Remember to address the underlying cause of the ulcer in order to promote wound healing.
- Alternatives include benzoic acid, hydrogen peroxide, and the use of sterile larvae (maggots).
- Be aware that application of this drug to an open area will lead to systemic absorption and possible adverse effects.

- The principal risk from these drugs is that of bleeding. See cautions above to identify those at particular risk.
    - See heparins (p. 109) for general advice on the management of major bleeding.
    - The action of fibrinolytic drugs cannot usually be reversed.
- The risk of bleeding is best established when they are used for myocardial infarction.
    - The absolute risk of haemorrhagic stroke from streptokinase is about 0.5–1%.
    - The risk from the other drugs (alteplase, reteplase, tenecteplase) is higher.
    - This increased risk must be set against the other risks from streptokinase.
- Steptokinase commonly causes hypotension when given for acute myocardial infarction. This adverse effect is less common with alteplase, reteplase, and tenecteplase.
    - For streptokinase, hypotension is related to the rate of infusion. If hypotension occurs, stop the infusion until the blood pressure recovers, then restart it at a lower rate.
- Allergic reactions to steptokinase are relatively common. It can also cause heart failure. These adverse effects are rare with the other thrombolytic drugs.
    - Allergy is characterized by rash, flushing, and uveitis. Stopping the infusion and restarting it a slower rate reduces these effects. Anaphylaxis is rare.
- Nausea and vomiting are common adverse effects of these drugs.

- Take care when giving these drugs to patients taking drugs that increase their risk of bleeding: warfarin, antiplatelet drugs, corticosteroids.
  - In many cases this increased risk will be justified, but ensure that you have considered it before prescribing the drug.

Safety and efficacy

- Patients receiving fibrinolytic drugs should have continuous cardiac monitoring and frequent measurements of pulse and blood presssure. Examine the patient for signs of bleeding.
- Resolution of acute ECG changes is usually used to assess the effectiveness of the fibrinolytic treatment. If the pain continues, or if the ECG evolves, seek cardiological advice.

- Warn patients that, although you have assessed them and feel that the potential benefits outweigh the risks, there is still a risk of bleeding, including stroke.
- Always ask the patient if they have received streptokinase in the past. If they have, use another thrombolytic drug.

Prescribing information: **Fibrinolytic drugs**

Most of the information given here relates to the use of these drugs in acute myocardial infarction. Seek expert advice for other indications.

Streptokinase

- 1 500 000 units by iv infusion over 1 hour.

Alteplase

- Accelerated regimen:
- 15 mg by iv injection, followed by
- 50 mg by iv infusion over 30 minutes, followed by
- 35 mg by iv infusion over 60 minutes.

Reteplase

- 10 units by iv injection over 2 minutes, followed 30 minutes later by
- 10 units by iv injection.

Tenecteplase

- By iv injection, 500–600 micrograms/kg (30–50 mg) over 10 seconds.

Pharmacology of drugs used to treat myocardial infarction

Symptomatic treatment

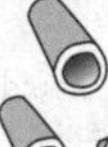

Glyceryl trinitrate – vasodilates, improving haemodynamics.

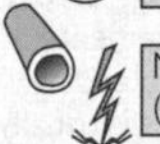

Morphine – relieves pain and vasodilates (reduces sympathetic activation).

Drugs used to treat the underlying pathophysiology (intracoronary clot)

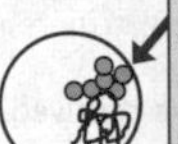

Antiplatelet drugs reduce platelet aggregation.

- Aspirin (given long-term)
- Clopidogrel (may be given long-term)
- Glycoprotein IIb/IIIa antagonists (e.g. abciximab, tirofiban)

- Fibrinolytic drugs break down formed clot.
- Anticoagulant drugs stop new clot forming.

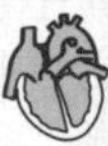

- β-adrenoceptor antagonists (beta-blockers) reduce myocardial oxygen demand; block neurohormonal activation (given long term).

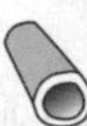

ACE inhibitors block neurohormonal activation (given long term).

Drugs used for secondary prevention

Lipid-lowering drugs (statins).

Smoking cessation (nicotine replacement therapy).

Antiarrhythmic drugs in those with established arrhythmias (see amiodarone, p. 100).

Patients with poor left ventricular function are at risk of embolus formation; they may benefit from anticoagulation.

Pharmacology of drugs used to treat heart failure

Symptomatic treatment

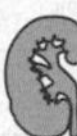

Loop diuretics cause salt and water loss. This alleviates breathlessness and oedema due to fluid overload, but stimulates the renin-angiotensin system.

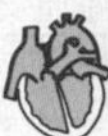

Cardiac glycosides (e.g. digoxin) have a positive inotropic effect, and can improve symptoms. They have not been shown to prolong life.

Drugs used to treat the underlying pathophysiology (neurohormonal activation)

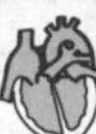

- ACE inhibitors block the formation of angiotensin II.
- Angiotensin receptor blockers block the action of angiotensin II.

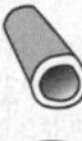

β-adrenoceptor antagonists (beta-blockers) block the actions of the activated sympathetic nervous system.

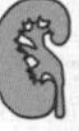

Spironolactone blocks the action of aldosterone in the kidney.

Drugs used for secondary prevention.
Heart failure is usually the result of ischaemic heart disease.

Antiplatelet drugs (aspirin).

Lipid-lowering drugs (statins).

Smoking cessation (nicotine replacement therapy).

Antiarrhythmic drugs in those with established arrhythmias (see amiodarone, p. 100).

Patients with poor left ventricular function are at risk of embolus formation. They may benefit from anticoagulation.

Notes
- Nitrates are given for the relief of angina. They can also be given with the vasodilator hydralazine for the treatment of severe intractable heart failure (specialist use).
- Phosphodiesterase inhibitors (milrinone and enoximone) can improve symptoms in the short term, but they increase mortality during long-term therapy.

Nitrate drugs

Nitric oxide donors

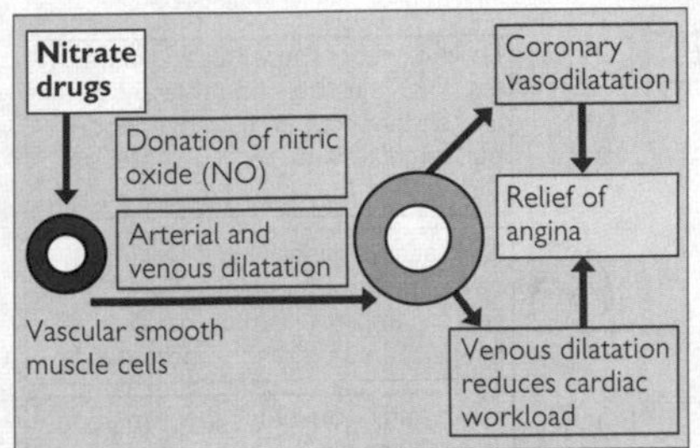

Drugs in this class

- Glyceryl trinitrate
- Isosorbide mononitrate*
- Isosorbide dinitrate*

*Available in modified-release formulations

- Treatment and prevention of angina.
- Treatment of acute left ventricular failure.

- Nitrates are first-line treatments for the symptoms of angina but do not affect the course of the underlying disease.
- They cause vasodilatation; this can be hazardous in some patients:
  - Patients who are hypovolaemic (severe hypotension).
  - Patients with cardiac disease such as hypertrophic cardiomyopathy or mitral stenosis.
  - Patients with bleeding (e.g. following head trauma or cerebral haemorrhage).
- No dosage adjustment is usually required in renal or hepatic insufficiency.
- Avoid these drugs during pregnancy; the effects on blood pressure can affect placental blood flow.

Treatment of angina (see teaching point below)

- Glyceryl trinitrate is given as sublingual tablets or spray for the symptomatic relief of angina. It acts within a few minutes and lasts for 20–30 minutes.
  - If the patient has predictable angina on exertion, they can take the glyceryl trinitrate beforehand to prevent angina.
- If the first dose of glyceryl trinitrate does not relive the angina, advise the patient to take a second dose after 5 minutes. If this does not relieve their symptoms, they should seek urgent medical attention.
- Glyceryl trinitrate can relieve symptoms of angina at rest or on minimal exertion, but these are symptoms of unstable disease; advise the patient to seek urgent medical attention.
- Glyceryl trinitrate is most useful for intermittent symptoms. Glyceryl trinitrate is relatively unstable; the sublingual tablets have a limited shelf-life. Advise the patient to dispose of any unused tablets after 3 months, and obtain a fresh supply. The spray formulation lasts longer, but check the expiry date.
- If the patient has frequent symptoms, a modified-release formulation that acts over a longer period may be suitable. Remember that nitrates do not affect the disease process; ensure that the patient has been adequately investigated.

- If nitrates are given repeatedly, patients rapidly become tolerant to their effects (within 24 hours). It is important to have a nitrate-free period of at least 4–8 hours during the day.
  - Immediate-release formulations should usually be given at 08.00 and 14.00, to give a nitrate-free period overnight. The timing of the doses can be altered to coincide with the patient's symptoms, but they should not be given 12 hours apart.
  - Modified-release formulations are usually formulated to provide relief over an 18-hour period.
  - Remove nitrate patches to provide a nitrate-free period (usually overnight).
  - Avoid giving intravenous glyceryl trinitrate for long periods.
- Nitrates by intravenous infusion are used in the treatment of acute coronary syndromes for symptomatic relief and because they lower blood pressure. Intravenous nitrates are sometimes given to control severe hypertension before thrombolysis.

Acute left ventricular failure

- Diuretics are the mainstay of treatment of acute left ventricular failure, but they require adequate renal function to work. They also take time to act. Intravenous nitrates can be given to reduce cardiac preload.
  - Intravenous nitrates are particularly useful if the patient has poor or absent renal function, as diuretics may not work. It takes time to arrange dialysis to remove fluid.
  - Intravenous nitrates cannot be used if the patient has cardiogenic shock; a further reduction in blood pressure may be fatal.

- The adverse effects of nitrates are related to their vasodilator properties.
  - The most common is a throbbing headache; this may improve with time.
  - Other common adverse effects include dizziness, postural hypotension, and tachycardia.
  - Hypotension is the most serious adverse effect; take care to titrate the dose to minimize the risk of falls.
- Prolonged intravenous administration can cause methaemoglobinaemia; this is rare.
- Avoid prolonged intravenous administration; the patient will become tolerant to the effects of the drug.

- Drug interactions are uncommon.
- These drugs will potentiate the actions of other drugs that lower blood pressure.
  - Do not give sildenafil (Viagra®) to patients taking nitrates; there is a risk of severe hypotension.
- Nitrates can increase the excretion of heparin; this may reduce its effect.
- Drugs with antimuscarinic effects, causing a dry mouth, will reduce the absorption of nitrates that are given sublingually.

Safety and efficacy

- Review the patient's clinical status regularly. Patients with severe angina may be very limited by their disease. An assessment of their ability to carry out activities of daily living is often of more use than how far they can walk.
- Symptomatic treatment is only one aspect of the treatment of angina; see below.
- Measure the lying and standing blood pressures regularly.

- Make sure that the patient knows that this treatment is for acute chest pain.
- Make sure the patient knows to seek medical attention urgently if the symptoms change or are unrelieved by the nitrate.
- Warn the patient that nitrates can cause a headache.
- Explain the importance of storing these drugs correctly. Glyceryl trinitrate tablets should be kept in a glass bottle with a foil-lined lid. The bottle should not contain cotton wool (which absorbs the drug). Obtain a fresh supply of tablets every 8 weeks.

Prescribing information: **Nitrate drugs**

Many modified-release formulations of these drugs are available; the following immediate-release formulations are given as examples.

Treatment of angina

- Glyceryl trinitrate sublingual tablet, 500 micrograms, as required. (Also available in 300 microgram and 600 microgram tablets.)
- Isosorbide mononitrate tablet, initially 10 mg bd (see above for timings).
  - Usual maintence dose 20–40 mg bd.
  - May be increased to 120 mg, in divided doses.
  - May be reduced to 5 mg bd if the patient develops a headache.
- Isosorbide dinitrate tablet, initially 10 mg bd
  - May be increased to 120 mg, in divided doses.

Intravenous formulations

- Glyceryl trinitrate 50 mg in 50 mL 0.9% saline ('normal saline')
- Or isosorbide dinitrate 0.1% (1 mg/mL) (also available as 0.05% (0.5 mg/mL)).
- Infuse at 0.5–10 mL/hour according to the blood pressure and symptoms.
  - Start the infusion slowly and increase gradually to achieve the optimal effect.
  - Usually maintain the systolic blood pressure at about 90–100 mmHg.

TEACHING POINT Treatment of angina

Risk factors for coronary artery disease	
• Smoking	• Hypertension
• Hyperlipidaemia	• Diabetes mellitus

- Angina is the symptom experienced when the myocardium is ischaemic, usually as a result of coronary artery disease. Classically, angina is a dull, tight, central chest pain that may radiate to the neck and left arm. Some patients do not have classical symptoms, but recognize other symptoms as angina.
- The first-line treatment for angina is a beta-blocker given regularly, and a nitrate given as required to relieve the pain.
- Coronary artery disease is usually the cause of angina; patients need to be advised how to adjust their lifestyle to modify their risk factors (e.g. smoking, diet, exercise). Patients with angina should also be given an antiplatelet drug (e.g. aspirin) and a cholesterol-lowering drug (e.g. a statin).
- Once a diagnosis of angina has been made, the patient should have their risk of myocardial infarction assessed. This is usually by means of an exercise tolerance test with electrocardiographic monitoring. An alterative is a cardiac nuclear perfusion scan.
- Those at high risk should be assessed for coronary angiography, with a view to percutaneous intervention or bypass grafting. Some patients are at low risk, and others do not have lesions amenable to intervention. For these patients optimization of pharmacotherapy, in combination with lifestyle changes, is indicated.
- Many patients are adequately treated with a beta-blocker and nitrate alone. Beta-blockers are recommended as they have beneficial effects on vascular growth and function.
- Some patients are unable to take a beta-blocker, or their symptoms are inadequately controlled. Consider a calcium channel blocker for these patients. The most commonly prescribed are the dihydropyridines (e.g. amlodipine, nifedipine). Verapamil and diltiazem lower heart rate; this may be beneficial if tachycardia is a feature. Verapamil should not be given to patients taking beta-blockers (risk of severe hypotension and asystole).
- Reassess patients with severe, intractable symptoms. Is the diagnosis correct and treatment optimal?
- For those with persistent symptoms who need symptomatic relief, consider a long-acting (modified-release) nitrate formulation and/or nicorandil.

Nicorandil

Potassium channel activator

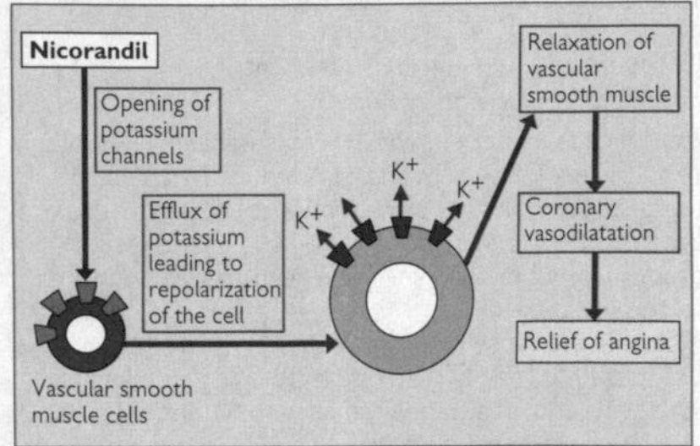

Treatment of angina

See nitrate drugs, p. 137

- Treatment and prevention of angina.

- Nicorandil is not a treatment for acute angina or acute coronary syndromes.
- Avoid nicorandil in patients with acute myocardial infarction or acute heart failure.
- Avoid nicorandil in patients with hypotension; it can lower the blood pressure.
- No dosage adjustment is usually required in renal or hepatic insufficiency.
- There is no information as to the safety of nicorandil during pregnancy; avoid it unless absolutely essential.

- Symptomatically, nicorandil is of similar efficacy to other drugs used to treat angina, but it is not thought to alter the underlying disease process.
- Its place in the treatment of chronic angina is still being established. It is most commonly used for patients who have symptoms despite maximal first-line and second-line antianginal treatment.
  - Make sure that these patients do not have coronary lesions amenable to surgical intervention or angioplasty.

- Nicorandil is usually well tolerated.
- Headache is common early in treatment, but tolerance often develops.
- Nicorandil can also cause nausea, flushing, and vomiting.
- In high dosages, nicorandil can cause hypotension and tachycardia.
- Rare adverse effects include oral ulceration, myalgia, and hypersensitivity (e.g. angio-oedema).

- Drug interactions are uncommon.
- Patients taking nicorandil should not also take sildenafil (Viagra®), as this combination can cause severe hypotension.

Safety and efficacy

- Review the patient's clinical status regularly. Patients with severe angina may be very limited by their disease. An assessment of their ability to carry out activities of daily living is often of more use than how far they can walk.
- Measure the lying and standing blood pressure regularly.

- Make sure the patient knows that this treatment is for the long-term control of their angina, rather than an acute treatment for chest pain.

Prescribing information: **Nicorandil**

Treatment and prevention of angina

- By mouth, initially 10 mg bd.
  - May be reduced to 5 mg bd if the patient develops a headache.
- Titrate the dose to optimal effect.
  - Usual daily dose 10–20 mg bd, but may be increased to 30 mg bd.

Beta-adrenoceptor antagonists ('beta-blockers')

Competitive antagonists at beta-adrenoceptors

- These drugs are classified according to their relative selectivity for β_1 adrenoceptors. Selective β_2 antagonists are not clinically useful, as they block bronchodilatation.
- The actions of beta-adrenoceptor agonists are illustrated below. Antagonists will block these actions. Some of these drugs exhibit partial agonist activity; this is called intrinsic sympathomimetic activity. The Table 2.1 gives guidance on the selection of a beta-blocker drug.

β_1 agonists

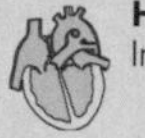

Heart
Increased force and rate of contraction

β_2 agonists

Arteries and veins
Dilatation, mainly in skeletal muscle

Bronchial Muscle
Relaxation

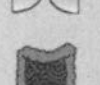

Gastrointestinal tract
Relaxation

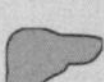

Liver and Pancreas
Glycogenolysis, gluconeogenesis, lipolysis

Uterus
Relaxation

Detrusor muscle
Relaxation

- Treatment of hypertension:
  - First-line option for the treatment of essential hypertension.
  - Specialist use in the medical treatment of aortic dissection (labetalol).
  - Specialist use with α-adrenoceptor antagonists in the preoperative treatment of phaeochromocytoma.
- Coronary artery disease.
  - Prophylaxis against angina.
  - Adjunct to the treatment of, and following myocardial infarction.
- Treatment of arrhythmias.
  - Especially those following myocardial infarction.
  - SVT and AF.
- Treatment of stable heart failure.
- Symptomatic relief of hyperthyroidism (see carbimazole, p. 416).
- Symptomatic relief of severe anxiety/panic.
- Prophylaxis against migraine headache.
- Treatment of glaucoma (topical).
- Treatment of benign essential tremor.

- Selectivity for receptor subtypes is always relative, and these drugs should not be given to patients with asthma.
- Note that many patients with COPD do not have a reversible (bronchospastic) component to their disease. Do not deny them treatment with beta-blockers without formally assessing whether they have a reversible component. Record the results of lung function tests clearly, so that they are available if an acute event occurs (e.g. unstable angina).

- Do not give these drugs to patients with 2nd or 3rd degree heart block.
- Do not give these drugs to patients with acute or unstable heart failure.
- These drugs are not contraindicated in patients with diabetes, but they can mask the physiological responses to hypoglycaemia. They do not block sweating, which can be the only sign of hypoglycaemia in a diabetic patient taking a beta-blocker. Avoid giving them to patients who have frequent episodes of hypoglycaemia.
- Do not give these drugs with verapamil; there is a risk of asystole or a catastrophic fall in cardiac output.
- Avoid giving these drugs to women who are pregnant, unless absolutely necessary. They can cause intrauterine growth retardation, fetal bradycardia, and hypoglycaemia.

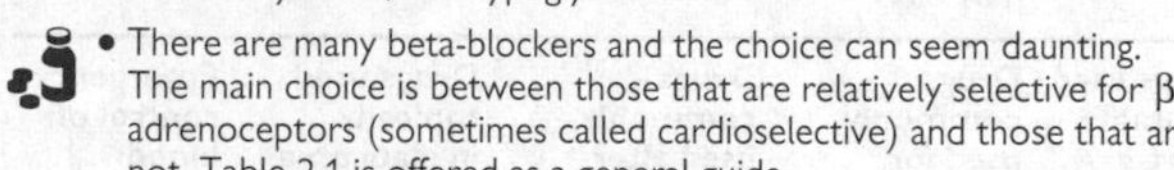

- There are many beta-blockers and the choice can seem daunting. The main choice is between those that are relatively selective for β_1 adrenoceptors (sometimes called cardioselective) and those that are not. Table 2.1 is offered as a general guide.
- Do not stop treatment with a beta-blocker suddenly. Rebound symptoms can be severe, including precipitation of an acute coronary syndrome.

Hypertension

- Current guidelines suggest choosing an ACE inhibitor, a beta-blocker, a calcium channel blocker, or thiazide diuretic as first-line treatment of essential hypertension (British Hypertension Society Guidelines (2004) *Br Med J*, **328**:634–40).
  - A beta-blocker is particularly suitable for patients with risk factors for coronary artery disease.
- See teaching point below for information on the emergency treatment of hypertension.

Prophylaxis against angina

- Nitrate drugs relieve the symptoms of angina, but antiplatelet drugs (e.g. aspirin) and beta-blockers provide prophylaxis against the pathophysiological basis of the disease.
- Assess the patient's risk. This is usually done by an exercise tolerance test.

Myocardial infarction

- Beta-blockade can be an important adjunct to thrombolytic and antiplatelet drugs in the treatment of acute coronary syndromes, but see note below.
- Beta-blockers have an established important role in the prevention of cardiac and vascular remodelling following myocardial infarction.
- There is a debate as to the relative importance of very early treatment with beta-blockers in patients with myocardial infarction. Seek specialist local guidance.

Table 2.1

Non-selective beta-blockers	**β_1-selective beta-blockers**	**Relatively water-soluble drugs**[1]	**Drugs with peripheral vasodilator properties**[2]	**Drugs with 'intrinsic sympathomimetic activity' (partial agonists)**[3]
Propranolol	Atenolol, betaxolol, bisoprolol, metoprolol, nevibolol	Atenolol, celiprolol, nadolol, sotalol	Labetolol, celiprolol, carvedilol, nevibolol	Oxprenolol, pindolol, acebutolol, celiprolol
Drugs used for stable heart failure	**Drugs commonly used for arrhythmias**	**Drugs commonly used after myocardial infarction**	**Drugs used topically in glaucoma**	**Emergency control of blood pressure (see below)**
Bisoprolol, carvedilol, metoprolol	Esmolol (short-acting, used intravenously); sotalol (also has class III antiarrhythmic actions)	Atenolol, metoprolol	Betaxolol, carteolol, levobunolol, metipranolol, timolol	Labetalol (also has alpha-adrenoceptor blocking actions)

[1]These penetrate the CNS poorly, so cause fewer vivid dreams and less sleep disturbance. They are excreted by the kidneys, so the dose must be reduced in renal insufficiency.

[2]The clinical importance of these properties has not been clearly established. Carvedilol is recommended for the treatment of stable heart failure.

[3]These drugs cause less bradycardia. The clinical importance of this has not been clearly established.

Heart failure

- Used correctly, beta-blockers can prolong life and improve symptoms in heart failure of all grades of severity.
- Like ACE inhibitors, beta-blockers act by inhibiting neurohormonal activation. Unless contraindicated, the patient should already be taking an ACE inhibitor.
- The initial dosages of beta-blockers are much lower than those for other indications.
- Only start this treatment when the patient is stable. Do not start treatment with beta-blockers if the patient has symptomatic bradycardia or hypotension.
- See recommended procedure below.

Treatment of arrhythmias

- Beta-blockers can be useful in the treatment of (tachy)arrhythmias in the peri-infarction period.
- A short-acting beta-blocker such as esmolol can be used for the treatment of acute SVT. See adenosine (p. 78) for alternatives.
  - Longer-acting drugs have a role in prophylaxis against SVT.
- Beta-blockers will reduce the heart rate in patients with AF.
  - Always consider whether cardioversion would be more appropriate. This can be electrical (DC shock) or chemical (options include flecainide, verapamil, amiodarone).
  - If the patient has established AF, or if cardioversion has been ineffective, there are several other options for rate control. These include digoxin and a calcium channel blocker (e.g. diltiazem).
- Sotalol also has class III antiarrhythmic actions (see amiodarone, p. 100); it is only used for treating arrhythmias.
  - It is more effective than lidocaine for the treatment of sustained ventricular tachycardia.
  - It will prolong the QT interval, and so carries a risk of inducing the arrhythmia torsade de pointes (see antihistamines, p. 610).

Hyperthyroidism

- A non-selective beta-blocker can provide symptomatic relief in severe hyperthyroidism, but is not a treatment for the underlying disease.
  - When the diagnosis is thyroiditis, treatment with a beta-blocker until the inflammation has subsided may be all that is required.

Prophylaxis against migraine

- There are many choices for prophylaxis against migraine headache; a beta-blocker can be useful in some patients.
- Seek specialist assessment for patients who require regular prophylaxis.

Treatment of glaucoma (see p. 605 for guidance)

- Topical beta-blockers are a first-line treatment for glaucoma.
  - Systemic absorption of these drugs can be significant and can cause adverse effects (e.g. bronchospasm).
  - The prostaglandin analogue, latanoprost, is an alternative first-line choice (see prostaglandins, p. 450).

- The most important adverse effect of these drugs is bronchoconstriction. They are contraindicated in patients with asthma. If treatment with a beta-blocker is absolutely essential, use one of the β_1-selective drugs, although selectivity is always a relative term (see teaching point in adrenoceptor agonists, p. 195). This should only be initiated in hospital, and with very close monitoring.
- Common adverse effects are cold limbs and peripheries (including Raynaud's phenomenon), and a feeling of tiredness. These may be intolerable for some patients.
- There has been concern that beta-blockers worsen diabetic control, but there is little objective evidence of this. The burden of cardiovascular disease is very great in these patients so this potential disadvantage is usually outweighed by the cardiovascular benefits. However, they mask some of the symptoms of hypoglycaemia and may not be helpful in patients with a high risk of attacks of hypoglycaemia.

- Beta-blockers have an important trophic role in chronic heart failure; however, they are negatively inotropic and can precipitate or worsen heart failure. Follow the guidance given above.
- Beta-blockers that penetrate the CNS will cause sleep disturbance and nightmares.
- These drugs can cause erectile impotence, but so do many of the diseases for which they are used. Discuss this with your patient so that you can identify whether the drug is likely to be responsible or not.
- Labetalol can cause liver damage. This risk is usually acceptable if it is used for the emergency control of blood pressure; it is rarely used for long-term treatment.

- Do not use beta-blockers with verapamil; there is a risk of asystole or a catastrophic reduction of cardiac output. Do not give intravenous verapamil for at least 8 hours after a beta-blocker was last given.
- Beta-blockers will augment the action of any other drugs that lower heart rate or blood pressure.
- Sotalol prolongs the QT interval. Avoid giving it with other drugs that prolong the QT interval.

Safety and efficacy

- Measure the pulse and blood pressure to avoid over- or undertreatment.
  - Do this at rest and after mild exercise (e.g. running on the spot for 10 seconds); beta-blockers prevent exercise-induced tachycardia and rise in blood pressure.
  - Patients given beta-blockers intravenously should have continuous cardiac monitoring.
- The outcome measure for most indications is the prevention of future events. This can be difficult to monitor, so careful assessment of the risks versus benefits before treatment begins is essential.

- Warn the patient that they may experience tiredness and cold hands, but that this may improve with time, if they can tolerate it.
- Warn the patient of the risk of erectile impotence.
  - There is no evidence that warning patients of this adverse effect makes it more likely to occur.
  - These drugs can cause impotence, but so do many of the diseases for which they are used. Discuss this with your patient before treatment so that you can identify whether the drug is likely to be responsible or not.
  - Since the introduction of sildenafil (Viagra®), patients are more willing to talk about impotence.

Prescribing information: **Beta-blockers**

There are many beta-blockers; the following are given as examples.

Atenolol

- Hypertension, treatment of angina, arrhythmias.
  - By mouth, 50–100 mg daily.

Propranolol

- Thyrotoxicosis (adjunct).
  - By mouth, initially 40 mg 3 or 4 times daily; higher doses may be required.
- Anxiety with symptoms such as palpitation, sweating, and tremor.
  - 40 mg once daily, increased to 40 mg 3 times daily if necessary.

Metoprolol

- Early intervention within 12 hours of myocardial infarction.
  - By intravenous injection, 5 mg every 2 minutes to a maximum of 15 mg.
  - Followed after 15 minutes by 50 mg *by mouth*, every 6 hours for 48 hours.
  - Maintenance, 200 mg daily in divided doses. Consider switching to a once-daily drug (e.g. atenolol) for maintenance treatment.

Sotalol

- Treatment of arrhythmias
  - *By mouth*, initially 80 mg daily in 1 or 2 divided doses.
  - Increase gradually at intervals of 2–3 days to a usual dose of 160–320 mg daily in 2 divided doses.
  - Higher doses (480–640 mg daily) can be given under specialist supervision for life-threatening ventricular arrhythmias.

Timolol

- Treatment of glaucoma
  - Eye drops, apply twice daily to affected eye(s).
  - Note that there are two different concentrations, 0.25% and 0.5%.

TEACHING POINT Procedure for starting a beta-blocker in heart failure (bisoprolol is given as an example)

- Unless contraindicated, the patient should already be taking an ACE inhibitor.
- Patients should be stable. They should not need inotropic support and should have no signs of marked fluid retention.
- Start with a very low dose.
  - Initially, 1.25 mg once daily (in the morning) for 1 week.
- Titrate slowly up to the maintenance dose.
  - 2.5 mg once daily for 1 week, then 3.75 mg once daily for 1 week, then 5 mg once daily for 4 weeks, then 7.5 mg once daily for 4 weeks, then 10 mg once daily.
- The maximum dose is 10 mg daily.
- Transient worsening of heart failure, hypotension, or bradycardia can occur.
- Observe the patient for 2–3 hours after initiation and each dose increase.
- Reduce the dose if symptoms develop. Reconsider titrating upwards once the patient has stabilized again.
- If the drug has to be stopped, aim to do this over 1–2 weeks, if possible.

TEACHING POINT Emergency treatment of hypertension

It is rarely necessary to reduce blood pressure very rapidly. Indeed, very rapid reduction can precipitate watershed ischaemia in the CNS (causing a stroke).

Accelerated phase (malignant) hypertension

- If the patient has accelerated phase hypertension, the diastolic blood pressure is typically 130–140 mmHg or more. Bedrest alone is effective. Begin treatment by mouth with either a β_1 beta-blocker (e.g. 5 mg of bisoprolol) or a calcium channel blocker (e.g. 5 mg of amlodipine).
- The aim is to reduce diastolic blood pressure by 20–30 mmHg in the first week. The target diastolic blood pressure of 80–85 mmHg can be achieved over the coming months.
- Very occasionally, blood pressure needs to be reduced urgently. Indications for this include:
  - Hypertensive encephalopathy.
  - Eclampsia (pre-eclampsia with fits); deliver the baby if possible. See also magnesium (p. 550).
  - Acute hypertensive left ventricular failure.
  - Dissecting aortic aneurysm.

Management

- Labetalol by iv infusion is the drug of choice, but do not give for phaeochromocytoma (see alpha-adrenoceptor blockers, (p. 472)).
  - Initially, 2 mg/min. Adjust rate of infusion according to response.
- Sodium nitroprusside is an alternative, but requires continuous arterial blood pressure monitoring because of its short half-life and unpredictable effects on blood pressure.

Angiotensin converting enzyme inhibitors (ACE inhibitors)

Inhibitors of dipeptidyl carboxypeptidase enzymes (e.g ACE, kininase)

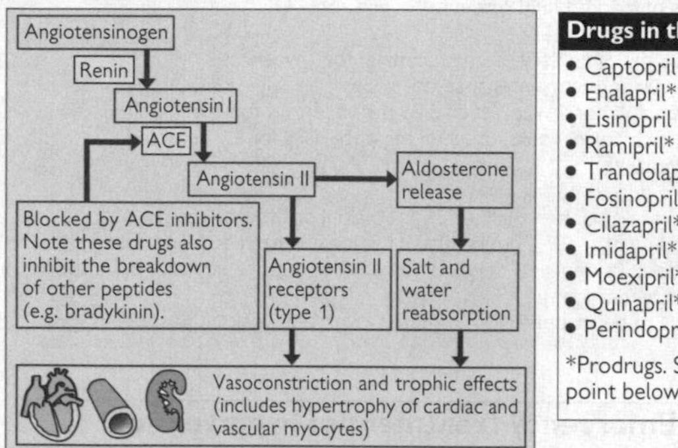

Drugs in this class

- Captopril
- Enalapril*
- Lisinopril
- Ramipril*
- Trandolapril*
- Fosinopril*
- Cilazapril*
- Imidapril*
- Moexipril*
- Quinapril*
- Perindopril*

*Prodrugs. See teaching point below.

- Treatment of hypertension.
- Prevention of cardiac remodelling following myocardial infarction.
- Treatment and prevention of diabetic nephropathy (in type I diabetes).
- Treatment of heart failure.

- Contraindicated in pregnancy; blocking the effect of angiotensin can cause birth defects.
- Can cause severe renal impairment in patients with renovascular disease — avoid.
- ACE inhibitors cause vasodilatation and can precipitate a fall in blood pressure in patients with a fixed cardiac output: aortic stenosis, mitral stenosis, and hypertrophic cardiomyopathy. Seek expert advice before using in these groups.
- ACE inhibitors that are given as prodrugs (see list above) require transformation to their active metabolites in the liver. These drugs may be less effective in patients with hepatic insufficiency (see below).

Notes on the use of ACE inhibitors

- The ACE inhibitors have been available for considerably longer than the angiotensin receptor blockers (ARBs), and have a larger evidence base. An ACE inhibitor would usually be the first choice for the indications given above.
- ACE inhibitors also inhibit bradykinin metabolism. This is thought to be responsible for the dry persistent cough that causes some patients to be unable to tolerate an ACE inhibitor. ARBs only block the angiotensin receptor, so they do not usually cause a cough.
- The evidence from clinical trials is that higher doses of these drugs are more effective than lower ones. Aim to titrate the dose to the maximum that is well tolerated. Take responsibility for doing this; do not assume that others will.
- Although these drugs have benefits that may be independent of blood pressure, they do lower the blood pressure. If the systolic blood pressure is below 100 mmHg, consider carefully whether these potential benefits outweigh the risk of hypotension.

Hypertension

- British Hypertension Society guidelines suggest that an ACE inhibitor, beta-blocker, calcium channel blocker, or thiazide diuretic should be first-line choices for the treatment of hypertension.
- ACE inhibitors are less likely to be effective in low-renin hypertension, which is common among Afro-Caribbean patients.
- An ACE inhibitor may be a particularly good choice for patients with diabetes (see below).
- Titrate the dose to the desired reduction in blood pressure. Note that in clinical trials most patients required a second drug (usually a thiazide diuretic) in order to achieve their target blood pressure.

Treatment following myocardial infarction

- There is good evidence that treatment with an ACE inhibitor reduces detrimental cardiac and vascular remodelling following myocardial infarction.
- Begin treatment as soon as is practicable after the infarct (see notes on heart failure below).

Heart failure

- ACE inhibitors are pivotal to the treatment of heart failure; they improve symptoms and prolong life.
- The introduction of an ACE inhibitor in a patient who is unstable or undergoing a heavy diuresis is potentially hazardous. Stabilize the patient first; if the patient has severe heart failure, admit to hospital for initiation of ACE inhibitor treatment.
- It is recommended that diuretics be withdrawn for 24–48 hours before an ACE inhibitor is started. They can be restarted once treatment has been initiated, but note that diuretic requirements may be lower.
- Give a small initial dose (e.g. captopril 6.25 mg, enalapril 2.5 mg). Give this when the patient is in bed and measure the blood pressure. This first dose may be associated with a transient fall in blood pressure, which may be cardiovascularly significant. This usually occurs within 4 hours of the dose.
- Hypotension with the first dose of an ACE inhibitor is not a contraindication to further treatment, but it should be a warning to proceed carefully.
- Increase the dose, at intervals of 2 weeks, to achieve the maximum tolerated.
- ACE is not the only enzyme than can convert angiotensin I to angiotensin II. Some patients treated with ostensibly adequate doses of ACE inhibitors show evidence of reactivation of the renin/angiotensin system, and they have a poor prognosis. The best therapeutic intervention for these patients has not been established, but is the subject of clinical trials.

Treatment and prevention of diabetic nephropathy

- ACE inhibitors have a beneficial effect in delaying the progression of nephropathy in patients with type I diabetes. This effect seems to be independent of their effects on blood pressure, but this is controversial.
- There is debate about the extent to which these results also apply to patients with type II diabetes. Trials of angiotensin receptor blockers have shown efficacy in type II diabetes. Most clinicians do not distinguish between type I and type II diabetes, because the cause of the damage is thought to be very similar.

Patients at high risk of vascular disease

- The detrimental trophic effects of angiotensin have been highlighted by the HOPE trial. This showed that treatment with an ACE inhibitor conferred considerable benefit on patients who were at a high risk of vascular disease but who had not yet had an event. (HOPE trial, *New Engl J Med* (2000), **342**:145–53.)
- The drug used in the HOPE trial was ramipril, but there is no evidence that this drug has any special properties that other drugs in the class do not share. The most important factor is the maximum dose tolerated.

- The most common adverse effect is hypotension, particularly if the intravascular volume has been depleted by diuretics. If possible, stop diuretic treatment 2 days before starting an ACE inhibitor.
- A small deterioration in renal function is often seen on starting these drugs. The long-term benefits usually outweigh this disadvantage. Patients with renovascular disease are at risk of severe progressive renal impairment, leading to insufficiency. Measure the renal function and stop the drug if it continues to deteriorate.
- These drugs can cause hyperkalaemia; this is rare if they are used on their own, but see interactions below.
- Hypersensitivity, characterized by angio-oedema can be caused by these drugs but is rare.
  - They can cause anaphylactoid reactions (see acetylcysteine, p. 625) during dialysis with high-flux polyacrylnitrile membranes, or low density lipoprotein apheresis with dextran sulfate. Withhold the drug during these treatments.
- Dry cough is common (about 20% of patients). It is thought to result from reduced breakdown of bradykinin in the bronchial mucosa. This may be intolerable; see patient information notes below.

- ACE inhibitors potentiate the actions of other drugs that lower blood pressure.
- These drugs can cause hyperkalaemia; the risk is greater if the patient is given a potassium-sparing diuretic. Although this combination should usually be avoided, there is a special case for the use of low-dose spironolactone with ACE inhibitors in patients with heart failure. See spironolactone (p. 186).
- Avoid NSAID drugs; they antagonize the hypotensive action of these drugs and can cause renal impairment.
- Treatment with diuretics increases the risk of hypotension (especially severe first-dose hypotension) due to ACE inhibitors. See above for advice on the safe use of these drugs in heart failure.

Safety

- Measure renal function 4 days and 2 weeks after starting these drugs.
- Measure renal function 1 week after increasing the dose.
- Measure the plasma potassium if the patient is also taking a potassium-sparing drug. See interactions above.
- Measure the blood pressure.

Efficacy

- This will depend on the indication. Aim to achieve the maximum tolerated dose.
- Advise the patient about the importance of attending for blood tests to measure renal function.

- These drugs can cause a dry persistent cough. This may be intolerable for some, but many are able to tolerate it if they know the benefits these drugs have. If the patient cannot tolerate the cough, consider treatment with an angiotensin receptor blocker. Sodium cromoglicate occasionally relieves the cough caused by ACE inhibitors.

Prescribing information: **Angiotensin converting enzyme inhibitors**

Many drugs are available; captopril, enalapril, lisinopril, and ramipril are given as examples.

Captopril

- By mouth, initial dose 6.25 mg.
- Needs to be given three times daily to give 24-hour cover.
- May be increased to 12.5 mg tds, 25 mg tds, and a maximum of 50 mg tds.
- Consider a once-daily drug for long-term treatment.

Enalapril

- By mouth, inital dose 2.5 mg
- Should be given twice daily for 24-hour cover.
- May be increased to 5 mg, 10 mg, 20 mg, and a maximum of 40 mg daily, in divided doses.

Lisinopril

- By mouth, initially 2.5 mg daily.
- May be increased to 10 mg, 20 mg, and a maximum of 40 mg daily (In hypertension).
- Usual maintenance dose 10–20 mg daily.

Ramipril

- By mouth, initially 2.5 mg daily.
- May be increased to 5 mg, then to a maximum of 10 mg daily.

TEACHING POINT Prodrugs

- Prodrugs are drugs that are not pharmacologically active in the form in which they are administered (usually by mouth).
- A prodrug must undergo some form of chemical conversion to form the active drug. The most common pathway of activation is by cytochrome P450 enzymes in the liver, but see below for other examples (for more information on cytochrome P450 enzymes see flecainide and erythromycin, pp. 91 and 347).
- Advantages and disadvantages of prodrugs are summarized below.

Disadvantages	Advantages
The requirement for activation in the liver can slow the onset of action of the drug.	The distribution of the prodrug may be better. For example, dopamine given by mouth is of no value in treating Parkinson's disease, it does not enter the brain. Its precursor L-dopa does enter the brain, where it is metabolized to dopamine.
Other drugs may interact with the cytochrome P450 enzymes responsible for the activation of the drug. For example, the antiplatelet drug clopidogrel is a prodrug. It is metabolized by CYP 3A4 to produce the active form. A metabolite of atorvastatin, atorvastatin acid, competes with clopidogrel for occupation of the enzyme-binding site in CYP 3A4, reducing the activation of clopidogrel. In this way, atorvastatin reduces the antiplatelet action of clopidogrel in a dose-dependent manner.	The prodrug may be better absorbed than the drug. For example, the antiviral drug aciclovir is relatively poorly and unreliably absorbed when taken by mouth. The prodrug valaciclovir is better absorbed, resulting in more predictable plasma concentrations when it is given by mouth.
Organ insufficiency (e.g. liver cirrhosis) can reduce activation and render prodrugs ineffective.	A prodrug can be used to target the site of action. For example, olsalazine is a dimer of 5-aminosalicylic acid; it is cleaved by bacteria in the lower bowel to release 5-aminosalicylic acid.

Angiotensin receptor antagonists/blockers (ARBs)

Antagonists at the angiotensin II receptor (type 1)

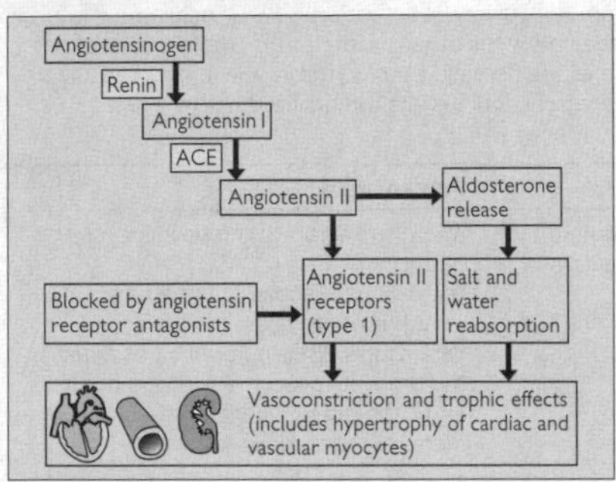

Drugs in this class

- Candesartan
- Eprosartan
- Irbesartan
- Losartan
- Telmisartan
- Valsartan

- Treatment of hypertension.
- Treatment and prevention of diabetic nephropathy.
- There is some evidence that these drugs are useful in the treatment of heart failure.

- Contraindicated in pregnancy; blocking the effect of angiotensin can cause birth defects.
- Can cause severe renal impairment in patients with renovascular disease — avoid.
- ARBs cause vasodilatation and can precipitate a fall in blood pressure in patients with a fixed cardiac output: aortic stenosis, mitral stenosis, and hypertrophic cardiomyopathy. Seek expert advice before using in these groups.
- Dosages of valsartan, losartan, and candesartan should be reduced in hepatic insufficiency (see below).

Notes on the use of ARBs

- The ACE inhibitors also block the actions of angiotensin; they have been available for considerably longer than ARBs, and have a larger evidence base. An ACE inhibitor would usually be the first choice for the indications given above.
- ACE inhibitors also inhibit bradykinin metabolism and this is thought to be responsible for the dry persistent cough that some patients find intolerable. ARBs only block the angiotensin receptor, so they do not usually cause a cough.
- The major use of ARBs is in patients who are unable to tolerate an ACE inhibitor owing to cough. It has also been suggested that they may have a role in combination with ACE inhibitors, but this has yet to be demonstrated in large-scale clinical trials.

Hypertension

- British Hypertension Society guidelines suggest that an ACE inhibitor, beta-blocker, calcium channel blocker, or thiazide diuretic should be first-line choices for the treatment of hypertension (British Hypertension Society Guidelines, *Br Med J* (2004), **328**: 634–40).
- ARBs are less likely to be effective in low-renin hypertension; this is common among Afro-Caribbean patients.

- An ACE inhibitor or ARB may be a particularly good choice for patients with diabetes (see below).
- Titrate the dose to the desired reduction in blood pressure. Note that in clinical trials most patients required a second drug (usually a thiazide diuretic) in order to achieve the target blood pressure.

Treatment and prevention of diabetic nephropathy
- Irbesartan and losartan, like the ACE inhibitors, have a beneficial effect in delaying the progression of nephropathy in patients with type II diabetes. This effect may be independent of their effects on blood pressure.
- Titrate the dose to the maximum tolerated. Aim for 100 mg losartan daily or 300 mg irbesartan daily.

Heart failure
- The VALHEFT trial failed to show a mortality advantage from the addition of valsartan to existing heart failure therapy when that therapy included an ACE inhibitor or beta-blocker.
- However, subgroup analysis did suggest benefit in those not taking an ACE inhibitor or beta-blocker. An ARB, such as valsartan, may be useful in patients unable to tolerate an ACE inhibitor. Aim for the highest tolerated dose, such as valsartan 160 mg twice daily. (VALHEFT (Cohn *et al*) *New Engl J Med* (2001), **345**: 1667–75.)
- The precautions that apply to the initiation of ACE inhibitors in patients with heart failure also apply to the initiation of ARB treatment (see starting an ACE inhibitor section).

- The most common adverse effect is hypotension, particularly if the intravascular volume has been depleted by diuretics. If possible, stop diuretic treatment 2 days before starting these drugs.
- A small deterioration in renal function is often seen on starting these drugs. The long-term benefits usually outweigh this disadvantage. Patients with renovascular disease are at risk of severe progressive renal impairment leading to failure. Measure renal function and stop the drug if it continues to deteriorate.
- These drugs can cause hyperkalaemia; this is rare if they are used on their own, but see interactions below.
- Hypersensitivity, characterized by angio-oedema, can be caused by these drugs, but is rare.

- ARBs will potentiate the actions of other drugs that lower blood pressure.
- These drugs can cause hyperkalaemia; the risk is greater if the patient is given a potassium-sparing diuretic. Although this combination should usually be avoided, there is a special case for the use of low-dose spironolactone with angiotensin receptor blockers in patients with heart failure. See spironolactone (p. 186).
- Avoid NSAIDs; they antagonize the hypotensive action of ARBs and can cause renal impairment.
- Treatment with diuretics increases the risk of hypotension.

Safety
- Measure renal function 4 days and 2 weeks after starting these drugs. Measure renal function 1 week after increasing the dose. Measure the plasma potassium concentration if the patient is also given a potassium-sparing drug (see interactions above).
- Measure the blood pressure.

Efficacy

- This will depend on the indication. Aim to achieve the maximum tolerated dose.
- Advise the patient of the importance of attending for blood tests to measure renal function.

Prescribing information: **Angiotensin receptor antagonists**

Losartan

- By mouth, 50 mg daily.
- May be increased in increments of 25 mg daily to a maximum of 100 mg daily.
- Reduce the initial dose to 25 mg daily in renal or hepatic insufficiency.

Irbesartan

- By mouth, 150 mg daily.
- May be increased to a maximum of 300 mg daily.
- Reduce the initial dose to 75 mg daily in renal insufficiency.

Candesartan

- By mouth, initially 4 mg daily; increase to 8 mg daily if tolerated.
- May be increased to a maximum of 16 mg daily.
- Reduce the initial dose to 2 mg daily in renal or hepatic insufficiency.

Valsartan

- By mouth, initially 80 mg daily.
- May be increased to a maximum of 160 mg daily.
- Reduce the initial dose to 40 mg daily in renal or hepatic insufficiency.

TEACHING POINT Trough to peak ratio

- One of the goals of antihypertensive therapy is to achieve 24-hour control.
- If there is considerable inter-dose variability, the concentration at the trough may be inadequate.
- One way of expressing the inter-dose variability of a drug is in terms of the trough to peak ratio (usually expressed as a percentage). As it is a ratio, it does not give information as the absolute magnitude of an effect.
- If a drug is still fully effective at its trough concentration, the trough to peak ratio is of limited value. The lower the percentage value, the greater the time during which the patient may experience inadequate control.
- It is also important to examine exactly what is being compared. Many antihypertensive drugs have a poor correlation between plasma concentration and therapeutic effect, and so it is only really helpful to give trough to peak ratios for outcome measures (blood pressure).

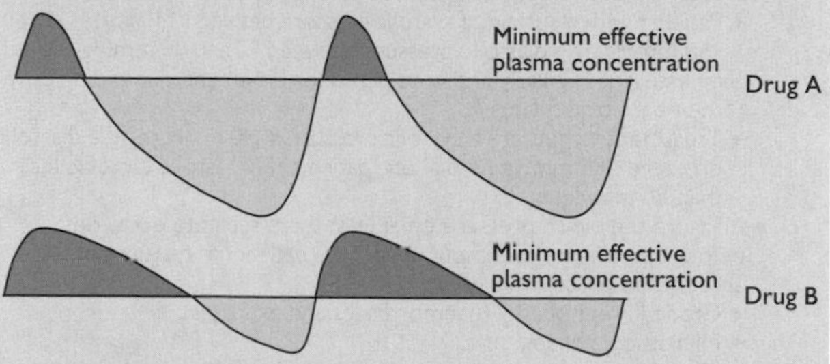

Comparison of two drug regimens

- The plasma concentration of drug A is above the minimum effective concentration (horizontal line) for only a short period. The ratio of trough to peak will be a low percentage, indicating that control may be inadequate.
- Drug B has a higher trough to peak ratio and may be a more suitable drug choice.
- The position of the horizontal bar (minimum effective plasma concentration) is critical; if this were below the trough concentration for either drug, the trough to peak ratio would be clinically meaningless.

An approach to the treatment of hypertension

- Based on the British Hypertension Society Guidelines (*Br Med J* 2004; **328**: 634–40).
- Blood pressure is a continuous variable. Guidelines suggest various cut-offs for treatment. These are practically useful, but remember that they are artificial.
- Hypertension is an important contributing factor to cardiovascular disease including stroke and renal impairment.
- Both the systolic and diastolic blood pressures contribute to the risk. The pulse pressure (systolic pressure–diastolic pressure) may prove to be the most important determinant of risk.
  - Treatment is recommended for patients with a sustained systolic blood pressure above 160 mmHg or a diastolic pressure above 100 mmHg.
  - Patients with a sustained systolic pressure between 140 and 150 mmHg or a diastolic pressure between 90 and 99 mmHg should be assessed regularly and considered for treatment, depending on their cardiovascular risk.
  - Treatment targets are a systolic pressure <140 mmHg and a diastolic pressure <85 mmHg (in diabetic patients the diastolic target is less than 80 mmHg).
- Measure the blood pressure on at least three separate occasions before deciding on treatment, unless the patient has features of accelerated phase hypertension:
  - Grade III retinopathy (haemorrhages and exudates).
  - Microscopic haematuria.
  - Microangiopathic features on the blood film (fragmented red blood cells and a low platelet count).
  - The diastolic blood pressure is commonly >130 mmHg.
  - Clinical features include encephalopathy and heart failure.
- See beta-blockers (p. 147) for guidance on the emergency treatment of hypertension.

Treatment

- Non-pharmacological interventions:
  - Reduce weight if the patient is obese.
  - Avoid excess alcohol intake (blood pressure increases linearly with alcohol intake over 20 units/week).
  - Reduce salt intake (advise the patient to avoid very salty foods (e.g. junk foods) and adding salt in cooking or at the table).
  - Take regular exercise (defined as 20 minutes of exercise sufficient to cause sweating, 3 times per week).

Choice of drug

- The British Hypertension Society suggests that an ACE inhibitor, beta-blocker, calcium channel blocker, or diuretic should be the first-line choice.
- Certain drugs may be indicated in some patients, for example:
  - ACE inhibitors and angiotensin receptor blockers in patients with diabetic renal disease.
  - Alpha-adrenoceptor blockers in patients with refractory hypertension.
  - Calcium channel blockers in patients of Afro-Caribbean origin with low-renin hypertension.
  - Alpha methyldopa for hypertension during pregnancy.

- See individual articles for more information on these drugs.
- See metformin (p. 409) for more information on the treatment of hypertension in patients with diabetes mellitus.
- Begin treatment with a low dose. If this is only partially effective, increase the dose.
- If the drug is not well tolerated or ineffective, add another class of antihypertensive drug. For example:
  - ACE inhibitor and diuretic.
  - Beta-blocker and calcium channel blocker.
- If this is ineffective add another drug; e.g. ACE inhibitor (or beta-blocker), calcium channel blocker, and diuretic.
- Assess the patient's overall cardiovascular risk and treat as necessary; consider:
  - Smoking cessation.
  - Lipid profile (statin treatment).
  - Antiplatelet therapy (aspirin).

Pharmacology of drug treatments for hypertension

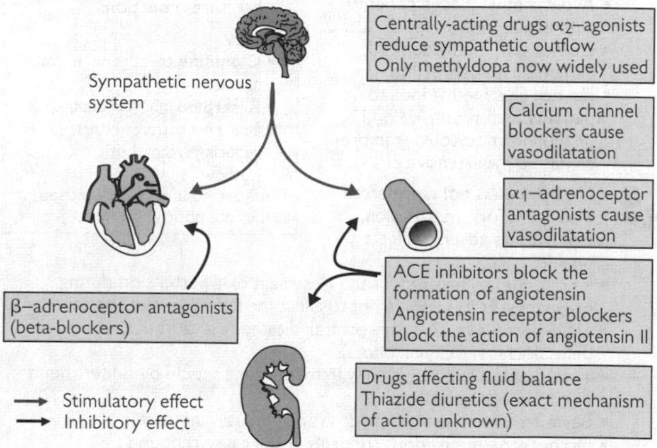

Methyldopa (alpha-methyldopa)

Centrally-active antihypertensive drug

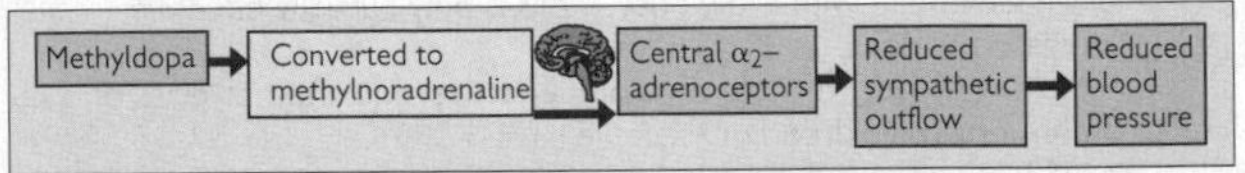

- Treatment of hypertension.
  - Usually reserved for the treatment of hypertension during pregnancy.

- Patients with renal insufficiency are more sensitive to the sedative and hypotensive effects of methyldopa; begin treatment with a lower dose.
- Avoid methyldopa in patients with active liver disease.
- Do not give methyldopa to patients with depression.
- Do not give methyldopa to patients with porphyria or a phaeochromocytoma (can precipitate a hypertensive crisis).

Note on other centrally-acting antihypertensive drugs

Moxonidine An imidazoline receptor antagonist. It acts in the ventral medulla to reduce sympathetic outflow. It can be used when other drugs are inappropriate or have not achieved the target blood pressure reduction.

Others

- **Clonidine** α_2-adrenoceptor agonist.
- **Reserpine** inhibits reuptake of amine neurotransmitters, reducing sympathetic outflow.

These are no longer widely used, as they are poorly tolerated.

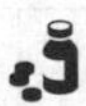

- Methyldopa is not a preferred treatment for hypertension, owing to its adverse effects profile.
- It continues to be used for the treatment of hypertension during pregnancy, as it is known not to affect the fetus. Most of the other antihypertensive drugs are contraindicated (e.g. diuretics, beta-blockers, ACE inhibitors).
- Treatment of hypertension with methyldopa should be under the direction of a specialist.
- Begin treatment with a low dose and gradually increase it.
- Do not stop methyldopa suddenly; it can cause rebound hypertension.

- Adverse effects are less common if the total daily dose is below 1 g.
- Sedation and tiredness are very common. Tolerance can develop, but not in all patients.
- Methyldopa causes a dry mouth in 40% of patients.
- Methyldopa can cause diarrhoea.
- Methyldopa can cause a positive direct Coomb's test in 20% of patients.
  - However, autoimmune haemolytic anaemia is less common (about 2%).
  - Take care as this can interfere with the crossmatching of blood.
- Rare but serious adverse effects include:
  - Hepatitis; this is most common during the first 4 weeks of treatment.
  - A lupus-like syndrome (see procainamide, p. 85).

- Methyldopa enhances the effect of other drugs that lower the blood pressure.
- Do not give it with monoamine oxidase inhibitor antidepressants, and take care with other antidepressants; the hypotensive effect is enhanced.
- Do not give with lithium; this can cause neurotoxicity without changing the plasma lithium concentration.
- Methyldopa enhances the effect of sympathomimetic drugs (including salbutamol given by infusion).

Efficacy

- Women who become hypertensive during pregnancy must be monitored closely.
    - Measure the blood pressure regularly.
    - Dip the urine for protein.
- Measure liver function tests if the patient develops any signs or symptoms of hepatitis.

- Warn the patient that methyldopa can cause drowsiness that can interfere with skilled motor tasks (e.g. driving).
- Alcohol enhances the sedative effect of methyldopa.

Prescribing information: **Methyldopa**

Hypertension

- By mouth, initially 250 mg tds.
- Can be gradually increased to a maximum total daily dose of 3 g.

Calcium channel blockers (see also individual sections)

Inhibitors of the influx of calcium into cells

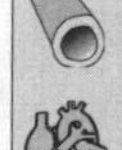

The contraction of vascular smooth muscle cells depends on influx of calcium into the cell in response to depolarization. Inhibition of this influx of calcium causes vasodilatation. These drugs have differential effects on the heart and peripheral vasculature, depending on their chemical structures (see box).

Groups of calcium channel blockers

Dihydropyridines
- Typified by nifedipine
- Principally affect the peripheral vasculature

Phenyalkylamines
- Typified by verapamil
- Principally affect the heart

Benzthiazepines
- Typified by diltiazem
- Affect the heart and peripheral vasculature

The three classes of calcium channel blockers are listed in the box above. Each class is discussed in its own separate section:
- Dihydropyridines, p. 164.
- Phenylalkylamines, p. 170.
- Benzthiazepines, p. 168.

TEACHING POINT Modified-release formulations: advantages and disadvantages

- Many drugs are removed rapidly from the body, either by metabolism in the liver or excretion via the kidneys. As a result, their duration of action is short. In many cases, one wants a drug to act throughout the day (e. g. in the treatment of hypertension). In order to give 24-hour cover, the drug will have to be taken several times throughout the day (see below). Ideally, the dose should be evenly spaced, but this is often impractical, and so the drug is taken at mealtimes.
- Patients are less likely to take their medicines correctly if they need to be taken several times daily. Many drugs are presented as modified-release formulations to reduce the frequency of administration.
- The drug is released slowly and evenly over the course of the day from a modified-release formulation and so only needs to be taken once or twice daily (see figure below).
    - This advantage needs to be weighed against the potential disadvantages.
- It takes time for a steady state to be achieved with a modified-release formulation.
- It is therefore generally good practice to start treatment with an immediate-release formulation and to use this to titrate to the optimal dose for that patient.
- Having defined the optimal dose you may want to consider changing to a modified-release formulation for maintenance treatment.
- This is not always straightforward, as the milligram doses of immediate-release and modified-release formulations are rarely equivalent.
- Similarly, modified-release formulations differ from manufacturer to manufacturer, so one cannot assume that the same milligram doses of two modified-release formulations will have the same pharmacodynamic effect.
    - For example, lithium, theophylline, and nifedipine modified-release formulations are not interchangeable.
    - Prescribe these drugs by brand name to be sure of consistency.
- Switching to a modified-release formulation may require a further period of dosage adjustment to optimize treatment.
- Once you have given a patient a modified-release formulation of a drug, the effects will last for many hours. This is potentially hazardous if toxicity occurs.
- It is worth noting that most modified-release formulations are under patent and may be more expensive than immediate-release alternatives.

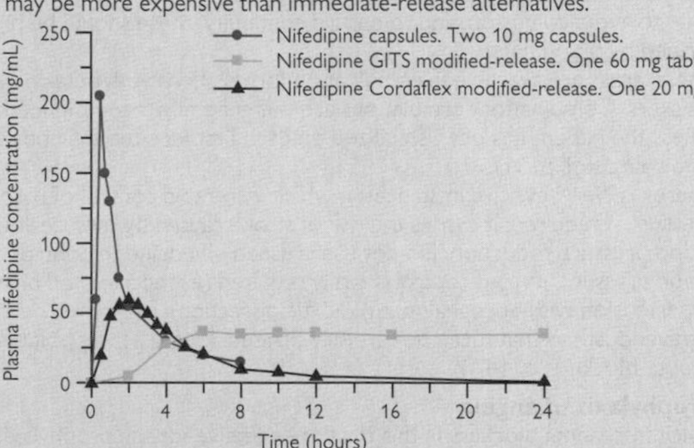

Plasma nifedipine concentrations following oral dosage with three different formulations of nifedipine (one normal formulation and two different modified-release formulations). The drug in each case is the same, but the pharmacokinetic characteristics of each formulation are very different.
(Redrawn from data in Chung M *et al. Am J Med* 1987; **83**(6B): 10-14. and Nemes *et al. Int J Clin Pharm Ther* 1998; **36**: 263-9.)

Dihydropyridines (nifedipine-like)

- Treatment of hypertension.
- Prophylaxis of angina.
- Symptomatic treatment of Raynaud's syndrome.
- Prophylaxis of migraine (specialized use, unlicensed).
- Nimodipine is used for the prevention and treatment of ischaemic neurological deficits after subarachnoid haemorrhage.

Drugs in this class

- Amlodipine
- Felodipine
- Isradipine
- Lacidipine
- Nicardipine
- Nifedipine
- Nimodipine
- Nisoldipine

- Avoid in pregnancy and breastfeeding (teratogenic in animals; excreted in breast milk).
- These drugs are vasodilators; they can cause severe hypotension in patients with a fixed cardiac output (e.g. aortic stenosis, mitral stenosis).
- Do not use soon after myocardial infarction (within 1 month) or if the patient has unstable/uncontrolled angina.
- Reduce the dose in severe hepatic insufficiency.

- Use a once-daily (modified-release) formulation of nifedipine. The immediate-release formulation can cause an exaggerated fall in blood pressure and reflex tachycardia (see teaching point).
- Nicardipine, amlodipine, felodipine, and modified-release nifedipine may be a better choice in patients with heart failure, as they do not reduce myocardial contractility.

Treatment of hypertension

- Calcium channel blockers are among the first-line drugs advised in the British Hypertension Society Guidelines (*Br Med J* 2004; **328**: 634–40).
- Calcium channel blockers are useful in the treatment of low-renin hypertension; this is more common in patients of Afro-Caribbean origin.
- Many branded modified-release formulations of these drugs are available; to avoid confusion, and to ensure continuity, these should be prescribed by brand name.
- These drugs are available in combination formulations with beta-blockers. Combination formulations are not generally recommended, unless the patient has been stabilized on each first (see teaching point in misoprostol, p. 31).
- There are very few circumstances in which very rapid control of blood pressure is required; it carries the risk of stroke caused by over-zealous blood pressure reduction. Do not use crushed nifiedpine to control blood pressure. If rapid control is really required (e.g. accelerated phase hypertension with encephalopathy, aortic dissection), use a drug intravenously so that it can be carefully titrated. (See teaching point in beta-blockers, p. 147.)

Prophylaxis of angina

- Calcium channel blockers in this class are effective for the prophylaxis of angina. However, they should not be used when the patient is unstable (angina or heart failure), as the vasodilating action may make matters worse.

Nimodipine following subarachnoid haemorrhage

- Start treatment as soon as possible after the haemorrhage.
- Available as an intravenous infusion if the patient is unable to take tablets.
- Monitor the blood pressure closely during treatment, especially when given intravenously.
- Treatment should continue for a minimum of 5 days and a maximum of 21 days.

- Adverse effects that are the result of vasodilatation are common (1–10% of patients): flushing, headache, and peripheral oedema.
  - Diuretics can be used for the peripheral oedema, but one should reconsider treatment when having to prescribe one drug to treat an adverse effect of another.
- These drugs cause gum hyperplasia rarely.

Safety and efficacy

- Measure the blood pressure. The frequency required will depend on the clinical circumstances (see nimodipine above).
- Be aware that the maximum effect on blood pressure may not occur for some days or weeks after a maintenance dosage has been established, especially with modified-release formulations.

- These drugs will augment the effect of other drugs that lower blood pressure. Take care when adding them to existing treatment.
- These drugs increase plasma digoxin and ciclosporin concentrations; measure the plasma concentrations of these drugs after achieving a maintenance dose.
- The metabolism of these drugs (except amlodipine) is affected by grapefruit juice. Advise the patient to avoid grapefruit juice (see teaching point in antihistamines, p. 610).

- Warn the patient about the possibility of ankle swelling or headache. Explain that these effects may improve over time.
- Advise the patient to avoid drinking grapefruit juice, as it may increase the risk of adverse effects.

Prescribing information: **Dihydropyridines**

Nifedipine

- Immediate-release nifedipine is not recommended (see below).
- Many modified-release formulations are available for the treatment of hypertension. Doses are not equivalent between different modified-release formulations. See individual manufacturers' information for dosage ranges.

Amlodipine

- Treatment of hypertension or angina.
  - By mouth, initially 5 mg once daily; increase to a maximum of 10 mg once daily.

Felodipine

- Treatment of hypertension
  - By mouth, initially 5 mg (elderly 2.5 mg) daily in the morning.
  - The usual maintenance dose is 5–10 mg daily.
  - Dosages above 20 mg daily are rarely needed.
- Prophylaxis of angina.
  - By mouth, initially 5 mg daily in the morning; increase if necessary to 10 mg daily.

Nimodipine for prevention and treatment of ischaemic neurological deficits after subarachnoid haemorrhage

- Prevention
  - *By mouth*, 60 mg every 4 hours, starting within 4 days of subarachnoid haemorrhage and continued for 21 days.
- Treatment
  - *By intravenous infusion* via central catheter. 1 mg/hour initially, increased after 2 hours to 2 mg/hour, provided there is no severe fall in blood pressure.
  - Patients with unstable blood pressure, or who weigh less than 70 kg, should begin with 500 micrograms/hour.
  - Continue intravenous infusion for at least 5 days (maximum 14 days).
  - In the event of surgical intervention during treatment continue for at least 5 days after surgery.
  - If the subarachnoid haemorrhage was caused by trauma, continue the intravenous infusion for 7–10 days, then complete a 21-day course by mouth.

TEACHING POINT Immediate-release nifedipine and excess mortality

- Immediate-release nifedipine is rapidly absorbed and after an oral dose has its maximal effect on blood pressure within 1-2 hours. It is also rapidly metabolized in the liver and so has a rapid offset of action.
- To achieve 24-hour blood pressure control immediate-release nifedipine needs to be given three times daily.
- Long-term clinical trials have shown that despite ostensibly good blood pressure control, treatment with immediate-release nifedipine is associated with excess mortality. This is because the rapid onset and offset of action leads to oscillations in the blood pressure when measured over the whole day. Rapid falls in blood pressure cause a reflex tachycardia. The rapidly changing heart rate and blood pressure lead to an excess of cardiovascular events because many of these patients have underlying coronary disease.
- Nifedipine is a useful drug for the treatment of hypertension, but it should be given as a modified-release formulation. Modified-release formulations are not associated with excess mortality.
- Crushed immediate-release formulations have been used to lower blood pressure rapidly. This is potentially hazardous and should not be done. Once the dose has been given, you have no control over the rate and extent of the blood pressure fall. If the blood pressure needs to be lowered rapidly give a rapidly-acting drug (e.g. a nitrate or labetalol) by intravenous infusion so that the effect can be carefully titrated (see teaching point in beta-blockers, p. 147).

Benzthiazepines (diltiazem)

- Prophylaxis of angina.
- Treatment of hypertension.

- Avoid in pregnancy and breastfeeding (experimental evidence of teratogenicity; enters breast milk).
- Diltiazem is negatively inotropic; avoid using in patients with heart failure.
- Diltiazem also affects cardiac conduction; avoid using it in patients with 2nd or 3rd degree heart block or sick sinus syndrome.
- Begin with lower doses if the patient has liver or renal insufficiency.

- Diltiazem combines the features of the other classes of calcium channel blockers. It is a vasodilator and slows intracardiac conduction.
- The major use of diltiazem is in the treatment of angina. The negative chronotropic effect can be especially useful in patients with ischaemic heart disease.

Treatment of angina

- Although diltiazem is negatively inotropic, this effect is less marked than that of verapamil. It is uncommon for diltiazem to precipitate heart failure.
- To give 24-hour cover, immediate-release diltiazem needs to be given 3 times daily. Many modified-release formulations that also give 24-hour cover are available. To avoid confusion, and to ensure continuity of reproducible therapy, these should be prescribed by brand name.

- Adverse effects that are the result of vasodilatation are common (1–10% of patients): flushing, headache, and peripheral oedema.
- Hypotension can result from the negative inotropic and vasodilatory actions of diltiazem. Begin treatment with a low dose and titrate upwards. This will also reduce the risk of severe bradycardia.

Safety and efficacy

- When diltiazem is given intravenously the patient should have continuous cardiac monitoring and frequent measurement of blood pressure.
- When giving diltiazem by mouth, measure the blood pressure and heart rate before increasing the dose.

- Diltiazem will augment the effect of other drugs that lower blood pressure or reduce heart rate. Take care when adding it to existing treatment.
- Take care when considering co-prescribing diltiazem with beta-blockers, there is a risk of a significant reduction in cardiac output.
- Diltiazem increases plasma digoxin and ciclosporin concentrations; measure the plasma concentrations of these drugs after achieving a maintenance dose.
  - The dose of digoxin will usually need to be reduced by 25%.
  - The dose of ciclosporin will usually need to be reduced by 40%.

- Warn the patient that diltiazem can cause swelling of the ankles.

Prescribing information: **Diltiazem**

- Treatment of angina.
  - 60 mg 3 times daily (elderly, initially twice daily).
  - Can be increased if necessary to 360 mg daily.
- Modified-release formulations
  - See individual manufacturers' material for doses.
  - The same milligram dose of two different modified-release formulations may not be pharmacodynamically equivalent, so prescribe by brand name to ensure continuity of effect.

Phenylalkylamines (verapamil)

- Treatment and prevention of SVT.
- Treatment of hypertension.
- Prophylaxis of angina.

- Take care in pregnancy and breastfeeding (but no clear evidence of harm).
- Verapamil is negatively inotropic; avoid it in patients with known left ventricular impairment or heart failure (even if they are currently stable).
- The major action of verapamil is on cardiac conduction; avoid using it in patients with 2nd or 3rd degree heart block or sick sinus syndrome.
- Do not co-prescribe verapamil with beta-blockers; there is a risk of severe reduction of cardiac output (see drug interactions below for details).
- Reduce the dose in severe liver impairment.

- Although verapamil can be used for the treatment of hypertension and angina, there are more appropriate choices for these indications.
- The major use of verapamil is for the treatment and prevention of SVT.

Treatment of SVT

- Verapamil can be given intravenously to terminate SVT.
  - It should be given as a slow bolus injection over 2–3 minutes.
  - Ensure that adequate resuscitation facilities are immediately to hand and that the patient has continuous cardiac monitoring.
- See adenosine (p. 78) for guidance on the choice of drug to terminate SVT.
  - Verapamil can be useful in patients with asthma, in whom adenosine and beta-blockers should not be used.
- The decision about prophylactic (oral) treatment against SVT is a complex one. The frequency and severity of the SVT needs to be balanced against the efficacy and tolerability of drug treatment. Seek expert advice before committing a patient to long-term treatment. Not everyone who has an episode of SVT needs prophylactic drug treatment.

- The negative inotropic effect of verapamil can worsen cardiac failure; avoid using it in patients with impaired left ventricular function.
- Hypotension can result from the negative inotropic and vasodilatory actions of verapamil. Begin treatment with a low dose and titrate upwards. This will also reduce the risk of severe bradycardia.
- Gynaecomastia and gingival hyperplasia can be caused by long-term treatment.

Safety and efficacy

- When verapamil is administered intravenously the patient should have continuous cardiac monitoring and frequent measurement of blood pressure.
- When giving verapamil by mouth, measure the blood pressure and heart rate before increasing the dose.
- Ask the patient to keep a diary of episodes of SVT, so that you can assess the efficacy of treatment.

- Verapamil will augment the effects of other drugs that lower blood pressure or reduce heart rate. Take care when adding it to existing treatment.
- Do not co-prescribe verapamil with beta-blockers; there is a risk of severe reduction of cardiac output or asystole. Do not give intravenous verapamil for at least 8 hours after a beta-blocker was last given.

- Verapamil increases plasma digoxin and ciclosporin concentrations; measure the plasma concentrations of these drugs after achieving a maintenance dose.
  - The dose of digoxin will usually need to be reduced by 25%.
  - The dose of ciclosproin will usually need to be reduced by 40%.
- The metabolism of verapamil is affected by grapefruit juice (see teaching point in antihistamines, p. 610).

- Advise the patient to avoid drinking grapefruit juice, as it increases the risk of adverse effects.

Prescribing information: **Verapamil**

Supraventricular arrhythmias

Termination

- Treatment *by slow intravenous injection* over 2 minutes (3 minutes in elderly people), 5–10 mg.
- Give a further 5 mg after 5–10 minutes if required.

Prophylaxis

- Treatment *by mouth*, 40–120 mg 3 times daily.

Angina (but see notes above)

- 80–120 mg 3 times daily.

Hypertension (but see notes above)

- 240–480 mg daily in 2–3 divided doses.

Sites of action of diuretics

Diuretic drugs have different clinical uses, depending on their sites and mechanisms of action. See individual articles for guidance on the choice and appropriate use of diuretic drugs. Not all the drugs listed here are used therapeutically.

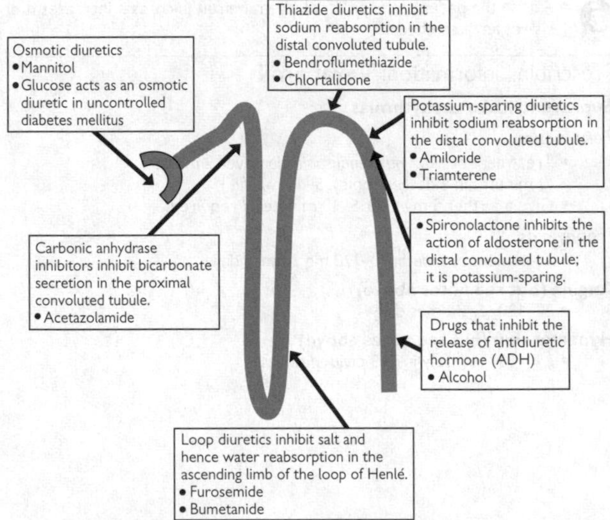

Notes on mannitol

- A hexahydric alcohol, related to mannose. It is filtered by the renal glomerulus, but is not reabsorbed; it therefore acts as an osmotic diuretic.
- Acts rapidly and is used in the emergency treatment of cerebral oedema and acute closed-angle glaucoma, but is not suitable for long-term treatment.
- Given by intravenous infusion; take care to avoid extravasation, as this can cause inflammation and thrombophlebitis.
- Emergency treatment of cerebral oedema (see p. 427 for more information):
  - 1 g/kg (5 mL/kg of a 20% solution) by rapid intravenous infusion.
- Emergency treatment of glaucoma before surgery:
  - 20% by slow intravenous infusion until the intraocular pressure has fallen to an acceptable value. The usual maximum total volume of mannitol that should be infused is 500 mL. This is a very specialized use; seek expert advice.

Treatment of pulmonary oedema

- The cardinal symptom of pulmonary oedema is severe breathlessness, due to fluid in the lung parenchyma. The volume of fluid can vary considerably. If the pulmonary oedema is acute, a small volume of fluid (about 100 mL) can be enough to cause severe symptoms; if however, the fluid has accumulated over several days or weeks, the volume in the lungs and pleural cavities can be very large (several litres).
- The priority of treatment is to provide adequate oxygenation of the blood. Immediate treatment is symptomatic, but if possible treat the underlying cause (see below).

Symptomatic treatments

- Sit the patient up. This improves ventilation–perfusion matching in the lungs.
- Give a high concentration of inspired oxygen by face mask, unless the patient is known to have chronic obstructive airways disease (see oxygen, p. 208).
- Diuretics. A loop diuretic (e.g. furosemide 40–80 mg) given by slow intravenous injection is often effective. Higher doses may be required if the patient has been taking large doses for long periods, as diuretic resistance can develop. The rapid initial action is due to pulmonary vasodilatation rather than diuresis, which comes later.
  - Remember that diuretics can only remove fluid from the intravascular space. It takes time for extravascular fluid to move into the intravascular space. Excessive doses of diuretics can cause hypotension, without relieving oedema.
  - Diuretics can only produce a diuresis if the patient has functioning kidneys. If diuretics do not work (e.g in chronic severe renal insufficiency or after acute tubular necrosis), a vasodilator drug (e.g. a nitrate) will temporarily relieve symptoms until fluid can be removed (e.g by dialysis). See nitrates (p. 134) for prescribing information.
- If the patient has bronchospasm, give a short-acting beta$_2$-adrenoceptor agonist (e.g. salbutamol).

Treatments for causes of pulmonary oedema

- If pulmonary oedema is due to left ventricular failure and if left ventricular function can be improved by treatment of the precipitating factor, the pulmonary oedema can be transient.

Common causes of acute left ventricular failure

- Myocardial infarction and ischaemia
  - Acute left ventricular failure is a poor prognostic feature. See p. 132 for an approach to the treatment of myocardial infarction.
  - Opiate drugs (e.g. morphine) have a vasodilator action; in addition to relieving pain, they can relieve the symptoms of pulmonary oedema.
  - Inotropic drugs, such as dobutamine, can improve left ventricular function in the short term, but may not affect the prognosis.
- Arrhythmias
  - A patient with impaired left ventricular function who develops AF can in turn develop acute left ventricular failure. Chemical or electrical cardioversion may be all that is required to relieve the symptoms.
- Valvular heart disease
  - Acute valvular insufficiency can precipitate acute left ventricular failure. Causes include myocardial infarction and infective endocarditis; emergency surgical intervention may be required.

Loop diuretics

Inhibitors of the $Na^+/K^+/Cl^-$ co-transporter

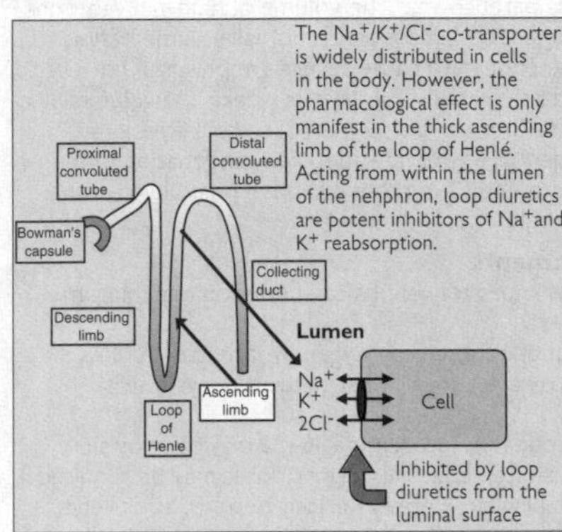

Drugs in this class

- Bumetanide
- Furosemide (frusemide)
- Torasemide

Furosemide is poorly absorbed, and bumetanide are torasemide may be preferable for long-term oral administration.

Etacrynic acid is an obsolete loop diuretic that has also been studied for its potential beneficial effects in the treatment of tumours.

- Loop diuretics are potent and act rapidly. They are used whenever a rapid diuresis is required, and in long-term therapy.
  - The most common indication is for the control of oedema, usually due to heart failure.
  - Note that diuretics improve symptoms in heart failure but do not reduce mortality.
  - They may also be used to promote a diuresis in acute renal insufficiency, but it is essential to ensure that the patient is adequately hydrated before using a diuretic in such cases.

- Loop diuretics act from within the lumen of the nephron. They will not work if the patient is anuric.
- Diuretics can cause severe hypokalaemia and hyponatraemia. Measure serum electrolytes before giving these drugs.
  - Avoid in people with hypokalaemia, or in whom hypokalaemia could have serious consequences (e.g. those taking digoxin).
  - Hypokalaemia can precipitate coma in patients with hepatic insufficiency.
- Loop diuretics are not useful in hypertension.
  - Consider a thiazide diuretic instead.
- Loop diuretics can precipitate gout.
  - Avoid in people with a history of gout. If treatment with a diuretic is necessary, give the patient allopurinol first.
- Can precipitate type II diabetes mellitus or worsen glucose control in diabetes mellitus.
  - Consider using an alternative drug.
- Co-administration with a loop diuretic results in a profound diuresis.
  - This may be desirable in refractory heart failure, but the combination should be avoided in other circumstances.
- These drugs are not used usually during pregnancy because of the risk of volume depletion.

Oedema

(see glucocorticoids, p. 427, and mannitol, p. 172, for treatment of cerebral oedema)

- Remember that in oedematous states most of the fluid is extravascular. Fluid can only be mobilized from these sites at a certain rate. Excessive diuresis will empty the intravascular space, leading to dehydration and hypotension.
  - The usual maximum target rate of fluid loss is one litre (one kg) per day.
- Patients with severe peripheral oedema also have an oedematous gut. This impairs absorption of these drugs, particulary furosemide.
  - Bumetanide and torasemide are better absorbed than furosemide, and may be better choices for oral administration in patients with severe oedema.
  - For patients with severe oedema, a continuous intravenous infusion will be more effective than a bolus dose.
- Patients become resistant to loop diuretics over time. The mechanism of this is complex, and may involve the hypertrophy of cells in the distal nephron. In practical terms, you may have to increase the dose over time to achieve the same effect. Patients taking diuretics in the long term may need high doses when they present acutely. By the same token, diuretic-naive patients presenting with, for example, acute heart failure due to myocardial infarction, may only need small doses.
  - Titrate the dose according to the clinical effect, not how unwell the patient is.
- Co-administration of a small dose of a thiazide or thiazide-like diuretic (usually metolazone) with a loop diuretic can produce a powerful diuresis in patients with oedema that is refractory to loop diuretics alone.
  - This requires close monitoring of electrolytes and fluid balance to avoid excessive diuresis.

Renal insufficiency

- These drugs have a role in oliguric renal insufficiency.
  - High doses are required.
  - Ensure that oliguria is not due to a pre-renal or post-renal cause.

Early or late

- Excessively rapid infusion of large doses of intravenous loop diuretics can cause ototoxicity, particularly if the patient has renal failure; furosemide is more ototoxic than bumetanide.
  - Rapid infusion does not improve the clinical effect, and slow infusion is often more effective.
  - Furosemide should be infused at a rate of no more than 4 mg/minute.
- Measure the plasma potassium concentration before initiating diuretic therapy.
- Other adverse effects include gastrointestinal disturbance, precipitation of attacks of gout, and rash.
- Loop diuretics can cause postural hypotension by reducing the circulating volume.

- Prior treatment with diuretics increases the risk of first-dose hypotension when starting treatment with ACE inhibitors (see ACE inhibitors, p. 148).
- Loop diuretics reduce the excretion of lithium.
  - Serum concentrations of lithium can rise.
  - Reduce the dose of lithium by a half initially and monitor serum lithium concentrations.

- Hypokalaemia resulting from diuretic treatment increases the risk of toxicity from digoxin and antiarrhythmic drugs.
- The risk of hypokalaemia is increased in patients taking theophylline.

Safety

- Ensure that the patient is not hypovolaemic before starting diuretic therapy.
- Measure plasma electrolytes before starting therapy, and on a regular basis while the patient is being stabilized on these drugs. There is very little evidence to suggest how often to measure the serum electrolytes of patients taking diuretics. The following is suggested as a practical approach.
  - Measure serum electrolytes before starting therapy and correct any hypokalaemia.
  - Measure the electrolytes again after 3–4 days and weekly thereafter, until the patient is stabilized on a dosage regimen.
  - If the patient is stable, it may be only necessary to measure electrolytes every 6 months thereafter.
  - Some patients require more frequent monitoring. In particular, increase the frequency of monitoring if a change in therapy is required or if the patient suffers an intercurrent illness or has renal impairment.
  - Patients receiving intravenous diuretic therapy should have their serum electrolytes measured every other day; some will require daily measurements.

Efficacy

- Monitor the patient's weight daily, as a measure of fluid loss.

- Compliance with diuretic therapy can be a problem; many patients find that the diuresis interferes with their daily activities. The diuretic action of these drugs lasts for about 6 hours. Discuss this with the patient and find the most convenient time for them to take their diuretics; this may not be first thing in the morning.
- Patients on established diuretic therapy are often able to adjust the dose according to their clinical status. This is helpful, as it encourages the patient to take the minimum effective dose.

Prescribing information: **Loop diuretics**

Furosemide

By mouth

- *Oedema* Initially 40 mg in the morning; maintenance 20 mg daily *or* 40 mg on alternate days; increase in resistant oedema to 80 mg daily or more.
- Do not give twice a day.
  - The kidney is refractory for 6–8 hours after an effective dose.
  - A second dose after 12 hours causes a diuresis overnight.
  - If the patient has an indwelling urinary catheter, twice daily administration (12 hours apart) may be acceptable.
- *Oliguria* Initially 250 mg daily; if necessary larger doses, increasing in steps of 250 mg, can be given every 4–6 hours to a maximum single dose of 2 g (rarely used).

By intramuscular injection or slow intravenous injection

- Initially 20–50 mg.

By intravenous infusion (by syringe pump if necessary)

- *Oliguria* Initially 250 mg over 1 hour (rate not exceeding 4 mg/minute). If a satisfactory urine output is not obtained in the subsequent hour, give a further 500 mg over 2 hours, then if there is no satisfactory response within the next hour, give a further 1 g over 4 hours. If there is still no response, dialysis will probably be required. An effective dose (up to 1 g) can be repeated every 24 hours.

Bumetanide

By mouth

- 1 mg in the morning; severe cases, increased up to 5 mg or more daily.
- In elderly patients, 500 micrograms daily may be sufficient.

By intravenous injection

- 1–2 mg, repeated after 20 minutes.

By intravenous infusion

- 2–5 mg over 30–60 minutes.

Torasemide

By mouth

- *Oedema* 5 mg once daily, preferably in the morning, increased if required to 20 mg once daily; usual maximum 40 mg daily.

TEACHING POINT Postural hypotension

- Remember that the blood pressure can be normal when measured with the patient sitting or lying. The principal feature of postural hypotension is that the blood pressure falls significantly on standing.
- Drugs are commonly responsible; examples include:
  - Drugs that cause dehydration (e.g. loop diuretics).
  - Drugs that lower blood pressure (e.g. thiazide diuretics, beta-blockers, ACE inhibitors, calcium channel blockers, alpha-blockers, centrally-acting antihypertensive drugs).
  - Vasodilators (e.g. nitrate drugs).
  - Drugs that cause adrenal insufficiency (e.g. abrupt corticosteroid withdrawal after long-term therapy).
  - Drugs that can affect CNS control of blood pressure (e.g. antipsychotic drugs, antidepressants).
  - Drugs that are sedative (e.g. antihistamines).
  - Elderly patients are most prone to this adverse effect of drugs.
- Other causes:
  - Autonomic neuropathy due to diabetes mellitus.
  - Venous insufficiency in the legs.

Treatment

- Identify the cause whenever possible. Withdraw or reduce the dose of any causative or contributory drugs.
- Advise the patient to stand up slowly, and in stages.
- Venous compression stockings can be of use if venous insufficiency is the cause.
- Reserve treatment with mineralocorticoids (fludrocortisone) for the most severely affected in whom other measures have been ineffective.
  - Fludrocorisone 50–300 micrograms by mouth, daily.

TEACHING POINT Drug names

- Drugs have several names, including a chemical name, a non-proprietary name, and one or more proprietary names.
- The recommended International Non-proprietary Name (rINN) is the name of the drug compound that is usually preferred. Many countries used to have their own names for drug compounds, some of which are more familiar than the recommended name (e.g. lignocaine is the old British Approved Name for lidocaine).
- Drugs are often grouped together in classes that share a similar name, to aid identification. For example, most beta-blocking drugs have the ending –olol (but beware, stanozolol is an anabolic steroid). Sometimes the chemical class name is cumbersome (e.g. thiazolidinediones); in these cases, the drug class referred to may be a nickname (e.g. 'the glitazones').
- Proprietary manufacturers give their drugs a brand name. This name need not reflect the drug class or chemical compound. In some cases, these brand names are more familiar than the rINN (e.g. Lasix®), but confusion can arise from similar sounding names. For this reason, prescribers are encouraged to use the rINN. The exception to this is when different formulations of the same drug have very different properties (e.g. modified-release formulations of lithium, theophylline, and nifedipine). In these cases, the brand should be specified as well as the rINN.

TEACHING POINT Potency of drugs

- A drug that is more potent than another exerts its pharmacodynamic effect at a lower concentration. A more potent drug does not necessarily have a larger maximum effect than a less potent drug. For example, bumetanide is a more potent inhibitor of sodium reabsorption in the ascending loop of Henlé than furosemide (compare their oral doses), but the maximum diuretic effects of these drugs are the same. Conversely, bumetanide and bendroflumethiazide are about equally potent as diuretics, but dose for dose bumetanide produces a larger effect.
- Usually the relative potency of two drugs is less important than their relative efficacy (see p. 10). However, sometimes a drug is more potent as a cause of adverse effects than another drug with equal therapeutic efficacy. For example, two antihistamines may have the same therapeutic efficacy in reducing the symptoms of hay fever, but at equivalent therapeutic doses one may produce more drowsiness than the other.

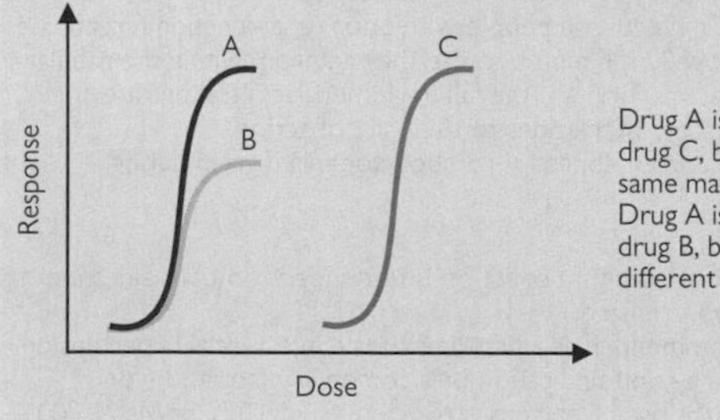

Drug A is more potent than drug C, but they have the same maximal efficacy. Drug A is as potent as drug B, but they have different maximal efficacies.

Thiazide and thiazide-like diuretics

Inhibitors of the Na^+/Cl^- co-transporter

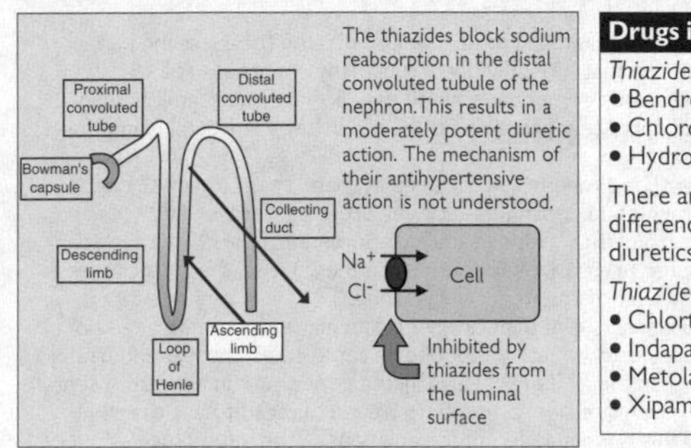

Drugs in this class

Thiazides
- Bendroflumethiazide
- Chlorothiazide
- Hydrochlorothiazide

There are no important differences among these diuretics.

Thiazide-like
- Chlortalidone
- Indapamide
- Metolazone
- Xipamide

- Treatment of hypertension.
- In combination with loop diuretics for the control of severe oedema in chronic heart failure.
  - This requires close monitoring.
- Specialized use in the treatment of nephrogenic diabetes insipidus.

- Thiazides can cause hypokalaemia.
  - Avoid in people with hypokalaemia, or in whom hypokalaemia could have serious consequences (e.g. those taking digoxin).
  - Hypokalaemia can precipitate encephalopathy in patients with hepatic insufficiency.
- Thiazides can precipitate gout.
  - Avoid in people with a history of gout. If treatment with a thiazide is necessary, give the patient allopurinol first.
- Thiazides can precipitate type II diabetes mellitus or worsen glucose control in diabetes mellitus.
  - Consider using an alternative drug.
- Co-administration with a loop diuretic results in a profound diuresis.
  - This may be desirable in refractory heart failure, but the combination should be avoided in other circumstances.
- Thiazides are ineffective in people with poor renal function (creatinine clearance below 30 mL/min) because they act from within the tubular lumen; in renal insufficiency, the fall in glomerular filtration rate reduces the access of thiazides to their site of action.
- Thiazides can cause neonatal thrombocytopenia if given during pregnancy.

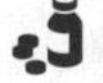

Hypertension
- Although their mechanism of action is not understood, thiazides are effective in hypertension.
- They are recommended as a first-line choice in essential hypertension, unless there is a contraindication or a compelling indication for another drug (British Hypertension Society Guidelines, *Br Med J*, 2004; **328**:634–40).

- Low doses are as effective as higher doses. Higher doses have a higher incidence of adverse effects.
- If the blood pressure is not adequately controlled by a low dose of a thiazide, a second agent should be considered, rather than increasing the dose.
  - Less than half of patients with hypertension will be adequately controlled with one drug.

Non-cardiac oedema

- Thiazides reduce oedema. However, they are not the best choice when a significant diuresis is required; a loop diuretic is a better choice.
- Do not use in idiopathic oedema; initial benefit is usually offset by tolerance and worsening oedema.

Heart failure

- Co-administration of a small dose of a thiazide or a thiazide-like diuretic (e.g. metolazone) with a loop diuretic can produce a powerful diuresis in patients with oedema refractory to loop diuretics alone.
- This requires close monitoring of electrolytes and fluid balance to avoid excessive diuresis.

Diabetes insipidus

- Thiazide and thiazide-like diuretics have a paradoxical antidiuretic action in nephrogenic diabetes insipidus.
  - Specialized use.
  - Suggested dose, chlortalidone 100 mg/day initially, reduced to 50 mg/day for maintenance.

Early

- All of these diuretics have the potential to cause hyponatraemia and hypokalaemia.
- Thiazides can precipitate acute attacks of gout.
- Thiazides can raise plasma lipid concentrations.
- Rashes are common, but usually mild.
- An allergic vasculitis is well described but rare.

Long-term

- Long-term treatment can cause hyperglycaemia and worsening of diabetic control.
- Thiazides can cause erectile impotence.
- Thrombocytopenia occurs rarely, owing to a direct effect on the bone marrow.

- NSAIDs interfere with the antihypertensive effect of thiazides.
- Note that prior treatment with diuretics increases the risk of first-dose hypotension when starting treatment with ACE inhibitors.
  - Suspend the diuretic for 2 days before starting an ACE inhibitor, and give the first dose of the ACE inhibitor when the patient is lying down (e.g. on going to bed). If this is not possible, admit the patient to hospital in order to start the ACE inhibitor.
- Thiazides reduce the excretion of lithium salts.
  - Serum concentrations of lithium can rise.
  - Reduce the dose of lithium by a half initially and monitor serum lithium concentrations.
- Hypokalaemia resulting from diuretic treatment increases the risk of toxicity from digoxin and antiarrhythmic drugs.
- The risk of hypokalaemia is increased in patients taking theophylline.

Safety

- Ensure that the patient is not hypovolaemic before starting diuretic therapy.
- Check plasma electrolytes before starting therapy and on a regular basis while the patient is being stabilized on these drugs. See loop diuretics (p. 174).

Efficacy

- Measure the patient's weight daily (as a measure of fluid loss) during the early stages of therapy for heart failure.

- Compliance with diuretic therapy can be a problem. Many patients find that the diuresis interferes with their daily activities. Discuss this with the patient and find the most convenient time for them to take their tablets. These drugs have a duration of action varying from 12 to 24 hours.

Prescribing information: **Thiazide diuretics**

Many thiazides are available. Only three (the best-established) are listed here.

Bendroflumethiazide (bendrofluazide)

- *Oedema*: initially 5–10 mg in the morning, daily or on alternate days.
- *Hypertension*: 2.5 mg in the morning; higher doses are rarely necessary.

Chlortalidone

- *Oedema*: up to 50 mg daily for a limited period.
- *Hypertension*: 25 mg in the morning; increasing the dose to 50 mg is rarely necessary.
- *Heart failure*: 25–50 mg in the morning, increased if necessary to 100–200 mg daily.

Metolazone

- *Oedema*: 5–10 mg in the morning, increasing if necessary to 20 mg daily in resistant oedema; maximum 80 mg daily.
- *Hypertension*: initially 5 mg in the morning; maintenance dose 5 mg on alternate days.
- *Heart failure*: suggested starting dose 2.5 mg 3 times per week, in combination with a loop diuretic; increase cautiously to desired effect.

Potassium-sparing diuretics (amiloride and triamterene)

Inhibitors of Na^+ channels in the distal convoluted tubule

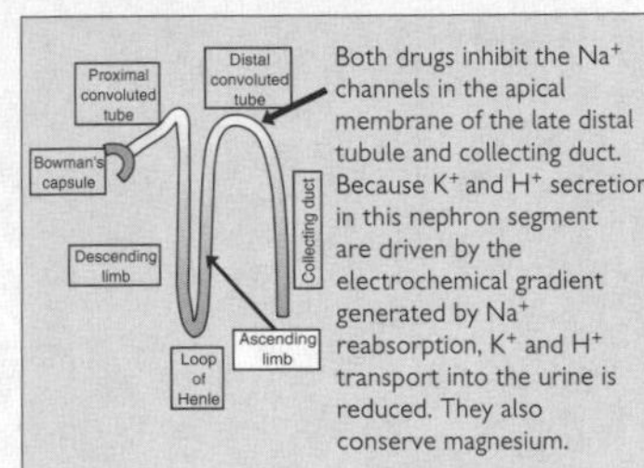

Both drugs inhibit the Na^+ channels in the apical membrane of the late distal tubule and collecting duct. Because K^+ and H^+ secretion in this nephron segment are driven by the electrochemical gradient generated by Na^+ reabsorption, K^+ and H^+ transport into the urine is reduced. They also conserve magnesium.

Drugs in this class

- Amiloride
- Triamterene
- (Spironolactone — see p. 186)

There are no important therapeutic differences between these two drugs.

Several combination formulations contain a potassium-sparing diuretic plus a loop diuretic or a thiazide diuretic. These include co-amilofruse (amiloride plus furosemide), co-amilozide (amiloride plus hydrochlorothiazide), and co-triamterzide (triamterene and hydrochlorothiazide).

Note ACE inhibitors also have a potassium-sparing effect.

- Although these drugs have diuretic action, their major use is in combination with thiazide or loop diuretics in order to conserve potassium.

- Potassium-sparing diuretics are not the most appropriate treatment for oedema; a loop diuretic is a better choice.
- Many patients given diuretics will not require a potassium-sparing diuretic. Do not give one unless the patient has or is at risk of hypokalaemia.
- Patients with renal insufficiency are at risk of hyperkalaemia. Potassium-sparing diuretics are not usually recommended in this group.
- Diuretics are best avoided in pregnancy; there is a risk of volume depletion.

- Consider for patients who develop, or are at risk of, hypokalaemia.
    - Often as a result of treatment with loop or thiazide diuretics, particularly in patients taking digoxin.
    - The potassium-sparing dose of these drugs is low.
- Many patients, particularly those with heart failure, will not require a potassium-sparing diuretic, as they should also be taking an ACE inhibitor, which has a potassium-sparing effect.
- Note that the aldosterone antagonist spironolactone (see p. 186), which has potassium-sparing effects, improves outcome in patients with heart failure when added to a diuretic and ACE inhibitor. The potassium-sparing diuretics, amiloride and tiamterene, have not been shown to have this effect; they do not affect aldosterone.

Combination formulations

Potassium-sparing diuretics with thiazides

- The routine addition of a potassium-sparing diuretic is not usually required for the treatment of hypertension, but may be useful in those who develop hypokalaemia with thiazide treatment.

Potassium-sparing diuretics with loop diuretics

- Patients should be established on a loop diuretic first; a potassium-sparing diuretic should only be added if required. If the patient is stable on a particular dose of a loop and a potassium-sparing diuretic, a combination product may be appropriate.
- The disadvantage of these combination products is that they are less flexible; changing the dose of one component will also alter the dose of the other component. For this reason they are really only suitable for patients who are stable on a fixed dose. (See misoprostol (p. 31) and co-phenotrope (p. 35) for more information.)

Early

- These drugs are usually well tolerated, but hypersensitivity reactions are reported uncommonly.

Late

- Triamterene inhibits dihydrofolate reductase and can cause folate deficiency, particularly in those with hepatic cirrhosis.
  - Consider spironolactone instead.
  - For the same reason, triamterene is not recommended in women who are pregnant or wish to become pregnant.
- Triamterene causes an interstitial nephritis rarely.
- Be aware that renal function may deteriorate over time, leading to hyperkalaemia in patients who were previously stable.

- There is a particular risk of hyperkalaemia when potassium-sparing diuretics are co-prescribed with:
  - ACE inhibitors or angiotensin receptor antagonists; this can be severe.
  - Ciclosporin and tacrolimus.
  - NSAIDs, especially indomethacin, which can worsen renal function and so cause hyperkalaemia.
  - Trimethoprim, which has potassium-sparing actions very like those of amiloride; use another suitable antibiotic.
  - Potassium supplements; do not co-prescribe.
- Triamterene has antifolate actions, avoid co-prescribing with:
  - Methotrexate.
  - Phenytoin.

Safety and efficacy

- Measure the plasma potassium concentration when starting a potassium-sparing diuretic, not only to ensure that it does not rise excessively, but also to ensure that the drug has the desired effect if the potassium was low (see also loop diuretics, p. 174). Taking a potassium-sparing diuretic is not a guarantee against hypokalaemia.

- Triamterene can cause the urine to fluoresce blue.

Prescribing information: **Potassium-sparing diuretics**

Amiloride

- With other diuretics, in congestive heart failure and hypertension, initially 5–10 mg daily.
- Cirrhosis with ascites, initially 5 mg daily.

Triamterene

- Initially 150–250 mg daily, reducing to alternate days after 1 week; taken in divided doses after breakfast and lunch; lower the initial dose when given with other diuretics.

Spironolactone

Aldosterone receptor antagonist

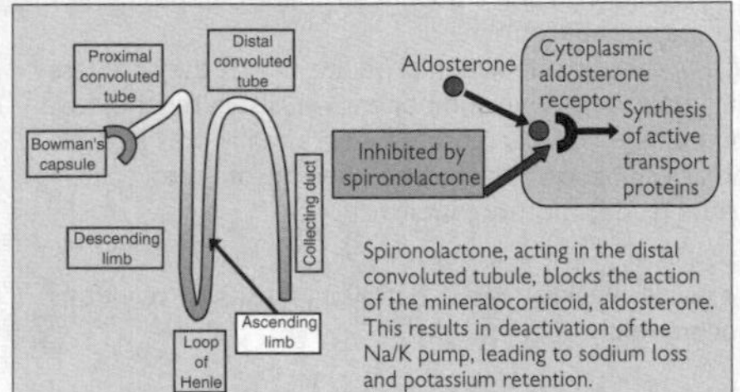

Other potassium-sparing diuretics

- Amiloride
- Triamterene

Note ACE inhibitors also have a potassium-sparing effect

- Control of ascites and oedema resulting from hepatic cirrhosis.
- Control of malignant ascites.
- As a potassium-sparing diuretic in heart failure.
- Symptomatic relief in the nephrotic syndrome.
- Diagnosis and treatment of primary hyperaldosteronism.

- Avoid in severe renal insufficiency.
  - Measure the serum potassium concentration before giving spironolactone.
- Avoid in pregnancy and breastfeeding.
- Avoid in Addison's disease.
- Do not combine with other potassium-sparing diuretics.

Ascites and oedema in hepatic cirrhosis

- Spironolactone is particularly useful for the secondary hyperaldosteronism associated with hepatic cirrhosis.
  - Exclude other causes of ascites (e.g. infection, malignancy).
  - Begin with a dose of 50 mg twice daily; build up gradually; maintenance doses in the range 200–400 mg/day.
  - Institute a low-salt diet (<0.5 g / day) and fluid restriction (<1.5 l /day).
  - Stop treatment if encephalopathy develops.

Malignant ascites

- Begin with a dose of 50 mg twice daily; build up gradually; maintenance doses in the range 200–400 mg/day.

Heart failure

- Spironolactone can be used as a potassium-sparing diuretic for patients taking loop diuretics who develop, or are at risk of developing, hypokalaemia.
- The antialdosterone action of spironolactone has particular benefits for patients with heart failure. Used in a low dose, in combination with loop diuretics and ACE inhibitors, spironolactone reduces mortality in patients with heart failure.

- The dose used is much lower than that used for a straightforward diuretic effect: 25 mg daily.
- Increasing the dose increases the risk of hyperkalaemia in these patients greatly, almost all of whom should also be taking an ACE inhibitor, which also has potassium-sparing effects.

Nephrotic syndrome

- Spironolactone is not a treatment for the underlying processes that cause the nephrotic syndrome. It should therefore only be used to alleviate oedema in patients for whom glucocorticoid treatment alone is insufficiently effective.

Primary aldosteronism (Conn's syndrome)

- Conn's syndrome is a rare cause of secondary hypertension, characterized by hypokalaemia; 75% of cases are due to a unilateral adrenal adenoma producing aldosterone.
- The antialdosterone action of spironolactone makes this drug useful as a diagnostic tool, as part of pre-surgical treatment, and for symptom palliation.
- This is a specialized use; seek expert advice.

Hirsutism

- This is an unlicensed specialized use; seek expert advice.

- Avoid giving spironolactone with other drugs that conserve potassium (e.g. potassium-sparing diuretics).
- Avoid giving potassium supplements to patients taking spironolactone.
- There is an increased risk of hyperkalaemia if ciclosporin and spironolactone are given together.
- NSAIDs can impair renal function and precipitate hyperkalaemia in patients taking spironolactone.
- The effect of digoxin is enhanced by spironolactone, which inhibits the renal excretion of digoxin.
- The excretion of lithium is inhibited by spironolactone.

Early

- Only use in low doses (25 mg/day) in those also taking ACE inhibitors. Higher doses are associated with a high risk of hyperkalaemia.
- Introduce and increase the dose gradually in those with hepatic cirrhosis. Avoid excessive diuresis, as this may lead to decompensation of liver function and hepatic encephalopathy.
- Nausea and abdominal discomfort are common with high doses, and it is often necessary to give doses of over 100 mg/day as two separate doses.

Late

- Spironolactone can cause painful gynaecomastia in men and breast enlargement in women. This effect usually resolves on stopping the drug.
- Occasionally, spironolactone in high doses can cause gastric ulceration.

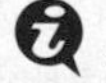

Efficacy

- In patients with ascites, aim for a mild diuresis, monitored by a weight reduction of no more than 0.5 kg/day.

Safety

- Measure the serum potassium concentration when starting spironolactone, not only to ensure that it does not rise excessively, but also to ensure that it has the desired effect if the potassium is low. Taking a potassium-sparing diuretic is not a guarantee against hypokalaemia.

Prescribing information: **Spironolactone**

Ascites and oedema in hepatic cirrhosis

- *By mouth* Begin with a dose of 50 mg twice daily. Build up gradually. Maintenance doses in the range 200–400 mg/day.

Malignant ascites

- *By mouth* Begin with a dose of 50 mg twice daily. Build up gradually. Maintenance doses in the range 200–400 mg/day.

Heart failure

- *By mouth* 25 mg daily.

Adrenoceptor agonists (sympathomimetics)

Agonists at α and β adrenoceptors

The body produces catecholamines peripherally from the adrenal medulla and sympathetic nerves. Dopamine and noradrenaline are also neurotransmitters in the CNS. Catecholamines have a large number of effects, characterized by the 'fight or flight reaction'. Synthetic sympathomimetics have differential effects by exploiting selectivity for different receptor subtypes (see teaching point below).

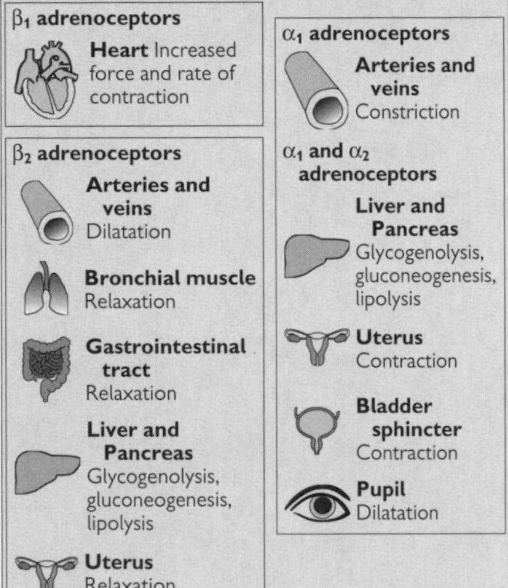

Drugs in this class

- Drugs acting on both α and β adrenoceptors: adrenaline, ephedrine
- Drugs acting predominantly on α adrenoceptors: noradrenaline, metaraminol, methoxamine
- Drug acting on β_1 and β_2 adrenoceptors: isoprenaline
- Drugs acting predominantly on β_1 adrenoceptors: dopamine, dobutamine
- Drugs acting predominantly on β_2 adrenoceptors: salbutamol, terbutaline, salmeterol (see pp. 214)
- Drugs acting predominantly in the CNS: amphetamines and anorectics (not considered further here)

- Treatment of shock.
  - Includes cardiopulmonary resuscitation and anaphylaxis.
  - Shock is a result of other pathological processes (e.g. myocardial infarction, sepsis); it is essential to treat these as well.

- Pregnancy. Remember that there are two circulations to consider, the mother's and the child's. The decision to use these drugs will depend on an assessment of the potential benefits and harms.
- Do not use these drugs to 'normalize the numbers'; use functional outcomes (e.g. urine output, level of consciousness).
- Avoid using sympathomimetics in patients with a phaeochromocytoma; they can induce a 'catecholamine storm'.
- These drugs always require individual dose titration, but there are no specific adjustments for renal or hepatic insufficiency.

Shock

- Selection of the most appropriate drug depends on the predominant clinical features. At its most basic level, shock can result from inadequate cardiac output (e.g. myocardial infarction) or from excessive peripheral vasodilatation (e.g. sepsis syndrome).
- An inotropic sympathomimetic is the most appropriate choice for the former case, and a vasoconstrictor sympathomimetic for the latter.
- All these drugs are given by intravenous injection or infusion. The duration of action of the synthetic drugs is often longer than that of the endogenous catecholamines. Give small doses initially and titrate the dose to optimal effect.
- It is easy to make mistakes when calculating and drawing up dosages on a mg/kg basis. Always check your calculations with someone else; use local dosage charts if these are available.
- For more information on giving drugs by variable rate intravenous infusion, see oxytocin (p. 455).
- These drugs should only be used when there is adequate medical and nursing supervision, such as in intensive care or coronary care wards.
- Use a central venous catheter when possible.

Adrenaline/epinephrine acts on both α and β adrenoceptors

- It is used on ICUs for its inotropic effects.
- It can be used for severe asthma unresponsive to selective β_2 agonists (e.g. salbutamol).
- Adrenaline is used intravenously for cardiopulmonary resuscitation.
- Adrenaline, given intramuscularly, is first-line treatment for anaphylaxis. The intravenous route is potentially hazardous and should not be used for this indication, unless there is expert supervision with adequate invasive monitoring; the subcutaneous route is unreliable because of variable absorption (see below).

Inotropic sympathomimetics

- The most common reason for hypotension is an inadequate intravascular volume. It is essential to ensure that the patient is adequately filled before giving these drugs.
- **Dobutamine** is selective for β_1 receptors in cardiac muscle; it increases contractility with little effect on heart rate.
- **Dopamine** given in low doses (5 micrograms/kg/min) causes vasodilatation and increases renal perfusion. It has traditionally been used in the treatment of incipient renal failure, but its efficacy has been questioned. Higher doses lead to vasoconstriction and can exacerbate heart failure.
- **Dopexamine** acts on β_2 receptors in cardiac muscle to produce a positive inotropic effect, and on peripheral dopamine receptors to increase renal perfusion; it is reported not to cause vasoconstriction.
- **Isoprenaline** is less selective and increases both heart rate and contractility. It is used only as a short-term emergency treatment of heart block or severe bradycardia. (see atropine (p. 201) for emergency treatment of bradycardia.)

Vasoconstrictor sympathomimetics

- These drugs will make the blood pressure rise, but perfusion of vital organs (especially the kidney) may fall. Blood pressure alone is not a direct measure of tissue perfusion.
- Remember other simple interventions, such as raising the foot of the bed.
- **Noradrenaline** is relatively selective for α-adrenoceptors. Its main use is in intensive care for the treatment of sepsis syndromes. Never give it through a peripheral vein, as it can cause severe ischaemia.
- **Methoxamine** and **metaraminol** are selective for α-adrenoceptors. Their principal use is in the treatment of hypotension that can result from spinal or epidural anaesthesia.
- **Ephedrine** is less selective and acts on both α and β adrenoceptors; it is therefore not commonly used but may be useful for treating of hypotension after spinal or epidural anaesthesia associated with bradycardia.

- Drugs in this class are classified according to their selectivity for receptor subtypes. Selectivity is always a relative term (see teaching point below). All of these drugs will produce effects through their actions on the other adrenoceptor subtypes, especially when used in high doses. See box above for the actions of adrenoceptor agonists.

- Catecholamines are metabolized by monoamine oxidase. Their actions will be greatly enhanced if the patient is taking a non-selective monoamine oxidase inhibitor (for depression). Note that the antibiotic linezolid is a non-selective monoamine oxidase inhibitor.
- Tricyclic antidepressants inhibit the reuptake of catecholamines into sympathetic neurons. Use very small doses of adrenoceptor agonists in patients taking these drugs.
- If a patient taking a beta-blocker is given a vasconstrictor sympathomimetic or mixed α and β adrenoceptor agonist (adrenaline), the α adrenoceptor actions will be unopposed, causing severe hypertension. Use very small doses in these patients and consider using a β_2 adrenoceptor agonist (e.g. intravenous salbutamol) as well. An alternative is to give glucagon; this increases cyclic AMP but does not act via adrenoceptors. This is an unlicensed indication and requires expert supervision (e.g. on the ICU). See also glucagon (p. 398).

Safety and efficacy

- The level of monitoring will depend on the clinical circumstances. The absolute minimum would be continuous cardiac monitoring and regular blood pressure measurement, but would usually include measurement of cardiac output and peripheral resistance with invasive blood pressure monitoring.
- Be clear about the clinical outcomes you are aiming for (e.g. urine output). These drugs have desirable and undesirable actions; do not use them to simply make the blood pressure reading 'normal'.

- Patients in critical care situations may be sedated or have a reduced level of consciousness. However, do not forget that they may still be able to hear and to feel pain. Explain what you are doing and take care to avoid unnecessary discomfort to the patient.

Prescribing information: **Adrenoceptor agonists**

Inotropic sympathomimetics

Dobutamine

- 2.5–10 micrograms/kg/min by intravenous infusion, adjusted according to response.

Dopamine

- 2–5 micrograms/kg/min by intravenous infusion. Higher doses not recommended (see above).

Dopexamine

- 500 nanograms/kg/min by intravenous infusion into a central or large peripheral vein.
- Can be increased to 1 microgram/kg/min, and further up to 6 micrograms/kg/min in increments of 0.5–1 microgram/kg/min at intervals of not less than 15 minutes.

Isoprenaline

- 0.5–10 micrograms/minute by intravenous infusion.

Adrenaline

- Cardiac arrest
  - 1 in 10 000 (100 micrograms/mL), a dose of 10 mL by intravenous injection, preferably through a central line.
  - If injected through a peripheral line, the drug must be flushed with at least 20 mL of sodium chloride 0.9% (to aid entry into the central circulation).

Anaphylaxis

  - 500 micrograms (0.5 mL adrenaline injection 1 in 1000).
  - The dose is repeated if necessary at 5-minute intervals according to blood pressure, pulse, and respiratory function.
  - A pre-filled syringe containing 300 micrograms (0.3 mL adrenaline injection 1 in 1000) can be given to patients at risk of anaphylaxis for immediate self-administration. Make sure that the patient and their family/carers know how and when to use it.

Vasoconstrictor sympathomimetics

Ephedrine

- For reversal of hypotension from spinal or epidural anaesthesia. Slow intravenous injection of a solution containing ephedrine hydrochloride 3 mg/mL, 3–6 mg (maximum 9 mg) repeated every 3–4 minutes to a maximum of 30 mg.

Metaraminol

- For reversal of hypotension from spinal or epidural anaesthesia, 15–100 mg by intravenous infusion, adjusted according to response.
- In emergency, 0.5–5 mg by intravenous injection followed by 15–100 mg by intravenous infusion, adjusted according to response.

Methoxamine

- For reversal of hypotension from spinal or epidural anaesthesia, 5–20 mg by intravenous infusion or slow intravenous injection.

Noradrenaline

- Intravenous infusion, via a central venous catheter, of a solution containing noradrenaline acid tartrate 80 micrograms/mL (equivalent to noradrenaline base 40 micrograms/mL) at an initial rate of 0.16–0.33 mL/minute, adjusted according to response.

TEACHING POINT Treatment of anaphylaxis

- Anaphylaxis is a rare but potentially fatal hypersensitivity reaction to drugs.
- It is IgE-mediated (see also anaphylactoid reactions, p. 625). The IgE crosslinks to mast cells, causing them to degranulate, releasing large amounts of inflammatory mediators, such as histamine. This sets off a cascade that leads to a very rapid inflammatory response, characterized by hypotension, rash, wheeze, and oedema—although not all may be present. This reaction usually occurs shortly after the drug has been given, but delayed reactions have occurred after up to 24 hours. Always think of anaphylaxis if a patient becomes unwell after they have been given a drug.
- The first-line treatment for anaphylaxis is 0.5 mg of adrenaline (0.5 mL of a 1:1000 solution) given by intramuscular injection into the lateral thigh. This can be repeated after 5 minutes, if required. Subcutaneous administration and administration into the arm is not recommended because of unreliable absorption.
- The patient may require cardiovascular support with intravenous fluids.
- Corticosteroids (e.g. 100 mg hydocortisone iv) and antihistamines (e.g. chlorphenamine (Piriton®) 10–20 mg iv) are useful adjunctive treatments, but are not life-saving.
- Do not forget to stop the drug if it is being given by infusion.
- Intravenous adrenaline can cause cardiac ischaemia; it should not be used unless adequate facilities are available (e.g. on the ICU). If it is used, intravenous adrenaline should be given as a dilute solution (e.g. 4 mg in 50 mL of saline), so that the dose can be titrated appropriately.
- Take note of the interactions of adrenaline with tricyclic antidepressants and beta-blockers, outlined above.

TEACHING POINT 'Selectivity'

A drug that is highly selective for a particular receptor subtype will bind to that receptor subtype at a much lower concentration (usually several orders of magnitude) than to other receptor subtypes. An appropriate concentration of drug will stimulate one receptor subtype but not the other. This is easy to achieve in an organ bath, but much less easy in the whole body. As you increase the concentration of a drug in order to achieve a larger effect, effects due to actions of the drug on the other receptor subtype will be seen. This is illustrated below, using a β_2 selective adrenoceptor agonist as an example. At concentration **X** the drug binds only to β_2 adrenoceptors, but the effect (bronchodilatation) is only two-thirds of the maximum. If the patient is very unwell, you will need to increase the dose to increase the bronchodilatation. At this higher concentration (**Y**) the β_1 adrenoceptors are also stimulated, causing tachycardia.

Selectivity is always relative and concentration-dependent. Whether you can achieve selectivity in a patient will depend on your ability to achieve a drug concentration that distinguishes between receptor subtypes in that patient, allowing for interindividual variability in the sensitivities of the different receptor subtypes. This is easier to achieve with an intravenous infusion than oral administration.

Note on 'affinity'. High-affinity drugs bind to receptors at low concentrations. Remember that the overall effect of the drug also depends on the potency of the drug (the ratio of signal to effect) and the interplay of other pharmacological and physiological control mechanisms. High affinity does not always mean that the drug will have a large effect.

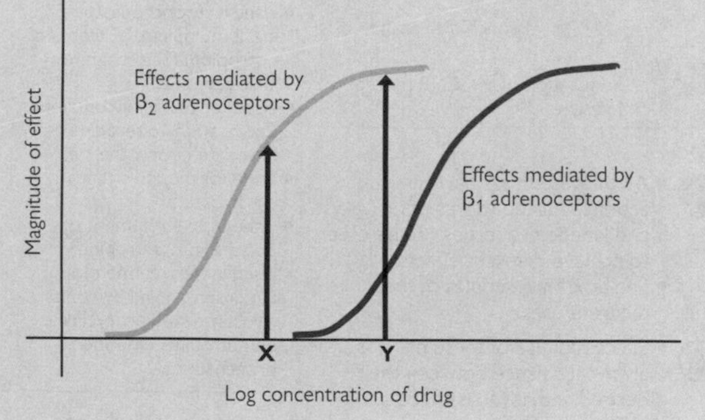

Muscarinic acetylcholine receptor antagonists (atropine and related compounds)

Antagonists at muscarinic acetylcholine receptors

These drugs are direct antagonists at the muscarinic receptor; they therefore have parasympatholytic actions.

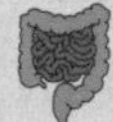
Relaxation of the smooth muscle in the bowel and bladder

Stimulation of bladder sphincter

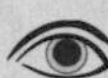
Pupil dilatation

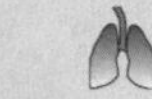
Reduced secretions: sweat, bronchi, mouth

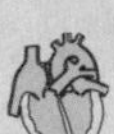
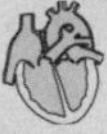
Increased heart rate

Bronchiolar dilatation

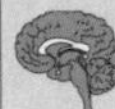
Stimulation of the CNS (except hyoscine)

Drugs in this class

- Used for relaxation of smooth bowel: e.g. hyoscine butylbromide, propantheline bromide, diciclоverine (dicyclomine).
- Used to dilate pupils: e.g. tropicamide, cyclopentolate.
- Used to reduce secretions perioperatively: e.g. atropine, hyoscine (scopolamine).
- Used to reduce secretions in palliative care: e.g. hyoscine hydrobromide and hyoscine butylbromide.
- Used to increase heart rate: e.g. atropine, glycopyrronium.
- Used as bronchodilators: e.g. ipratropium, oxitropium, tiotropium (See separate article, p. 222.)
- Used for urinary incontinence: Oxybutynin, tolterodine, flavoxate, propantheline.
- Used for motion sickness: e.g. hyoscine.
- Used in the treatment of poisoning: e.g. atropine.
- Used in the treatment of Parkinsonism and dystonias: e.g. benzhexol, procyclidine, benzatropine, biperiden, orphenadrine.

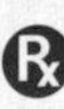

- All of these drugs have similar actions, but the routes of delivery and kinetic properties can be used to achieve different effects.
- See box for examples of the different uses.

- Successful use of these drugs is always a balance between their desired and adverse effects. Whether an effect is considered desired or adverse will depend on the indication.
- Remember the effect that these drugs can have on the heart; avoid them in patients with acute myocardial infarction, hyperthyroidism, or heart failure.
- These drugs are contraindicated in paralytic ileus and pyloric stenosis. Their effects on the bowel also make them unsuitable in gastro-oesophageal reflux disease, ulcerative colitis, and other causes of diarrhoea.
- Avoid them in patients with prostatic enlargement and closed angle glaucoma.
- These drugs should not be given to patients with myasthenia gravis, except to treat acute adverse effects caused by anticholinesterase inhibitors.

- People with Down's syndrome, the elderly, and children are more susceptible to the adverse effects of these drugs.

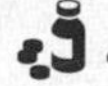

Relaxation of smooth bowel

- The quaternary amines hyoscine butylbromide and propantheline bromide are favoured for this indication. They are less lipid soluble, so cause fewer CNS effects. Because they are less lipid soluble, they are poorly absorbed when given by mouth, so are given parenterally (usually intravenously). Their major use is during radiological investigations to relieve spasm and improve the quality of the examination.
- Dicicloverine, hyoscine butylbromide, and propantheline are orally available drugs that are used to relieve bowel spasm associated with irritable bowel syndrome. Evidence for their efficacy is limited. Other muscarinic antagonists are not recommended, as they have marked systemic adverse effects.

Dilatation of pupils

- Relatively weak antimuscarinic drugs, such as tropicamide and cyclopentolate, are used topically to dilate the pupil as an aid to fundoscopy. Avoid using these drugs if the patient has had a head injury or requires neurological observation.
- Atropine 1% is given as eye drops to dilate the pupil and reduce the incidence of posterior synechiae in patients with uveitis.

Reduction of secretions

- This action of antimuscarinic drugs is useful during surgical procedures and the perioperative period. They can also reduce hypotension caused by anaesthetic drugs such as suxamethonium, halothane, and propofol. Hyoscine (scopolamine) has sedative and antiemetic actions. Make sure that the patient has adequate cardiovascular monitoring when these drugs are given.
- Antimuscarinic drugs are also given to reduce secretions in palliative care.

To increase heart rate (see teaching point below)

- Atropine and glycopyrronium can be used to increase the heart rate in symptomatic bradycardia.
- Do not treat the heart rate alone; if the patient is asymptomatic and has a heart rate above 40 beats per minute, no treatment is usually necessary.
- These drugs are of most use for the temporary bradycardias that can follow myocardial infarction, but a temporary pacemaker may be preferred.

Acute drug-induced dystonias

- Acute dystonias can be caused by antipsychotic, antiemetic, and antidepressant drugs.
- Other risk factors include young age, male sex, use of cocaine, and a history of acute dystonias.

Treatment

- Give biperiden 5 mg or procyclidine 5 mg.
- Intravenous administration is only necessary if the dystonia is life-threatening.
- Intramuscular administration is usually effective within 20 minutes. If it is not effective, second or third injections may be given at half-hour intervals.
- If the patient has an oculogyric crisis that does not respond to anticholinergic drugs, clonazepam 0.5–4 mg iv may be beneficial.
- After the dystonia has resolved, anticholinergic drugs should be given prophylactically for 4–7 days; the dose should be reduced gradually.

- These drugs are not effective in all cases (if the cause is unrelated to the actions of the vagus nerve).
- Urgently investigate the cause of the bradycardia. If the cause is 2nd or 3rd degree heart block, consider inserting a temporary pacing wire. An isoprenaline infusion may be used to stabilize the patient while the wire is inserted (see teaching point below).

Treatment of dystonias and Parkinsonism (especially drug-induced)

- Biperiden can be given parenterally for emergency treatment of acute dystonias. Procyclidine is given to reduce the extrapyramidal adverse effects of antipsychotic drugs. It is not effective for tardive dyskinesia (see antipsychotic drugs, p. 290).
- These drugs (list above) are occasionally used for the treatment of Parkinson's disease, especially in those with mild symptoms in whom tremor predominates. There are no important differences between the drugs that are used for this indication.

Treatment of travel/motion sickness

- Hyoscine hydrobromide is the most effective of the commonly available motion sickness treatments. It is available over the counter. A transdermal patch is also available on prescription. Remember that this needs to be applied several hours before travel and that hyoscine is sedative. Patients may feel drowsy for 24 hours after the patch has been removed. Advise patients not to drive after taking this drug.
- See teaching point in prochlorperazine (p. 67) for more information.

Treatment of poisoning

- Organophosphorus weedkillers and so-called 'nerve agent' gases are irreversible acetylcholinesterase inhibitors. Atropine can be given as an antidote. Take care to avoid exposing yourself to these drugs. Seek advice from the National Poisons Service on decontamination and treatment.
- Acetylcholinesterase inhibitors are given to reverse the effects of non-depolarizing muscle relaxants after anaesthesia (these drugs act on nicotinic acetylcholine receptors). Atropine and glycopyrronium are given to reduce the cardiovascular effects of the acetylcholinesterase inhibitors. Note that atropine has a shorter duration of action than several acetylcholinesterase inhibitors; continue to monitor the heart rate in the recovery room.
- Acetylcholinesterase inhibitors are given for the treatment of myasthenia gravis. These drugs should not be given to patients with myasthenia gravis, except to treat adverse effects of the acetylcholinesterase inhibitors.

Treatment of urinary incontinence

- Antimuscarinic drugs are effective for the treatment of detrusor instability, but not for stress incontinence. Stress incontinence is treated using non-drug methods.
  - Antimuscarinic drugs act by increasing bladder capacity and reducing involuntary contractions of the bladder.
- Adverse effects are common and usually dose-limiting.
- Begin treatment with a low dose and increase gradually to the maximum tolerated.
- The efficacy data are most robust for oxybutynin and tolterodine. Modified-release oxybutynin has similar efficacy to tolterodine.

- Adverse effects are almost inevitable (see above for list of actions).
- The most common are blurred vision, constipation, urinary retention.
- These drugs usually cause tachycardia and 'stimulant' CNS symptoms (confusion, hallucinations, and restlessness), but hyoscine hydrobromide reduces heart rate and causes sedation.
- These drugs reduce sweating; this may interfere with temperature control.

Safety and efficacy

- These drugs are given for short periods for most of their indications, and patients should be closely observed. Measure the patient's heart rate during long-term treatment.

- Many other drugs have antimuscarinic actions. These will be enhanced if the patient is also given an antimuscarinic drug. Drugs with marked antimuscarinic actions include tricyclic antidepressants, some antihistamines, and some antipsychotic drugs.
- These drugs antagonize the actions of some other drugs (e.g. the gastrointestinal effects of metoclopramide and domperidone).
- These drugs cause a dry mouth; this will impede the administration of drugs that are dissolved in the mouth (e.g. sublingual nitrates and 'melt' formulations of other drugs).

- Warn the patient about the common adverse effects of these drugs (see list above).
- Advise the patients that hyoscine hydrobromide can cause sedation, and that they should not drive after taking it.
- Patients who have had their pupils dilated will have blurred vision and should not drive until this has resolved.

Prescribing information: **Muscarinic acetylcholine receptor antagonists**

Atropine for bradycardia associated with anaesthesia (for emergency treatment see box below)

- By intravenous injection, 300–1000 micrograms.
- Increase the dose by 100 micrograms to achieve the desired effect.
- The dose may be repeated after 5 minutes if the initial response is inadequate.
- A dose of 3 mg is given as part of the algorithm for the treatment of non-VF/VT cardiac arrest.

Glycopyrronium for reduction of cardiac effects of acetycholinesterase inhibitors

- By intravenous injection, 200 micrograms per 1 mg of neostigmine.

Hyoscine hydrobromide for motion sickness

- By mouth, 300 micrograms 30 minutes before travel.
- Repeat the dose every 6 hours up to a total daily dose of 900 micrograms.
- This drug is available over the counter.

Palliative care

- Hyoscine **hydrobromide** 0.6–2.4 mg over 24 hours by subcutaneous infusion. This drug reduces respiratory secretions and has a sedative effect.
- Hyoscine **butylbromide** (note different drug and dose) 20–60 mg over 24 hours by subcutaneous infusion. This drug is less effective for secretions but is less sedative and relieves bowel spasm.

Pupil dilatation

- Tropicamide or cyclopentolate 0.5% eye drops, one drop.

Procyclidine for dystonia

- By mouth, 2.5 mg 3 times daily.
- Increased gradually to a usual maximum of 30 mg daily.
- In exceptional circumstances the maximum dose is 60 mg daily.

Biperiden for acute dystonia

- By intramuscular injection, 5 mg.
- See box above for more information.

Treatment of poisoning with insecticides and nerve gases

- Take care to avoid exposing yourself to the poisoning drug.
- Seek expert advice from the National Poisons Service.

Oxybutynin for detrusor instability

- 2.5 mg 2 or 3 times daily.
- Increase gradually to a maximum of 5 mg 4 times daily
- The elderly are more sensitive to the adverse effects of these drugs. Increase the dose more gradually and limit the maximum dose to 5 mg twice daily.
- By mouth, modified–release formulation.
  - Initially 5 mg daily, increased at weekly intervals to 30 mg daily.

Tolterodine for detrusor instability

- By mouth, 2 mg twice daily.
- Reduce the dose to 1 mg twice daily in the elderly.

TEACHING POINT Emergency treatment of bradycardia

- Heart rate is a continuous variable; the absolute rate is not the only factor you should consider. Ask if the heart rate is adequate to perfuse the body and maintain an adequate blood pressure.
- Transient symptomatic bradycardia is common after myocardial infarction. Intermittent atropine treatment is suitable for this, but if there is a less transient cause (e.g. 2nd or 3rd degree heart block) more definitive treatment will be required.

Symptomatic bradycardia

- Atropine is the initial treatment of choice.
  - Give 600–1200 micrograms by intravenous injection.
  - The dose may be repeated after 5 minutes if the initial response is inadequate. The maximum total recommended dose is 3 mg.
- Some patients will not respond; others will have recurrent episodes of bradycardia. These patients should have a temporary transvenous pacing wire inserted.
- This can take time to arrange and insert. If required, start an isoprenaline infusion or begin external cardiac pacing (this is uncomfortable) to support the cardiac output.

Isoprenaline infusion (now seldom used)

- Add isoprenaline 5 mg to 500 mL of dextrose (5%) or isotonic saline.
- Initially, infuse at a rate of 1 mL/min (10 micrograms/min).
- Adjust the rate of infusion to maintain the heart rate above 50 beats per minute.
- Isoprenaline acts on both β_1 and β_2 adrenoceptors; it carries a high risk of arrhythmia and is only suitable for short-term use while more definitive treatment is arranged.

Sildenafil (Viagra®)

Inhibitor of phosphodiesterase type V

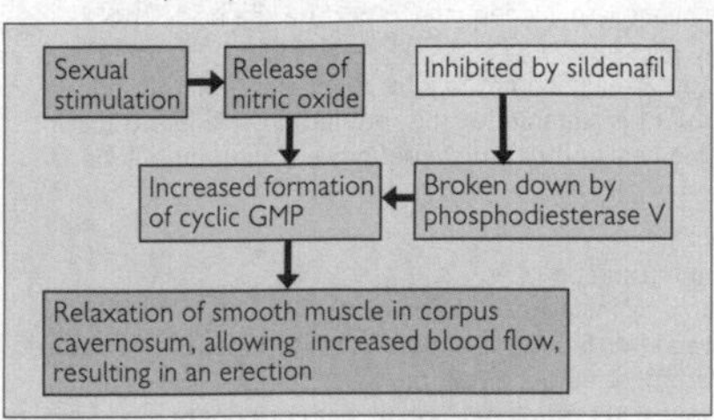

Drugs used to treat erectile dysfunction

- Alprostadil
- Apomorphine
- Sildenafil
- Tadalafil
- Vardenafil

There are restrictions on the prescription of these drugs on the NHS in the UK. See box below.

- Papaverine*
- Phentolamine*

*Unlicensed indication; specialist use only.

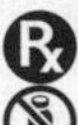

- Treatment of erectile dysfunction.

- Phosphodiesterase inhibitors have the potential to cause cardiovascular effects. Indeed, sildenafil was originally investigated as a potential treatment for angina. Avoid it if the patient has unstable cardiovascular disease, for example, recent myocardial infarction, recent stroke, or hypotension (<95/50 mmHg), is taking nitrate drugs (see below), or if sexual intercourse is inadvisable.
- Avoid sildenafil in patients who are at risk of priapism (leukaemia, multiple myeloma, sickle cell disease).
- Take care if the patient has a physical deformity of the penis (e.g. fibrosis, Peyronie's disease).
- Halve the dose in patients with moderate hepatic insufficiency; avoid it if the insufficiency is severe.
- Patients with renal insufficiency should be given half the usual dose.
- Do not combine drug treatments for erectile dysfunction.
- Sildenafil is taken as a recreational drug by men and women. There is no information about its safety in women who are pregnant.
- Sildenafil should not be given to men with certain inherited retinal disorders (see below).

- Sildenafil requires sexual stimulation in order to work (see mechanism of action).
- Investigate the cause of erectile dysfunction and if possible treat the underlying cause.
- Prescribing of these drugs in the NHS is limited; a specialist assessment is recommended (see box below).
- Begin with a low dose and increase this according to the response.
- Do not continue treatment if there is no response. Seek specialist advice.
- Remember that the patient should not take more than one dose every 24 hours.
- Sildenafil is not currently indicated for women. Remember that sildenafil is a treatment for erectile dysfunction, not an aphrodisiac.

- The most common adverse effects are headache (15% of patients), flushing (10%), and dyspepsia (5%).
- Phosphodiesterase type V is present in the eye. High doses of sildenafil can cause a coloured tinge to the vision. It can also cause painful red eyes.
  - Do not give sildenafil to patients with inherited disorders of phosphodiesterase that cause retinal degeneration.
  - In rare cases sildenafil can cause an increase in intraocular pressure.
- Sildenafil has been associated with cardiovascular events. It has been difficult to establish causality, because the patients in whom it is used are at a high risk of cardiovascular events. Note the cautions listed above before prescribing sildenafil.
- Sildenafil can rarely cause priapism (erection duration >4 hours) (see below for treatment).

- The combination of nitrates (and nicorandil) with sildenafil carries a risk of severe hypotension. Deaths have occurred as a result, and the combination should be avoided.
- Drugs that inhibit cytochrome P450 enzymes (e.g. erythromycin, ritonavir, cimetidine) increase the plasma concentration of sildenafil. Give half the usual dose initially.

Safety and efficacy

- Assess the patient carefully before giving this drug.
- Review the patient and adjust the dose as appropriate.
- Stop the drug if it is not effective.

- Grapefruit juice can increase the plasma concentration of sildenafil; warn the patient to avoid grapefruit juice.
- Advise the patient that the drug should be taken 1 hour before intercourse and that food will delay the onset of action.
- Warn patients for whom you prescribe a nitrate not to take sildenafil — it can be purchased via the internet.

Prescribing information: **Sildenafil**

- By mouth, initial dose 50 mg.
- Can be increased up to 100 mg if required.
- Only one dose to be taken in 24 hours.
- Note the dosage reductions mentioned above.

Safety and efficacy

TEACHING POINT Notes on erectile dysfunction

Causes

- Psychogenic, neurogenic, vascular, endocrine, and drug-induced.
- Drugs commonly cause erectile dysfunction:
  Antihypertensive drugs
  - Especially thiazide diuretics and beta-blockers

  Drugs that act on the CNS
  - Tricyclic antidepressants, SSRIs, antipsychotic drugs
  - Drugs used to treat Parkinson's disease

  Antihistamines
  Opioid drugs
  Cancer chemotherapy drugs
  Antiandrogen drugs (includes spironolactone) and LHRH receptor agonists

Remember that many of the diseases that these drugs are used to treat (e.g. heart failure) also cause erectile dysfunction. Treat the underlying cause whenever possible.

Limitations on prescribing in the NHS

- The UK government recommends that prescribing of drug treatments for erectile dysfunction in the NHS be limited to specialists within hospitals or primary care. The following groups may receive drug treatment for erectile dysfunction in the NHS:
  - Patients with diabetes mellitus, multiple sclerosis, Parkinson's disease, poliomyelitis, prostate cancer, severe pelvic injury, single-gene neurological disease, spina bifida, or spinal cord injury
  - Patients receiving dialysis for renal insufficiency
  - Patients who have had radical pelvic surgery, prostatectomy, kidney transplantation
  - Patients suffering severe distress, with disruption to normal social and occupational activities, a marked effect on mood, and disruption of interpersonal relationships

TEACHING POINT Treatment of priapism

- This is defined as an erection that persists for longer than 4 hours.
- Seek expert surgical advice.
- Try cooling the penis using ice packs, but do not apply ice directly to the skin.
- Consider aspiration using a 19–21 gauge butterfly needle inserted into the corpus cavernosum. Aspirate 20–50 mL of blood carefully.
- If this is unsuccessful, consider intracavernosal injections of very small amounts of a sympathomimetic, such as adrenaline.
  - This must be done very carefully, because systemic exposure to the drug can cause severe vasoconstriction in the coronary and cerebral vessels.
- Inject **10–20 micrograms** of adrenaline into the corpus cavernosum.
  - To do this, **dilute 0.1 mL of the 1:1000 adrenaline in 5 mL of isotonic saline**; inject only 0.5–1 mL at a time (10–20 micrograms).
- The injection can be repeated after 5-10 minutes. If this is unsuccessful, refer the patient for emergency surgical intervention.

Drugs that can cause priapism

- Alprostadil
- Apomorphine
- Chlorpromazine
- Heparin
- Hydralazine
- Papaverine
- Phentolamine
- Sildenafil
- Trazodone

Chapter 3

Respiratory system

Contents

Oxygen

An essential element

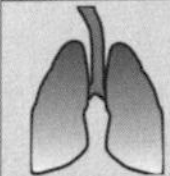

- Oxygen is an essential requirement for aerobic tissue respiration.
- Delivery depends on adequate ventilation, gas exchange, and circulatory distribution. A failure of any one of these causes tissue hypoxia and irreversible damage within 4 minutes.

Respiratory failure

A general term that describes ineffective gas exchange across the lungs by the respiratory system. The arterial blood gas measurement should be used to determine the presence of respiratory failure. A PaO_2 <8.0 kPa and/or $PaCO_2$ >6.6 kPa indicates respiratory failure.

- **Type I respiratory failure** is characterized by hypoxaemia with a low or normal $PaCO_2$. Examples of diseases that cause this pattern include pneumonia, and pulmonary embolism.
- **Type II respiratory failure** is characterized by hypoxaemia with a high $PaCO_2$. The most common cause of this pattern is chronic obstructive pulmonary disease.
- Do not forget non-respiratory causes of hypoxaemia; for example:
  - Reduced capacity of the blood due to anaemia.
  - Right to left shunting of blood in Eisenmenger's syndrome.
  - Low inhaled oxygen concentration at high altitude.

- Oxygen is indicated for the acute treatment of arterial hypoxaemia from any cause. Oxygen should be given if the PaO_2 falls below 8.0 kPa. Examples include:
  - Acute asthma
  - Acute myocardial infarction
  - Sickle cell crisis
  - Carbon monoxide poisoning
  - Venous thromboembolism
  - Fibrosing alveolitis
- Long-term oxygen therapy should also be considered for some patients with chronic hypoxaemia (see below).
- Oxygen is a drug and should be prescribed.

- Do not give oxygen near a naked flame or cigarette; there is a risk of explosion.
- Oxygen must be given in a controlled manner if the patient has type II respiratory failure (chronic obstructive pulmonary disease). See below for more information.

- Oxygen therapy can be life saving, but remember that it is not usually a specific treatment for the underlying cause of the hypoxaemia; treat this as well.
- Oxygen can be given by a simple face mask or nasal cannulae, but the inspired oxygen fraction varies with the rate and depth of the patient's respiration; whenever possible use a face mask with a Venturi attachment so that the inspired concentration of oxygen can be regulated precisely.
  - Nasal cannulae may deliver a lower than expected inspired concentration of oxygen if the patient breathes through the mouth.

- If a high concentration of oxygen is required, use a mask fitted with a reservoir. It is not usually possible to deliver an inspired concentration of oxygen that is consistently above 60% without assisted ventilation (continuous positive airways pressure (CPAP) ventilation or mechanical ventilation).
- Long-term oxygen therapy prolongs life in some patients with chronic hypoxia due to chronic obstructive pulmonary disease. The patient must be stable when assessed (not sooner than 4 weeks after an exacerbation), and arterial blood gas tensions should be measured on two occasions at least 3 weeks apart, while the patient is breathing air. Long-term oxygen therapy should be considered if:
  - The arterial P_aO_2 is less than 7.3 kPa.
  - The arterial P_aO_2 is 7.3–8 kPa and the patient has polycythaemia or evidence of pulmonary hypertension.
- Long-term oxygen therapy should also be considered for patients with:
  - Pulmonary malignancy with disabling dyspnoea.
  - Heart failure with a daytime P_aO_2 less than 7.3 kPa.
  - Other lung diseases (e.g. cystic fibrosis, interstitial lung disease) with hypoxaemia. Seek specialist advice.

- At high concentrations oxygen is toxic to tissues. Inspiration of a high concentration of oxygen (>80%) for more than 24 hours can cause tracheobronchitis and parenchymal lung damage. Use the lowest concentration of oxygen that maintains the patient's arterial oxygen concentration in the target range.
- Patients who have type II respiratory failure are chronically hypoxic. The rate and depth of their ventilatory effort is principally determined by the arterial oxygen concentration, rather than the carbon dioxide concentration (as it is in healthy people). If they are given a high inspired concentration of oxygen their respiratory effort will be suppressed. The arterial concentration of carbon dioxide rises and the patient becomes narcosed and may become apnoeic.

Oxygen delivery systems

Method	Flow rate	Inspired oxygen concentration
Low-flow mask*	6–10 L/min	Up to 60%
Nasal prongs*	1–2 L/min	24–30%
High-flow, jet-mixing (Venturi) mask	Depends on the equipment	24–60%
Non-rebreathing reservoir mask		Up to 90%
Anaesthetic face mask or endotracheal tube		Up to 100%

*Note that the inspired concentration delivered by these methods depends on the ventilatory minute volume.

Suggestions for initial oxygen dose

• Caridac or respiratory arrest	100%
• Hypoxaemia with $PaCO_2$ <5.3 kPa	40–60%
• Hypoxaemia with $PaCO_2$ >5.3 kPa	24% initially

- Patients with type II respiratory failure must be given oxygen by a method that allows the inspired concentration to be controlled (e.g. by mask with a Venturi attachment). If they are given unregulated oxygen (e.g. nasal cannulae, standard face mask), the inspired concentration of oxygen increases as the patient's ventilatory effort falls, producing a vicious circle leading to narcosis and apnoea.
  - These patients should usually be given either 24% or 28% oxygen, depending on their requirements and sensitivity to the increase in inspired oxygen concentration.
  - Remember that these patients are chronically hypoxic; it is unnecessary and potentially hazardous to try to raise their arterial oxygen concentration to normal. Take expert advice, but an oxygen saturation of around 85% may be adequate.
  - Not all patients with chronic obstructive airways disease have type II respiratory failure. Progressive severe narcosis from a high inspired concentration of oxygen can be avoided if the patient is monitored clinically and with arterial blood gas measurements. If you see a patient who is hypoxic and you do not know whether they have type II respiratory failure or not, give them enough oxygen to raise their arterial oxygen concentration to normal, but do not leave them unattended and measure their arterial blood gas concentrations.

Safety and efficacy

- In many circumstances pulse oximetry is adequate to monitor oxygen therapy. However, it is not suitable in the following circumstances:
  - *Carbon monoxide poisoning* The oximeter cannot distinguish oxyhaemoglobin from carboxyhaemoglobin, so the meter reading is misleading. Measure the arterial blood gas and carboxyhaemoglobin concentration. This is also true for methaemoglobinaemia.
  - *Type II respiratory failure* The pulse oximeter will measure arterial oxygenation, but it is also essential to know the arterial carbon dioxide concentration; this requires measurement of arterial blood gas concentrations.
- An oxygen saturation of 93% is approximately equivalent to an arterial oxygen concentration of 8 kPa. The oxygen concentration in blood falls rapidly at saturations below 92% because the steep part of the haemoglobin oxygen dissociation curve lies below this value.
  - Unless the patient is known to have structural lung disease, the oxygen saturation should always be above 92% and ideally should be 100%.
  - If a patient has acute asthma and the oxygen saturation falls below 92% at any time, this is an indication for assessment in the ICU; it signals that the patient is tiring or that current treatment is ineffective.
- Oxygen therapy should be stopped when arterial oxygenation is adequate with the patient breathing room air (PaO_2 >8 kPa; SaO_2 >90%), so long as the acid base status and clinical assessment is consistent with adequate tissue oxygenation.

- Warn the patient of the dangers of oxygen and naked flames. Ensure that no one in the room smokes while oxygen is in use. Patients with arterial hypoxaemia should discuss their requirements with the airline well in advance of any proposed travel.

Prescribing information: **Oxygen**

Acute oxygen therapy

- Specify the target oxygen saturation, range of inspired oxygen concentrations allowed, and mode of delivery.

Long-term oxygen therapy

- Oxygen concentrators are more economical for long-term treatment.
- The components of the system and accessories (e.g. face mask, humidifier) need to be prescribed. In the UK each region has an appointed supplier who will need to be contacted. Seek advice from a respiratory specialist or your health authority if you are considering long-term oxygen therapy.

Pharmacology of drugs used to treat asthma

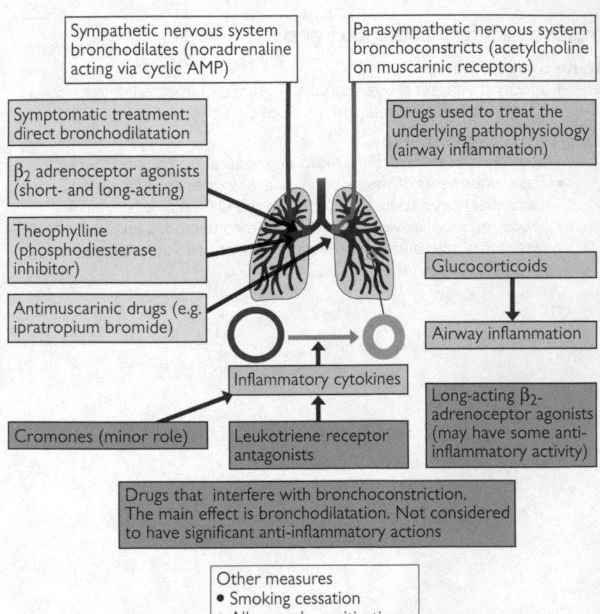

Guidelines for the treatment of asthma

- Global Initiative for Asthma (GINA)
  - *http://www.ginasthma.com/*
- British Thoracic Society/Scottish Intercollegiate Guidelines Network
  - *http://www.brit-thoracic.org.uk/sign/index.htm*

An approach to the treatment of COPD

- Global Initiative for Chronic Obstructive Lung Disease (GOLD). Guidelines at *http://www.goldcopd.com/*
- COPD is characterized by airflow limitation that is not fully reversible.
- Lung function tests show that:
  - FEV_1/FVC is less than 70%.
  - Post-bronchodilator FEV_1 is less than 80% of predicted.
- The most common cause of the inflammation that leads to COPD is exposure to tobacco smoke, although occupational exposures can also be important.
- The hallmark of COPD is a relentless and progressive decline in lung function owing to inflammation of the airways. None of the current drug therapies prevents this and so drug therapy is directed at reducing symptoms and complications.
- Smoking cessation is the only strategy that reduces this decline in lung function and must be a key treatment goal. See nicotine (p. 236) for advice on smoking cessation.

Symptomatic treatments

- Inhaled bronchodilating muscarinic receptor antagonists and β_2 adrenoceptor agonists are the mainstays of treatment
  - Long-acting inhaled β_2 adrenoceptor agonists are more effective and convenient than short-acting ones, but are more expensive.
- Theophylline is used as an additional bronchodilator in patients with more severe disease; it may have some anti-inflammatory action.
- Inhaled corticosteroids are not very effective and are only recommended in those with a FEV_1 less than 50% of predicted.
  - Recent studies with combination inhalers (corticosteroid + long-acting β_2 adrenoceptor agonists) have shown some benefit.
  - Avoid chronic treatment with systemic corticosteroids; the benefit/harm balance is unfavourable.

Other treatments

- Oxygen therapy has an important role in severe disease; see oxygen (p. 208) for more information.
- Patients with COPD should be vaccinated yearly against influenza to reduce the frequency of exacerbations.
- There is little evidence of benefit from mucolytic treatments.
- Antioxidant treatments may have a role, but this is still being evaluated.
- Cough may be a troublesome symptom, but is an important mechanism of mucus clearance; avoid the use of antitussives.
- Respiratory stimulants are not useful in the chronic treatment of COPD. See doxapram (p. 234) for more information.

Short-acting β_2 adrenoceptor agonists

Selective agonists at β_2 adrenoceptors

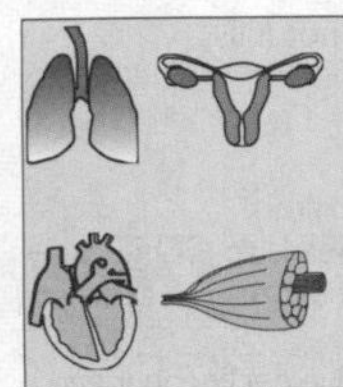

Agonist action at β_2 receptors has a number of actions (see adrenoceptor agonists, (p. 190). The clinically important actions are bronchodilatation and relaxation of the uterus. When used at higher doses, β_2 selectivity is lost, resulting in tachycardia and tremor

Drugs in this class

Used for relief or bronchospasm
- Salbutamol
- Terbutaline

Others
- Bambuterol
- Fenoterol
- Rimiterol

There are no important differences among these drugs. Salbutamol and terbutaline are the most commonly used.

Used to inhibit premature labour
- Salbutamol
- Ritodrine

- Relief of bronchospasm, both acute and chronic.
- Tocolytic (to halt premature labour).

- There are no specific contraindications.
- Allergy to short-acting β_2 agonists is rare.
- These drugs can be used for the relief of reversible airways obstruction in patients with COPD. The reversible component of this disease is often small, so these drugs will be limited in their effect. When the patient is well, perform lung function tests and determine the degree of reversibility.
- These drugs may be used during pregnancy. Note the tocolytic actions.
- No dosage adjustment is usually required in hepatic or renal insufficiency.

Acute bronchospasm
- Nebulized therapy is used most commonly, but a metered-dose inhaler (MDI) with a large-volume spacer device (e.g. 500 mL) can be used. See teaching point below for guidance on the treatment of acute asthma. See ipratropium (p. 225) for more information on large-volume spacer devices.
- Advantages of nebulized therapy:
  - Allows simultaneous oxygen therapy to be given.
  - Allows high doses to be given.
  - Allows continuous therapy, if required.
- Also available for intravenous/subcutaneous use in severe cases (in the ICU).

Chronic asthma
- An MDI is the most cost-effective initial choice.
  - Advise the patient to use it as required.
  - Monitor use and adjust therapy accordingly (see British Thoracic Society/Scottish Intercollegiate Guidelines Network Guidelines for details; *http://www.brit-thoracic.org.uk/sign/index.htm*).
  - Administration via a large-volume spacer reduces systemic exposure and increases the proportion delivered to the lungs.
  - β_2 adrenoceptor agonists are also available in a number of patented delivery devices and in dry-powder formulations. These may be suitable for patients who are unable to use an MDI correctly, but they are more expensive.
  - Ensuring that patients can use their inhalers correctly is very important; see long-acting β_2 agonists (p. 221) for the correct method.

- These drugs are available as combination inhalers with inhaled muscarinic antagonists. These inhalers may be convenient, but should only be used if the patient requires both drugs regularly and has previously been stabilized on a dosage regimen that is deliverable by the combination inhaler. See misoprostol (p. 31) for a discussion of the advantages and disadvantages of combination formulations.

Tocolytic
- Only initiate under specialist supervision. These drugs are given by intravenous infusion.
- These drugs are indicated for the inhibition of uncomplicated labour between 24 and 33 weeks.
- The greatest benefit is probably to allow time for corticosteroids to be given, and for transfer to a specialist unit.
- Alternatives include an oxytocin receptor antagonist (atosiban) or an NSAID (indometacin). Seek specialist advice.

Early
- The doses delivered by MDIs cause adverse effects only rarely. Nebulizers deliver much higher doses; a considerable proportion is absorbed through the nasal and buccal mucosae and is swallowed and absorbed. Selectivity at receptors is always relative; the large doses delivered by nebulizers or intravenously can cause tremor and tachycardia. In some patients, such as those with ischaemic heart disease, these drugs can cause tachyarrhythmias by actions on β_1 adrenoceptors.
- Note that nebulizer solutions are acidic and can cause paroxysmal bronchospasm rarely.

Late
- Increasing use of bronchodilators is a warning of worsening asthma. Review therapy before there is a crisis.

- Take care with other sympathomimetic drugs. Some of these (e.g. ephedrine) are available over the counter, and may be a component of some herbal remedies.

Efficacy
- Use peak expiratory flow rate (PEFR), pulse rate, and respiratory rate to guide the frequency of administration.

- Short-acting β_2 agonists only relieve the symptoms of asthma; they do nothing for the underlying pathology. In contrast, corticosteroids alter the course of the disease. Patients should be told that the short-acting adrenoceptor agonists are 'relievers' and that corticosteroids are 'preventers', in order to stress the different roles of these drugs in the treatment of asthma.
- Ensure that the patient knows how to use an inhaler device correctly. Ask them to show you how they use it. See long-acting β_2 agonists (p. 221) for correct inhaler technique.
- Ensure that the patient has a 'rescue plan' in case their symptoms worsen or they become unwell. Patients should be warned to seek medical help if they find that they need increasing doses of inhaled drugs to relieve symptoms.

Prescribing information: **Short-acting β_2 adrenoceptor agonists**

Salbutamol is given as an example

- *Aerosol inhalation* 100–200 micrograms (1–2 puffs) taken as required; for persistent symptoms up to 3–4 times daily. Review use regularly in those with increasing requirements.
  - Also available in CFC-free inhalers; warn patients that these may feel and taste different from their previous inhaler.
- Available in a number of dry-powder formats. Refer to the individual manufacturers' recommendations for correct use.
- *Inhalation of nebulized solution* Severe acute asthma, 2.5 mg or 5 mg, repeated as required to control symptoms. Review the treatment and clinical progress regularly.
  - Also used for chronic bronchospasm unresponsive to conventional therapy; seek specialist advice before starting long-term nebulizer therapy.
- *Intravenous infusion*
  - *Acute asthma* Specialized use. Ensure adequate supervision and monitoring. Usually reserved for use in high dependency/intensive care units. Initially, 5 micrograms/minute, adjusted according to response and heart rate; usually in the range 3–20 micrograms/minute.
  - *Treatment of premature labour* Specialized use. Initially, 10 micrograms/minute, rate increased gradually according to response at 10-minute intervals until contractions diminish, then increase the rate slowly until contractions cease (maximum rate 45 micrograms/minute); maintain rate for 1 hour after contractions have stopped, then gradually reduce by 50% every 6 hours; then by mouth, 4 mg every 6–8 hours.

TEACHING POINT Treatment of acute severe asthma in adults

(Also see British Thoracic Society/Scottish Intercollegiate Guidelines Network guidelines *http://www.brit-thoracic.org.uk/sign/index.htm*)

Features of acute severe asthma include: PEFR <33% of best, a respiratory rate >25 breaths/min, heart rate >100 beats/min, patient unable to complete sentences in one breath, a normal or high P_aCO_2.

- Give high-flow oxygen; nebulized therapy should be driven using oxygen.
- Give a short-acting β_2 agonist by nebulizer (e.g 2.5–5 mg salbutamol). If a nebulizer is not available, use a metered-dose inhaler with a spacer device. Adjust the frequency of administration according to the response. If the PEFR is below 50%, continuous therapy may be required initially.
- Give ipratropium bromide by nebulizer (0.5 mg every 4–6 hours).
- Give systemic steroids (e.g. hydrocortisone 100 mg iv). Make sure that you repeat the dose every 6–8 hours until the patient can take treatment by mouth (e.g. 40–50 mg prednisolone daily for at least 5 days).
- The routine administration of antibiotics is not recommended.

If the response to these initial treatments is poor seek expert advice; consider giving magnesium sulfate (1.2–2.0 g over 20 minutes by intravenous infusion).

Refer the patient for assessment by ICU if any of the following features are present:

- Poor respiratory effort/exhaustion (includes drowsiness and confusion).
- Worsening PEFR despite treatment.
- Arterial blood gas measurements show hypercapnia, hypoxia, or acidosis.

Long-acting β_2 adrenoceptor agonists

Selective agonists at β_2 adrenoceptors

- Like their short-acting counterparts, these drugs are selective agonists at β_2 adrenoceptors. They bind with high affinity and remain bound, resulting in a long duration of action. There is a debate as to whether these drugs have any clinically important anti-inflammatory action. In vitro this may be so, but it is important that patients understand that these drugs are for the relief of symptoms rather than prevention of disease.

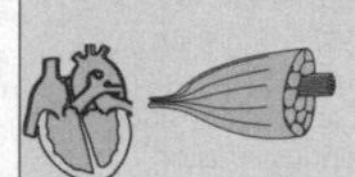

- These drugs are not usually used in high doses, but if they are β_2 selectivity is lost, resulting in tachycardia and tremor.

Drugs in this class

- Salmeterol
- Formoterol

Salmeterol has an onset of action that is slower than that of formoterol.

- Relief of chronic bronchospasm

- These drugs take too long to act to have a role in the treatment of acute asthma (see short-acting β_2 agonists, p. 214).
- These drugs can be used for the relief of reversible airways obstruction in patients with COPD. The reversible component of this disease is often small, so these drugs will be limited in their effect. When the patient is well, perform lung function tests and determine the degree of reversibility.
- β_2 agonists have tocolytic actions. Avoid these drugs in pregnancy unless the benefit outweighs the risk (see short-acting β_2 agonists, p. 214).
- No dosage adjustment is usually required in hepatic or renal insufficiency.

Chronic asthma

- The addition of a long-acting β_2 agonist is recommended in adults who have an inadequate response to low-dose inhaled steroids (equivalent of 200–400 micrograms beclomethasone daily).
  - Stage 3 of the British Thoracic Society/Scottish Intercollegiate Guidelines Network guidelines; *http://www.brit-thoracic.org.uk/sign/index.htm*
- If the response is inadequate, increase the dosage of inhaled steroid (equivalent of 800 micrograms beclomethasone daily).
- These drugs suppress symptoms, but steroid therapy should not be withdrawn as its anti-inflammatory action is still required for long-term control.
- These drugs are subject to a degree of tolerance, owing to agonist-induced receptor downregulation. Symptom control is usually maintained in chronic asthma, but it can reduce the efficacy of short-acting β_2 agonists if the patient has an acute deterioration.
  - This effect can be mitigated by giving intravenous steroids. In addition to their genomic actions, which take time to occur, they increase the numbers of adrenoceptors on the surfaces of cells.

- A metered-dose inhaler is the most cost-effective initial choice.
  - Administration via a large-volume spacer reduces systemic exposure and increases the proportion delivered to the lungs.
  - Long-acting β_2 adrenoceptor agonists are also available in a number of patented delivery devices and in dry-powder formulations. These may be suitable for patients unable to use an MDI correctly, but they are more expensive.
  - Ensuring that patients can use their inhalers correctly is very important; see over for the correct method.
  - These drugs are available as combination inhalers with inhaled corticosteroids. These inhalers may be convenient but should only be used if the patient requires both drugs and has previously been stabilized on a dosage regimen that is deliverable by the combination inhaler. See misoprostol (p. 31) for a discussion of the advantages and disadvantages of combination formulations.

Early

- The doses delivered by MDIs cause adverse effects only rarely.
  - Selectivity at receptors is always relative, so avoid large doses of these drugs, which can cause tremor and tachycardia. In some patients, such as those with ischaemic heart disease, these drugs can cause tachyarrhythmias by actions on β_1 adrenoceptors.
- Note that these drugs can cause paroxysmal bronchospasm rarely.

Late

- Increasing need for bronchodilators is a warning of worsening asthma. Review therapy before there is a crisis.

- Take care with other sympathomimetic drugs. Some of these (e.g. ephedrine) are available over the counter and may be components of some herbal remedies.

Efficacy

- Use PEFR and symptom scores to assess the effectiveness of your treatment regimen.
  - For example, ask whether asthma symptoms interfere with sleep or daily activities and whether the patient has symptoms every day.

- Long-acting β_2 agonists should not be used for acute symptoms.
- Ensure that the patient also has a short-acting β_2 agonist inhaler for use as required.
- Ensure that the patient knows how to use an inhaler device correctly.
- Ensure that the patient has a 'rescue plan' in case their symptoms worsen or they become unwell. Patients should be warned to seek medical help if they find that they need increasing doses of inhaled drugs to relieve symptoms.

Prescribing information: **Long-acting β_2 adrenoceptor agonists**

Salmeterol

- *Aerosol inhalation* 50 micrograms (2 puffs) bd taken regularly. Can be increased to 100 micrograms bd, if required.

Formoterol

- *Dry powder inhalation* 12 micrograms bd taken regularly. Can be increased to 24 micrograms bd, if required.

TEACHING POINT Correct use of a metered-dose inhaler

- Remove the cap from the mouthpiece and shake the inhaler vigorously.
- If you haven't used the inhaler for a week or more, or if it is the first time you have used it, spray it into the air first to check that it works.
- Sit up straight or stand up and lift the chin to open the airways.
- Take a few deep breaths and then breathe out gently. Immediately place the mouthpiece in your mouth and put your teeth around it (not in front of it and do not bite it), and seal your lips around the mouthpiece, holding it between your lips.
- Start to breathe in slowly and deeply through the mouthpiece. As you breathe in, simultaneously press down on the inhaler canister to release the medicine. One press releases one puff of medicine.
- Continue to breathe in deeply to ensure that the medicine gets into your lungs.
- Hold your breath for 10 seconds or for as long as you comfortably can, before breathing out slowly.
- If you need to take another puff, wait for 30 seconds, shake your inhaler again, then repeat the previous five steps.
- Replace the cap on the mouthpiece.

Bronchodilatory muscarinic receptor antagonists

Antagonists at muscarinic acetylcholine receptors

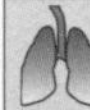

- The parasympathetic nervous system has a tonic bronchoconstricting action in the lungs. Therefore antagonists at muscarinic receptors have a bronchodilatory action. Systemic administration of anticholinergic drugs causes many adverse effects (see atropine, p. 196). These drugs are antagonists at M_2 and M_3 muscarinic receptors and are delivered directly to the lungs by inhalation. In addition, they are highly polar molecules; this reduces systemic absorption and associated adverse effects.
- The degree of bronchodilatation caused by these drugs is less than that from β_2 agonists. However, the relative contribution of the cholinergic system in COPD is greater than that in asthma. These drugs can therefore be particularly useful for symptomatic relief in COPD.

Drugs in this class

- Ipratropium
- Oxitropium
- Tiotropium

These drugs have different onsets of action. See text.

- Relief of acute and chronic bronchospasm.

- These drugs take time to act. However, they have a role in the treatment of acute bronchospasm, but must be used in conjunction with short-acting β_2 agonists.
- They can be used for the relief of reversible airways obstruction in patients with COPD. The reversible component of this disease is often small, so they will be limited in their effect. When the patient is well, perform lung function tests and determine the degree of reversibility.
- Although systemic exposure with these drugs is limited, take care in patients with urinary retention or closed-angle glaucoma.
- Not known to be harmful in pregnancy.
- No dosage adjustment is usually required in hepatic or renal insufficiency.

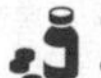

Chronic asthma

- Muscarinic receptor antagonists are indicated at Stage 4 of the British Thoracic Society guidelines for the treatment of chronic asthma. At this stage, the choice of additional treatment should be made by a specialist. There are several other options (long-acting β_2 agonists, leukotriene antagonists, methylxanthines). The most appropriate choice will depend on the individual's symptoms and disease (British Thoracic Society/Scottish Intercollegiate Guidelines Network guidelines; *http://www.brit-thoracic.org.uk/sign/index.htm*).
- These drugs suppress symptoms, but steroid therapy should not be withdrawn as its anti-inflammatory action is still required for long-term control.
- An MDI is the most cost-effective initial choice.
  - Administration via a large-volume spacer reduces systemic exposure and increases the proportion delivered to the lungs.

- Muscarinic receptor antagonists are also available in a number of patented delivery devices and in dry-powder formulations. These may be suitable for patients unable to use an MDI correctly, but they are more expensive.
- Ensuring that patients can use their inhalers correctly is very important; see long-acting β_2 agonists (p. 221) for the correct method.
- These drugs are available as combination inhalers with inhaled β_2 agonists. These inhalers may be convenient, but should only be used if the patient requires both drugs regularly and has previously been stabilized on a dosage regimen that is deliverable by the combination inhaler. See misoprostol (p. 31) for a discussion of the advantages and disadvantages of combination formulations.

Acute bronchospasm

- These drugs have a role in the treatment of acute bronchospasm. However, because they take time to act and cause less bronchodilatation than β_2 agonists, they should not be given on their own.
- Nebulized therapy is used most commonly, but an MDI with a large-volume spacer device can be used. See short-acting β_2 agonists (p. 217) for guidance on the treatment of acute asthma. See below for more information on large-volume spacer devices.
- Because the parasympathetic nervous system exerts a tonic action, there is little advantage to giving these drugs more often than 6 hourly.

COPD

- The contribution of the parasympathetic nervous system to bronchospasm in this disease is said to be greater than that in asthma. These drugs can therefore be particularly useful in patients with COPD.
- Nevertheless, much of the lung damage in COPD is irreversible, and drugs may be limited in their effects.

Onset and duration of action of bronchodilatory muscarinic receptor antagonists	
Ipratropium and oxitropium	Onset of action is over 30–60 minutes. Duration of action 3–6 hours. Usually given 3 times daily.
Tiotropium	Onset of action is over 30–60 minutes. Duration of action 24 hours. Usually given once daily.

Early

- The doses delivered by MDIs cause adverse effects only rarely.
  - These drugs can cause systemic anticholinergic adverse effects (e.g. blurred vision, dry mouth, urinary retention, glaucoma).
  - Note that these drugs can cause paroxysmal bronchospasm rarely.

Late

- Increasing use of bronchodilators is a warning of worsening asthma. Review therapy before there is a crisis.

- Take care with other anticholinergic drugs; these may potentiate the systemic adverse effects of these drugs.

Efficacy
- Use PEFR and symptom scores to assess the effectiveness of your treatment regimen.

- Muscarinic receptor antagonists should not be used alone for acute symptoms.
- Ensure that the patient also has a short-acting β_2 agonist inhaler for use as required.
- Ensure that the patient knows how to use an inhaler device correctly. Ask them to show you how they use the inhaler. See long-acting β_2 agonists (p. 221) for more information.
- Ensure that the patient has a 'rescue plan' in case their symptoms worsen or they become unwell. Patients should be warned to seek medical help if they find that they need increasing doses of inhaled drugs to relieve symptoms.

Prescribing information: **Bronchodilatory muscarinic receptor antagonists**

Ipratropium bromide
- *Aerosol inhalation* 20–40 micrograms (1–2 puffs) tds taken regularly.
  - May be increased to a maximum of 80 micrograms qds, if required.
  - Ensure that the patient derives additional benefit from higher dosages as they are more likely to cause adverse effects.

Tiotropium
- Delivered by proprietary dry-powder device; 18 micrograms once daily (delivered dose is 10 micrograms).

TEACHING POINT Large-volume spacer devices

- Metered-dose inhalers are the most cost-effective delivery devices, but only 7–20% of the delivered dose reaches the lungs. About 80% is deposited in the oropharynx. Any drug in the oropharynx will not improve symptoms, but it can be systemically absorbed and cause adverse effects (e.g. urinary retention from muscarinic receptor antagonists, fungal infection in the oropharynx from steroids).
- A large-volume spacer device offers several benefits:
  - It provides a holding chamber so that the patient does not have to breathe in at the very instant of pressing the metered-dose inhaler.
  - The jet of drug is delivered into the chamber and the aerosol is inhaled, rather than the jet of drug hitting the back of the throat. It is well established that the proportion of drug delivered to the lungs is increased when a large-volume spacer device is used.
  - Large particles that would not reach the lungs are deposited in the spacer device rather than in the oropharyx.
  - Any regular medication, especially inhaled corticosteroids, should be given via a large-volume spacer device.
- These devices are bulky and may be difficult to carry around all day. Advise the patient to use the large-volume spacer at home for their regular medication. If they are out, an extension device (a smaller alternative) will slow the aerosol jet and improve delivery to the lungs, but not as effectively as a large-volume spacer.
- Some patients cannot manage metered-dose inhalers despite adequate instruction. There are proprietary devices and dry-powder devices that may be easier to use. Remember that these are considerably more expensive, and deposition on the oropharynx with dry-powder devices is still around 60%. Reserve them for patients who really cannot manage a metered-dose inhaler.
- Large volume spacer devices can accumulate static charge, causing too much drug to stick to their sides. Advise the patient to wash the device every 4 weeks with washing-up liquid, and allow it to dry without wiping. Large-volume spacers should be replaced every 6–12 months.

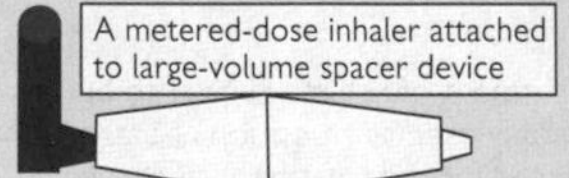

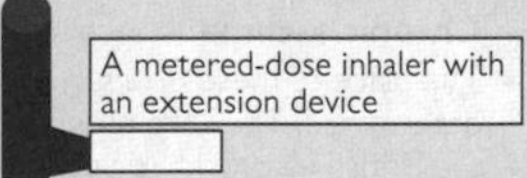

Leukotriene receptor antagonists

Antagonists at leukotriene LTC_4, LTD_4, and LTE_4 receptors

Drugs in this class
- Montelukast
- Zafirlukast

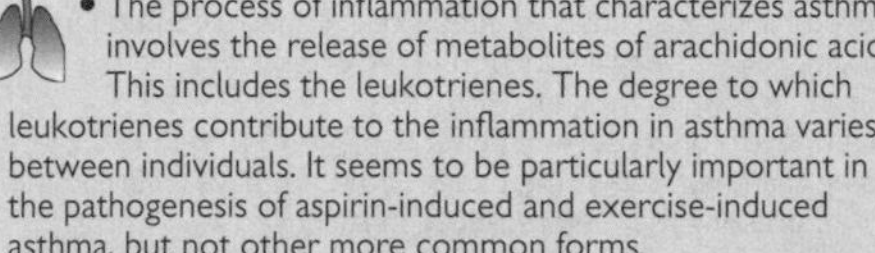

- The process of inflammation that characterizes asthma involves the release of metabolites of arachidonic acid. This includes the leukotrienes. The degree to which leukotrienes contribute to the inflammation in asthma varies between individuals. It seems to be particularly important in the pathogenesis of aspirin-induced and exercise-induced asthma, but not other more common forms.
- These drugs are antagonists of the leukotrienes LTC_4, LTD_4, and LTE_4. They are helpful in the control of chronic asthma, but they are less effective than corticosteroids. Whether they can be considered truly anti-inflammatory is a subject of debate. At present they should be considered as 'relievers'.

- Prophylaxis of asthma.

- These drugs take time to act and have no role in the treatment of acute asthma; see short-acting β_2 agonists (p. 217).
- These drugs are not currently licensed for the relief of reversible airways obstruction in patients with COPD. The reversible component of this disease is often small, so they are likely to be limited in their effect.
- No dosage adjustment is usually required in mild renal insufficiency.
- Evidence is limited in hepatic insufficiency; avoid in patients with established cirrhosis.
- These drugs have not been shown to be safe in pregnancy; avoid giving them unless essential.

Chronic asthma

- The place of these drugs in the treatment of asthma has yet to be determined. They are most commonly used as an option at Stage 4 of the British Thoracic Society guidelines for the treatment of chronic asthma. At this stage, the choice of additional treatment should be made by a specialist. There are several other options (long-acting β_2 agonists, muscarinic antagonists, methylxanthines). The most appropriate choice will depend on the individual's symptoms and disease (British Thoracic Society/Scottish Intercollegiate Guidelines Network guidelines; *http://www.brit-thoracic.org.uk/sign/index.htm*).
- Leukotriene antagonists suppress symptoms, but steroid therapy should not be withdrawn as its anti-inflammatory action is still required for long-term control.
- Unlike other treatments for asthma, these drugs are given by mouth. This may be convenient, but they should not be used in preference to other treatments that have better-established efficacy.
- Leukotriene antagonists have not been shown to be steroid-sparing (CSM advice).

- These drugs are usually well tolerated but can cause gastrointestinal disturbance.

- Churg–Strauss syndrome.
  - This syndrome, characterized by asthma, a systemic eosinophilic vasculitis, rhinitis, and sinusitis, has been associated with the use of these drugs. It is not clear whether they are the cause or whether they unmask existing disease. Nevertheless, a causative effect has not been excluded and precautions must be taken (see patient advice and monitoring sections below).
- Hypersensitivity phenomena including angio-oedema, rash, and transaminitis are rare.
- Very rarely these drugs can cause agranulocytosis.

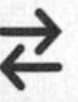

- These drugs can enhance the action of warfarin.

Efficacy

- Use PEFR and symptom scores to assess the effectiveness of your treatment regimen.
- Measure a full blood count, inflammatory markers, and liver function tests if the patient develops symptoms that could be due to the Churg–Strauss syndrome.

- Patients should be told that these drugs are for long-term prophylaxis against asthma, and that they should not be used for acute symptoms.
  - Ensure that the patient also has a short-acting β_2 agonist inhaler for use as required.
- Advise the patient to report immediately symptoms that could be due to the Churg–Strauss syndrome, for example:
  - A vasculitic rash.
  - Worsening of asthma symptoms.
- Ensure that the patient has a 'rescue plan' in case their symptoms worsen or they become unwell. Patients should be warned to seek medical help if they find that they need increasing doses of inhaled drugs to relieve symptoms.

Prescribing information: **Leukotriene receptor antagonists**

Montelukast

- *By mouth*, 10 mg daily, at bedtime.

Zafirlukast

- *By mouth*, 20 mg twice daily.

Cromones

Membrane stabilizing drugs

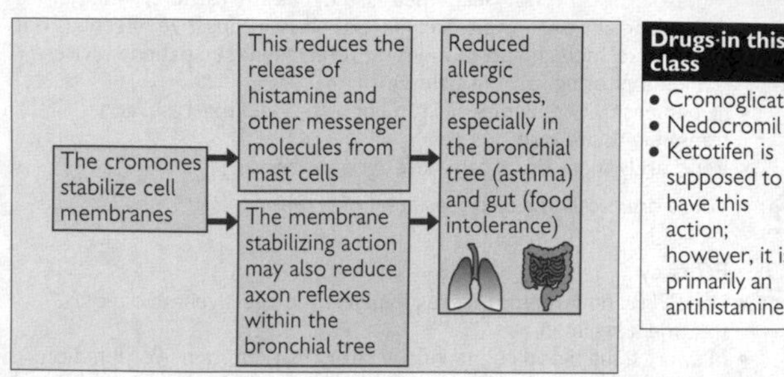

Drugs in this class

- Cromoglicate
- Nedocromil
- Ketotifen is supposed to have this action; however, it is primarily an antihistamine.

- Limited role in the prophylaxis of asthma in children.
- Prophylaxis against allergic rhinitis, allergic conjunctivitis.
- As an adjunct to avoidance in the treatment of food allergy.

- Cromones have no place in the treatment of acute asthma or anaphylaxis.
- Some formulations of these drugs contain benzalkonium chloride; some patients are allergic to this.
- There is no specific information on the safety of cromones in pregnancy.
- No dosage adjustment is usually required in renal or hepatic insuffuiciency.

Asthma

- These drugs reduce the frequency and severity of attacks when used in combination with inhaled β_2 adrenoceptor agonists (e.g. salbutamol) and inhaled steroids.
  - This effect is greater in children than adults. They are not recommended in adults.
  - These drugs have a role in the prevention of exercise-induced asthma provided they are taken half an hour before exercise.
- Cromones have no role in the acute treatment of asthma.
- Cromones are available as combination inhalers with β_2 adrenoceptor agonists. However, these are not recommended, as the two drugs have two different roles. Cromones are preventers, whereas β_2 adrenoceptor agonists are relievers.

Allergic rhinitis and conjunctivitis

- These drugs are available over the counter for treatment of these conditions.
- They provide some symptomatic relief but ensure that the diagnosis is correct.

Food allergy

- These drugs can have a role in genuine food allergy when the allergen is difficult to avoid.
- Ensure that the diagnosis is allergy and not intolerance or irritable bowel syndrome.

- Adverse effects are rare.
- A bitter taste is the most common adverse effect.

- As with any inhaled drug, these drugs can cause paradoxical bronchoconstriction.
- Some formulations of these drugs contain benzalkonium chloride; some patients are allergic to this.

- No clinically important drug interactions have been identified.

Efficacy

- Ensure that patients with asthma have regular follow-up and that they understand what to do if an exacerbation occurs.

- Make sure the patient and their carers (e.g. parents) understand the role of cromones in the treatment plan (preventer only).
- Ensure that the patient knows how to use an inhaler device correctly. Ask them to show you how they use the inhaler. See long-acting β_2 agonists (p. 221) for more information.

Prescribing information: **Cromones**

Sodium cromoglicate

- *Asthma prophylaxis* By aerosol inhalation, 10 mg (2 puffs) 4 times daily.
- *Exercise-induced asthma* By aerosol inhalation, 10 mg (2 puffs) half an hour before exercise.
- *Allergic conjunctivitis and rhinitis* Available over the counter as eye drops and nasal spray.
- *Food allergy* By mouth, 200 mg 4 times daily, before meals.

Nedocromil sodium

- *Asthma prophylaxis* By aerosol inhalation, 4 mg (2 puffs) 4 times daily.

Xanthine derivatives

Non-selective phosphodiesterase inhibitors

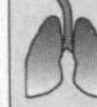

- The xanthine derivatives are inhibitors of phosphodiesterase. They reduce the breakdown of cyclic AMP, promoting bronchodilatation.
- This effect is not thought to account fully for the actions of theophylline. For example, theophylline also stimulates respiratory effort and is a purine receptor antagonist.
- Theophylline is subject to a large number of metabolic drug interactions and has a narrow therapeutic range. This limits its clinical usefulness.

Drugs in this class

- Theophylline
- Aminophylline*

*Aminophylline is 80% theophylline mixed with 20% ethylene diamine; this increases the solubility of theophylline, making it more suitable for intravenous injection.

- Treatment of reversible airways obstruction.

- Xanthines can be used for the relief of reversible airways obstruction in patients with COPD. The reversible component of this disease is often small, so they will be limited in their effect. When the patient is well, perform lung function tests and determine the degree of reversibility.
- Xanthines can cause cardiac arrhythmias; take particular care in patients with existing cardiac disease.
- Xanthines lower the seizure threshold; avoid them in patients with epilepsy.
- Xanthines are metabolized by the liver; reduce the dose in hepatic insufficiency.
- There is no specific dosage reduction in renal insufficiency but take care if it is severe. These patients are at greater risk of seizures.
- Xanthines have not been shown to be safe in pregnancy; avoid giving them unless essential. Use in the third trimester can cause neonatal irritability and apnoea.
- Theophylline is subject to large number of metabolic drug interactions; take care to check for these.

Acute bronchospasm

- Short-acting β_2 agonists are the first-line treatment of acute bronchospasm (see p. 214)
- Intravenous aminophylline has been used for the treatment of bronchospasm that is not responding rapidly to nebulized short-acting β_2 agonists, although systematic evidence of benefit is lacking.
  - Both drugs cause hypokalaemia, and the combination carries a high risk. Measure the plasma potassium concentration and be prepared to give potassium chloride.
  - Intravenous aminophylline is usually given as a loading dose followed by a continuous infusion. See below for dosage adjustments. Aminophylline is too irritant to be given by intramuscular injection.
  - Do not give the loading dose if the patient has been taking oral theophylline.
  - The patient must have close cardiac, biochemical, and clinical monitoring.

Chronic reversible airways obstruction

- These drugs are indicated at Stage 4 of the British Thoracic Society guidelines for the treatment of chronic asthma. At this stage, the choice of additional treatment should be made by a specialist. There are several other options (long-acting β_2 agonists, leukotriene receptor antagonists, muscarinic antagonists). The most appropriate choice will depend on the individual's symptoms and disease (British Thoracic Society/Scottish Intercollegiate Guidelines Network guidelines; *http://www.brit-thoracic.org.uk/sign/index.htm*).
- Theophylline commonly causes gastrointestinal adverse effects. These can be reduced by giving a modified-release formulation.
  - Modified-release formulations, given at night, can provide good symptom control in nocturnal asthma.
  - Prescribe modified-release formulations by brand name as they vary in their kinetics.
- These drugs suppress symptoms, but steroid therapy should not be withdrawn, as its anti-inflammatory action is still required for long-term control.
- Theophylline has a narrow therapeutic range. Plasma concentration monitoring is required; see below.

COPD (see p. 213)

- Theophylline is used as an additional bronchodilator in patients with severe disease, and may have some anti-inflammatory action.

- CNS stimulant effects may be the first to appear. These include nervousness, fine tremor, and anxiety.
- Gastrointestinal adverse effects are very common, they are characterized by nausea and vomiting.
- High doses can cause cardiac arrhythmias. This effect is potentiated by concomitant use of β_2 agonists.
- Higher doses can cause convulsions.

- See monitoring section below for a list of drugs that affect the plasma theophylline concentration.
- There is an increased risk of arrhythmias and hypokalaemia when xanthines are given with β_2 agonists and other sympathomimetics.
- There is an increased risk of convulsions when xanthines are given with antibiotics that lower the seizure threshold (e.g. quinolones).

Drugs and factors that INCREASE plasma theophylline concentration	Drugs and factors that DECREASE plasma theophylline concentration
Acute illness (e.g. infection, cardiac failure)	Cigarette smoking
Cimetidine	St John's wort
Ciprofloxacin (quinolone antibiotics)	Antiepileptic drugs (phenytoin, carbamazepine, barbiturates)
Erythromycin/clarithromycin (macrolide antibiotics)	Antiviral drugs (e.g. ritonavir)
Oral contraceptives	
Fluvoxamine (SSRI)	
Antifungal drugs (itraconazole, ketoconazole)	
Calcium channel blockers (e.g. diltiazem, verapamil)	

Safety

- Measure the plasma theophylline concentration:
    - During acute treatment
        - When the patient has a history of prior therapy with theophylline and you are contemplating intravenous treatment for an acute exacerbation. Do not give a loading dose. Use the concentration to calculate the infusion rate.
        - If the response to treatment is inadequate. The purpose is to guide the rate of infusion.
    - During chronic therapy when control is inadequate or toxicity is suspected.
- The target range is 10–20 micrograms/mL (55–110 micromol/L); see barbiturates (p. 264) for more information on the measurement of the plasma concentrations of drugs.
- Sampling time:
    - During intravenous infusion take the sample after 8–12 hours, but stop the infusion for 15 minutes before the sample is taken to allow plasma concentration equilibration. Do not forget to restart the infusion while you are waiting for the result.
    - During chronic therapy, take the sample 8–12 hours after the last dose.
- Relationship between dose and plasma concentration:
    - During intravenous treatment, an additional loading dose of 1 mg/kg will raise the plasma concentration by about 2 micrograms/mL.
    - During oral treatment, an additional daily dose of 200 mg will raise the plasma concentration by about 5 micrograms/mL.

Efficacy

- If used acutely, measure the PEFR, pulse, and respiratory rate to guide the rate of administration.
- If used chronically, measure the PEFR and symptom scores to assess the effectiveness of your treatment regimen.

- When xanthines are used chronically, patients should be told that these drugs are for long-term prophylaxis against asthma, and that they should not be used for acute symptoms.
    - Ensure that the patient also has a short-acting β_2 agonist inhaler for use as required.
- Ensure that the patient has a 'rescue plan' in case their symptoms worsen or they become unwell. Patients should be advised to seek medical help if they find that they need increasing doses of inhaled drugs to relieve symptoms.

Prescribing information: **Xanthine derivatives**

Theophylline

- By mouth, 125–250 mg tds. See above for monitoring information.
- If a modified-release formulation is required, prescribe by brand name as they vary in their kinetics.
    - The amount of drug per tablet varies with formulation.

Aminophylline

- Loading dose (see notes above) by intravenous injection over 20 minutes, 5 mg/kg.
- Continuous intravenous infusion, usual initial dose 500 **micrograms**/kg/hour.
  - Adjust according to response and plasma concentration (see above).
- The following are suggested alternative rates of continuous infusion for common clinical situations.
  - *Co-existing COPD* 600 **micrograms**/kg/hour.
  - *Hepatic insufficiency* 100–500 **micrograms**/kg/hour.
  - *Concomitant drugs that* ***increase*** *plasma theophylline concentrations* 300 **micrograms**/kg/hour.

Doxapram

Non-specific CNS stimulant (analeptic drug)

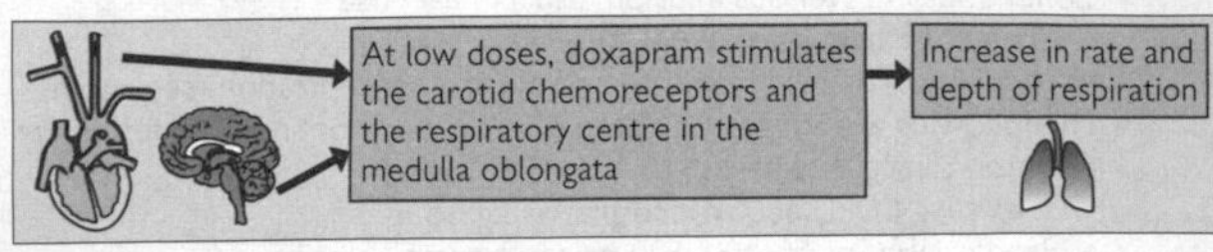

- Limited role in the short-term treatment of ventilatory failure in patients with COPD.
  - Doxapram has no role in the treatment of asthma.

- Doxapram is not an appropriate treatment when intubation and mechanical ventilation is indicated.
- Do not use doxapram if there is physical obstruction to the airway.
- Avoid this drug in pregnancy, unless absolutely essential.
- Doxapram is a non-specific stimulant; avoid giving it to patients with coronary artery disease or uncontrolled hypertension.

- Doxapram will only make the patient breathe more. Its role has largely been replaced by mechanical and assisted ventilation (IPPV and CPAP).
- Doxapram is only likely to be useful when there is an acute problem that may improve:
  - When ventilatory failure is due to hypercapnia. As ventilation increases, so the CO_2 will fall and the patient's own ventilatory effort will increase.
  - When there is ventilatory failure due to bronchial secretions; the improvement in ventilatory effort may allow the patient to cough these up.
  - Do not use this drug when there is no real possibility of improvement.
- Doxapram has no role in the treatment of chronic ventilatory failure.
- Doxapram is not the most appropriate choice for ventilatory failure after anaesthesia. Reverse the cause (e.g. opiate toxicity) rather than stimulating respiration.
  - Doxapram can be useful for the treatment of buprenorphine poisoning.
  - Buprenorphine is an opioid partial agonist, and so the opioid antagonist naloxone is less effective.
  - Doxapram can be used to stimulate respiratory effort until the effects of buprenorphine wear off.
- Doxapram should only be given when there is close supervision and monitoring of the patient.

- Doxapram is a non-specific stimulant; adverse effects are dose related and common and fall into two categories:
  - Cardiac: tachycardia and arrhythmias.
  - CNS: dizziness, restlessness, tremor, and convulsions.

- The action of doxapram is potentiated by other CNS stimulants (e.g. MAOIs).
- Theophylline can potentiate the CNS actions of doxapram.
- Avoid sympathomimetic drugs; the combination can cause severe hypertension.

Safety and efficacy

- These patients should be closely supervised. Measure the respiratory rate and oxygen saturation frequently. Supplement this with arterial blood gas measurements to tailor the treatment. Change the rate of infusion to achieve a balance between the respiratory and non-specific stimulant actions.
  - As the patient begins to improve, slow the rate of infusion.

- These patients are critically ill and doxapram is rarely life-saving. Ensure that the patient is comfortable.

Prescribing information: **Doxapram**

Acute ventilatory failure

- By intravenous infusion, 1.5–4.0 mg/min adjusted according to response.
- This drug is available ready mixed (doxapram hydrochloride 2 mg/mL in glucose 5%) in a 500 mL infusion bag.

Nicotine

Agonist at nicotinic acetylcholine receptors

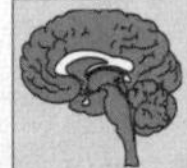

Nicotine products provide a replacement for the nicotine in tobacco. They reduce some of the cravings associated with stopping smoking. Once the patient has stopped smoking, nicotine replacement therapy can be withdrawn slowly.

- An adjunct to motivational support in patients who want to stop smoking.

- Take care if the patient has cardiovascular disease, although the risk from nicotine replacement therapy is much lower than that from smoking.
- Take care if the patient has diabetes mellitus or hyperthyroidism.
- Nicotine crosses the placenta. It is not recommended during pregnancy, although it may be less harmful than continuing to smoke; women should be encouraged to stop without pharmacological intervention.
- Avoid nicotine replacement in patients with phaeochromocytoma; it can precipitate a crisis.

Smoking cessation

- Nicotine replacement therapy can be bought over the counter without prescription.
- Nicotine replacement therapy is an adjunct to motivational support in smoking cessation, not a replacement for it. Assess the patient's level of motivation and social support.
- The effectiveness of nicotine replacement therapy is similar to that of amfebutamone, but because it is safer it is preferred.
- Nicotine replacement therapy will not abolish cravings; nor will it address the social aspects of smoking behaviour.
- Nicotine replacement therapy is available as chewing gum, a transdermal patch, an inhaler, a nasal spray, lozenges, and sublingual tablets.
- The use of gum is best established.
  - If the patient smokes <20 cigarettes/day use 2 mg of gum.
  - If they smoke >20/day use 4 mg of gum.
  - Chew the gum as required. Usual usage is around 8–12 gums daily.
  - Reduce the amount of gum chewed as able.
- Treatment is usually for a maximum of 3 months.

- Nicotine is not subject to any major drug interactions.

- Serious adverse effects are rare.
- Nicotine replacement therapy can cause angio-oedema and urticaria.
- It can rarely precipitate AF.
- Nicotine patches can cause local hypersensitivity reactions.

Safety and efficacy

- Suitable patient selection is essential. Motivational support is vital.

- Explain that nicotine helps with smoking cessation but will not abolish cravings.

Prescribing information: **Nicotine**

Smoking cessation

- Available over the counter.
- See above for a suggested regimen.

Amfebutamone (bupropion)

Inhibitor of the re-uptake of noradrenaline and dopamine in central monoaminergic neurons

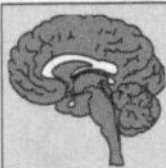

Amfebutamone, an amphetamine derivative, was originally developed as an atypical antidepressant drug. The mechanism by which it aids smoking cessation is not known. It probably involves an adaptive response within the brain to changes in monoaminergic neurotransmission.

Nicotine replacement therapy is first-line treatment for smoking cessation

(See p. 236).

- An adjunct to motivational support in patients who want to stop smoking.

- Amfebutamone is contraindicated in patients with:
  - Epilepsy (it lowers the seizure threshold). Take care in those at risk of seizures (e.g. those who drink excess alcohol).
  - Eating disorders.
  - CNS tumors.
- Limit the daily dose to 150 mg in those with hepatic or renal insufficiency.
- The safety of amfebutamone in pregnancy has not been established; it is not recommended.
  - Women who smoke should be encouraged to stop before becoming pregnant. If they are already pregnant, encourage them to give up without pharmacological intervention.

Smoking cessation

- Amfebutamone is an adjunct to motivational support in smoking cessation, not a replacement for it. Assess the patient's level of motivation and social support.
- NICE offers the following advice for the use of amfebutamone.
  - It should be offered only to those who commit to a specific quit date.
  - Initial treatment should be for 3–4 weeks. Treatment should only be continued if the patient is not smoking.
  - There is no evidence to recommend combining amfebutamone with nicotine.
- Treatment with amfebutamone increases the number of patients abstinent at one year from about 9% to 19%.
- The effectiveness of nicotine replacement therapy is very similar, but because it is safer it is preferred.

- Avoid giving amfebutamone with any drugs that lower the seizure threshold: antidepressant drugs, antimalarial drugs, antipsychotic drugs, quinolone antibiotics, theophylline, sedative antihistamines, systemic corticosteroids, excess alcohol, tramadol.
- Adverse effects are common and can be serious.

- CNS effects are common.
  - Insomnia is very common; advise the patient not to take amfebutamone during the late evening.
  - Other effects include agitation and anxiety.

- Amfebutamone can cause seizures and hallucinations. These are rare (1 in 1000 patients), but remember that this drug is given to individuals who would be considered 'healthy'.
- Hypersensitivity reactions occur in 3% of patients. They are severe in 0.1% (including the Stevens–Johnson syndrome).
- Amfebutamone can cause hypertension.

Safety and efficacy

- Suitable patient selection is essential. Do not expose patients who are unlikely to succeed in stopping smoking to the potential risks from this drug.
- Motivational support is essential.

- Explain that amfebutamone helps with smoking cessation but will not abolish cravings.
- Make sure that the patient knows amfebutamone can cause seizures. Smoking causes long-term morbidity and mortality, but a seizure can have a major effect on a patient's ability to live and work today. The risk may well be justified, but the patient must be aware of it before treatment starts.
- Amfebutamone can cause drowsiness that will interfere with skilled motor tasks (e.g. driving).

Prescribing information: **Amfebutamone**

Smoking cessation

- Start amfebutamone 2 weeks before the agreed quit date. Initially 150 mg daily. Increase to 150 mg twice daily after 6 days

Chapter 4

Central nervous sytem

Contents

Carbamazepine

Anticonvulsant

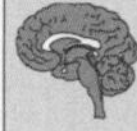

Carbamazepine is structurally related to the tricyclic antidepressants. Its precise mechanism of action is unknown, but it opens potassium channels and prolongs the time that the fast sodium channels are in the inactive state. This stabilizes membranes, reducing the initiation and propagation of action potentials. These effects are seen in the brain and peripheral nervous system.

- Treatment of epilepsy. Drug of choice for:
  - Simple and complex partial seizures.
  - Tonic-clonic secondarily generalized seizures.
- Treatment of trigeminal neuralgia.
- Prophylaxis of manic-depressive illness (specialized use).
- Symptomatic treatment of postherpetic neuralgia and diabetic neuropathy (unlicensed uses).

Treatment of epilepsy (based on NHS Prodigy guidelines www.prodigy.nhs.uk)

See teaching point under benzodiazepines (p. 269) for acute treatment of seizures.

Treatment of partial seizures (simple, complex, with or without secondary generalization)

- *Preferred monotherapy* Carbamazepine, sodium valproate, or lamotrigine (more costly).
- *Alternative monotherapy* Phenytoin, phenobarbital, or primidone. These are less often used, owing to their poor adverse effects profile, and to dose titration difficulties with phenytoin.
- If combination drug treatment is necessary, the current options are combination of the preferred monotherapies or use of the newer drugs (gabapentin, tiagabine, topiramate, or vigabatrin).

Treatment of generalized seizures (primary generalized tonic-clonic seizures, myoclonic seizures, absences)

- *Preferred monotherapy* Sodium valproate is effective against all the generalized seizures. Myoclonic and absence seizures are made worse by carbamazepine.
- *Alternative monotherapies* Depend on seizure type.
- *Primary generalized tonic-clonic* Carbamazepine or lamotrigine (more costly).
- *Absence* Ethosuximide or lamotrigine (unlicensed use).
- *Myoclonic* Clonazepam or lamotrigine (unlicensed use).
- If combination drug treatment is necessary, this is usually with those drugs used for monotherapy. Of the newer antiepileptic drugs, only lamotrigine and topiramate are currently licensed for add-on treatment of primary generalized tonic-clonic seizures.

- Pregnancy
  - There is an increased risk of neural tube defects in the children of mothers taking carbamazepine. Counsel women about this and seek specialist advice for women with epilepsy considering pregnancy.
  - Give folic acid supplements (5 mg/day).
  - There is a risk of neonatal bleeding with carbamazepine; prophylactic vitamin K_1 is recommended for the mother before delivery (as well as for the neonate).
- Patients with liver disease metabolize carbamazepine more slowly.
- Avoid in porphyria (see teaching point below).
- Avoid in patients with a history of bone marrow depression (see adverse effects).

- Do not use intravenously in people with evidence of heart block (2nd degree or higher), unless the patient has a pacemaker.
- When using carbamazepine for epilepsy, avoid drugs that lower the seizure threshold (e.g. amfebutamone, tricyclic antidepressants, MAOIs, SSRIs).

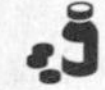

Epilepsy

- Carbamazepine is given by mouth for the long-term control of seizures. It is not used for acute control of seizures. See benzodiazepines (p. 269) for guidance on this.
- Begin treatment with a low dose and increase gradually (100–200 mg every 2 weeks).
- Different formulations have different properties; avoid switching formulations.
- Use the plasma drug concentration to help you determine the optimal maintenance dose.
  - Carbamazepine induces its own metabolism (see teaching point below).
  - In practical terms, this means that a dose that was adequate on day 1 may not be by day 14.
  - It takes about 2 weeks for carbamazepine to reach a new steady state after a dosage change. Any plasma drug concentration you measure before 2 weeks can be misleading.
- If monotherapy is ineffective at maximum tolerated doses, introduce an alternative drug slowly without tapering the first. If the patient has a good response to the second drug, gradually withdraw the original drug. Only 10% of patients require two or more drugs to control their epilepsy.
- Avoid abrupt withdrawal of carbamazepine, as this can precipitate rebound seizures.
  - If the drug needs to be withdrawn, taper the dose over a period of weeks under cover of another antiepileptic drug.

Trigeminal neuralgia (see also gabapentin (p. 674) for treatment of neuropathic pain)

- Begin with a low dose to minimize the incidence of adverse effects.
- If used early, carbamazepine reduces the severity and frequency of attacks.
- Use the lowest effective dose.
- Can be combined with a tricyclic antidepressant.

Bipolar disorder

- Carbamazepine can be effective in the treatment of bipolar disorder in patients who are unresponsive to lithium. It seems to be especially useful in those with rapidly cycling disease (more than four episodes per year). This is a specialized use and it should only be instituted under expert supervision.

- Adverse effects are common; these can be reduced by giving the drug in divided doses, giving a modified-release formulation, and by altering the times at which the patient takes the tablets.
- Carbamazepine can cause leukopenia. This can be severe and progressive. It affects about 6% of patients, usually within the first few months of treatment. Withdraw the drug if the patient becomes leukopenic.
- The most common adverse effect is a generalized erythematous rash; this is usually transient, but it can be intolerable.

- CNS adverse effects (drowsiness, impaired balance, and paraesthesia) affect half of patients given carbamazepine.
- Visual symptoms (diplopia and blurred vision) are common when the daily dose exceeds 1200 mg.
- Carbamazepine can cause SIADH (see vasopressin (p. 478) for more information).

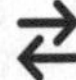

- Carbamazepine interacts with many drugs (see teaching point below); the most important are given here.
- Carbamazepine can lower the plasma concentration of many other antiepileptic drugs (see below for a list). Most patients do not need two drugs for control of epilepsy (see how to use above).
- Carbamazepine increases the rate of metabolism of oestrogens and progestogens; this can render oral contraceptives ineffective. Advise women to use additional (barrier) methods of contraception.
- Carbamazepine increases the rate of metabolism of immune modulators such as ciclosporin and tacrolimus. Measure the plasma concentrations of these drugs to ensure that they remain within the target range (see teaching point below).
- Carbamazepine increases the rate of metabolism of warfarin, reducing its anticoagulant effect. Measure the INR more regularly until a new steady state has been established.
- Avoid co-prescribing with St John's wort, which is an enzyme inducer.

Efficacy

- The usual target plasma concentration for optimum response is 13–42 micromol/L (4–10 microgram/mL).
- Remember that this is target concentration range; it will not apply to all patients and is not a guarantee of success. Ask the patient to keep a record of any seizures.
- Take the blood sample immediately before the next dose is due.
- Wait 2 weeks after a dosage change before taking a sample for plasma concentration measurement (see barbiturates, p. 264).

Safety

- The manufacturers recommend monitoring of blood counts and liver function tests. The adverse effects that this will detect are uncommon and a monitoring regimen with an adequate detection rate has not been devised. Advise the patient to report any symptoms consistent with leukopenia immediately (see below). Have a low threshold for measuring a full blood count.

- Always ensure that the patient is aware of the law regarding seizures and driving (see lamotrigine, p. 261).
- Advise the patient to seek immediate medical attention if symptoms such as fever, sore throat, mouth ulcers, unexplained bruising, or bleeding develop.
- Warn the patient that carbamazepine can interact with many medicines; advise them to check with their prescriber before starting or stopping any medication.
- Warn women of child-bearing age that the oral contraceptive may not be effective and that they must take additional contraceptive precautions.

Prescribing information: **Carbamazepine**

Treatment of epilepsy

- Initially, 100–200 mg by mouth, 1–2 times daily.
- Increase slowly to usual maintenance dose of 0.8–1.2 g daily, in divided doses (in some cases 1.6–2.0 g daily may be needed).

Trigeminal neuralgia

- Initially, 100 mg 1 or 2 times daily.
- Increase gradually according to response; the usual dose is 200 mg 3 or 4 times daily.

Prophylaxis of bipolar disorder unresponsive to lithium (specialized use)

- Initially, 400 mg daily in divided doses.
- Increase until symptoms are controlled; the usual dosage range is 400–600 mg daily.

TEACHING POINT Drugs and porphyria

- The porphyrias are a group of rare disorders of haem biosynthesis. Each type is associated with an abnormality of an enzyme in the haem biosynthetic pathway.
- Many drugs can trigger an attack of prophyria; other precipitating factors include:
  - Alcohol
  - Malnourishment
  - Infection
- Drugs that precipitate porphyria are inducers of cytochrome P450 in the liver. Cytochrome P450 contains haem. Induction leads to an exaggerated response of δ-amino laevulininc acid synthase and over-production of porphobilinogen and its metabolic products.

Drugs to avoid in porphyria

This is not an exhaustive list, check individual articles and the BNF before prescribing any drug for a patient with porphyria.

- Alcohol
- Some anaesthetic gasses (e.g. halothane)
- Some antibiotics (e.g. rifampicin, sulfonamides)
- Some ACE inhibitors
- Barbiturates
- Carbamazepine
- Dapsone
- Female sex hormones (oestrogens, progestogens)
- Furosemide
- Methyldopa
- Some NSAIDs
- Sulfonylureas
- Theophylline

TEACHING POINT Drugs that induce their own metabolism

- Carbamazepine is metabolized in the liver by the group of cytochrome P450 isoenzymes called CYP 3A4. This is the largest and most important of the isoenzyme groups, and it is responsible for the metabolism of many drugs.
- Carbamazepine induces this group of isoenzymes over a period of about 2 weeks. With repeated administration, the rate of metabolism of carbamazepine increases as the amount of metabolizing enzymes increases. The half-life of carbamazepine is around 65 hours after a single dose, but falls to around 20 hours during long-term administration.
- If the patient takes a fixed daily dose of carbamazepine, the plasma concentration will fall with time. A dose that adequately controls a patient's seizures may not be adequate 2 weeks later (see illustration below).
- This process is very complex, and a kinetic model would need to take into account the changing kinetics of the drug and changing kinetics of the metabolizing isoenzymes. In practice it is not possible to generate such models for the individual; it is therefore necessary to have more empirical guidance.
- From a practical point of view, one needs to ask two questions:
  - Will the dose of the inducing drug still be adequate once steady state has been reached?
  - Will the inducing drug affect the metabolism of another drug, such that it might become ineffective?
- Measure the plasma carbamazepine concentration 2 weeks after starting the drug or changing the dose. This will usually give sufficient time for a steady state to be reached. The same applies to phenytoin, the other commonly prescribed drug that also induces its own metabolism by CYP 3A4.
- Several other drugs are also metabolized by CYP 3A4; these are: Be prepared to increase the doses of these drugs. Take particular care with the oral contraceptive, immune modulators, and drugs used to treat HIV infection. Unfortunately there is no simple rule that tells you by how much the dose will need to be altered.

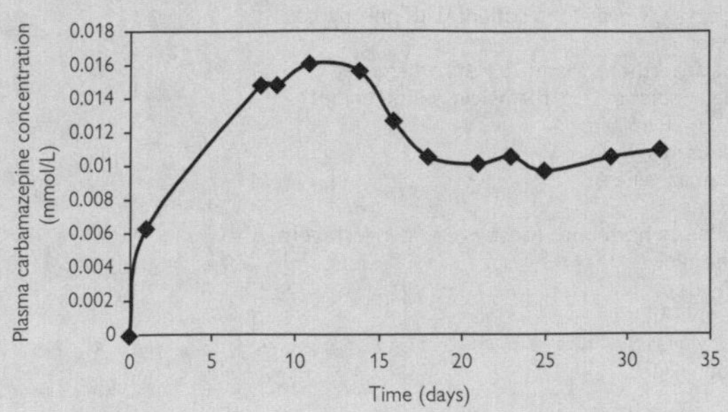

Redrawn using data from Lai A A *et al*, *Clin Pharmacol Ther*, 1978; **24**: 316-23.

Drugs that induce their own metabolism by CYP 3A4
- Carbamazepine
- Phenytoin
- Barbiturates
- Rifampicin
- St John's wort

Drugs that are metabolized by CYP 3A4 (These drugs are subject to interactions when co-prescribed with drugs that induce or inhibit CYP 3A4)	**Examples**
• Macrolide antibiotics	Erythromycin, clarithromycin (not azithromycin)
• Antiarrhythmic drugs	Quinidine
• Benzodiazepines	Diazepam, midazolam
• Immune modulators	Ciclosporin, tacrolimus
• HIV protease inhibitors	Indinavir, ritonavir, saquinavir
• Calcium channel blockers	Amlodipine, nifedipine, felodipine, diltiazem, verapamil
• HMG CoA reductase inhibitors	Simvastatin. atorvastatin (not fluvastatin, pravastatin)
• Anticoagulants	Warfarin

Phenytoin

Sodium channel blockade; modulation of GABA-ergic neurotransmission

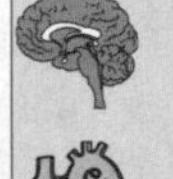

- In the **brain,** phenytoin inhibits the initiation and propagation of action potentials. The exact mechanism is unknown, but it involves sodium channel blockade and potentiation of GABA-ergic pathways. This results in seizure control, but also CNS depression.
- In the **heart,** the blockade of fast sodium currents has a lidocaine-like antiarrhythmic effect.
- Phenytoin was once used in the treatment of cardiac glycoside-induced arrhythmias, but this is now obsolete.

Note on fosphenytoin

- Fosphenytoin is a prodrug of phenytoin. It can be given more rapidly by intravenous infusion than phenytoin.
- Intravenous infusion requires close cardiac monitoring.
- Seek expert advice before using this drug.
- Note that the prescription should state the dose in terms of phenytoin sodium equivalents (fosphenytoin 1.5 mg approximately equivalent to phenytoin 1 mg).

- Treatment and prevention of generalized tonic-clonic seizures and partial seizures.
- Used rarely as second-line treatment for trigeminal neuralgia.

- Caution in pregnancy.
  - There is an increased risk of neural tube defects in children of mothers taking phenytoin, owing to the antifolate effect of phenytoin.
  - Counsel women about this, seek specialist advice for women considering pregnancy, and ensure folic acid supplementation (5 mg/day).
  - There is a risk of neonatal bleeding with phenytoin; prophylactic vitamin K_1 is recommended for the mother before delivery (as well as for the neonate).
- Toxic effects occur at lower doses in patients with liver disease.
- Avoid abrupt withdrawal of phenytoin; it can precipitate rebound seizures.
- Phenytoin can cause coarse facies, acne, hirsutism, and gingival hyperplasia.
  - Consider alternatives in young patients who may have to take the drug for many years.
  - Good oral hygiene reduces the risk of gingival hyperplasia.
- Avoid in porphyria.
- Do not use intravenously in those with heart block (2nd degree or complete).

Epilepsy

- Used orally for the long-term control of seizures.
- Used intravenously in patients in whom rapid control is required (e.g. status epilepticus).
- Do not give phenytoin intramuscularly; it precipitates at the site of injection.
- Phenytoin has non-linear kinetics (for explanation, see over).
  - In practical terms, this means that relatively small increases in dose can lead to large increases in plasma concentrations, and therefore effect.

- Increase the dose slowly, in small steps, and measure the plasma concentration to guide you (see below).
- The initial dose is usually 150–300 mg daily (3–4 mg/kg).
  - Increase gradually (in 25–50 mg steps) to a usual maintenance dose of 200–500 mg daily.
  - Do not increase the dose more often then every 2–3 weeks.
- Intravenous infusion for status epilepticus: 15 mg/kg infused slowly (less than 50 mg per minute).
  - Maintenance doses of 100 mg required every 6–8 hours.
  - Use the plasma concentration to guide dose and frequency.
- Fosphenytoin is a prodrug of phenytoin, used parenterally when oral phenytoin therapy is not possible; seek specialist advice (see box above).

Early

- Acute toxicity is associated with slurred speech, nystagmus, blurred vision, nausea, vomiting, and mental confusion.
- Phenytoin blocks sodium channels and can therefore cause cardiovascular and CNS depression, especially when given intravenously. Ensure that the patient has close nursing support and cardiac monitoring.
- Intravenous phenytoin causes local venous irritation; give it into an adequately large vein (e.g. antecubital) or via a central line.
- Phenytoin can cause a number of skin problems, ranging from a mild measles-like rash to the Stevens–Johnson syndrome. Phenytoin must be withdrawn and not restarted if the more severe manifestations are observed. Careful reintroduction is possible if the rash is mild.
- At high doses phenytoin can interfere with insulin release, resulting in hypoglycaemia (and hence seizures).
  - Phenytoin can precipitate non-ketotic hyperglycaemia (HONK).
- Haematological effects include megaloblastic anaemia, leukopenia, thrombocytopenia, agranulocytosis, and aplastic anaemia.
  - The manufacturers recommend regular blood tests, but these have not been shown to be predictive.
  - Teach the patient to recognize the symptoms and check a full blood count if suspicious.

Late

- Long-term treatment can result in coarse facies, acne, hirsutism, and gingival hyperplasia.
- Phenytoin can interfere with the metabolism of vitamin D, resulting in rare cases of rickets and osteomalacia.
- Phenytoin has an antifolate effect (see above).

- See box below for list of drug interactions. See also teaching point about protein binding interactions.
- Phenytoin is an inducer of liver enzymes (see teaching point in carbamazepine, p. 246). It can therefore increase the metabolism of other drugs.
  - The induction of liver enzymes by phenytoin occurs over a period of 10–14 days, after which a new equilibrium develops. Measure the plasma concentration 2 weeks after a change in the drug regimen.
- The metabolism of phenytoin can be affected by other drugs.
  - These metabolic interactions occur at the time the other drug is introduced and can occur even before a new equilibrium is established.

- Always check before stopping or starting a drug in a patient taking phenytoin.

The most common and important drug interactions are marked in **bold**. Other antipepileptic drugs are in italics.

Drugs that can increase serum phenytoin concentrations (increased risk of toxicity)
- **Amiodarone**, aspirin, antifungal agents (e.g. itraconazole), cimetidine, chloramphenicol, chlordiazepoxide, diazepam, diltiazem, H_2 receptor antagonists, isoniazid, metronidazole, methylphenidate, nifedipine, omeprazole, oestrogens, phenothiazines, phenylbutazone, salicylates, sulfonamides, tolbutamide, trazodone.

Drugs that decrease serum phenytoin concentrations (risk of seizures)
- *Carbamazepine*, sucralfate, *vigabatrin.*

Drugs that can increase or decrease serum phenytoin concentrations
- *Phenobarbital, sodium valproate*, antineoplastic agents, ciprofloxacin.

Other interactions
- Many antidepressants lower the seizure threshold.
- Antifolate effect increased by **pyrimethamine, co-trimoxazole, trimethoprim**; this can cause anaemia.

Drugs whose effects are altered by phenytoin
- Reduced effect of: antifungal agents, antineoplastic agents, antiviral agents, **ciclosporin**, clozapine, corticosteroids, doxycycline, *ethosuximide*, furosemide, methadone, oestrogens, **oral contraceptives**, quinidine, rifampicin, repaglinide, sertindole, theophylline, thyroxine, **vitamin D**.
- The effect on **warfarin** is variable; monitor the INR closely.

Efficacy
- The usual target plasma concentration for an optimum response is 40–80 micromol/L (10–20 mg/L); see barbiturates (p. 264) for more information on the measurement of the plasma concentration of drugs.
- The target is lower in chronic renal insufficiency (as low as 20–40 micromol/L in severe renal insufficiency) because of reduced protein binding.

Safety
- Be aware that small changes in dose, the introduction or withdrawal of other drugs, and missed doses can result in significant changes in plasma concentration.
  - This can manifest as a loss of therapeutic effect (seizures) if the concentration falls, or by the appearance of toxic features if the concentration rises.
- Have a low threshold for checking a full blood count if any haematological abnormality is suspected.

- Always ensure that the patient is aware of the law regarding seizures and driving (see lamotrigine, p. 261).
- Advise the patient to seek immediate medical attention if symptoms such as fever, sore throat, mouth ulcers, unexplained bruising, or bleeding develop.
- Advise good oral hygiene, which will reduce the risk of gingival hyperplasia.
- Warn the patient that phenytoin can interact with many medicines; advise them to check with their prescriber before starting or stopping any medication.

Prescribing information: **Phenytoin**

By mouth

- Initially, 3–4 mg/kg/day *or* 150–300 mg/day (as a single dose or in two divided doses).
- Increase gradually as necessary (with plasma phenytoin concentration monitoring).
- Usual dose 200–500 mg/day (exceptionally, higher doses can be used).

By slow intravenous injection or infusion for status epilepticus

- 15 mg/kg at a rate not exceeding 50 mg/minute, as a loading dose.
- With blood pressure and ECG monitoring.
- Maintenance doses of about 100 mg should be given thereafter at intervals of every 6–8 hours, monitored by measurement of plasma concentrations; rate and dose should be reduced according to weight.
- To avoid local venous irritation each injection or infusion should be preceded and followed by an injection of sterile isotonic saline through the same needle or catheter.

TEACHING POINT Non-linear kinetics (zero-order kinetics)

- Phenytoin is metabolized in the liver by hydroxylation. The enzyme system responsible becomes saturated at concentrations of phenytoin within the target range. An increase in dose can therefore result in an unexpectedly large rise in plasma concentration (see illustration), as the liver cannot increase the rate at which it metabolizes the drug (hence the term non-linear kinetics). The rate of elimination of phenytoin changes with changing concentration and so the traditional concept of half-life does not apply.
- In order to avoid these problems, the daily dose of phenytoin should be increased gradually (in steps of 25–50 mg) and the plasma concentration should be checked once a new equilibrium has been reached (usually 14 days after the dose change).
- Note that starting or stopping another drug that alters the metabolism of phenytoin can have the same effect as changing the dose. Always check before changing the medication of a patient taking phenytoin, and measure the serum phenytoin concentration 5–7 days later.
- Drugs that exhibit non-linear kinetics are difficult to administer safely. However, phenytoin is the only example of a commonly prescribed drug with these kinetic properties within or near the therapeutic dosage range.
- Alcohol also has non-linear kinetics, and is eliminated at a rate of about 6 g/h at almost all doses. This explains why the blood alcohol concentration may still be above the legal limit for driving the morning after a bout of heavy drinking.

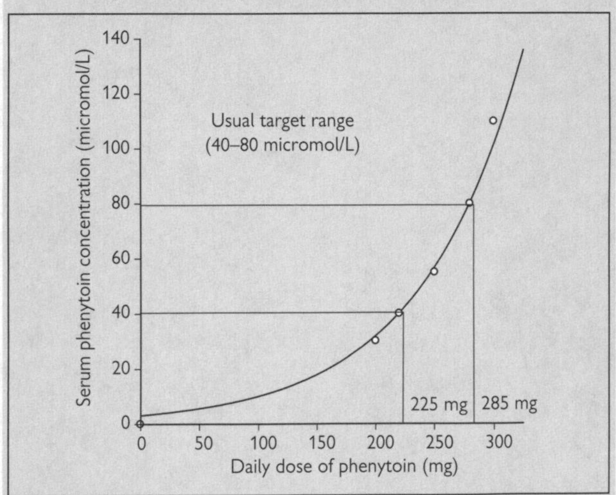

The relation between the serum phenytoin concentration and the daily dose. In this patient, the range of doses associated with the target range of serum concentrations (40–80 micromol/L) was 225–285 mg/day.

TEACHING POINT Plasma protein binding displacement drug interactions

- A drug that has a higher affinity for protein binding sites than another drug could displace the other drug, leading to a sudden rise in the unbound fraction of the second drug and possible toxicity.
- In practice, such interactions are almost never seen, because the plasma concentration of the displacing drug would have to rise very fast (e.g. by rapid intravenous injection), and because redistribution and an increase in the rate of clearance of the displaced drug usually compensate for the protein displacement.
- However, such interactions can lead to misinterpretation of plasma drug concentrations.
    - Phenytoin is highly protein bound; it also has a low hepatic extraction ratio. This means that the proportion of the drug that is cleared from the blood by each passage through the liver is small (other examples include warfarin and tolbutamide). The rate of clearance of the drug depends on the unbound fraction of the drug. By contrast, if a drug has a high hepatic extraction ratio, the rate of blood flow though the liver is the rate limiting factor.
    - If phenytoin is displaced from its protein binding sites by another drug, the unbound fraction in the plasma increases, but so does the rate of metabolism of the drug. Over time a new equilibrium will be reached; the unbound *fraction* will remain higher, but the total concentration of drug in plasma will be lower, so the unbound *concentration* will be the same as it was before the interaction occurred.
- In common with most plasma drug assays, the assay for phenytoin measures the total phenytoin concentration; it does not distinguish between bound and unbound fractions. The total phenytoin concentration after the addition of the second drug will be lower; this could be misinterpreted as subtherapeutic if the plasma concentration is taken in isolation. It is essential to interpret plasma concentrations according to the patient's condition; in this case it would be expected that the patient would be stable, so the dose does not need to be changed. So, when measuring plasma phenytoin concentrations, also measure the plasma albumin concentration and renal function, since hypoalbuminaemia and chronic renal insufficiency reduce the protein binding of phenytoin.

Sodium valproate

Anticonvulsant

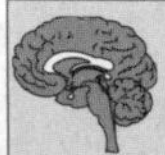

The exact mechanism of action of valproate is not known. Valproate enhances GABA-ergic neurotransmission by several mechanisms. For example, it reduces GABA breakdown and, by inhibiting GABA transaminase, increases the sensitivity of GABA receptors.

- Treatment of epilepsy. Indicated for all forms, but particularly useful for:
  - Primary generalized seizures.
  - Myoclonic seizures.
- May also be used for:
  - Atypical absence seizures.
  - Atonic and tonic seizures.

- Caution in pregnancy. There is a 2% risk of neural tube defects, abnormalities of the face, and limb abnormalities in children of mothers taking valproate.
  - Counsel women about this.
  - Seek specialist advice in women considering pregnancy.
  - Ensure folic acid supplementation (5 mg daily).
- Sodium valproate can cause liver toxicity; avoid it in patients with acute or chronic liver disease.
- Reduce the dose in patients with any degree of renal insufficiency.

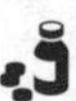

Epilepsy

- Valproate is given orally for the long-term control of seizures.
  - It can be given intravenously for acute control of seizures, as an alternative to a phenytoin infusion.
    - For guidance on this, see treatment of status epilepticus in benzodiazepines (p. 269).
    - See prescribing notes below.
- Begin treatment with a dose of 300 mg twice daily.
  - The dose can be titrated rapidly upwards, increasing by 200 mg daily at intervals of 3 days.
  - The usual maintenance dose is 2 g daily (also see prescribing notes).
- If monotherapy is ineffective at maximum tolerated doses, introduce an alternative drug slowly without tapering the first. If the patient has a good response to the second drug, gradually withdraw the original drug. Only 10% of patients require two or more drugs to control their epilepsy.
- Avoid abrupt withdrawal of valproate as this can precipitate rebound seizures.
  - If valproate needs to be withdrawn, taper the dose over a period of weeks under cover of another antiepileptic drug.
  - Emergency withdrawal may be necessary if serious skin or haematological adverse effects occur.

Treatment of epilepsy

- See teaching point under benzodiazepines (p. 269) for treatment of acute seizures.
- See carbamazepeine (p. 242) for more information.

Note on related drugs

Valproic acid
This is said to have a 1:1 dose relation with valproate. In addition to its use in the treatment of epilepsy, valproic acid has a licence for the treatment of acute mania associated with bipolar disorder. This is a specialized use; seek expert guidance.

Divalproex sodium (valproate semisodium)
This drug is indicated for the treatment of manic episodes associated with bipolar disorder. Seek expert advice.

- Adverse effects are common.
- Gastrointestinal adverse effects are very common, usually characterized by nausea and vomiting.
  - These are most common early in treatment and can be mitigated by using an enteric-coated formulation and giving the drug with food.
  - These adverse effects usually improve with time.
- Sodium valproate causes oedema and weight gain; warn the patient.
- Valproate can cause liver toxicity; this is rare but potentially fatal.
  - Young patients and those with organic or degenerative brain disease are at greatest risk.
  - Follow the monitoring guidance below.
- Adverse effects due to excessive dose include ataxia, tremor, and reduced co-ordination.
- Rare but serious adverse effects include thrombocytopenia (and other blood disorders) and pancreatitis.
- Sodium valproate can cause transient hair loss; note that the regrowth may be curly.

- Valproate interacts with fewer drugs than some other antiepileptic drugs.
- Valproate can interact with phenytoin, and the effect is unpredictable; avoid the combination when possible.
- Valproate increases the effect of phenobarbital and primidone.
- Antipsychotic drugs, chloroquine, and antidepressant drugs reduce the effect of valproate.

Efficacy

- Plasma concentration measurement is not routinely recommended, as there is a poor correlation with clinical effect. It can be used to confirm that the patient is taking the drug if control is poor.
- Efficacy must be judged on the basis of seizure frequency and adverse effects.

Safety

- Measure liver function tests every 2 months for the first 6 months of treatment. If these are abnormal, withdraw the drug.
- Have a low threshold for measuring a full blood count. Advise the patient to report immediately any symptoms consistent with bone marrow toxicity (see below).
- Ensure that the patient is aware of the law regarding seizures and driving (see lamotrigine, p. 261).

- Advise the patient to seek immediate medical attention if symptoms such as fever, sore throat, mouth ulcers, unexplained bruising, or bleeding develop.
- Advise the patient to seek immediate medical attention if they become jaundiced.
- Advise women of child-bearing age to seek advice before trying to become pregnant, so that an expert opinion can be sought.

Prescribing information: **Valproate**

Treatment of epilepsy

- By mouth, initially 300 mg bd.
- Increase by 200 mg daily at intervals of 3 days.
- The usual maintenance is 2 g daily (20–30 mg/kg), in divided doses.
  - This may be increased to 2.5 g daily if required.

Treatment of status epilepticus

- See benzodiazepines (p. 269) for guidance.
- By intravenous injection over 3–5 minutes, 400–800 mg (up to 10 mg/kg).
- Followed by an intravenous infusion of up to 2.5 g daily.

TEACHING POINT Epilepsy, antiepileptic drugs, and teratogenicity

- Most women with epilepsy will have a normal pregnancy and delivery, an unchanged seizure frequency, and a greater than 90% chance of a normal baby.
  - If a mother with epilepsy is not taking treatment, there is a small increase in the incidence of abnormalities such as cleft palate and spina bifida. Paternal epilepsy has no effect.
  - Infants born to women receiving anticonvulsant drugs have at least double the risk of being born with an anomaly or malformation.
- Most malformations are minor and form part of what appears to be a fetal anticonvulsant syndrome.
  - The incidence varies between 1% and 11% in infants of mothers taking antiepileptic drugs, compared with 2.3% in the general population.
  - The most common features include hypertelorism, an abnormal midface, epicanthic folds, microcephaly, transverse palmar creases, and minor skeletal abnormalities.
  - More serious malformations include spina bifida and congenital heart disease. The latter can be detected *in utero* using ultrasound.
- All the older antiepileptic drugs (carbamazepine, sodium valproate, phenytoin, phenobarbital) are teratogenic. Some newer antiepileptic drugs (e.g. gabapentin and lamotrigine) have not been shown to be teratogenic, but experience is limited.
- Anticonvulsant drugs may be teratogenic for several reasons. Some have actions on folate metabolism; others form epoxides, free radical intermediates, and arene oxides.
- The risk of an abnormal fetus is related to the number and dosage of the anticonvulsant drugs. The risk is increased significantly if the mother is taking several drugs, especially if sodium valproate forms part of the combination.
- Carbamazepine therapy carries a slightly lower risk when compared with valproate, phenytoin, or phenobarbital. However, if seizure control is good, it is probably best to leave the treatment unchanged, provided a single anticonvulsant is used.
- High-dose folate supplements should be given before conception and throughout the pregnancy.
- Always seek expert advice if a woman with epilepsy is considering becoming pregnant.

Lamotrigine

Anticonvulsant

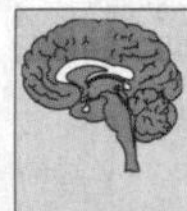

The exact mechanism of action of lamotrigine is not known. It is thought to act as a use-dependent blocker of voltage-gated sodium channels, thus inhibiting the release of exitatory neurotransmitters (e.g. glutamate).

Treatment of epilepsy

- See teaching point under benzodiazepines (p. 269) for treatment of acute seizures.
- See carbamazepine, p. 242.

- Treatment of epilepsy. Can be used as monotherapy for:
  - Partial seizures.
  - Tonic-clonic primarily generalized seizures.
  - Tonic-clonic secondarily generalized seizures.
  - Seizures associated with Lennox–Gastaut syndrome.

- Pregnancy.
  - Experience with lamotrigine is limited.
  - In general, good control of epilepsy outweighs the risks.
  - Counsel women about this; seek specialist advice for women considering pregnancy.
- Halve the dose in patients with moderate hepatic insufficiency. Reduce to a quarter if the insufficiency is severe.
- Metabolites of lamotrigine can accumulate and cause adverse effects in patients with moderate to severe renal insufficiency.

Epilepsy

- Lamotrigine is given orally for the long-term control of seizures.
  - It is not used for control of acute seizures; see benzodiazepines (p. 269) for guidance on this.
- Begin treatment with a low dose and increase gradually (25–50 mg every 2 weeks).
- If monotherapy is ineffective at maximum tolerated doses, introduce an alternative drug slowly without tapering the first. If the patient has a good response to the second drug, gradually withdraw the original drug. Only 10% of patients require two or more drugs to control their epilepsy.
- Avoid abrupt withdrawal of lamotrigine, as this can precipitate rebound seizures.
  - If the drug needs to be withdrawn, taper the dose over a period of weeks under cover of another antiepileptic drug.
  - Emergency withdrawal may be necessary if serious skin or haematological adverse effects occur.

- Adverse effects are common.
- Skin reactions are common and usually occur within the first 8 weeks of treatment. A maculopapular erythematous rash occurs in 10% of patients. The drug should be withdrawn if this occurs, especially if there are systemic (flu-like) symptoms. This is because more serious reactions also occur (1 in 1000 patients); these include Stevens–Johnson syndrome and a syndrome of fever, malaise, eosinophilia, and arthralgia.
- Lamotrigine can cause bone marrow toxicity; this is rare but can be serious (aplastic anaemia).

- CNS adverse effects are common. These include dizziness, nervousness, tremor, and confusion.
- Specific effects on the eye include diplopia, blurred vision, and a painful red eye.
- Gastrointestinal adverse effects are also common, usually characterized by nausea and vomiting.

- Other antiepileptic drugs
  - Lamotrigine can raise the plasma concentration of carbamazepine; the risk of adverse effects is increased.
  - Sodium valproate increases the lamotrigine concentration; halve the initial dose and dose increments.
  - Enzyme-inducing antiepiletic drugs lower lamotrigine concentrations (see carbamazepine teaching point (p. 246) for more information); double the initial dose.
- Tricyclic antidepressant drugs and mefloquine antagonize the anticonvulsant action of lamotrigine; avoid these combinations.

Efficacy

- Plasma concentration measurement is not used.
- Efficacy must be judged on the basis of seizure frequency and adverse effects.

Safety

- The manufacturers recommend monitoring of blood counts, blood clotting, and liver function tests. The adverse effects that this will detect are uncommon, and a regimen with an adequate detection rate has not been devised. Advise the patient to immediately report any symptoms consistent with bone marrow toxicity (see below). Have a low threshold for measuring a full blood count.

- Always ensure that the patient is aware of the law regarding seizures and driving (see below).
- Advise the patient to seek immediate medical attention if symptoms such as fever, sore throat, mouth ulcers, unexplained bruising, or bleeding develop.
- Advise the patient to seek immediate medical attention if a rash develops.
- Warn the patient that lamotrigine can interact with many medicines; advise them to check with their doctor or pharmacist before starting or stopping any medication.
- Advise women of child-bearing age to seek advice before trying to become pregnant, so that an expert opinion can be sought.

Prescribing information: **Lamotrigine**

Treatment of epilepsy

- By mouth, initially 25 mg daily for 14 days.
- Increase to 50 mg daily for 14 days.
- Increase by 50–100 mg at intervals of 14 days, to a usual maintenance dose of 100–200 mg daily, in divided doses.
- In rare cases, doses of 500 mg daily have been used.
  - If combined with valproate, halve these doses.
  - If combined with enzyme-inducing drugs, twice the dose may be required, but take care with the titration.

TEACHING POINT Epilepsy and fitness to drive

- The legal basis of fitness to drive lies in the EC Directives on driver licensing, the Road Traffic Act 1988, and subsequent regulations, including in particular the Motor Vehicles (Driving Licences) Regulations 1999.
- Because this is the subject of legislation, prescribers should take care to limit themselves to advising their patients of the rules, and not to try to interpret them. Epilepsy is the most common cause of collapse while driving, but there are rules governing loss of consciousness from any cause (see adenosine, p. 81).
- It is the responsibility of patients to inform the DVLA about their medical condition. Respect for patient confidentiality usually prohibits healthcare professionals from disclosing information about patients to a third party such as the DVLA. However, recent changes in the case law in the UK allow this confidence to be broken if you have reason to suspect that a patient is driving when they should not. The need to protect the public overrides the individual's rights in this case.
- The rules below apply to Group 1 drivers; the rules for Group 2 drivers (e.g. heavy goods vehicles, passenger service vehicles) are much more strict; seek advice from the DVLA.
- Remind patients that they should contact their insurance company as well as the DVLA. Failure to do so could invalidate their insurance.

The current epilepsy regulations for Group 1 entitlement

- A person who has suffered an epileptic attack whilst **awake** must refrain from driving for **one** year from the date of the attack before a driving licence may be issued.

OR

- A person who has suffered an attack whilst **asleep** must also refrain from driving for **one** year from the date of the attack, unless they have had an attack whilst asleep more than three years ago and have not had any awake attacks since that asleep attack.

AND

- In any event, the driving of a vehicle by such a person should not be likely to cause danger to the public.
- For more information see *www.dvla.gov.uk*

Barbiturates

CNS depressants

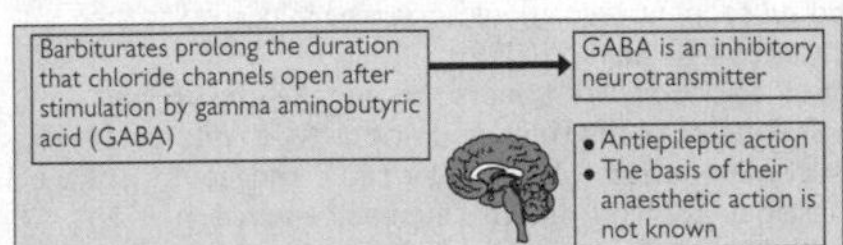

Drugs in this class

Short-acting
- Thiopental

Intermediate-acting
- Amobarbital
- Butobarbital
- Quinalbarbital

Long-acting
- Phenobarbital
- Primidone (metabolized to phenobarbital)

- These drugs are now very limited in use.
- Only thiopental for induction of anaesthesia is widely used.
- Intermediate-acting barbiturates are only used for severe intractable insomnia in patients who are already taking barbiturates.
  - Patients should not be started on these drugs de novo.
- Long-acting barbiturates have a limited role in the treatment of epilepsy.

- With the exception of thiopental, these drugs are all controlled drugs.
- Dependency and tolerance readily occur with long-term use of these drugs. They are also dangerous in overdose. For these reasons they are not usually recommended.
- Avoid them in people with respiratory disease; they can cause respiratory depression.
- Avoid barbiturates in people with hepatic insufficiency; they can precipitate decompensation and coma.
- Avoid barbiturates in severe renal insufficiency.
- These drugs should not be given during pregnancy:
  - They can cause congenital defects and vitamin K deficiency in the newborn. The latter can cause haemolytic disease of the newborn.
  - Neonates can also suffer withdrawal symptoms.
- Avoid these drugs in porphyria.

Thiopental for anaesthesia
- This is an effective anaesthetic, but it has no analgesic actions.
- It acts for a short time because it is rapidly distributed around the body; redistribution occurs later because of release from fat stores.
- It is irritant; make sure the vein for injection is patent.

Phenobarbital for epilepsy
- Phenobarbital has a limited role in the treatment of epilepsy. Primidone is largely metaboliized to phenobarbital. These drugs are effective for both tonic-clonic and partial seizures, but there are safer alternatives.
- Barbiturates are not first-line treatment for their other indications; there are safer alternatives.
- But do not stop these drugs suddenly:
  - This can cause rebound insomnia, anxiety, tremor, and convulsions.
  - The withdrawal syndrome can be fatal.

- Most of the adverse effects of these drugs are the result of long-term use and do not apply to single doses of thiopental.
- Tolerance to these drugs develops rapidly. They also commonly cause dependence.

- Barbiturates have a hangover effect.
- The most common adverse effects are dizziness and ataxia.
- Excessive doses can accumulate, causing respiratory depression.
- High dosages can also cause paradoxical excitement and confusion.
- Long-term use of these drugs can cause a megaloblastic anaemia.
  - Treat this with folic acid.
- These drugs are very dangerous in overdose, owing to respiratory depression.
- Hypersensitivity phenomena, including skin blisters, are relatively common.

- Barbiturates are subject to a large number of drug interactions because they are potent inducers of liver enzymes (see carbamazepine, p. 246).
- Barbiturates can lower the plasma concentration of many other antiepileptic drugs.
- Barbiturates increase the rate of metabolism of oestrogens and progestogens; this can render the oral contraceptive pill ineffective. Advise women to use barrier methods of contraception.
- Barbiturates can increase the rate of metabolism of immune modulators, such as ciclosporin and tacrolimus. Measure the plasma concentrations of these drugs to ensure that they remain within the target range (see teaching point below).
- Barbiturates can increase the rate of metabolism of warfarin, reducing the anticoagulant effect. Measure the INR more regularly until a new steady state has been established.
- Avoid co-prescribing with St John's wort.

Safety and efficacy

- Plasma concentration measurement is recommended if phenobarbital is given long-term.
  - The target plasma concentration is 15–40 mg/L (60–80 micromol/L); see below for more information about measurement of the plasma concentration of drugs.
  - This is limited in its usefulness because patients become tolerant to the effects of barbiturates.
  - Primidone is metabolized to phenobarbital; measure the phenobarbital concentration.

- Warn the patient that these drugs cause drowsiness that may interfere with skilled motor tasks (e.g. driving).
  - Patients with epilepsy must be made aware of the law regarding driving.
- Warn patients that the effect of alcohol is enhanced by barbiturates.
- Warn female patients that these drugs may render the oral contraceptive pill ineffective.

Prescribing information: **Barbiturates**

- The use of thiopental for anaesthesia is specialized.
- Barbiturates are not generally recommended for their other indications. Detailed prescribing information is not given.

TEACHING POINT

Plasma drug concentration target ranges

- Measurement of the plasma concentration of drugs is only practically useful in certain circumstances:
  - When there is difficulty in evaluating therapeutic or toxic effects clinically.
    - For example, it is simpler and clinically more helpful to measure the blood pressure when a beta-blocker is given for hypertension.
  - When there is a clear relation between plasma concentration and effect.
    - For example, toxicity from phenytoin is almost universal at plasma concentrations above 80 micromol/L. By contrast, the plasma concentration of sodium valproate correlates poorly with its antiepileptic effect.
  - When the drug has a low toxic to therapeutic ratio.
  - The drug should not be metabolized to active metabolites.
    - If the drug has active metabolites, interpretation of a single plasma concentration becomes impossible.
- The target concentration range gives an indication of the concentrations over which the drug is likely to be therapeutic, or over which adverse effects are less common. A plasma drug concentration within this range is not a guarantee of therapeutic efficacy or absence of adverse effects. The plasma concentration must be used in conjunction with clinical observations to individualize a patient's therapy.
- Some patients are more prone to the adverse effects of drugs (e.g. elderly people); the target range for these patients may well be lower than for others.
- Remember that the plasma concentration is a dynamic measure that depends on the pharmacokinetic properties of the drug. This has practical implications:
  - Plasma concentrations measured before a steady state has been reached can be misleading (see amiodarone (p. 103) for more information about steady state and the half-life of a drug).
  - The time at which the sample is taken is important; see below for more information.
- The table opposite gives examples of drugs for which plasma concentration measurement is of proven benefit; see individual articles for more information.

Drug	Sample timing	Reason for plasma concentration measurement	Target concentration range
Aminoglycoside antibiotics (e.g. gentamicin)	Peak 15 mins after the end of an intravenous infusion; trough just before the next dose	Ototoxicity is related to the trough concentration	Peak <12 mg/mL Trough <2 mg/mL
Carbamazepine	2 weeks after changing the dose	Carbamazepine induces its own metabolism (see carbamazepine, p. 246)	17–42 micromol/L
Phenytoin	14 days after a dose change	Pheytoin has zero-order kinetics (see phenytoin, p. 252)	40–80 micromol/L (10–20 mg/L)
Digoxin	At least 6 hours after the last dose	Digoxin is excreted by the kidneys; renal function can vary with intercurrent illness or concomitant medications (e.g. NSAIDs)	1.0–2.6 nmol/L
Ciclosporin	Immediately before a dose	Low concentrations increase the risk of transplant rejection; high concentrations cause nephrotoxicity	125–200 ng/mL (whole blood)
Lithium	Exactly 12 hours after the previous dose	Lithium excretion is affected by sodium balance	0.4–1.0 mmol/L
Theophylline	During chronic therapy; 8–12 hours after the previous dose	Theophylline has a narrow therapeutic range; drug interactions are common	10–20 micrograms/mL

Benzodiazepines

Hypnotics and anxiolytics

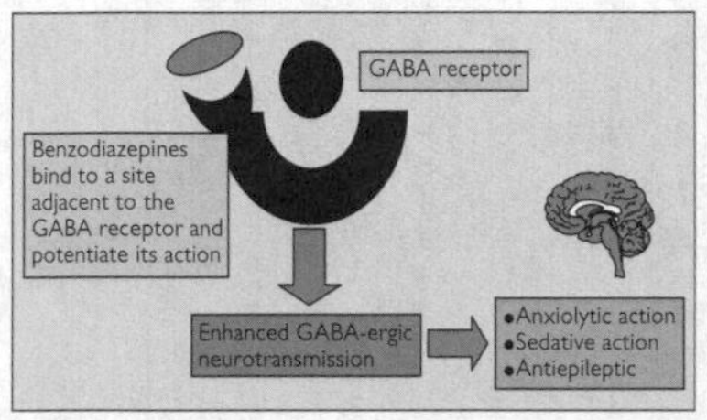

Drugs in this class (with approximately equivalent dosages

Long-acting	
• Diazepam	5 mg
• Lorazepam	0.5 mg
• Nitrazepam	5 mg
• Chlordiazep-oxide	15 mg
Short-acting	
• Oxazepam	15 mg
• Temazepam	10 mg
• Lormetazepam	0.5–1.0 mg
• Loprazolam	0.5–1.0 mg
Used for epilepsy	
• Clobazam	
• Clonazepam	

- Treatment of anxiety, and premedication before operations and procedures.
- Short-term use for night sedation.
- Sedation for procedures.
- Treatment of seizures.
- Skeletal muscle relaxant to relieve muscle spasm.
- Adjunct to the treatment of alcohol withdrawal.

- The sedative effect can be dangerous in patients with respiratory insufficiency, sleep apnoea syndrome, or myasthenia gravis.
- Benzodiazepines can precipitate decompensation in patients with hepatic insufficiency.
- They can be subject to abuse. Temazepam gel-filled capsules can be melted and injected and cannot be prescribed in the NHS. Temazepam and flunitrazepam (Rohypnol®) are subject to special legal constraints. A controlled drug prescription is required for flunitrazepam, but not for temazepam. Think carefully whether another drug would be appropriate before prescribing these drugs.
- Avoid regular use of these drugs in pregnancy; they can cause withdrawal symptoms in the newborn.

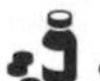

Anxiety

- The CSM advises using the smallest possible dose for the shortest possible time. Benzodiazepines are not an appropriate treatment for mild anxiety.
- Benzodiazepines do not have an antidepressant action and are not a treatment for psychosis.
- Shorter-acting drugs, such as oxazepam or lorazepam, may be preferred over longer-acting ones; they have less of a hangover effect. However, these drugs carry a greater risk of withdrawal symptoms — see box below.

Insomnia

- The CSM advises that benzodiazepines should only be used when the insomnia is 'severe, disabling, or subjecting the patient to extreme distress'.

- Chronic insomnia is rarely helped by benzodiazepines. They are more effective for:
  - Transient insomnia in those who normally sleep well but are subject to a disrupting event (e.g. an operation or jet lag). Give 1 or 2 doses of a short-acting benzodiazepine.
  - Short-term insomnia associated with a specific event (e.g. illness or bereavement). Keep treatment to less than 1 week.
- Do not take more than 1 dose per night.

Seizures

- Benzodiazepines are first-line treatment for the termination of seizures and status epilepticus. See teaching point.
- Most benzodiazepines are not suitable for the long-term control of epilepsy; their effect wears off rapidly (tachyphylaxis).
- Benzodiazepines are used for the treatment and prophylaxis of febrile convulsions. This is a specialized use; seek expert advice.
- Clonazepam and clobazam are used for the long-term treatment of tonic-clonic seizures, partial seizures, or as an adjunctive treatment. This a specialized use and their effect abates with time.

Premedication and sedation

- Diazepam and lorazepam have a long duration of action. They are not the most suitable choice for premedication, especially for day-case surgery. Consider temazepam instead.
- Midazolam has amnesic properties and can produce profound sedation. This can be used to advantage for some procedures and for sedation on intensive care, but take care when mild sedation is all that is required.
- Intravenous diazepam can be used for the severely agitated, such as those withdrawing from alcohol (see below).
- See antipsychotic drugs (neuroleptic drugs) (p. 295) for guidance on the management of the acutely agitated patient.

Treatment of muscle spasm

- Benzodiazepines have a limited role in the treatment of muscle spasm. See baclofen (p. 588).
- Benzodiazepines are not appropriate for acute muscle spasm associated with an acute injury.

Alcohol withdrawal

- Chlordiazepoxide is the benzodiazepine of choice for treatment of alcohol withdrawal. It is safer than clomethiazole, which should only be used for in-patients.
- Use a rapidly-reducing dosage regimen (see prescribing information), but titrate the dose to the patient's clinical state.
- Do not give benzodiazepines if the patient is still drinking alcohol.
- Intravenous diazepam can be used for severe agitation if withdrawal is taking place in hospital (see prescribing information). Diazepam should not be used if the patient has hepatic encephalopathy, cirrhosis, or alcoholic hepatitis; it can induce coma.

- Benzodiazepines can cause respiratory distress and even arrest, especially when given intravenously.
  - Ensure that adequate resuscitation facilities are available.
  - Do not use the GABA antagonist flumazenil when diazepam has been used for control of seizures; it can cause intractable seizures.

- CNS adverse effects are common: ataxia, confusion, and drowsiness. In a few patients benzodiazepines cause paradoxical aggression.
- Dependency, both psychological and physical, is common with prolonged use. Avoid prolonged treatment.

- Benzodiazepines potentiate the effect of any other CNS depressant (including alcohol).
- Drugs such as erythromycin, ketoconazole, fluconazole, and itraconazole inhibit the metabolism of benzodiazepines, and so potentiate their action.

Safety and efficacy

- Ensure that adequate resuscitation facilities are available whenever giving a benzodiazepine intravenously.

- Benzodiazepines are very useful drugs when used selectively for short periods. Only prescribe short courses and review the patient rather than issue a repeat prescription.
- Warn the patient about the sedative effects.
- When using benzodiazepines to aid alcohol withdrawal, make sure that patients understand that they must not drink alcohol while taking these drugs; it is dangerous and defeats the purpose of giving them.

Prescribing information: **Benzodiazepines**

Diazepam

- *Anxiety* By mouth, 2 mg 3 times daily, increased if necessary to 15–30 mg daily in divided doses. Use half the adult dose in elderly people.
- *Severe agitation, especially in those withdrawing from alcohol* 10–20 mg intravenously over 1–2 minutes. Repeated if necessary with 5 mg every 5 minutes until the patient is calm.
- *Seizures* By intravenous injection, 10–20 mg at a rate of 0.5 mL (2.5 mg) per 30 seconds.
- *Seizures* By rectal solution, 500 micrograms/kg. Tubes available contain 2.5 mg, 5 mg, 10 mg, and 20 mg, depending on the manufacturer.

Lorazepam

- *Seizures* By intravenous injection, 2–4 mg.

Temazepam

- *Insomnia (short-term use)* 10–20 mg at bedtime.

Nitrazepam

- *Insomnia (short-term use)* 5–10 mg at bedtime.

Chlordiazepoxide (see also below)

- *Alcohol withdrawal* By mouth, 10–50 mg 4 times daily, gradually reducing over 7–14 days.

TEACHING POINT Guidelines for the withdrawal of benzodiazepines

- Abrupt withdrawal can cause confusion, convulsions, and psychosis in severe cases.
- The more common withdrawal syndrome is one of insomnia, anxiety, sweating, appetite loss, disturbed sleep, and vivid dreams.
- These symptoms are very similar to those for which the benzodiazepine may have been prescribed in the first place, and are commonly misinterpreted as a recurrence of symptoms, leading to a repeat prescription for benzodiazepines.
- Withdrawal symptoms can occur within a few hours for short-acting drugs, but up to 3 weeks after cessation for the long-acting ones.
- For patients who have been taking benzodiazepines for a long time, it is advised that the dose be reduced by 2.0–2.5 mg (diazepam equivalents) every 2 weeks.
    - If symptoms occur, maintain the current dose until the patient improves. This can take weeks.
    - The process can take a very long time (months) and you should warn the patient of this.
    - Beta-blockers should only be used if other measures fail.
    - Antidepressants should only be used when there is a clear diagnosis of depression or panic disorder.
    - Do not use antipsychotic drugs during benzodiazepine withdrawal.

TEACHING POINT Treatment of status epilepticus

- Status epilepticus is defined as a seizure that lasts for more than 30 minutes, or when repeated seizures occur over 30 minutes without full recovery in between.
- Whenever a seizure continues for longer than a few seconds you should aim to stop it as soon as possible.
- Give intravenous glucose 1–2 mL/kg if the seizure is due to hypoglycaemia.
    - If the patient is withdrawing from alcohol, give B vitamins first (e.g. Pabrinex®, 1 pair of ampoules).
- A benzodiazepine is the first-line drug treatment, but do not forget other basic measures such as securing the airway (place the patient in the recovery position; do not put anything in their mouth) and giving oxygen.
- Give either:
    - Lorazepam 0.07 mg/kg (usually 4 mg in adults) by intravenous injection over 2 minutes. Repeat the dose once after 10–20 minutes, if required, *or*
    - Diazepam 10–20 mg by injection over 2–4 minutes. Maximum dose 40 mg.
    - If intravenous access is not possible, diazepam is available as a solution for rectal administration.
    - Note that the emulsion formulation (Diazemuls®) is less irritant than other formulations for intravenous administration.
- Ensure that adequate resuscitation facilities are available; in particular, be prepared to deal with respiratory compromise as a result of benzodiazepine use.
- If the seizure continues beyond 10 minutes, give intravenous phenytoin.
    - If the patient has not been taking phenytoin, the loading dose is 18 mg/kg (usual adult dose 1.0–1.5 g) by intravenous infusion (50 mg/min). Flush the line after infusion.
    - If the patient has been taking phenytoin consider either:
        - A lower loading dose (10 mg/kg; 500 mg –1.0 g total) *or*
        - Another drug, such as sodium valproate.
- If this is unsuccessful, transfer to ITU and seek expert advice.

TEACHING POINT

Chlordiazepoxide dosage regimen for alcohol withdrawal in hospital

- Patients should begin treatment as soon as they are able to tolerate oral medication. This regimen sedates for 1–2 days (the period of greatest risk), but then rapidly tails off over the next 3–4 days.
- There is a risk of fits as the dose is reduced.
- Do not sedate for too long; patients sedated for more than 2 days are at risk of chest infections.
- Some of these patients will have liver dysfunction. Review the dose carefully (twice daily) to avoid over-sedation.
- A maximum of 24 hours' supply may be prescribed on discharge

Day	Regular dose	As required
Day 1	20 mg qds	10 mg prn, max 200 mg daily
Day 2	20 mg qds	10 mg prn, max 200 mg daily
Day 3	20 mg tds	
Day 4	20 mg bd	
Day 5	20 mg bd	
Day 6	STOP	

Clomethiazole (chlormethiazole)

Similar in action to, but pharmacologically distinct from, benzodiazepines

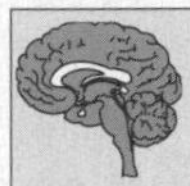

The mechanism of action of clomethiazole is not known. It has sedative and anxiolytic properties that are similar to those of the benzodiazepines.

Treatment of alcohol withdrawal

- See benzodiazepines, p. 267.

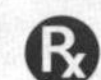

- Hypnotic for short-term use (in elderly people).
- Adjunct to the treatment of alcohol withdrawal.
  - Clomethiazole should only be used for withdrawal taking place as an in-patient. It is potentially hazardous if the patient continues to drink alcohol. Consider chlordiazepoxide as an alternative.

- The sedative effect can be dangerous in patients with respiratory insufficiency, sleep apnoea syndrome, or myasthenia gravis.
- The intravenous formulation can cause marked respiratory depression and should not be used.
- Clomethiazole can precipitate decompensation in patients with hepatic insufficiency (cirrhosis).
- Clomethiazole is potentially hazardous if the patient continues to drink alcohol.
- Clomethiazole can be habit-forming and lead to dependency.
- Patients with renal insufficiency are more sensitive to the effects of this drug; reduce the dose.
- Avoid clomethiazole during pregnancy; it can affect fetal development (limited information).

Insomnia

- Clomethiazole can be used as a hypnotic for short-term use. It may be of particular use in elderly people, as it has little hangover effect.
- See benzodiazepines (p. 266) for further guidance on the use of hypnotic drugs.

Alcohol withdrawal

- Clomethiazole is no longer the drug of choice in alcohol withdrawal. Consider chlordiazepoxide instead.
- The capsules may be used, but only by in-patients. The intravenous formulation causes marked respiratory depression and should not be used.

- Clomethiazole can cause respiratory depression.
  - Ensure that adequate resuscitation facilities are available.
- Nasal irritation and sneezing are common.
- Other adverse effects include conjunctival irritation, headache, nausea, and vomiting.
- Dependency can occur with prolonged use. Avoid prolonged treatment.

- Clomethiazole potentiates the effects of other CNS depressants (including alcohol).

Safety and efficacy

- Clomethiazole can be useful when used selectively for short periods. Only prescribe short courses and review the patient rather than issue a repeat prescription.

- Warn the patient about the sedative effects.
- When using clomethiazole to aid alcohol withdrawal, make sure that the patient understands that they must not drink alcohol while taking the drug; it is dangerous and defeats the purpose of giving it.

Prescribing information: **Clomethiazole**

Insomnia

- Short-term use for severe insomnia, 1 or 2 capsules at bedtime (1 capsule contains 192 mg clomethiazole)
- Alternatively, 5–10 mL syrup (250 mg/5 mL)

Alcohol withdrawal

- Specialist use, use local protocol.

Benzodiazepine-like hypnotics

These drugs are not benzodiazepines chemically, but bind to the same receptor

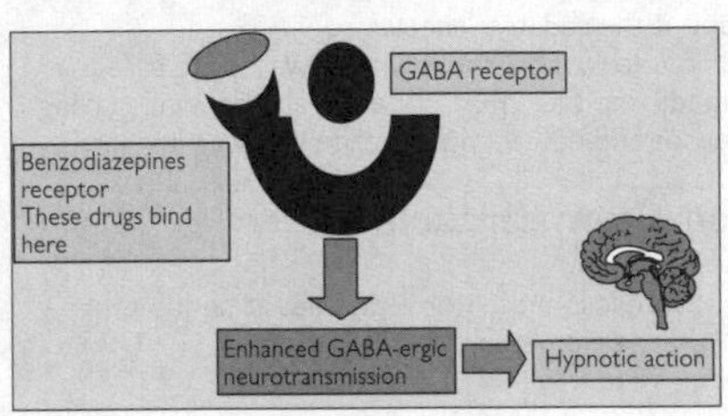

Drugs in this class
All are short-acting
• Zaleplon
• Zolpidem
• Zopiclone

- Short-term treatment of insomnia.

- These hypnotics are not effective for the other indications for which benzodiazepines are used.
- The sedative effect can be dangerous in patients with respiratory insufficiency, sleep apnoea syndrome, or myasthenia gravis.
- Halve the dose in elderly people.
- Pregnancy and breast feeding — insufficient evidence to recommend use.

Insomnia

- Chronic insomnia is rarely helped by treatment with hypnotics. They are more effective for:
  - Transient insomnia in those who normally sleep well but are subject to a disrupting event (e.g. an operation or jet lag). Give 1 or 2 doses.
  - Short-term insomnia associated with a specific event (e.g. illness or bereavement). Keep treatment to less than 1 week.
- These drugs are not licensed for long-term treatment.
- Take a single dose at night if unable to sleep.

- Reported adverse effects include drowsiness, headache, weakness, and dizziness.
- These drugs are prone to cause confusion in the elderly; halve the dose.
- There is emerging evidence of dependence with long-term use in some patients. Do not use long-term.

- Drugs such as erythromycin, ritonavir, and cimetidine inhibit the metabolism of these drugs and so potentiate their action. See erythromycin (p. 347) for more information.

Safety and efficacy

- These may be useful drugs when used selectively for short periods. Only prescribe short courses and review the patient rather than issue a repeat prescription.

- Warn the patient about the sedative effects.

Prescribing information: **Benzodiazepine-like hypnotics**

Zaleplon

- *Insomnia* By mouth, 10 mg at night. Halve the dose in the elderly.

Zolpidem

- *Insomnia* By mouth, 10 mg at night. Halve the dose in the elderly.

Zopiclone

- *Insomnia* By mouth, 7.5 mg at night. Halve the dose in the elderly.

Tricyclic antidepressants

Inhibitors of the reuptake of noradrenaline (norepinephrine) and serotonin (5-HT) in central monoaminergic neurons

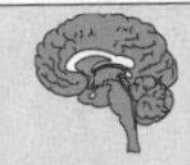

- Although the pharmacological actions of these drugs are well described, the mechanism by which they have an antidepressant effect is not fully understood. It appears to involve adaptive responses within the brain to the changes in monaminergic neurotransmission.

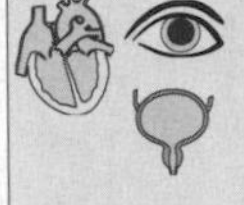

- These drugs also have central and peripheral anticholinergic effects. These are responsible for many of the adverse effects caused by tricyclic antidepressants.

- Some tricyclic antidepressants are also H_1 histamine receptor antagonists. This may be responsible for the drowsiness caused by some of these drugs.

Tricyclic antidepressants and related drugs

Sedative
- Amitriptyline
- Clomipramine
- Dosulepin (dothiepin)
- Doxepin*
- Maprotiline
- Mianserin*
- Trazodone*
- Trimipramine

Less sedative
- Amoxapine
- Imipramine
- Lofepramine*
- Nortriptyline

*Drugs with fewer anticholinergic effects.

- Treatment of depression (especially of the endogenous type).
- Treatment of panic disorder.
- Treatment of nocturnal enuresis (unlicensed indication).
- Treatment of painful diabetic neuropathy (unlicensed indication).
- Prophylaxis against migraine headache (unlicensed indication).

- Do not use with monoamine oxidase inhibitors (MAOIs), especially tranylcypromine.
  - Wait 2–3 weeks after stopping an MAOI before starting a tricyclic antidepressant, and vice versa.
- Tricyclic antidepressants have anticholinergic effects; consider alternatives in patients with prostatic enlargement or closed-angle glaucoma.
- Be aware that tricyclic antidepressants lower the seizure threshold.
- Take care if the patient has hepatic insufficiency; the sedative effects of these drugs are enhanced.
- No dosage reduction is usually required if the patient has renal insufficiency.
- These drugs are used during pregnancy, but they can cause neonatal tachycardia and irritability.

Depression
- All of these drugs take about 2 weeks before they begin to work. Consider additional emergency treatment, such as electroconvulsive therapy, if this delay poses an unacceptable risk to the patient.
- Given that these drugs are thought to act by adaptive effects, rather than via a direct pharmacological action, combination formulations and modified-release formulations are not recommended.

- Choose a sedative or less sedative drug depending on how agitated the patient is.
- Advise patients to take their tablets last thing at night; this will minimize the impact of anticholinergic effects.
- Improvement in sleep is often the first benefit of treatment; other symptoms take longer to improve.
- These drugs are potentially fatal in overdose; limit the quantities prescribed on each occasion and review the patient before issuing a repeat prescription. (See below for treatment of tricyclic antidepressant overdose.)
  - Amoxapine, desipramine, and dothiepin appear to be associated with the highest risk of death when taken in overdose (*BMJ* 2002, 325:1332–3).
- Withdraw these drugs slowly:
  - Over 4 weeks if the patient has taken a short course.
  - Over 6 months after long-term maintenance treatment.

Treatment of panic disorder

- Starting treatment with a tricyclic antidepressant can cause a transient worsening of symptoms. Start with a low dose and increase gradually.

Treatment of noctural enuresis (imipramine, amitriptyline, nortriptyline)

- Note that the use of an enuresis alarm is first-line treatment.
- Do not use in children under 7 years old.
- Treatment is not usually continued for more than 3 months.

Treatment of painful diabetic neuropathy — see gabapentin (p. 674) for more information

- Other classes of antidepressant do not appear to be effective.

Prophylaxis against migraine

- This is a second-line option.
- Note that this a prophylactic treatment. Other drugs are required once the headache has occurred.

- Anticholinergic adverse effects are common: dry mouth, blurred vision, constipation, difficulty with micturition.
  - Tolerance to these effects develops; it is worth encouraging patients to persevere with treatment if possible.
- Tricyclic antidepressants are associated with cardiac toxicity, especially in overdose.
  - This is characterized by tachycardia, ventricular arrhythmias, and heart block; prolongation of the QT interval correlates well with the severity of toxicity.
- Tricyclic antidepressants lower the seizure threshold.
- Hypotension occurs in up to 20% of patients treated with tricyclic antidepressants.
- Tricyclic antidepressants can cause the syndrome of inappropriate ADH secretion, resulting in hyponatraemia with confusion.
  - The elderly are especially likely to develop this adverse effect.

- These drugs enhance the sedative effect of other drugs (e.g. alcohol, antihistamines, opioids).
- They increase the risk of arrhythmias when given with drugs that prolong the QT interval (e.g. amiodarone, sotalol, antipsychotic drugs).
- Do not give these drugs with MAOIs (unless under specialist supervision).

- Take care when giving tricyclic antidepressants with other drugs that stimulate the CNS (e.g. entacapone, selegiline, sibutramine).
- Take care if the patient has epilepsy; tricyclic antidepressants lower the seizure threshold and increase the metabolism of common antiepileptic drugs.
- Tricyclic antidepressants can cause the serotonin syndrome, especially when they are co-prescribed with other drugs that affect serotonin metabolism (see SSRIs, p. 283).
- Do not give these drugs with the antimalarial drugs lumefantrine and Artemisia derivatives.

Safety

- Pharmacological intervention is only part of the treatment for depression. Regular clinical assessment is important to ensure that the patient is improving.
- Measure the plasma electrolytes if the patient becomes confused; tricyclic antidepressants can cause hyponatraemia through inappropriate ADH secretion.

Efficacy

- 10–20% of patients fail to respond. Treatment with an inadequate dose is responsible for a proportion of these. Review the dose if the patient is not responding.
  - The caveat to this is that elderly people may not be able to tolerate large doses, owing to the anticholinergic effects.

- Explain to the patient that these drugs will not work instantly, that it may take weeks before the first benefits are seen, and that it may be some months before they recover.
- Warn the patient about anticholinergic adverse effects. Explain that many patients become tolerant to these after a short period, allowing them to continue treatment.
- Explain that the tablets are only part of the treatment; psychological support is also important.
- These drugs may cause drowsiness that will interfere with skilled motor tasks (e.g. driving).

Prescribing information: **Tricyclic antidepressants**

There are many drugs in this class; the following are given as examples.

Amitriptyline

- *Depression* Initially 75 mg (elderly and adolescents 30–75 mg) daily in divided doses *or* as a single dose at bedtime, increased gradually as necessary to 150–200 mg.
- *Nocturnal enuresis* Children 7–10 years, 10–20 mg; 11–16 years, 25–50 mg at night.
- *Other indications* See how to use section.

Clomipramine

- *Depression* Initially 10 mg daily, increased gradually as necessary to 30–150 mg daily in divided doses *or* as a single dose at bedtime; maximum 250 mg daily. Elderly, initially 10 mg daily, increased carefully over about 10 days to 30–75 mg daily.
- *Phobic and obsessional states* Initially 25 mg daily (elderly 10 mg daily), increased over 2 weeks to 100–150 mg daily.

Imipramine

- *Depression* Initially up to 75 mg daily in divided doses, increased gradually to 150–200 mg (up to 300 mg in hospital patients). Up to 150 mg may be given as a single dose at bedtime. Elderly, initially 10 mg daily, increased gradually to 30–50 mg daily.
- *Nocturnal enuresis* Children 7 years, 25 mg; 8–11 years, 25–50 mg; over 11 years, 50–75 mg at bedtime.

Lofepramine

- *Depression* 140–210 mg daily in divided doses. Elderly people may respond to lower doses.

TEACHING POINT Treatment of tricyclic antidepressant overdose

- Deliberate overdose of tricyclic antidepressants is common and is responsible for a significant proportion of the fatal overdoses in the UK.
- The toxicity of tricyclic antidepressants in overdose is principally related to their effects on the heart.
  - Adrenergic and anticholinergic effects (tachycardia and arrhythmias).
  - Quinidine-like delays in cardiac conduction (prolonged QT interval).
  - Direct myocardial depression.
- **Clinical features of tricyclic antidepressant overdose**
  - Anticholinergic features: hot dry skin, dry mouth and tongue, dilated pupils, and urinary retention.
  - Cardiac features: the most common finding is a sinus tachycardia. ECG features include prolongation of the PR and QT intervals; in very severe poisoning the ECG may be bizarre.
  - CNS features: drowsiness is common and can very rapidly progress to coma with respiratory arrest. Fits occur in over 5% of cases.
- **Management summary** (refer to your local poisons centre for the latest guidelines)
  - Be prepared to intubate and ventilate the patient if necessary. Institute continuous cardiac monitoring.
  - Give activated charcoal (50 g) by mouth or nasogastric tube if more than 4 mg/kg has been ingested within 1 hour, provided the airway can be protected. A second dose of charcoal (50 g) should be considered after 2 hours in patients with central features of toxicity. Give multiple-dose activated charcoal if a modified-release formulation has been ingested.
    - Forced diuresis, haemodialysis, and haemoperfusion are of no proven value.
  - Resist the temptation to treat arrhythmias with drugs. Arrhythmias are best treated by correction of hypoxia and acidosis.
  - Even in the absence of acidosis, sodium bicarbonate 50 mmol should be given iv to an adult with arrhythmias or significant ECG abnormalities (500 mL of 1.26% sodium bicarbonate contains 75 mmol, and 50 mL of 8.4% contains 50 mmol). The mechanism of action of bicarbonate is to alter binding of tricyclic antidepressants to the myocardium. Further doses may be required depending on clinical response.
  - Control convulsions with intravenous diazepam (0.1–0.3 mg/kg body weight) or lorazepam (4 mg). Do not use phenytoin.

Selective serotonin reuptake inhibitors (SSRIs)

Inhibitors of the reuptake of serotonin (5-HT) in central monoaminergic neurons

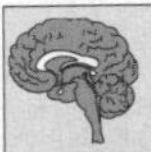

- Although the pharmacological actions of these drugs are well described, the mechanism by which they have an antidepressant effect is not fully understood. It appears to involve an adaptive response within the brain to the changes in serotoninergic neurotransmission.
- Unlike the related tricyclic antidepressants, these drugs do not have marked central and peripheral anticholinergic effects.

Drugs in this class

- Fluoxetine
- Paroxetine
- Fluvoxamine
- Sertraline
- Citalopram
  - Escitalopram is an isomer of citalopram

- Treatment of depression (especially of the endogenous type).
- Treatment of panic disorder (paroxetine, citalopram) and social phobias (paroxetine).
- Treatment of obsessive-compulsive disorder (fluoxetine, fluvoxamine, paroxetine).
- Treatment of bulimia nervosa (fluoxetine).
- Treatment of generalized anxiety and post-traumatic stress disorder.

- Do not use with MAOIs, especially tranylcypromine
  - Wait 2–3 weeks after stopping an MAOI before starting an SSRI, and vice versa.
- SSRIs can have a stimulant effect; they are contraindicated in bipolar depression and mania.
- Although the SSRIs have few anticholinergic effects, take care in patients with prostatic enlargement or closed-angle glaucoma.
- The use of SSRIs is not recommended in patients receiving electroconvulsive therapy, but this is a risk/benefit decision that should be taken by the specialist treating the patient. SSRIs lower the seizure threshold.
- The manufacturers advise that these drugs should only be given during pregnancy if they are essential. There is no evidence of toxicity.
- Halve the dose or avoid these drugs in severe hepatic or renal insufficiency.

Depression

- SSRIs are no more effective antidepressants than tricyclic drugs, but they are better tolerated. In addition, they are considerably less cardiotoxic in overdose.
- Like the tricyclic antidepressants, they take about 2 weeks before they begin to work. Consider additional emergency treatment, such as electroconvulsive therapy, if this delay poses an unacceptable risk to the patient (but see cautions above).
- The differences between the SSRIs are not great, but the following factors may be taken into account:
  - Rapid onset of action required: avoid fluoxetine. Fluoxetine has a slower onset of action than the other SSRIs; however, the long half-life may be an advantage when compliance is erratic.
  - Paroxetine and fluvoxamine are slightly less well tolerated than the other SSRIs.
  - When there are concomitant medications that have the potential to interact, citalopram or sertraline may be the best choice.

Other indications

- The other indications for the use of SSRI should be reserved for specialist use following a thorough assessment and consideration of other therapeutic options. SSRIs are not appropriate for mild anxiety or shyness.

- Adverse effects are very common (57% of patients), but in most cases they are mild and transient.
- Gastrointestinal adverse effects are common: nausea, constipation, diarrhoea, dry mouth, and dyspepsia.
- Headache.
- SSRIs can cause 'stimulant' CNS symptoms: agitation, anxiety, tremor, akathisia, nervousness, and insomnia.
- Hyponatraemia caused by a syndrome of inappropriate ADH secretion (SIADH) is especially likely in the elderly.
- Hypersensitivity phenomena and vasculitis are rare.
- The SSRIs can cause the serotonin syndrome; this is uncommon when they are used on their own, but is much more common when the patient is taking another drug that affects serotonin metabolism (see teaching point below).
- There has been a suggestion of increased aggression or suicidal ideation with SSRIs. There is thought to be an increased risk of suicide in children under 18; they are not recommended in this age group.
    - All the SSRIs can be associated with agitation and restlessness (akathisia).
- Withdrawal reactions are relatively common, particularly with paroxetine.
    - Withdraw over 4 weeks if the patient has taken a short course.
    - Withdraw over 6 months if they have been on long-term maintenance treatment.
- There is some evidence that SSRIs increase the risk of gastrointestinal bleeding, but the risk is small.

- Do not give SSRIs with an MAOI (unless under specialist supervision).
- Take care when giving these drugs with other drugs that can stimulate the CNS (e.g. 5-HT_1 agonists ('triptans'), entacapone, selegiline, sibutramine, lithium, tramadol).
- Take care if the patient has epilepsy; SSRIs lower the seizure threshold and can increase the metabolism of common antiepileptic drugs.
- Do not give these drugs with the antimalarial drugs lumefantrine and Artemisia derivatives.
- The SSRIs interact with the cytochrome P450 enzymes. This is greatest for fluoxetine, fluvoxamine, and paroxetine; less for sertraline; and least for citalopram.
- SSRIs can cause the serotonin syndrome, especially when they are co-prescribed with other drugs that affect serotonin metabolism (see teaching point below).

Safety and efficacy

- Pharmacological intervention is only part of the treatment for depression. Regular clinical assessment is important to ensure that the patient is improving.
- Measure the plasma electrolytes if the patient becomes confused. SSRIs can cause hyponatraemia.

- Explain to the patient that these drugs will not work instantly; it may take weeks before the first benefits are seen, and it may be some months before they recover.
- Explain that the tablets are only part of the treatment; psychological support is also important.
- Warn the patient that adverse effects are common, but are usually mild and transient.
- These drugs may cause drowsiness that will interfere with skilled motor tasks (e.g. driving).

Prescribing information: **SSRIs**

Fluoxetine

- *Depression* 20 mg daily, increased after 3 weeks to 60 mg daily, if necessary

Citalopram

- *Depression* 20 mg daily as a single dose in the morning or evening, increased if necessary to a maximum of 60 mg daily. Elderly, maximum 40 mg daily.

Fluvoxamine

- *Depression* Initially 50–100 mg daily, increased if necessary to a maximum of 300 mg daily. If giving over 100 mg, divide the dose.

Paroxetine

- *Depression* Usually 20 mg each morning; if necessary increased gradually in steps of 10 mg to a maximum of 50 mg daily. In elderly people, 40 mg daily.

Sertraline

- *Depression* Initially 50 mg daily. This is also the usual maintenance dose, but it may be increased if necessary by increments of 50 mg over several weeks to a maximum of 200 mg daily.

TEACHING POINT The serotonin syndrome

The serotonin syndrome is a potentially fatal consequence of excessive serotonergic neurotransmission. It can be confused with the neuroleptic malignant syndrome, as there are some features in common, but as the table below shows there are some key differences.

Feature	Serotonin Syndrome	Neuroleptic Malignant Syndrome
Neuroleptic drugs	0	+++
Serotonergic drugs	+++	0
Hyperactivity	+++	0
Clonus	+++	0
Tremor	+++	+
Shivering	+++	0
Hyper-reflexia	+++	0
Rapid onset	+++	0
Leaden rigidity	0	+++
Bradykinesia	0	+++
Stupor/ mutism	0	+++
CPK activity	++	+++
Hallucinations	+	++

Drugs that can cause the syndrome

- SSRIs
- Serotonin precursors (tryptophan)
- Serotonin agonists (the 'triptans', buspirone, and LSD)
- Serotonin releasers (MDMA/ecstasy, amphetamines, amphetamine-like compounds, sibutramine)
- MAOIs
- Others (chlorphenamine, pethidine, cocaine, tramadol, levodopa, bromocriptine, lithium, St John's wort)

- The serotonin syndrome is rare when only one serotonergic drug is used, but the risk is greatly increased when two or more are used. A list is given above; note that some are not obvious and so are more likely to be co-prescribed.
- Management is largely supportive.
  - There is little trial evidence to guide management in more severe cases; contact your local poisons information centre for specific advice.
  - Treat fits with diazepam.
  - Dantrolene and cooled iv fluids may be used for the features of malignant hyperthermia.
  - Other treatments, such as chlorpromazine, cyproheptadine, and propranolol, are more controversial. Seek expert advice before using these drugs.

Venlafaxine

Inhibitor of the reuptake of serotonin (5-HT) and noradrenaline

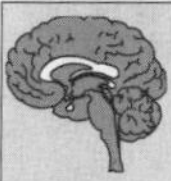

- Although the pharmacological actions of this drug are well described, the mechanism by which it has an antidepressant effect is not fully understood. It appears to involve an adaptive response within the brain to the changes in neurotransmission.
- Venlafaxine has fewer anticholinergic adverse effects than tricyclic antidepressant drugs.

Other antidepressant drugs

- Tricyclic antidepressant drugs
- Selective serotonin reuptake inhibitors (SSRIs)
- Mirtazapine* (presynaptic α_2 antagonist)
- Nefazodone* (SSRI and serotonin receptor antagonist)
- Reboxetine* (noradrenaline reuptake inhibitor)
- Tryptophan* (amino acid)

*Specialist use; not considered further here.

- Treatment of depression (especially of the endogenous type).
- Treatment of generalized anxiety.

- Do not use with MAOIs, especially tranylcypromine.
- Wait 2–3 weeks after stopping an MAOI before starting an SSRI, and vice versa.
- Although venlafaxine has few anticholinergic effects, take care in patients with prostatic enlargement or closed-angle glaucoma.
- Venlafaxine lowers the seizure threshold.
- Avoid venlafaxine in patients with severe hypertension, recent myocardial infarction, or unstable cardiac disease.
- There is no information on the safety of venlafaxine in pregnancy; avoid using it.
- Avoid venlafaxine in severe hepatic or renal insufficiency.

Depression

- Venlafaxine is not usually used as first-line treatment of depression. Consider a tricyclic antidepressant or SSRI.
- Venlafaxine is increasingly used as adjunctive therapy in severe or resistant cases. Seek a specialist opinion before using it in this way.
- Avoid abrupt withdrawal.

- Gastrointestinal adverse effects are common, especially nausea.
- Venlafaxine can cause hypertension.
- Hypersensitivity phenomena (e.g. urticaria) are uncommon, but can be severe. Stop the drug if they occur.
- Venlafaxine can cause the serotonin syndrome; this is uncommon when it is used on its own, but is much more common when the patient is taking another drug that affects serotonin metabolism (see teaching point in SSRI, p. 283).

- Take care if the patient has epilepsy; venlafaxine lowers the seizure threshold and increases the metabolism of some antiepileptic drugs.
- Venlafaxine can cause the serotonin syndrome, especially when it is co-prescribed with other drugs that affect serotonin metabolism.
- Avoid giving this drug with sibutramine; there is an increased risk of CNS toxicity.

Safety and efficacy

- Pharmacological intervention is only part of the treatment of depression. Regular clinical assessment is very important to ensure that the patient is improving.
- Measure the blood pressure if the daily dose exceeds 200 mg.

- Explain to the patient that venlafaxine will not work instantly; it may take weeks before the first benefits are seen, and it may be some months before recovery is complete.
- Explain that the tablets are only part of the treatment; psychological support is also important.
- Advise the patient to seek medical advice if they develop a rash while taking this drug.
- Venlafaxine may cause drowsiness that will interfere with skilled motor tasks (e.g. driving).

Prescribing information: **Venlafaxine**

Depression

- By mouth, 37.5 mg twice daily.
- Can be increased to 75 mg twice daily after several weeks, if required.
- The maximum dose in severe cases is 375 mg daily (in divided doses), but the patient should not be maintained on this dose.

Monoamine oxidase inhibitors (MAOIs)

Inhibitors of the enzyme monoamine oxidase

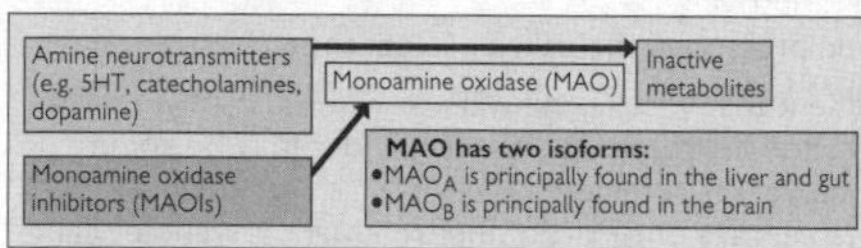

Drugs in this class

- Non-selective MAOIs
  - Phenelzine, isocarboxazid, tranylcypromine, iproniazid
- Inhibitor of MAO$_A$
  - Moclobemide (reversible)
- Inhibitor of MAO$_B$
  - Selegiline

Note that linezolid (an antibiotic) is also a non-selective, reversible MAOI.

- Second-line treatment of depression (non-selective inhibitors and moclobemide).
  - Especially if there are phobic or other atypical symptoms (e.g. hysteria).
- Treatment of Parkinson's disease (selegiline).

- Avoid these drugs in patients with cerebrovascular disease; they are more susceptible to adverse effects.
- Avoid them in patients with established cardiac disease, hypertension, or arrhythmias.
- They can cause CNS stimulation; avoid them in patients with a history of psychotic illness.
- The non-selective MAOIs can cause idiosyncratic liver damage; avoid them in patients with hepatic insufficiency.
- There is little evidence of harm from these drugs during pregnancy, but use them only when the likely benefits are compelling.

Treatment of depression

- These drugs are potentially hazardous; see adverse effects below. Their use is usually restricted to patients unresponsive to other treatments. For these reasons they should be initiated and monitored by a specialist.
- Phenelzine and isocarboxazid cause less CNS stimulation than tranylcypromine and iproniazid; they are therefore the usual drugs of choice.
- It may take 2–3 weeks for an effect of these drugs to be apparent, and 4–6 weeks for the effect to be maximal.
- They are sometimes used in combination with other antidepressant drugs (tricyclic drugs and SSRIs); this increases the incidence of serious adverse effects and should only be done under the supervision of a specialist.
  - Wait 14 days after stopping an MAOI before starting another antidepressant drug, and vice versa.
- When withdrawing these drugs, do so slowly.

Parkinson's disease *(selegiline)*

- Treatment with selegiline has become controversial, because of evidence that it can increase mortality during long-term treatment. This remains a subject of debate and should be balanced against any potential benefit from improved symptomatic control that may result from treatment.
- Selegiline is usually used with levodopa to reduce the end-of-dose deterioration in control.

    - When these drugs are used together, the dose of levodopa must be reduced by 10–50%.
- Selegiline is also used early in treatment to delay the time when levodopa is required.
    - There is little evidence that early treatment with selegiline has any effect on the overall progression of the disease.

- Adverse effects from these drugs are very common.
- CNS effects include dizziness, over-stimulation, insomnia, agitation, and anxiety.
- They may also have autonomic effects: dry mouth, blurred vision, postural hypotension, and blurred vision.
- Gastrointestinal adverse effects include nausea and vomiting.
- They can cause hyponatraemia, resulting in confusion and seizures.
- They are most commonly remembered because they can cause the tyramine ('cheese') reaction.
    - Note that selegiline does not cause this adverse effect, and that it is less common with moclobemide.
    - The tyramine reaction is characterized by severe hypertension, headache, palpitation, sweating, nausea, and vomiting. It can be fatal.
    - It occurs as a result of ingestion of tyramine-rich foods or co-administration of other drugs that potentiate aminergic neurotransmission (see teaching point below).
    - This reaction makes these drugs potentially hazardous and limits their clinical use.

- The incidence of adverse effects is more common when these drugs are given with other antidepressant drugs. This should only be done under specialist supervision.
- These drugs can cause the serotonin syndrome (see SSRIs, p. 283) when given with other drugs that potentiate serotonin neurotransmission; these include pethidine, sibutramine, amfebutamone (bupropion), and 5-HT_1 agonists (the triptans). Avoid these drugs.
- They can potentiate the action of oral hypoglycaemic drugs (mechanism unknown); avoid the combination.
- Co-administration of certain drugs and foods can result in the tyramine reaction. Avoid these drugs. See box below for a list.

Safety and efficacy

- Depression
    - It is recommended that patients taking these drugs be reviewed every 1–2 weeks initially and then every 4 weeks for the duration of treatment (usually 6 months).
    - If the patient becomes confused or has a seizure, measure the plasma sodium concentration.
- Parkinson's disease
    - Initial dose titration will require regular review, especially if the patient is also taking levodopa.
- Warn patients that these drugs can interfere with skilled motor tasks, especially driving.
- Give patients taking non-selective MAOIs a warning card containing advice on how to avoid the tyramine reaction.

Prescribing information: **MAO inhibitors**

Depression

- *Moclobemide* Initially 150 mg bd; increased as required, up to 600 mg daily.
- Although phenelzine and isocarboxazid are preferred over tranylcypromine and iproniazid, they should only be used by specialists; detailed prescribing information is not given.

Parkinson's disease

- *Selegiline* By mouth, either 10 mg daily, or 5 mg at breakfast and 5 mg at midday. Consider an initial dose of 2.5 mg in the elderly.

Drugs and foods that can precipitate the tyramine reaction in patients taking MAOIs (*not* selegiline or moclobemide)

Drugs	Tyramine-rich foods
• Other amine drugs ◆ Ephedrine, pseudoephedrine (note that these are common components of many decongestant cough and cold cures) • Dopamine receptor agonists ◆ Levodopa, pergolide, ropinirole, cabergoline, lisuride, apomorphine • Direct sympathomimetics ◆ Beware lidocaine with adrenaline • Indoramin	• Cheese (especially cheddar) ◆ Not cottage or cream cheeses • Meat and yeast extracts ◆ E.g. Oxo®, Bovril®, Marmite®, Vegemite® • Some red wines • Hung game and poultry • Pickled herring • Broad beans • Alcoholic and dealcoholized beverages

Antipsychotic/neuroleptic drugs

Antipsychotic/neuroleptic drugs

Dopamine receptor antagonists

These drugs are dopamine receptor type 2 (D_2) antagonists. →

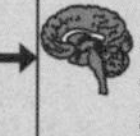

This is probably the basis of their acute sedative/tranquillizing effect. The antipsychotic effect is probably an adaptive response to the antidopaminergic actions.

These drugs also have anticholinergic, antihistaminic, and α-adrenergic actions. The contribution of these to their antipsychotic effect is not known, but they do cause adverse effects.

Note on atypical antipsychotic drugs
These drugs are relatively weak dopamine receptor antagonists. They have greater effects at other receptors (e.g. clozapine is an α-adrenoceptor, 5-HT_2, and histamine receptor antagonist; risperidone is a 5-HT_2 receptor antagonist).

- Sedative and tranquillizing effects.
  - Treatment of severe anxiety, acute mania, or psychosis.
  - Sedation in acute confusional states.
  - Premedication before general anaesthesia.
  - As an adjunct to analgesia in palliative care.
    - See prochlorperazine (p. 62) for antiemetic actions.
- Treatment of chronic schizophrenia.
- Occasionally used for treatment of intractable hiccup.

- Do not use sedative drugs inappropriately. They are not suitable for patients you find difficult or who suffer with dementia. The elderly are particularly sensitive to the effects of these drugs; give small initial dosages.
- Do not give these drugs to patients with a lowered level of consciousness.
- Antipsychotic drugs have anticholinergic effects; avoid them in patients with urinary retention or closed-angle glaucoma.
- Antipsychotic drugs can cause cardiac arrhythmias, usually by prolonging the QT interval. The risk is greatest with droperidol, haloperidol, thioridizine, and sertindole.
- Do not use these drugs in patients with hepatic insufficiency; they can induce hepatic coma.
- Patients with renal insufficiency are more sensitive to the actions of these drugs; use smaller initial doses.
- Do not use antipsychotic drugs in patients with Parkinsonian symptoms; the antidopaminergic actions can worsen these.
- Antipsychotic drugs can lower blood pressure; avoid them in patients with hypotension.
- Do not use antipsychotic drugs in patients with phaeochromocytoma; they can precipitate a hypertensive crisis.

Example drugs in this group

- Phenothiazines
  - Chlorpromazine
  - Prochlorperazine
  - Thioridizine
- Thioxanthenes
  - Flupenthixol
  - Clopentixol
- Butyrophenones
  - Haloperidol
- Atypical antipsychotic drugs
  - Risperidone
  - Clozapine
  - Olanzapine
  - Quetiapine
  - Sertindole

- Antipsychotic drugs vary in the degree of sedation they cause. Those that cause less sedation tend to have more marked extrapyramidal or anticholinergic effects.
  - Very sedative (e.g. chlorpromazine).
  - Moderately sedative but marked antimuscarinic actions (e.g. thioridazine). (Thioridazine limited to specialists only now, owing to a high risk of arrhythmias.)
  - Less sedative but marked extrapyramidal actions (e.g. prochlorperazine).
  - Haloperidol — high risk of extrapyramidal effects but causes less hypotension.

Acute treatment

- The doses of these drugs are lower when they are given by intramuscular injection than by mouth. This is particularly true if patients are very physically active (agitated), as this will increase the speed of absorption from the muscle.
- Review the dose daily to avoid over-sedation.
- Antipsychotic drugs are more effective for the acute psychotic symptoms of schizophrenia, rather than chronic withdrawal symptoms.
- They are a specific treatment for schizophrenia, but not for any other diagnoses. They can provide a window of time in which to assess and investigate an acutely unwell patient. Always consider the underlying cause for the patient's symptoms and treat that, if it is possible.
- See teaching point below for guidance on the management of the acutely agitated patient.

Anaesthesia

- These drugs have been used for premedication, but benzodiazepines are now preferred.
- Droperidol is a useful antiemetic, but has been withdrawn because it prolongs the QT interval.

Hiccup

- Remember that hiccup is a symptom of diaphragmatic irritation, not a diagnosis.
- Ideally the cause should be treated, but when this is not possible, consider a small dose of haloperidol.

Use of antipsychotic drugs in palliative care (see also p. 654)

- Haloperidol can be used in a dose of 1.5 mg daily by mouth, or twice daily if required. Haloperidol is effective for most chemical causes of vomiting (e.g. hypercalcaemia, renal failure).
- Levomepromazine (methotrimeprazine) causes sedation in about 50% of patients. It can be given by subcutaneous infusion at a dose of 25–200 mg/24 hours. Lower doses (5–25 mg/24 hours) can be effective and cause less sedation.

Treatment of chronic schizophrenia

- The choice of drug for long-term treatment should be made by a specialist.
- Treatment is often by depot injection, which improves compliance but can be associated with a higher risk of extrapyramidal adverse effects than treatment by mouth.

- Depot injections release the drug slowly; they are not appropriate for the treatment of acute symptoms. See calcium channel blockers (p. 163) for more information on modified-release formulations.
  - Zuclopenthixol is used for patients with aggression and agitation.
  - Note that several of the depot injections contain sesame oil; check that the patient is not allergic to this.
- Some patients benefit from a dose of antipsychotic drug that is above the licensed maximum. The Royal College of Psychiatrists offers the following guidance:
  - Antipsychotic drugs above their licensed maximum dose should only be used under the direct supervision of a specialist.
  - Consider alternative or adjuvant treatments first.
  - Do not increase the dose more rapidly than weekly.
  - If there has been no additional benefit after 3 months at the higher dose, reduce the dose and consider alternatives.
  - Patients are at greater risk of adverse effects at these higher dosages. They should have formal monitoring of body temperature, blood pressure, pulse, and ECG.
- Do not withdraw antipsychotic drugs suddenly.
- ⚠ All of these drugs cause sedation to a greater or lesser degree. Tolerance to this can develop with time.
- Antipsychotic drugs can cause the neuroleptic malignant syndrome.
  - This is characterized by fever, anorexia, rigidity, lowered level of consciousness, and autonomic disturbances (tachycardia, hyperthermia), and can be fatal.
  - Stop the drug immediately. There are no established effective treatments, but cooling, bromocriptine (a dopamine receptor agonist), and dantrolene (see p. 590) can be helpful.
  - The syndrome usually lasts 5–7 days.
- Extrapyramidal (antidopaminergic) adverse effects are common.
  - Acute dystonias can develop after only a few doses.
  - Akathisia tends to develop if large initial dosages are used.
  - Parkinsonian symptoms develop gradually.
    - This group of symptoms can be treated with procyclidine.
  - Tardive dyskinesia is most commonly associated with prolonged use, but can occur after short-term treatment.
    - This is characterized by involuntary dyskinetic movement of the jaw, lips, and trunk.
    - It can persist despite withdrawal of the drug.
    - There are no established effective treatments, but some manufacturers suggest that the effect can be mitigated by withdrawal of the drug as soon as the first symptoms appear.
  - The young, elderly, and debilitated are at greatest risk.
- The antidopaminergic actions can also cause prolactin release, leading to galactorrhoea, gynaecomastia, and menstrual disturbances.
- The anticholinergic actions can cause dry mouth, blurred vision, and urinary retention.
- Antipsychotic drugs can cause dizziness, but are also used to treat acute vertigo (see prochlorperazine, p. 62).
- Hypersensitivity phenomena, such as photosensitive rash, are common.

- These drugs can cause cardiac arrhythmias, usually by prolonging the QT interval. The risk is greatest with droperidol, haloperidol, thioridizine, and sertindole.
- Antipsychotic drugs can cause hypotension, especially in hypovolaemic patients. Take care postoperatively.
- Antipsychotic drugs can lower body temperature.
- Antipsychotic drugs increase the risk of thromboembolism about 3-fold, probably through an action on platelets; the atypical drugs probably do not do this.
- Rare adverse effects include blood dyscrasias and liver toxicity (jaundice).
    - Clozapine carries a particular risk of agranulocytosis (see below).
- Long-term treatment can cause corneal opacities and pigmentation of the cornea, conjunctiva, and retina.

- Antipsychotic drugs potentiate the actions of other sedating drugs (e.g. alcohol).
- Antipsychotic drugs potentiate the actions of other drugs that lower the blood pressure.
- Avoid giving them to patients taking other drugs that can prolong the QT interval (this includes tricyclic antidepressant drugs). See teaching point in antihistamines (p. 610).
- The risk of neurotoxicity from lithium is increased when it is given with these drugs.
- Avoid giving these drugs with other drugs that can cause agranulocytosis.
- Avoid giving them with others that increase the risk of thromboembolism (e.g. oestrogens).

- Perform an ECG before starting treatment with antipsychotic drugs. Measure the QT interval and consider if it is prolonged. Note the guidance on monitoring given above if the patient is given a dose above the licensed maximum.
- Consider thromboprophylaxis if the patient is at increased risk (e.g. admitted to hospital for surgery).
- Measure a full blood count, liver function tests, and creatine kinase (CK) if the patient develops an unexplained fever or infection.

Special precautions for the use of clozapine

- Clozapine is a useful atypical antipsychotic, but it is associated with a significant risk of agranulocytosis.
- All patients given clozapine must be enrolled in the national monitoring scheme (Clozaril® Patient Monitoring Scheme).
- Patients must have a full blood count weekly for the first 18 weeks of treatment, every fortnight up to 1 year, and monthly thereafter.

- Warn the patient that these drugs cause sedation that may interfere with skilled motor tasks (e.g. driving).
- Warn the patient that they may develop a photosensitive rash; advise them to use a sun-block.
- Advise the patient to seek medical attention if they develop an unexplained fever or infection.
- Chlorpromazine can cause contact sensitization. Advise patients and carers not to crush the tablets, and to avoid unnecessary handling of the drug.

Prescribing information: **Antipsychotic drugs**

- Many drugs are available; chlorpromazine and haloperidol are given as examples.
- See prochlorperazine (p. 62) for antiemetic actions of these drugs.
- Detailed information is not given for the chronic treatment of schizophrenia; this should be under the direction of a specialist.

Chlorpromazine

- Schizophrenia and other psychoses, mania, short-term adjunctive management of severe anxiety, psychomotor agitation, excitement, and violent or dangerously impulsive behaviour.
  - By mouth, initially 25 mg 3 times daily.
    - The usual maintenance dose is 75–300 mg daily.
    - Up to 1 g daily may be required in psychoses.
  - By intramuscular injection, 25–50 mg every 6–8 hours.
    - 20–25 mg chlorpromazine hydrochloride by intramuscular injection is equivalent to 40–50 mg of chlorpromazine by mouth.
  - Halve the initial dose in elderly or debilitated patients.

Haloperidol

- Schizophrenia and other psychoses, mania, short-term adjunctive management of psychomotor agitation, excitement, and violent or dangerously impulsive behaviour.
  - By mouth, initially 1.5–3 mg 2 or 3 times daily.
    - 3–5 mg 2 or 3 times daily in severely affected or resistant patients.
    - In resistant schizophrenia up to 30 mg daily may be needed.
  - By intramuscular or intravenous injection, initially 2–10 mg.
    - Then every 4–8 hours, according to the response.
    - The total maximum dose is 18 mg.
  - Halve the initial dose in elderly or debilitated patients.
- Intractable hiccup.
  - By mouth, 1.5 mg 3 times daily adjusted according to the response.

TEACHING POINT

Guidelines for pharmacological intervention for severely disturbed behaviour in adult in-patients

The following is intended as a guide only, seek expert assistance.

- Your first priority is your own safety and the safety of other staff. Summon sufficient help and do not intervene when you are at risk.
- In many cases non-drug interventions, such as talking-down, distraction, or seclusion will suffice.
- If this is unsuccessful consider:
  - Lorazepam, 2–4 mg by mouth. If the patient is unwilling to take oral medication lorazepam can be given by intramuscular or intravenous injection.
  - If the patient has psychotic symptoms, consider giving haloperidol, 5–10 mg by intramuscular injection. This should not normally be repeated.
  - Lorazepam may be repeated, but allow at least 30 minutes between doses. The usual maximum is 16 mg in 24 hours.
- Ensure that adequate resuscitation facilities are available, including facilities for mechanical ventilation.
- The purpose of these interventions is to calm the patient so that they can be adequately assessed, not to render them unconscious.

Lithium

Alkali metal element

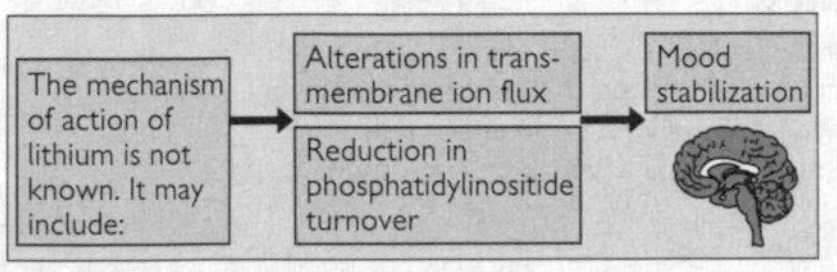

Treatment of mania

- Initial treatment with benzodiazepines.
- If severe, consider neuroleptic and atypical antipsychotic drugs.
- Lithium takes several days (7–10) to act.
  - It may be started once the patient is stable, or during the initial phase under neuroleptic 'cover'.
- Other drugs used for prophylaxis against mania:
  - Carbamazepine.
  - Valproic acid.

Oral therapy (lithium carbonate or lithium citrate)

- Treatment of mania.
  - To reduce mood swings in bipolar disorder.
- Adjunctive treatment of resistant, recurrent depression.
- Prophylaxis against cluster headache (unlicensed use).

Topical therapy (lithium succinate)

- Treatment of seborrhoeic dermatitis (see box).

- Lithium can cause sodium depletion. Avoid it in patients with cardiac disease or Addison's disease.
- Lithium is excreted by the kidneys. Its use in patients with mild or moderate renal insufficiency requires close monitoring (see below). Avoid lithium if the patient has severe renal insufficiency.
- Lithium is possibly teratogenic (congenital heart disease). This risk must be weighed against the effect of severe mood swings. Avoid lithium when mothers are breastfeeding.
- Avoid lithium if the patient has hypothyroidism.

- The decision to treat with lithium and subsequent supervision should be under the direction of a specialist.
- The systemic availability of lithium differs from different formulations; prescribe lithium by brand name and do not switch between formulations.
- Lithium is given initially in divided doses but a once-daily formulation is favoured for long-term treatment.
- Diarrhoea, vomiting, and intercurrent illnesses can alter the excretion of lithium. Be prepared to reduce the dose or to suspend treatment if these occur.
- Suspend treatment with lithium 24 hours before major surgical procedures.
- When withdrawing lithium, do so slowly, over a period of weeks. This reduces the risk of relapse.

- Adverse effects from lithium are common. These include: gastrointestinal disturbance, fine tremor.
- Lithium is excreted by the kidney and can cause impairment of urine concentration by blocking the action of antidiuretic hormone (ADH) and by long-term tubulointerstitial damage. This nephrogenic diabetes insipidus causes polydipsia and poluria.
  - In some cases, this will cause weight gain and oedema.

- Lithium can exacerbate psoriasis.
- Lithium can cause a goitre; hypothyroidism is more common than hyperthyroidism.
- Long-term use increases the risk of thyroid dysfunction and can cause mild cognitive and memory impairment.
- Intoxication by lithium is characterized by blurred vision, worsening gastrointestinal symptoms, drowsiness, ataxia, and a coarse tremor. Suspend the drug and measure the serum concentration.
- Features of severe toxicity (usual serum concentration >2 mmol/L) include hyper-reflexia, convulsions, psychosis, syncope, and renal insufficiency. This can be fatal; see below for guidance.

- Lithium toxicity is more common if body sodium is depleted; take great care if lithium is given with diuretics.
- Combination with high doses of neuroleptic drugs can cause a neurotoxic syndrome.
- Lithium can cause the serotonin syndrome, especially when given with MAOIs or SSRIs; (see SSRIs, p. 283).
- The renal clearance of lithium is reduced by drugs that impair renal function (e.g. ACE inhibitors, angiotensin receptor blockers, and NSAIDs).
- Methyldopa increases the risk of toxicity from lithium.

Safety

- The usual target serum concentration of lithium is 0.4–1.0 mmol/L; see barbiturates (p. 261) for more information on the measurement of the plasma concentration of drugs.
  - The target may be lower in the elderly.
- Lithium takes about 3 days to reach a new steady state after a dosage change.
  - Measure the concentration exactly 12 hours after the last dose.
  - A result from a sample taken at another time after the dose may not be comparable.
  - Once the patient is stable, many psychiatrists measure the serum concentration every 3 months.
  - However, there is another school of thought that advises measuring the serum concentration only when it is likely to change (e.g. at times of sodium depletion or intercurrent illness).
  - Choose your method of monitoring depending on how well the patient can be expected to recognize when problems arise.
- If the patient is given lithium long-term, they should have their thyroid function measured every 6–12 months.
- Treatment for longer than 3–5 years is not usually recommended, unless there are clear benefits.

- Give the patient a lithium advice card.
- Warn the patient that changes in dietary sodium (salt) can affect the lithium concentration. Advise them to avoid large changes in dietary salt intake and to maintain an adequate fluid intake.
  - Patients with diarrhoea or vomiting should suspend their lithium.

Prescribing information: **Lithium**

- Systemic availability varies between formulations. Prescription of lithium should be under the direction of a specialist.
- Detailed prescribing information is not given.

TEACHING POINT Treatment of poisoning by lithium

- Prevention is important; monitor the serum concentration (see above).
- Symptoms and signs of moderate toxicity (lithium concentration >1.5 mmol/L): Blurred vision, worsening gastrointestinal symptoms, drowsiness, ataxia, and a coarse tremor.
- Symptoms and signs of severe toxicity (lithium concentration >2 mmol/L): Hyper-reflexia, convulsions, psychosis, syncope, and renal insufficiency.
- Lithium toxicity can be fatal.
- Most cases of toxicity are due to a change in the handling of lithium in patients taking long-term lithium.
  - See drug interactions and patient advice notes above.
- Most of the treatment is supportive.
  - Activated charcoal does not adsorb lithium.
  - Consider haemodialysis or whole bowel irrigation for severe cases.
  - Discuss your treatment plan with your local poisons information service.

Pharmacology of drugs used to treat Parkinson's disease

The triad that is clinically known as parkinsonism (tremor, rigidity, and hypokinesia) results from deficient dopaminergic neurotransmission in the nigrostriatal tracts. In Parkinson's disease this is due to loss of dopaminergic cells in the substantia nigra. Chemicals such as the pethidine analogue MPTP (1-methyl 4-phenyl 1,2,3,6-tetrahydropyramine) can destroy dopaminergic cells. Drugs can cause parkinsonism by direct effects on dopaminergic neurotransmission (e.g. antipsychotic drugs) or by modulating other systems that in turn affect dopaminergic systems (e.g. the striatal cholinergic system).

Drug treatment for Parkinson's disease is based on four principles:

- Replacing dopamine (e.g. levodopa).
- Mimicking the actions of dopamine (e.g. dopamine receptor agonists).
- Causing the release of more dopamine (e.g. apomorphine).
- Modulating cholinergic neurotransmission (e.g. acetylcholine receptor antagonists).

Drug treatments for Parkinson's disease are depicted pictorially below.

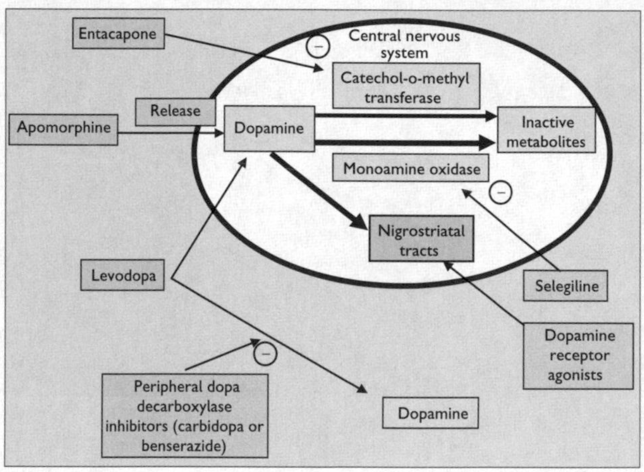

Levodopa (L-dopa)

Dopamine precursor

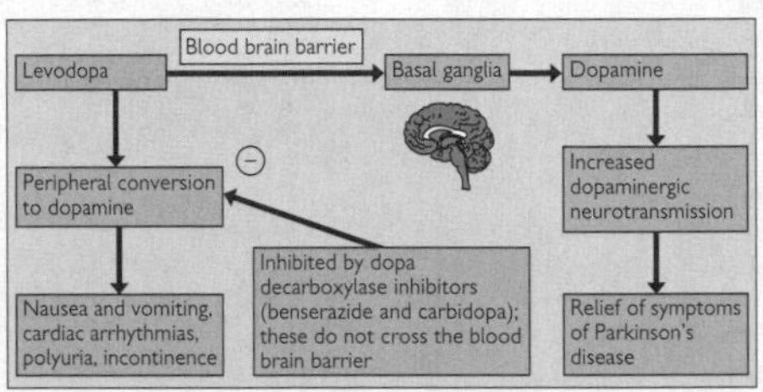

Drugs in this class

- Levodopa
- Levodopa *plus* benserazide
  - Co-beneldopa (Madopar®)
- Levodopa *plus* carbidopa
  - Co-careldopa (Sinemet®)

Administration of levodopa alone is not recommended, because of peripheral adverse effects. Formulations that contain a peripheral dopa-decarboxylase inhibitor (co-careldopa and co-beneldopa) should be used.

- Treatment of Parkinson's disease.
  - Levodopa should not be used for Parkinsonism caused by neuroleptic drugs or other dopamine receptor antagonists (see procyclidine, p. 196).

- Levodopa can only be beneficial if the patient still has a reasonable number of functioning dopaminergic neurons. It is less effective in elderly people, those with post-encephalitic Parkinson's disease, and those with long-standing disease.
- Do not give levodopa alone.
- Avoid levodopa in patients with psychiatric disease or dementia. The elderly are at particular risk of confusion caused by levodopa.
- Levodopa can be arrhythmogenic; avoid it in patients with established cardiac or cerebrovascular disease.
- Avoid levodopa in patients with glaucoma.
- No dosage adjustment is usually required for patients with renal or hepatic insufficiency.
- Levodopa has shown toxicity in animal studies of pregnancy; avoid it in pregnant women whenever possible.

- Levodopa is most effective for bradykinesia and rigidity; it has relatively little effect on tremor.
- Because dopaminergic neuron loss is usually progressive, the effect of levodopa diminishes with time. Some patients are less likely to benefit from levodopa; see above.
- 10–20% of patients are unresponsive to levodopa.
- Begin treatment with a low dose; increase this every 2–3 days until the optimal effect is achieved.
- 'End-of-dose effect'
  - The benefit from levodopa lasts for a shorter and shorter time. Consider giving a modified-release formulation, more frequent administration, or reducing dietary protein intake (amino acids compete with levodopa for uptake in the ileum).
- 'On/off effect'
  - This refers to debilitating fluctuations in performance that some patients experience. The 'off' periods of akinesia can last 2–4 hours and are unrelated to the dose of levodopa. Consider treatment with apomorphine, a dopamine receptor agonist given by subcutaneous infusion (seek specialist advice).

- Adverse effects are common and are due to the effects of dopamine on the CNS and periphery.
- CNS effects are commonly dose-limiting.
  - Confusion, especially in the elderly.
  - Involuntary movements.
  - Psychiatric effects: euphoria, agitation, anxiety.
- Peripheral effects (reduced but not abolished by peripheral dopa decarboxylase inhibitors).
  - Nausea and vomiting. This can be reduced by taking levodopa with meals. If severe consider giving domperidone (a dopamine receptor antagonist that does not cross the blood brain barrier).
  - Cardiac arrhythmias and hypotension.
  - Difficulty with micturition, polyuria, incontinence.

- The effect of levopdopa is enhanced by MAOIs. With the exception of selegiline, these should be withdrawn 2 weeks before starting levodopa.
- Neuroleptic drugs are dopamine receptor antagonists; they reduce the effect of levodopa.
- There is a risk of cardiac arrhythmias if the patient is given volatile liquid anaesthetics, such as halothane.
- Levodopa enhances the effect of any drugs that lower blood pressure.
- Avoid giving with amfebutamone; there is an increased risk of serious adverse effects.

Safety and efficacy

- The final dose of levodopa is usually a compromise between motor performance and the tolerability of adverse effects.
- Levodopa has a gradual onset of action over 6–18 months. There may then be a period of relative stability lasting 1–2 years, followed by a gradual decline.
- Measure the blood pressure; take care to avoid hypotension.
- Depression is common in patients with Parkinson's disease; ask the patient about mood and treat appropriately.

- Advise the patient that improvements will be gradual.
- Levodopa may interfere with the performance of certain skilled tasks, such as driving. Patients with Parkinson's disease should contact the DVLA and their insurers.
- Some patients taking levodopa find they fall asleep very quickly; they should be warned about this as it can be hazardous.

Prescribing information: **Levodopa**

Levodopa

- Giving levodopa alone is not recommended.

Co-beneldopa (levodopa plus benserazide)

- By mouth, initially 50 mg of levodopa 3 times daily (tablet size is 62.5 mg, as it contains 12.5 mg of benserazide). Increase by 100 mg levodopa once or twice weekly to usual maintenance dose of 400–800 mg of levodopa daily, in divided doses (after meals).

Co-careldopa (levodopa plus carbidopa)

- By mouth, initially 50 mg of levodopa 3 times daily (tablet size is 62.5 mg as it contains 12.5 mg of carbidopa). Increase by 100 mg levodopa once or twice weekly to usual maintenance dose of 400–800 mg of levodopa daily, in divided doses (after meals).
  - A daily dose of 70–100 mg of carbidopa is required to inhibit peripheral dopa decarboxylase fully.

Dopamine receptor agonists

Agonists at dopamine D_2 receptors

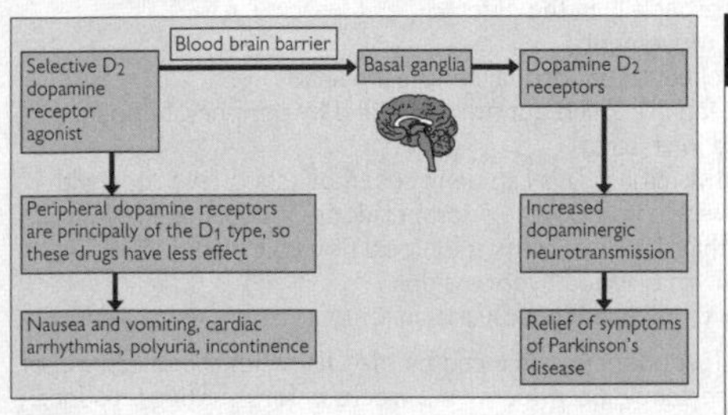

Drugs in this class

- Ergotamine derivatives
  - Bromocriptine
  - Cabergoline
  - Lisuride
  - Pergolide
- Related drugs
  - Ropinirole
  - Apomorphine (D_1, D_2 agonist)
  - Amantadine
  - Rimantadine
  - Pramipexole (D_2, D_3 agonist)

- Treatment of Parkinson's disease.
  - These drugs should not be used for Parkinsonism caused by neuroleptic drugs (see procyclidine, p. 196).
- Bromocriptine has other specialized uses; see box.
- Amantadine has a limited role in the treatment and prophylaxis of influenza infection; (see guanosine derivatives, p. 366).

Note on bromocriptine

- Reduces prolactin release from the pituitary in hyperprolactinaemia.
- Paradoxical action in acromegaly reduces the release of growth hormone.
- These are specialized uses; seek expert advice.

- These drugs are not usually first-line choices for the treatment of Parkinson's disease; consider levodopa instead.
- Avoid dopamine receptor agonists in patients with psychiatric disease or dementia. The elderly are at particular risk of confusion.
- Dopamine receptor agonists can be arrhythmogenic; avoid them in patients with established cardiac or cerebrovascular disease.
- Reduce the dose of ropinirole and cabergoline in patients with severe hepatic insufficiency.
- Reduce the dose of amantadine in patients with moderate renal insufficiency; avoid ropinirole in patients with severe renal insufficiency.
- Avoid these drugs in women who are pregnant; there is some evidence of toxicity in animals for some of these drugs. The manufacturers of pergolide advise that it should only be used if the potential benefit outweighs the risk.

- These drugs are usually reserved for patients:
  - With long-standing disease.
  - Unresponsive to levodopa.
  - Unable to tolerate levodopa.
  - With severe on/off reactions.
  - As an adjunct to levodopa.
- Initially give small doses frequently; this reduces adverse effects.
- Apomorphine should only be given by specialists. It is given for disabling 'on/off' symptoms.
  - Treatment needs to be initiated as an in-patient.
  - Give domperidone for 2 days before starting apomorphine.
  - Hypotension is very common at the start of treatment.
  - Apomorphine can be given by subcutaneous injection or infusion.

- Adverse effects are common and are due to the effects of dopamine on the CNS and periphery.
- CNS effects; these are commonly dose-limiting.
  - Confusion, especially in the elderly.
  - Involuntary movements.
  - Psychiatric effects: euphoria, agitation, anxiety.
- Peripheral effects
  - Nausea and vomiting. This can be reduced by taking these drugs with meals. If severe consider giving domperidone (a dopamine receptor antagonist that does not cross the blood-brain barrier).
  - Cardiac arrhythmias and hypotension.
    - Hypotension is particularly common.
  - Difficulty with micturition, polyuria, incontinence.
- All the ergotamine derivatives (see box above) can cause pulmonary, retroperitoneal, and pericardial fibrosis.
- Apomorphine can cause haemolytic anaemia.

- Neuroleptic drugs are dopamine receptor antagonists; they will reduce the effects of these drugs.
- These drugs will enhance the effect of any drugs that lower blood pressure.
- Avoid giving with amfebutamone; there is an increased risk of serious adverse effects.
- Metoclopramide antagonizes the effects of these drugs.
- Oestrogens increase prolactin secretion; avoid oestrogen-containing contraceptives if the patient has hyperprolactinaemia.

Safety and efficacy

- The CSM advises that patients taking ergotamine-derivative dopamine agonists 'should be monitored for progressive fibrotic disorders'.
- In practical terms we suggest:
  - Measure the ESR, urea, and electrolytes and perform a chest X-ray before treatment.
  - Consider lung function tests if the patient has a history of lung disease or is a smoker.
  - Repeat the tests if there is any change in the patient's condition.
- If the patient is given apomorphine, it is recommended that they have a blood film examination and measurement of bilirubin every 6 months.
- The final dose of these drugs is usually a compromise between motor performance and the tolerability of adverse effects.
- Measure the blood pressure; take care to avoid hypotension.
- Depression is common in patients with Parkinson's disease; ask the patient about mood and treat appropriately.

- These drugs may interfere with the performance of certain skilled tasks, such as driving. Patients with Parkinson's disease should contact the DVLA and their insurer.
- Some patients taking these drugs find that they fall asleep very quickly; they should be warned about this, as it can be hazardous.

Prescribing information: **Dopamine receptor agonists**

Bromocriptine and pergolide are given as examples.

Bromocriptine

- Parkinson's disease, by mouth with food.
  - Initially, 1.25 mg at night for 1 week.
  - Increase to 2.5 mg daily for second week.
  - Increase to 2.5 mg twice daily for third week.
  - Increase to 2.5 mg 3 times daily for fourth week.
  - Increase dose by 2.5 mg every 3–14 days as tolerated. Usual maintenance dose 10–40 mg daily, in divided doses.
- Acromegaly
  - Usual maintenance dose 20 mg daily; note how much larger the dose is than the dose used in Parkinson's disease.

Pergolide

- By mouth, take with food.
  - Initially, 50 micrograms at night on day 1.
  - Then 50 micrograms twice daily on days 2–4.
  - Increase by 100–250 micrograms daily every 3 or 4 days (given as 3 divided doses), up to 1.5 mg by day 28.
  - May be increased by 250 micrograms daily, up to a maintenance dose of 2.0–2.5 mg daily (in divided doses).

Entacapone

Entacapone

Inhibitor of catechol-o-methyl transferase

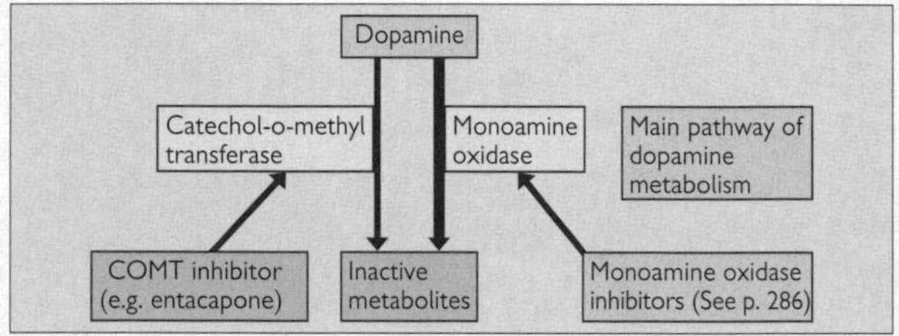

- Adjunctive treatment of Parkinson's disease.
  - Should not be used for Parkinsonism caused by neuroleptic drugs (see procyclidine, p. 196).

- This drug is not a first-line choice for the treatment of Parkinson's disease; consider levodopa instead.
- Avoid entacapone in patients with phaeochromocytoma; it can precipitate a hypertensive crisis.
- Avoid entacapone in patients with severe hepatic insufficiency.
- No dosage reduction is usually required if the patient has renal insufficiency.
- There is no evidence about the safety of this drug during pregnancy.

- Entacapone is usually reserved for patients with debilitating 'end-of-dose' effects (see levodopa, p. 302) and those who are poorly controlled by levodopa.
  - The dose of levodopa will usually need to be reduced by between 10% and 30% if the patient is taking entacapone.

- Adverse effects are common and are due to the effects of dopamine on the CNS and periphery.
- CNS effects, including dizziness, are commonly dose-limiting.
- Peripheral effects include nausea and vomiting.
- Entacapone can cause hepatitis; this is rare.

- The effect of warfarin is increased by entacapone (mechanism not known).
- The effect of sympathomimetic drugs is increased.
- The risks of adverse effects due to MAOIs, tricyclic antidepressants, and SSRIs are increased.

Safety and efficacy

- Patients taking entacapone usually have severe symptoms; they should therefore have regular clinical review to adjust their treatment regimen.
- Depression is common in patients with Parkinson's disease; ask the patient about mood and treat appropriately.

- Entacapone can interfere with the performance of certain skilled tasks, such as driving. Patients with Parkinson's disease should contact the DVLA and their insurers.
- Warn the patient that entacapone may turn the urine a red/brown colour.

Prescribing information: **Entacapone**

- Parkinson's disease
  - 200 mg with each dose of levodopa (with a dopa decarboxylase inhibitor).
  - Maximum dose 2 g daily.

Acetylcholinesterase inhibitors

Inhibitors of the breakdown of acetylcholine

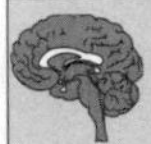

- These drugs increase cholinergic neurotransmission, both muscarinic and nicotinic.
- In the brain, this increases cholinergic neurotransmission.

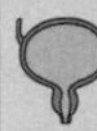

- The smooth muscle of the bowel is stimulated and the sphincters of the bowel and bladder relax.

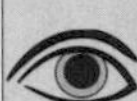

- In the eye, they cause pupillary constriction and open the canal of Schlemm.

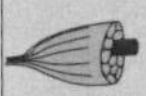

- Skeletal muscle is depolarized (contracts).

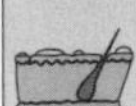

- Secretions are increased (sweat, saliva, and bronchial).

- The drugs in this class are not interchangeable; see how to use section for information on drug selection.
- Diagnosis and treatment of myasthenia gravis.
- Treatment of Alzheimer's-type dementia.
- Reversal of curare-like muscle block in anaesthesia.
- Reversal of pupillary dilatation after the use of drugs such as cyclopentolate.
- Relief of postoperative urinary retention and upper motor neuron lesion neurogenic bladder.

- Note that organophosphates (e.g. parathion) are irreversible acetylcholinesterase inhibitors.
- Avoid systemic treatment (tablets) in pregnancy and breastfeeding, asthma/COPD (increased secretions and bronchospasm), and cardiovascular disease (bradycardia and hypotension).
- Dosage adjustments are not usually required in hepatic or renal insufficiency.

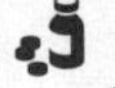

Myasthenia gravis (edrophonium, neostigmine, pyridostigmine, distigmine)

- Edrophonium only lasts for 5 minutes and is used for the diagnosis of myasthenia.

Drugs in this class

The treatment of Alzheimer's disease
- Donepezil
- Rivastigmine
- Galantamine

The treatment of myasthenia gravis
- Neostigmine
- Distigmine
- Edrophonium
- Pyridostigmine

Lambert-Eaton Myasthenic Syndrome (LEMS)

- A syndrome clinically similar to myasthenia gravis caused by autoantibodies against voltage-gated calcium channels.
- 60% of patients with this syndrome have a non-small-cell lung cancer; surgical removal of the tumour can improve symptoms temporarily.
- Immunosuppressive drugs are usually not indicated.
- 3,4-diaminopyridine enhances the release of acetylcholine from the presynaptic nerve terminals by inhibiting voltage-gated potassium channels; it has a role in the symptomatic treatment of LEMS. Seek specialist advice.

- Neostigmine lasts for 4 hours. It can be given parenterally (sc or im), in which case one-tenth of the oral dose should be given.
- Pyridostigmine is a less potent drug but has a long duration of action. It can be especially useful for weakness experienced on waking.
- Distigmine has the longest duration of action, but it also carries the greatest risk of a cholinergic crisis and is rarely used.

Treatment of Alzheimer's-type dementia (donepezil, rivastigmine, galantamine)

- See NICE guidance overleaf.
- Benefit is seen in about half the patients treated.

Anaesthesia (edrophonium, neostigmine)

- Used to reverse neuromuscular block due to non-depolarizing neuromuscular blockers (neostigmine).
- Neostigmine lasts for 20–30 minutes. Ensure that the patient is closely monitored, as the effect of the non-depolarizing blocker can outlast the effect of the acetylcholinesterase inhibitor.
- Premedicate the patient with atropine or glycopyrronium to avoid bradycardia and increased bronchial secretions.
- Edrophonium is used to differentiate myasthenia gravis from dual (depolarizing and non-depolarizing) block (e.g. due to suxamethonium). It will reverse any non-depolarizing component. If there is significant improvement with edrophonium, give neostigmine.

Neurogenic bladder (distigmine)

- Not recommended for relief of postoperative acute urinary retention, as cardiac adverse effects can be hazardous.
- Can be beneficial for upper motor neuron lesion neurogenic bladder (specialized use).

- The adverse effects of these drugs are related to their cholinergic actions.
  - Muscarinic: abdominal cramps, bradycardia, sweating, hypersalivation, and increased bronchial secretions.
    - These effects can be reversed by atropine; have it available when starting treatment for myasthenia.
  - Nicotinic: muscle cramps.
- The incidence of adverse effects can be minimized by starting at a low dose and gradually titrating the dose up.
- An excessive dose can lead to a 'cholinergic crisis', characterized by depolarizing muscle block.
- Treatment with these drugs increases the risk of convulsions (central cholinergic effect).

- Several drugs antagonize the action of neostigmine and pyridostigmine: aminoglycoside antibiotics, clindamycin, chloroquine, hydroxychloroquine.

Efficacy

- Myasthenia gravis. Treatment is usually limited by the patient's ability to tolerate the adverse effects.
- Alzheimer's disease. See NICE guidance box for details.

- Myasthenia gravis. Ensure that the patient understands the treatment, so that they are able to titrate the dose to achieve a maximal therapeutic effect.

- Alzheimer's disease. Ensure that the patient is likely to be able to comply with treatment, as it will not be effective with intermittent administration. The benefits from therapy are modest; ensure that the patient, family, and carers understand this.

NICE guidance on the use of acetylcholinesterase inhibitors as adjunctive treatment for Alzheimer's disease

Relates to the use donepezil, rivastigmine, and galantamine.

- The patient must have no worse than mild to moderate dementia, with a mini-mental state examination (MMSE) score greater than 12 points.
- The diagnosis of Alzheimer's-type dementia should be made in a specialist clinic. Assessment should include:
  - Cognitive, global, and behavioural scoring.
  - Activities of daily living.
  - Likelihood of compliance with treatment.
- Care may be shared by the specialist and general practitioner.
- The patient should be assessed 2–4 months after the maintenance dose is established. Treatment should only continue if:
  - There is improvement, or no deterioration in the MMSE score *and*
  - There is behavioural or functional improvement.
- Treatment should be reassessed every 6 months. It should normally only be continued while the MMSE score remains above 12 and there is a worthwhile effect on behavioural or functional factors.

Prescribing information: **Acetylcholinesterase inhibitors**

The following are offered as examples.

Myasthenia gravis

- *Edrophonium* Diagnosis of myasthenia gravis, by intravenous injection, 2 mg followed after 30 seconds (if no adverse reaction has occurred) by 8 mg.
  - In adults without suitable veins, by intramuscular injection, 10 mg.
- *Neostigmine bromide* 15–30 mg by mouth at suitable intervals throughout the day; total daily dose usually 75–300 mg.
  - By subcutaneous or intramuscular injection, *neostigmine metilsulfate* 1.0–2.5 mg at suitable intervals throughout the day (usual total daily dose 5–20 mg).

Alzheimer's disease

- *Donepezil* 5 mg once daily at bedtime, increased if necessary after 1 month to 10 mg daily. Maximum 10 mg daily.
- *Galantamine* Initially 4 mg twice daily for 4 weeks, increased to 8 mg twice daily for 4 weeks. Maintenance dosage usually 8–12 mg twice daily.
- *Rivastigmine* Initially 1.5 mg twice daily, increased in steps of 1.5 mg twice daily at intervals of at least 2 weeks according to response and tolerance. Usual dosage range 3–6 mg twice daily. Maximum 6 mg twice daily.

Anaesthesia

- *Edrophonium* Brief reversal of neuromuscular blockade in diagnosis of dual block. By intravenous injection over several minutes, 500–700 micrograms/kg (after or with atropine sulfate 600 micrograms).

- *Neostigmine* Reversal of non-depolarizing neuromuscular blockade. By intravenous injection over 1 minute, 50–70 micrograms/kg (maximum 5 mg) after or with atropine sulfate 0.6–1.2 mg.

Neurogenic bladder

- *Distigmine* 5 mg daily or on alternate days, half an hour before breakfast (specialized use).

Serotonin 5-HT_1 receptor agonists ('triptans')

Antimigraine drugs

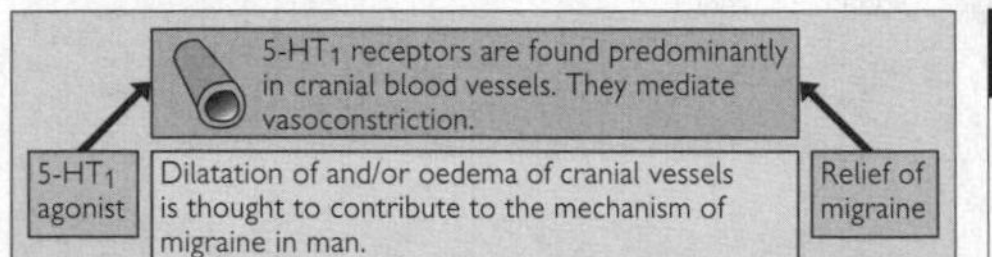

Drugs in this class

- Almotriptan
- Eletriptan
- Naratriptan
- Rizatriptan
- Sumatriptan
- Zolmitriptan

- Treatment of acute migraine headache.
  - These drugs are the recommended treatment for patients who do not respond to simple analgesia.
  - See teaching point, p. 317.
- One of these drugs (sumatriptan) has been shown to be useful in the treatment of cluster headache (see below).

- Triptans cause vasoconstriction. Do not give them to patients with coronary artery disease, uncontrolled hypertension, or a previous stroke or transient ischaemic attack (TIA). They are contraindicated in familial hemiplegic migraine.
- Triptans are excreted by both the kidneys and liver. Do not give them to patients with severe hepatic or renal insufficiency.
- There is little information about the safety of these drugs in pregnancy. The manufacturers recommend that they should only be used when the benefit outweighs the risk.
- Some of the drugs in this class (almotriptan, naratriptan, and sumatriptan) contain a sulfonamide component. Do not give these drugs to patients with hypersensitivity to sulfonamides.

- Triptans are effective for the treatment of acute migraine headache, but they are not used for prophylaxis against migraine (see teaching point below and pizotifen, p. 318).
- Do not give these drugs to patients in whom the diagnosis is not known.
- These drugs should be taken as soon as symptoms begin to develop.
  - Several formulations are available: tablets, sublingual melts, intranasal spray, and subcutaneous injection.
  - Administration by subcutaneous injection is the most effective route, but this is very expensive and not usually justified.
  - Take care to avoid intravenous injection which can cause coronary ischaemia.
- A second dose can be taken after 2 hours if the response to the first dose is incomplete.
- If the patient does not obtain any relief at all from the first dose, it should not be repeated. Consider alternatives.

Note on cluster headache

- Cluster headache does not usually respond to conventional analgesics.
- Sumatriptan, given by subcutaneous injection, is effective for acute cluster headache. An alternative is 100% oxygen, given at the start of an attack.
- Patients with frequent headaches should be assessed by a specialist.

- These drugs cause vasoconstriction. This can lead to:
  - Transient rises in blood pressure.
  - Coronary artery constriction. Do not give these drugs to patients with coronary artery disease or Prinzmetal's (variant) angina (coronary vasospasm).
- These drugs can cause sensations of tingling, heat, heaviness, flushing, and weakness.
- They can also produce a sense of pressure in various part of the body (e.g. throat or chest). This may be related to their vasoconstrictive effects; beware coronary vasoconstriction.
- Hypersensitivity reactions are rare.

- Ergotamine compounds also cause vasoconstriction. They have been used for the treatment of migraine but are no longer recommended. Do not give triptans with ergotamine derivatives.
- Some triptans are in part metabolized by monoamine oxidase. Do not give sumatriptan, rizatriptan, or zolmitriptan to patients taking an MAOI.
- The following drugs inhibit the metabolism of the triptans; avoid the combination.
  - Erythromycin, clarithromycin.
  - Antifungal drugs such as itraconazole and ketoconazole.
  - HIV protease inhibitors such as indinavir and ritonavir.

Efficacy

- Ensure that the diagnosis is migraine and review the patient to ensure that the treatment has been effective. If the treatment was ineffective or only partially effective, consider another drug or formulation.

- Warn the patient that both migraine and these drugs can cause dizziness that may interfere with skilled motor tasks (e.g. driving). Patients should not drive when they have a migraine headache.

Prescribing information: **5-HT$_1$ receptor agonists**

There are several options: sumatriptan, naratriptan, and rizatriptan are given here as examples.

Sumatriptan

- By mouth, 50 mg. Can be repeated after not less than 2 hours. Maximum dose 300 mg in 24 hours.
- By subcutaneous injection, 6 mg. Can be repeated once after not less than 1 hour.
- By intranasal spray, 20 mg (1 spray). Can be repeated once after not less than 2 hours.

Naratriptan

- By mouth, 2.5 mg as soon as possible after onset. Can be repeated after 4 hours. Maximum dose 5 mg in 24 hours.

Rizatriptan

- By mouth, 10 mg. Can be repeated once after not less than 2 hours.

TEACHING POINT Treatment of acute migraine headache

- Prevention is important; advise patients to avoid triggers (e.g. tiredness, certain foods).
- First-line treatment is simple analgesia.
  - Consider paracetamol, aspirin, or an NSAID.
  - An antiemetic, such as metoclopramide or domperidone, can be useful if nausea and vomiting are prominent features.
- In many cases this will be sufficient, especially if the patient recognizes early symptoms and responds.
- First-line treatment is insufficient in some patients. Others develop symptoms very rapidly, before conventional analgesics can respond.
  - Consider a 5-HT_1 receptor agonist for these patients.
  - If the drug is effective, they should take it as the migraine develops (e.g. when the aura occurs), not try simple analgesia first.
- Ergotamine drugs have been used for the treatment of migraine. They are effective but carry a very high risk of adverse effects. They are no longer recommended, but they may be used by some specialists in rare cases.

Pizotifen

Serotonin 5-HT receptor antagonist

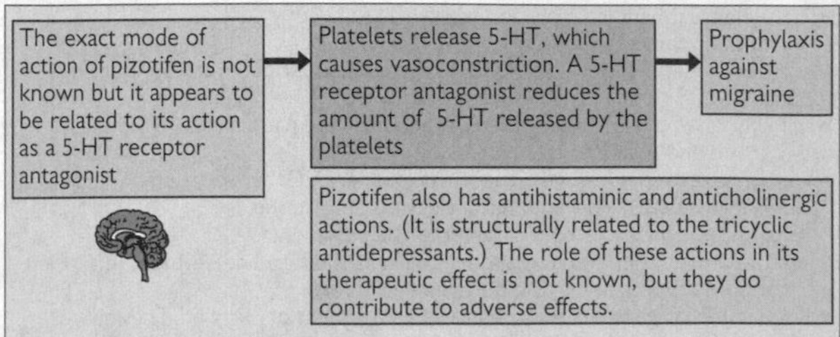

- Prophylaxis against migraine headache.

Drugs used for the prophylaxis of migraine

- Pizotifen
- Beta-adrenoceptor antagonists (beta-blockers)
- Tricyclic antidepressants
- Used rarely: sodium valproate, cyproheptadine, methysergide

- Pizotifen has anticholinergic actions; avoid it in patients with prostatic enlargement or a history of closed-angle glaucoma.
- There are no dosage adjustments for hepatic or renal insufficiency.
- There is little information about the safety of pizotifen in pregnancy. The manufacturers recommend that it should only be used when the benefit outweighs the risk.

- Pizotifen is effective for prophylaxis against migraine, but it is not used for the treatment of acute migraine headache (see triptans, p. 317, for more information).
- Do not give pizotifen to patients in whom the diagnosis is not known.
- All of the drugs used for prophylaxis of migraine commonly cause adverse effects. Patients who suffer frequent migraine headaches, and for whom prophylaxis is being considered, should be assessed by a specialist.
  - Patients with occasional headache do not need prophylaxis.
- Pizotifen causes drowsiness, but tolerance develops with time. Start with a low dose and give it at night.

- Pizotifen causes drowsiness. See note above.
- Pizotifen stimulates appetite and can cause weight gain. This limits its usefulness.
- The anticholinergic actions of pizotifen can cause nausea, dry mouth, and urinary retention, and can precipitate glaucoma.

- The sedative actions of other drugs (e.g. alcohol) can be enhanced if the patient is also given pizotifen.

- Ensure that the diagnosis is migraine, and review the patient to ensure that the treatment is effective. If not, consider another drug.
- Measure the patient's weight; pizotifen can cause weight gain.

- Warn patients that migraine and pizotifen can cause dizziness and drowsiness that may interfere with skilled motor tasks (e.g. driving). Patients should not drive when they have a migraine headache.

Prescribing information: **Pizotifen**

Prophylaxis against migraine headache

- By mouth. Initially 500 micrograms at night.
- Increase gradually as tolerated. Usual maintenance dose 1.5 mg at night.
- Maximum dose 3 mg at night.

Chapter 5

Infections

Contents

Penicillins

β-lactam antibiotics

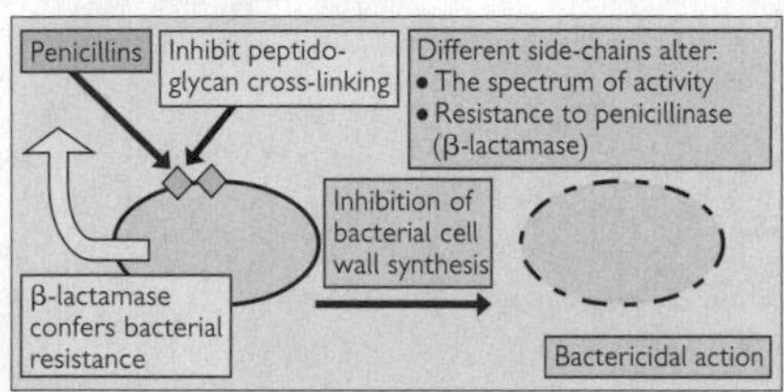

Drugs in this class

- Penicillinase (β-lactamase)-sensitive penicillins
  - Benzylpenicillin (penicillin G, parenteral)
  - Penicillin V (phenoxymethyl penicillin, oral)
- Penicillinase-resistant penicillins
  - Flucloxacillin
- Broad-spectrum penicillins
  - Ampicillin
  - Amoxicillin
  - Co-amoxiclav (amoxicillin plus clavulanic acid; Augmentin®)
- Antipseudomonal penicillins
  - Piperacillin (with tazobactam; Tazocin®)
  - Ticarcillin (plus clavulanic acid)

- Widely-used antibiotics with good penetration of body tissues and fluids.
  - Relatively poor penetration of CSF unless the meninges are inflamed (e.g. meningococcal meningitis).
- Flucloxacillin is given for infections due to staphylococci, as most produce β-lactamase.
  - Commonly used for the treatment of endocarditis and cellulitis.
- The broad-spectrum penicillins cover Gram-positive bacteria (e.g. enterococci) and some Gram-negative bacteria, but are susceptible to β-lactamase.
  - Commonly used for chest and urinary tract infections.
  - Resistance to these drugs is common amongst staphylococci and *E. coli*.
  - Co-amoxiclav has better coverage of these resistant bacteria.
- The antipseudomonal penicillins (carboxypenicillins) should be reserved for the treatment of infections due to *Pseudomonas aeruginosa*.
  - They may be used in combination with an aminoglycoside antibiotic, as they have synergistic actions.
  - Commonly used for the treatment of neutropenic sepsis and endocarditis.

- Allergy to penicillin is common (1–10% of patients).
  - Those with a history of true allergy to penicillin should not be given any β-lactam antibiotic, including cephalosporins, the carbapenems, and co-amoxiclav.
  - A non-confluent rash affecting only a small area or occurring >72 hours after starting the penicillin does not usually represent an allergic reaction; cephalosporins and carbapenems are not subsequently contraindicated.

Clavulanic acid and tazobactam

These are inhibitors of β-lactamase. Compound formulations with a penicillin can overcome β-lactamase-mediated resistance. However, not all resistance is β-lactam-mediated. For example, penicillin-resistant pneumococci and gonococci have other resistance mechanisms.

- Penicillins accumulate in renal insufficiency. High dosages can cause cerebral irritation.
  - Antibiotic solutions for intravenous injection contain large amounts of electrolytes (Na^+ and K^+); these will also accumulate in renal insufficiency.
  - Avoid intrathecal injection of penicillins.
- Penicillins are not known to be harmful in pregnancy, but avoid clavulanic acid, unless it is essential.

- Always consider the likely causative organisms when treating infection empirically.
- Avoid using a broad-spectrum drug when one with a narrow spectrum will cover the causative organism.
- Using a broad-spectrum antibiotic increases the risk of antibiotic-associated diarrhoea (see cephalosporins, p. 331).

Methicillin-Resistant *Staphylococcus aureus* (MRSA)

- These organisms commonly cause hospital-acquired infection and are increasingly common in the community as well.
- They are resistant to all β-lactams, including flucloxacillin.
- Consider MRSA as a causative organism if a patient becomes unwell in hospital or does not respond to conventional treatment.
- To avoid infection of other patients, discuss appropriate eradication and treatment regimens and precautions with your microbiology and infection control teams.

- Hypersensitivity is relatively common. An urticarial rash occurs in 1–10% of patients. Anaphylactic reactions are much less common (0.05% of patients).
  - A significant number of patients develop a rash that is not directly due to the penicillin. This may be due to the disease or a viral infection (e.g. Epstein–Barr virus).

Penicillin hypersensitivity

- *IgE antibody-mediated reactions* Reactive degradation products of the penicillin molecule combine with a protein carrier and act as haptens. The clinical spectrum that results ranges from a mild local reaction to anaphylactic shock.
- *Non-IgE antibody-mediated reactions* Modification of erythrocyte surface components due to binding of β-lactams or their metabolic products can cause the formation of antierythrocyte antibodies, resulting in a Coombs'-positive haemolytic anaemia.

- Penicillins can cause cerebral irritation and convulsions. The use of high dosages in patients with renal insufficiency increases the risk.
- Eradication of the patient's normal flora can cause:
  - Superinfection by *Candida* in the oropharynx. This is most common in the elderly and debilitated.
  - Antibiotic-associated diarrhoea. Avoid broad-spectrum drugs unless essential.
- Penicillins commonly cause diarrhoea by different mechanisms (see cephalosporins, p. 331).
- Penicillins can cause cholestatic jaundice. The risk is greatest with flucloxacillin and formulations containing clavulanic acid.
  - Elderly patients and those treated for longer than 2 weeks are at greatest risk.
  - The jaundice can appear several weeks after the drug has been stopped.

- Rare adverse effects include:
  - Coombs'-positive haemolytic anaemia and thrombocytopenia.
  - Interstitial nephritis.
  - Hypernatraemia and hyperkalaemia in patients with renal insufficiency (see above).

- If a penicillin causes diarrhoea, this may reduce the effectiveness of the oral contraceptive owing to reduced absorption; warn the patient.
- Penicillins reduce the excretion of some NSAIDs by reducing tubular secretion.

Safety and efficacy

- Measures of clinical improvement are the most important, but inflammatory markers such as the CRP and ESR are often helpful; remember that very occasionally penicillins can cause fever.
- Whenever possible, take cultures before staring antibiotic treatment. Check the sensitivities of the causative organism. Discuss any unusual results with a microbiologist.
- Measure the patient's renal function and liver function tests, especially if long-term treatment is required (>7 days).

- Warn the patient of the risk of rash and other hypersensitivity phenomena.
- Warn female patients that if they develop diarrhoea the oral contraceptive may be ineffective.

Prescribing information: **Penicillins**

There are many formulations of these drugs. The following are given as examples. Dosages and duration of treatment will depend on the indication. Check your local antibiotics policy.

Benzylpenicillin

- By intramuscular injection or slow intravenous injection/infusion, usual dosage range 2.4–4.8 g daily in 4 divided doses.

Flucloxacillin

- By mouth, 250–500 mg every 6 hours. Give at least 30 minutes before food.
- By intramuscular injection, 250–500 mg every 6 hours.
- By slow intravenous injection/infusion, 0.25–2.0 g every 6 hours.

Ampicillin

- By mouth, 0.25–1.0 g every 6 hours. Give at least 30 minutes before food.
- By intramuscular injection, 500 mg every 4–6 hours.
- By slow intravenous injection/infusion, 500 mg every 4–6 hours.

Amoxicillin

- By mouth, 250–500 mg every 8 hours.
- By intramuscular injection, 500 mg every 8 hours.
- By slow intravenous injection/infusion, 0.5–1.0 g every 8 hours.

Co-amoxiclav (Augmentin®)

- By mouth, 250 mg amoxicillin and 125 mg clavulanic acid in a single tablet; 1 tablet 3 times daily.
- Double the dose of amoxicillin (but not clavulanic acid) in severe infections.

Piperacillin (with tazobactam)

- By slow intravenous injection/infusion, usually 4.5 g every 6 hours.

Carbapenems

β-lactam antibiotics

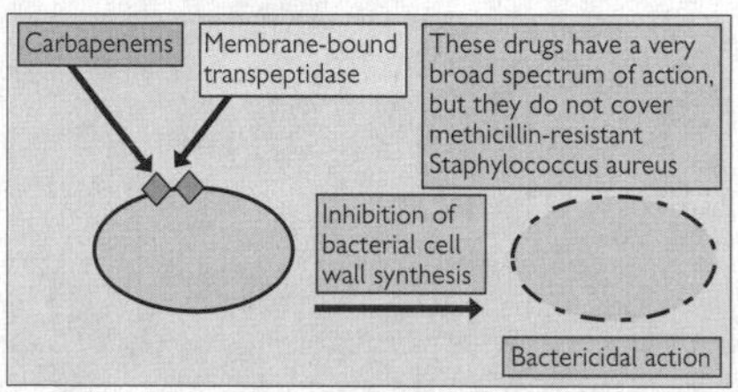

Drugs in this class

- Imipenem
  - Plus cilastatin, which blocks the renal metabolism of imipenem, increasing its duration of action
- Meropenem
- Ertapenem

Related β-lactam

- Aztreonam (a monobactam). Specialist use only. Gram-negative but not Gram-positive cover.

- These drugs have a very broad spectrum of activity.
  - Aerobic and anerobic, Gram-positive and Gram-negative organisms.
  - The spectrum includes *Pseudomonas spp.*
  - These drugs do not cover methicillin-resistant *Staphylococcus aureus* (MRSA).
  - Meropenem has slightly better Gram-negative activity.

- Those with a history of allergy to penicillin should not be given any β-lactam antibiotic, including cephalosporins, the carbapenems, and co-amoxiclav. The incidence of cross-reaction is about 50%.
  - A non-confluent rash affecting only a small area or occurring >72 hours after starting the penicillin does not usually represent an allergic reaction.
- These drugs accumulate in renal insufficiency.
  - The dose of imipenem or meropenem should be reduced as follows:
    - Mild insufficiency, reduce the frequency from every 8 hours to every 12 hours.
    - Moderate insufficiency, halve the usual dose and give every 12 hours.
    - Severe insufficiency, halve the usual dose and give every 24 hours.
  - Antibiotic solutions for intravenous injection contain a large amount of electrolytes (Na^+ and K^+); these will also accumulate in renal insufficiency.
- Avoid these drugs if the patient has epilepsy; the risk of fits is greater with imipenem.
- These drugs are not known to be safe in pregnancy. There is some evidence of toxicity from imipenem in animals.

- Always consider the likely causative organisms when treating infection empirically.
- Avoid using a broad-spectrum drug when one with a narrow spectrum will cover the causative organism.
- Using a broad-spectrum antibiotic increases the risk of antibiotic-associated diarrhoea (see cephalosporins, p. 331). It also selects for resistant organisms (see glycopeptides, p. 335).
- These drugs have a very broad spectrum, but they are not appropriate in most settings when likely causative organisms are known.
  - Most hospitals restrict their use to places where infection by a wide range of resistant organisms is possible (e.g. on the ICU).

- Do not forget that these drugs do not cover methicillin-resistant *Staphylococcus aureus* (MRSA).
- Discuss the case with a specialist in infection before using these drugs.

- Hypersensitivity is relatively common. This is usually characterized by a rash, which can be severe.
- Carbapenems lower the seizure threshold. The risk is greater with imipenem, which is not recommended for the treatment of meningitis.
  - They can also cause confusion.
- Carbapenems can cause antibiotic-associated diarrhoea (see cephalosporins, p. 331).
- Carbapenems can cause abnormalities of liver function tests.
- Carbapenems can cause a positive Coombs' test; haemolytic anaemia is rare.

- The risk of seizures is increased if imipenem is given with ganciclovir; avoid this combination.

Safety and efficacy
- Measures of clinical improvement are the most important, but inflammatory markers such as the CRP and ESR are often helpful.
- Whenever possible, take cultures before starting antibiotic treatment. Check the sensitivities of the causative organism. Discuss any unusual results with a microbiologist.
- Measure the patient's renal function and liver function. Reduce the dose as outlined above in renal insufficiency.

- Check that the patient is not allergic to penicillins before giving these drugs.

Prescribing information: **Carbapenems**

Dosages and duration of treatment will depend on the indication. Check your local antibiotics policy.

Imipenem (with cilastatin)
- By intravenous infusion, usual dose 500 mg (of imipenem) tds or qds.
- See above for dosage adjustments in renal insufficiency.
- Higher doses may be required; seek microbiological advice.

Meropenem
- By intravenous infusion, 500 mg tds.
- See above for dosage adjustments in renal insufficiency.
- Higher doses may be required; seek microbiological advice.

Cephalosporins and cephamycins

β-lactam antibiotics

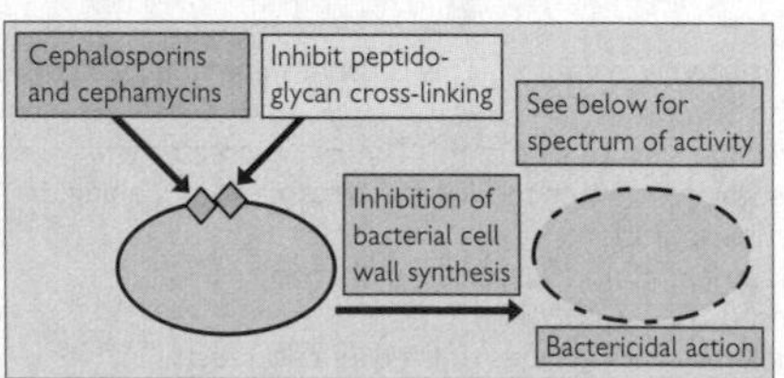

Drugs in this class

First-generation
- Principally Gram-positive cover (but not *Enterococcus spp.*)
  - cefradine, cefazolin, cefalexin, cefadroxil

Second-generation
- Improved Gram-negative cover but at the expense of Gram-positive cover
  - cefuroxime, cefaclor, cefamandole, cefprozil

Third-generation
- Greater Gram-negative cover, but less Gram-positive cover, especially *Staph. aureus*
  - cefotaxime and ceftriaxone
  - ceftazidime (covers *Pseudomonas* but has minimal Gram-positive cover)

Other cephalosporins
  - cefpirome
  - cefixime
  - cefpodoxime, covers respiratory tract pathogens

Cephamycin
  - cefoxitin (has some anaerobic activity)

- Widely-used antibiotics with good penetration to body tissues and fluids.
  - Relatively poor penetration to CSF unless the meninges are inflamed.
  - See box and penicillins (p. 322).
  - Cefotaxime is commonly used as a first-line drug for the treatment of meningitis (a notifiable disease — see antituberculosis drugs (p. 361) for more information).
  - Commonly used for surgical prophylaxis (see below).

- Those with a history of allergy to penicillin should not be given any β lactam antibiotic, including cephalosporins, the carbapenems, and co-amoxiclav.
  - A non-confluent rash affecting only a small area or occurring more than 72 hours after starting the penicillin does not usually represent an allergic reaction.
- These drugs can accumulate in renal insufficiency.
  - Antibiotic solutions for intravenous injection contain a large amount of electrolytes (Na^+ and K^+); these will also accumulate in renal insufficiency.
  - As a rule of thumb, give the usual initial dose but reduce subsequent doses by half in renal insufficiency.
- These drugs are not known to be harmful in pregnancy, but avoid them unless they are essential.
- Avoid these drugs if the patient has porphyria.

- The word 'cef' is commonly used to describe these drugs. Do not do this. Be specific about the cephalosporin to which you are referring. These antibiotics do not have the same spectrum of activity and mistakes have been made.
- Always consider the likely causative organisms when treating infection empirically.

- Avoid using a broad-spectrum drug when one with a narrow spectrum will cover the causative organism.
  - Cephalosporins are probably some of the most inappropriately used antibiotics.
- Using a broad-spectrum antibiotic increases the risk of antibiotic-associated diarrhoea (see below).
  - Cephalosporins are now the most common cause of antibiotic-associated diarrhoea.
  - See notes below; limit intravenous treatment to the shortest possible time.

Note on prophylactic antibiotic treatment

- The prophylactic use of antibiotics (commonly a cephalosporin plus metronidazole) has an important role in the prevention of postoperative infection. If, however, the patient develops a postoperative infection, it is unlikely that the organism responsible will be sensitive to the antibiotics used for prophylaxis. Take appropriate cultures and discuss a change in antibiotic regimen with a microbiologist or specialist in infection.
- Do not continue prophylactic antibiotic treatment for inappropriately long periods.

- Hypersensitivity is relatively common. An urticarial rash occurs in 5% of patients. Anaphylactic reactions are much less common.
- Eradication of the patient's normal flora can cause:
  - Superinfection by *Candida* in the oropharynx. This is most common in the elderly and debilitated.
  - Antibiotic-associated diarrhoea. Avoid broad-spectrum drugs unless essential.
  - Cephalosporins commonly cause diarrhoea by different mechanisms (see box below).
- Cephalosporins can cause abnormalities of liver function tests, and frank hepatitis.
- Rare adverse effects include:
  - Coombs'-positive haemolytic anaemia.
  - Bone marrow suppression (thrombocytopenia).
  - Interference with the action of clotting factors, causing haemorrhage.
  - Hypernatraemia and hyperkalaemia in patients with renal insufficiency (see above).

- The risk of drug interactions is small.
- Cephalosporins can potentiate the effect of warfarin, but the effect is inconsistent. Some can cause bleeding disorders.
- Antacids may reduce the absorption of these drugs given by mouth.

Safety and efficacy

- Measures of clinical improvement are the most important, but inflammatory markers such as the CRP and ESR are often helpful.
- Whenever possible, take cultures before starting antibiotic treatment. Check the sensitivities of the causative organism. Discuss any unusual results with a microbiologist.
- Measure the patient's renal function and liver function tests, especially if long-term treatment is required (>7 days).
- Cephalosporins can give a false-positive urine glucose test and Coombs' test.

- Warn the patient of the risk of rash and other hypersensitivity phenomena.
- Warn female patients that if they develop diarrhoea the oral contraceptive pill may be ineffective.

Prescribing information: **Cephalosporins and Cephamycins**

There are many drugs and formulations. Their uses and spectra of activity are not equivalent. The following are given as examples. Dosages and duration of treatment will depend on the indication. Check your local antibiotics policy.

- **Cefalexin** for urinary tract, respiratory tract, sinus, skin, and soft tissue infections by sensitive organisms.
  - By mouth, 250 mg qds or 500 mg bd.
- **Cefuroxime**, second-generation drug, commonly used for surgical prophylaxis.
  - By slow intravenous injection/infusion, 750 mg tds.
  - Dose may be doubled in severe infections.
- **Ceftriaxone**, third-generation drug, commonly used for treatment of meningitis.
  - By slow intravenous injection/infusion, 2 g bd for meningitis, otherwise once daily.
  - Lower doses may be appropriate.
- **Ceftazidime**, third-generation drug with activity against *Pseudomonas*.
  - By slow intravenous injection/infusion, 1 g tds.
  - Dose may be doubled in severe infection.
- **Cefotaxime**, third-generation drug with a broad spectrum.
  - By slow intravenous injection/infusion, 1 g bd.
  - May be increased up to 12 g daily (in divided doses in severe infection).

TEACHING POINT Antibiotic-associated diarrhoea

- Antibiotics can cause diarrhoea in several ways:
  - They alter bowel flora, which can cause diarrhoea.
  - Alteration of the bowel's normal flora can allow overgrowth of other organisms, such as *Clostridium difficile*. This overgrowth can cause a diarrhoeal illness ranging in severity up to pseudomembranous colitis.
  - Some antibiotics (penicillins) can cause diarrhoea due to a hypersensitivity reaction; this is rare.
- The increasing use of broad-spectrum antibiotics has made this condition very common in hospitals. Clindamycin was the first antibiotic to be associated with pseudomembranous colitis, but cephalosporins are now the most common cause of dirahhoea due to *Clostridium difficile*. Consider carefully whether a narrow-spectrum antibiotic would suffice, before you start a broad-spectrum antibiotic.
  - The elderly and debilitated are at greatest risk. The risk increases with prolonged courses of antibiotics, but it can appear after only a single dose.
  - The most severe form of antibiotic-associated diarrhoea, pseudomembranous colitis, is not a trivial disease. It can be fatal, especially in those who are already frail. Furthermore, it prolongs hospital stays by up to 10 days, increasing the risk of other hospital-acquired infection and placing a considerable burden on resources.
  - *Clostridium difficile* is diagnosed by identification of its toxin in the stool. The toxin can be present after the diarrhoea has subsided and presence of the toxin alone is not grounds for treatment; however, infection control procedures should be followed.

Prevention is as important as treatment

- Review the current antibiotic regimen.
  - Avoid broad-spectrum drugs, unless they are essential.
  - Limit intravenous antibiotic treatment to the shortest possible time.
- Follow universal precautions when attending to and examining patients.
- Take care to avoid cross-contamination from those known to be infected.

Treatment

- Supportive measures are essential. Ensure that the patient has an adequate fluid intake.
- Follow infection control procedures carefully.
- Metronidazole is the first-line treatment.
  - By mouth, 400 mg tds for 7 days.
- If this is ineffective, consider treatment with vancomycin.
  - By mouth, 125 mg every 6 hours, for 7–10 days.
- In a small number of severe cases this will not be sufficient. Seek expert advice. Options include re-establishment of the normal gut flora with lactobacillus (although trial evidence of efficacy is poor).

Glycopeptide antibiotics

Antibiotics

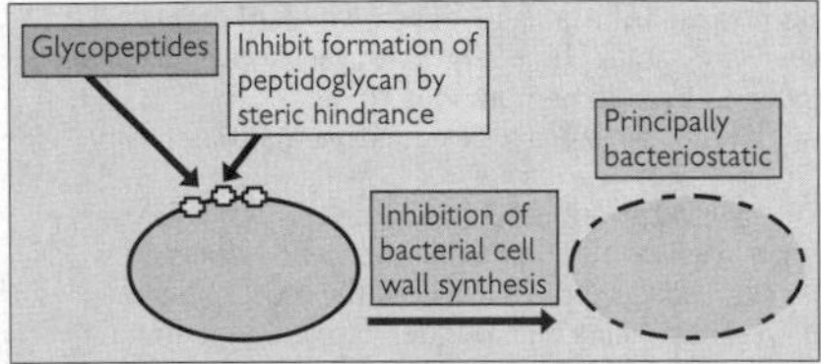

Drugs in this class

- Vancomycin
- Teicoplanin

Treatment of multiresistant bacteria

See teaching point below.

- Treatment of infection by Gram-positive cocci, especially multiresistant staphylococci (e.g. MRSA).
  - These drugs have no activity against Gram-negative bacteria.
- Given into the peritoneal cavity for the treatment of peritonitis in patients receiving peritoneal dialysis (CAPD) (unlicensed indication).
- Treatment of antibiotic-associated diarrhoea (vancomycin, given by mouth).

- Glycopeptides are not absorbed in significant amounts when given by mouth. They must be given by intravenous infusion if systemic exposure is required.
  - Systemic administration is not suitable for the treatment of antibiotic-associated diarrhoea. In this case treatment must be given by mouth.
- Glycopeptides are excreted by the kidney. They are given to patients with renal insufficiency, but close serum concentration monitoring is required.
- Glycopeptides are not known to be safe in pregnancy; avoid using them parenterally unless essential.

- Always consider the likely causative organisms when treating infection empirically.
- Reserve glycopeptides for treatment of infections either known to be, or suspected to be, due to multiresistant organisms (see teaching point below).
- The standard dose of 1 g twice daily is often excessive in elderly patients; reduce to 750 mg twice daily and measure the serum concentration early (see below).
- Rapid intravenous injection can cause the 'red man syndrome' due to histamine release, characterized by fever, chills, rash, and hypotension. Give glycopeptides by intravenous infusion over 60–90 minutes.

Antibiotic-associated diarrhoea

- Vancomycin is a second-line treatment, usually reserved for those patients who have failed to respond to a course of treatment with metronidazole. See cephalosporin (p. 331) for guidance on the treatment of antibiotic-associated diarrhoea.

- Glycopeptides are excreted by the kidney and can be nephrotoxic. Take particular care and monitor the serum concentration closely in patients with renal insufficiency.
  - Glycopeptides can also be ototoxic.

- Excessively rapid infusion can cause the 'red man syndrome' (see above). Give these drugs by slow infusion.
- Hypersensitivity is relatively common. This is most commonly characterized by a rash, which can be severe.
- Occasionally glycopeptides can cause neutropenia, agranulocytosis, or thrombocytopenia.

- The risk of nephrotoxicity and ototoxicity is increased if these drugs are given with aminoglycosides, loop diuretics (e.g. furosemide), or ciclosporin.
- Colestyramine antagonizes the action of vancomycin when it is given by mouth.

Safety and efficacy

- Measures of clinical improvement are the most important, but inflammatory markers such as the CRP and ESR are often helpful.
- Whenever possible, take cultures before starting antibiotic treatment. Check the sensitivities of the causative organism. Discuss any unusual results with a microbiologist.
- Measure the patient's renal function before and during treatment. Measure a full blood count especially if long-term treatment is required (more than 7 days).

Serum concentration measurement

- Trough concentrations are most helpful; aim for a trough concentration of 5–10 mg/L.
  - If renal function is normal, take the sample after the third dose.
- Plan when you will be taking serum samples for measurement and liaise with your laboratory to ensure that they will be able to process the samples at the times you request. This is especially important at weekends.
- If the patient's renal function is normal give the dose after taking the sample for measurement. Use the result to adjust the size of the next dose.
- If the patient's renal function is not normal, wait for the result before giving the next dose of vancomycin.
- If you are unsure, take advice about dosage adjustment. Vancomycin acts by time-dependent killing, so it is usually better to reduce the dose than to increase the dosage interval.

- Warn the patient of the risk of rash and other hypersensitivity phenomena.

Note on time-dependent versus concentration-dependent antibacterial action

- The mechanisms of action of antibiotics vary considerably. The ways in which they act may depend on the peak concentration of antibiotic (concentration-dependent killing) or on the length of time over which the bacteria are exposed to the drug (time-dependent killing).
- The aminoglycosides are examples of the former, the glycopeptides of the latter.
- This is why the dosage regimens and associated monitoring are very different for these two classes of antibiotics. See the monitoring sections for further information.

Prescribing information: **Glycopeptide antibiotics**

The following are given as examples. Dosages will depend on the indication and renal function. Check your local antibiotics policy.

Vancomycin

- By intravenous infusion over 60–90 minutes, usual dose 1 g every 12 hours.
  - Take note of advice above and adjust according to serum trough concentration.
- By mouth, for antibiotic-associated diarrhoea, 125 mg every 6 hours for 7–10 days.

Teicoplanin

- By slow intravenous infusion, 400 mg every 12 hours.
  - Take note of advice above and adjust according to serum trough concentration.
  - Dose may be reduced to 200 mg every 12 hours after 3 doses.

TEACHING POINT Multiresistant organisms

- The emergence of multiresistant organisms is a major public health challenge. They are most common in hospital, where broad-spectrum antibiotics are widely used (e.g. intensive care units), but there is an increasing incidence of multiresistant organisms in the community.
- Some of these organisms are resistant to all classes of antibiotics.
- The ability to treat multiresistant organisms can give the impression that antibiotics such as vancomycin are better and more powerful than conventional drugs, such as the penicillins. This impression is false; these antibiotics have a limited spectrum of activity and are relatively difficult to use. If your patient has a penicillin-sensitive organism, a penicillin is a much better and safer choice. Selection of resistant organisms is driven by the use of broad-spectrum antibiotics. Use a narrow-spectrum antibiotic if you know the causative organism. Reserve drugs such as vancomycin for those patients at risk from multiresistant organisms; inappropriate use will drive the selection of more and more resistant organisms. For example, vancomycin-resistant enterococci (VRE) and staphylococci (VRSA) are emerging.
- Infection control procedures (isolation, hand washing, etc.) are as important as the appropriate antibiotic selection in the fight against multiresistant organisms.

Other antibiotics used for the treatment of multiresistant organisms.

- Always discuss the case with a microbiologist before using these drugs.

Linezolid

- An oxazolidinone antibiotic. Has activity against methicillin-resistant *Staphylococcus aureus* (MRSA) and vancomycin-resistant enterococci.
- This drug is a reversible MAOI; see MAOIs (p. 286) for further information.
- The CSM has warned that linezolid can cause myelosuppresion; monitor the full blood count closely.

Quinupristin with dalfopristin

- A mixture of streptogramin antibiotics that have activity against MRSA. They are not active against *Enterococcus faecalis* or Gram-negative organisms.
- This combination can prolong the QT interval.

Tetracyclines

Antibiotics

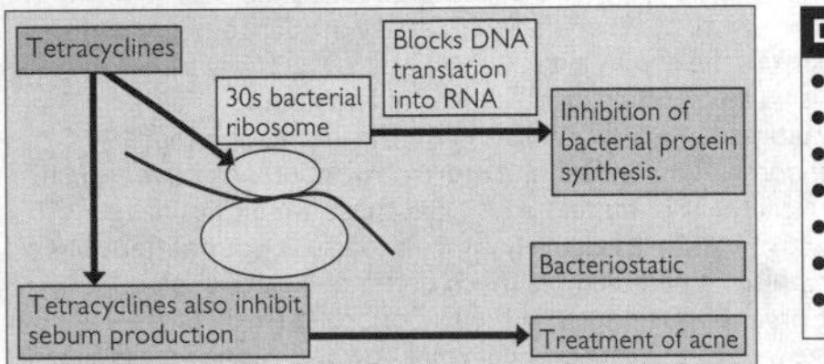

Drugs in this class

- Tetracycline
- Oxytetracycline
- Doxycycline
- Minocycline
- Demeclocycline
- Chlortetracycline
- Lymecycline

- These drugs have a broad spectrum but their clinical usefulness is now limited by widespread resistance. However, they are still the drugs of choice for infection by intracellular organisms:
  - Chlamydiae (non-specific urethritis, psittacosis, trachoma).
  - Rickettsiae (e.g. Q fever).
  - Brucellae (with streptomycin or rifampicin).
  - Spirochaetes (*Borrelia burgdorferi*–Lyme disease).
- Tetracyclines are also used to treat acne.
- Demeclocycline is used to treat the syndrome of inappropriate ADH (SIADH). See also lithium (p. 478).
- Doxycycline is used as prophylaxis against malaria (see antimalarials, p. 382).

- Avoid tetracyclines in patients with myasthenia gravis or systemic lupus erythematosus. They can worsen muscle weakness.
- Avoid tetracyclines if the patient has diabetes insipidus; they can exacerbate it.
- Tetracyclines can worsen hepatic and renal function; avoid them in patients with renal or hepatic insufficiency.
- Do not give tetracyclines to children; they are deposited in teeth and can cause dental yellowing and hypoplasia.
- For the same reason, do not give these drugs to women who are pregnant or who are breastfeeding.
  - Tetracyclines can be deposited in the bones and teeth of women and children.

- The absorption of tetracyclines is markedly inhibited by divalent and trivalent cations, with which they form chelates:
  - Milk and milk products.
  - Zinc, iron, magnesium, and aluminium.
  - Take tetracyclines with plenty of water 30 minutes or more before food. Avoid taking them with milk or antacids or supplements that contain the elements listed above.
- Diagnosis of the infections above may require specialized investigations; seek advice from a microbiologist or infectious diseases specialist.
- Demeclocycline reduces the sensitivity of the collecting ducts to antidiuretic hormone (ADH); this induces diabetes insipidus. This effect is sometimes used to treat the syndrome of inappropriate ADH (SIADH). See lithium (p. 478) for diagnostic criteria.

Treatment of acne (see teaching point below)

- Tetracyclines can be given by mouth or by topical application for this indication.
- Topical application has lower systemic exposure and so a lower risk of effects on bones and teeth.
- Bacterial resistance is increasing, so limit the use of tetracyclines to patients with moderate acne with an inflammatory component.
    - Use a non-antibiotic antimicrobial (e.g. benzoylperoxide) when possible.
- Do not use different oral and topical antibiotics at the same time.
- Tetracyclines improve acne but take time to act and do not abolish it.
    - Some improvement may be seen within 4–6 weeks, but it can take 8–12 weeks before full improvement is seen.

- Adverse effects are more common with systemic than with topical administration.
- Nausea and vomiting are common. Tetracyclines can cause oesophageal irritation; they should be taken with plenty of water (not milk).
- Tetracyclines are excreted by the kidneys and can cause nephrotoxicity. Avoid them if the patient has renal insufficiency. Nephrotoxicity is more likely if the patient is dehydrated from vomiting or diuretic drugs. Ensure that the patient remains well hydrated.
    - Doxycycline does not cause nephrotoxicity.
    - Demeclocycline can cause nephrogenic diabetes insipidus (see above).
    - Some of the breakdown products of tetracyclines are nephrotoxic. Do not use out-of-date drugs.
    - Tetracyclines can cause a rise in the blood urea concentration without a rise in creatinine. Take care; this can falsely suggest that the patient has renal insufficiency.
- Hypersensitivity to tetracyclines is relatively common. Demeclocycline commonly causes a photosensitive rash.
    - These drugs can cause irreversible pigmentation of the skin; this is more common with prolonged use.
- Tetracyclines are deposited in developing teeth, causing yellowing. They can also cause dental hypoplasia.
- Tetracyclines can cause 'benign' intracranial hypertension ('pseudotumor cerebri'). This is rare but potentially serious; the term 'benign' is misleading.
    - Ask the patient about headache and visual disturbance and withdraw the drug if these occur.
- Tetracyclines can cause blood disorders (anaemia, thrombocytopenia), but these are rare.
- Minocycline can cause a systemic lupus erythematosus-like syndrome; this is rare.

- Avoid milk and minerals that chelate tetracyclines (see above for a list).
- Drugs that induce cytochome P450 enzymes increase the metabolism of tetracyclines, reducing their action. See carbamazepine (p. 246) for more information.
- These drugs increase the effect of warfarin; measure the INR and reduce the warfarin dose if appropriate.

- Doxycycline increases blood ciclosporin concentrations.
- Do not give tetracyclines with retinoids (also used for acne); the risk of intracranial hypertension is increased.

Safety and efficacy

- Measures of clinical improvement are the most important, but inflammatory markers such as the CRP and ESR are often helpful if these drugs are used to treat infection.
- Whenever possible, take cultures before starting antibiotic treatment. Some of the organisms that tetracycline are used to treat require special culture conditions; discuss this with a microbiologist. Check the sensitivities of the causative organism.
- Measure the patient's renal function (urea and creatinine), taking note of the factors discussed above.
- If treatment is to extend beyond 6 months, measurement of liver function tests and inflammatory markers is recommended. Examine the patient, looking for irreversible skin pigmentation.

- Warn the patient that topical tetracyclines can stain clothing.
- Warn the patient to avoid milk, mineral supplements, and some other drugs (see list above) whilst taking tetracyclines.
- Advise the patient to report any persistent headaches or visual disturbances promptly.

Prescribing information: **Tetracyclines**

There are many formulations of these drugs. The following are given as examples. Dosages and duration of treatment will depend on the indication. Check your local antibiotics policy.

Tetracycline for infection

- By mouth, 250 mg every 6 hours.
- May be increased to 500 mg every 6 hours.

Demeclocycline for treatment of SIADH

- By mouth, initially 0.9–1.2 g daily, in divided doses.
- Usual maintenance dose 600–900 mg.

Minocycline for acne

- By mouth, 100 mg daily (dose may be divided).

TEACHING POINT Treatment of acne

- Acne occurs when excess oil (sebum) production combined with dead skin cells clogs pores. Bacterial growth in the pores causes red inflamed pimples, pus-filled whiteheads, or blackheads.
- Acne is more common
  - In adolescents
  - In men
  - In greasy skin
  - In unwashed skin
  - During menstruation
  - If anabolic steroids are used
  - If pores are blocked by cosmetics
- Simple measures, such as regular washing (antibacterial soaps do not increase efficacy) and exposure to natural sunlight may be all that is required for mild acne.
- Acne can be scarring; severe acne should be treated early to prevent severe scarring.
- All treatments take time to act.

Mild or moderate acne

- Topical treatment is usually sufficient. A non-antibiotic antimicrobial, such as benzoylperoxide or azelaic acid, is usually preferred, owing to increasing emergence of antibiotic resistance.
  - Consider treatment with a topical antibiotic if there has been no response after 2 months of treatment.
- Topical antibiotics (erythromycin, clindamycin, or tetracycline) should be reserved for patients with an inflammatory component.
  - Adverse effects from these topical formulations are uncommon.
- If these treatments are ineffective, consider treatment with a topical retinoid.
  - These take several months to act and are likely to cause redness of the skin and peeling.
  - Do not apply these drugs to large areas of the skin. Avoid exposure to UV light. Use a sunscreen if exposure to the sun is unavoidable.
  - These drugs are contraindicated during pregnancy. See retinoids (p. 612) for more information.

Moderate to severe acne

- A proportion of patients do not respond to topical treatments.
- Consider systemic treatment in these cases.
- First-line choices are oral antibacterials, such as tetracyclines (see above) or erythromycin. Erythromycin can be used in younger patients, but bacterial resistance is widespread. Topical anticomedonal treatment (e.g. benzoylperoxide) can be continued, but do not use different topical and systemic antibiotics at the same time (increases resistance).
  - Trimethoprim is a second-line option for resistant acne; treatment should be supervised by a specialist.
  - Co-pryndiol (an antiandrogen plus an oestrogen) is a second-line option for women with acne. It is contraindicated in pregnancy and increases the risk of thromboembolism. The antiandrogen action may improve hirsutism.
- Oral retinoids are reserved for treatment of the most severe acne; they can only be prescribed by consultant dermatologists. See retinoids (p. 612) for more information.

Aminoglycoside antibiotics

Antibiotics

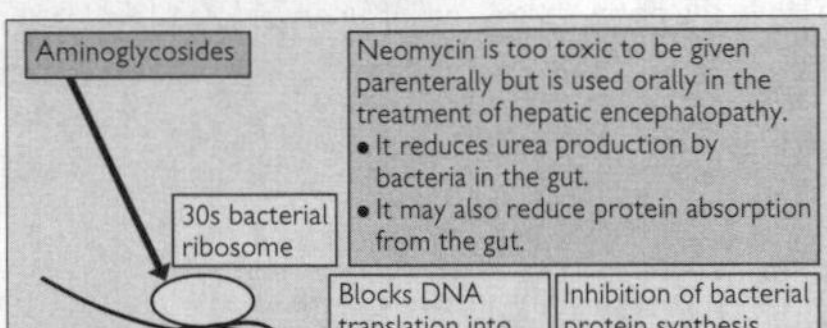

Drugs in this class

- Gentamicin*
- Neomycin
- Netilmicin
- Tobramycin*
- Amikacin*
- Kanamycin
- Streptomycin
  - Used almost exclusively for the treatment of *Mycobacterium tuberculosis* (TB). See antituberculosis drugs, p. 358.

*Drugs with activity against *Pseudomonas aeruginosa*

- These drugs are most commonly given for serious Gram-negative infections.
- They have some action against some Gram-positive bacteria. For example, they act synergistically with penicillins in the treatment of staphylococcal endocarditis. The penicillin breaks the cell wall, allowing the aminoglycoside to enter.
  - Gentamicin is the usual drug of choice.
  - Amikacin is usually reserved for gentamicin-resistant Gram-negative bacteria.
  - Tobramycin is given by nebulizer for treatment of *Pseudomonas aeruginosa* in patients with cystic fibrosis.
  - Neomycin is too toxic for parenteral administration; it is given orally for gut clearance (sterilization) (e.g. as part of the treatment of hepatic encephalopathy).
  - These drugs penetrate the chest and abscesses poorly.

- Aminoglycosides can interfere with neuromuscular transmission; avoid them in patients with myasthenia gravis.
- Aminoglycosides are excreted by the kidney. They are given to patients with renal insufficiency, but close serum concentration monitoring is required if repeated doses are used.
- Avoid aminoglycosides during pregnancy whenever possible; there is a risk of damage to the baby's vestibular and auditory nerves.

- Aminoglycosides are not absorbed from the gut; they must be given parenterally.
  - Tobramycin can be given by nebulized solution.
- Aminoglycosides are given in two ways:
  - As a single large dose, usually once daily according to the regimen outlined below.
  - For their synergistic action with another antibiotic (see above) (e.g. in the treatment of endocarditis). In this case, the drug is given as a smaller dose 2 or 3 times daily.

- Hypersensitivity is relatively common. A rash occurs in 5% of patients.
  - Streptomycin can cause contact dermatitis; wear gloves when handling it.
- Aminoglycosides can be ototoxic and nephrotoxic. The risk is related to the trough concentration rather than the peak concentration. Make sure the serum concentration has fallen below 2 mg/L before giving another dose.

- Aminoglycosides can have a neuromuscular blocking action, especially when given in large doses.
- Neomycin can cause superinfection of the pharynx and gut with yeasts and fungi.
- Aminoglycosides can cause antibiotic-associated diarrhoea, but this is uncommon.
- Tobramycin can cause bronchospasm and haemoptysis when given by nebulizer.

- The risk of nephrotoxicity is increased if aminoglycosides are given with loop diuretics (e.g. furosemide), antifungal drugs (e.g. amphotericin), cytotoxic drugs, and ciclosporin.
- Neomycin reduces vitamin K absorption, potentiating the effect of warfarin. Neomycin also reduces the absorption of digoxin.
- Aminoglycosides potentiate the effects of neuromuscular blocking drugs.

Safety and efficacy

- Measures of clinical improvement are the most important, but inflammatory markers such as the CRP and ESR are often helpful.
- Whenever possible, take cultures before starting antibiotic treatment. Check the sensitivities of the causative organism. Discuss any unusual results with a microbiologist.
- Measure the patient's renal function (including tobramycin given by nebulizer).

Gentamicin

- Plan when you will be taking serum samples for measurement, and liaise with your laboratory to ensure that they will be able to process the samples at the times you request. This is especially important at weekends.
- Measure the serum concentration and adjust the dose and interval as appropriate.
    - For twice or three times daily dosing:
        - Measure the serum concentration after 3 doses if renal function is normal. If renal function is abnormal, measure the concentration earlier.
        - The peak concentration should be taken 1 hour after the dose has finished being given, and should be in the range 5–10 mg/L.
        - The trough concentration should be taken just before the next dose and should be less than 2 mg/L.
    - A nomogram for once-daily dosing is given on p. 343
- Seek advice for target ranges of other aminoglycosides.

- Warn the patient of the risk of rash and other hypersensitivity phenomena.

Prescribing information: **Aminoglycoside antibiotics**

There are many formulations of these drugs. The following are given as examples. Dosages will depend on the indication and renal function. Check your local antibiotics policy. See azathioprine (p. 515) for more information on giving drug dosages by body weight.

Gentamicin

- Once daily regimen, see box below
- Twice or three times daily regimen. By intramuscular injection or slow intravenous injection/infusion, usual dose range 60–80 mg twice daily.

Amikacin

- By intramuscular injection or slow intravenous injection/infusion, 15 mg/kg daily in 2 divided doses
- May be increased to 22.5 mg /kg daily in 3 divided doses.

Netilmicin

- By intramuscular injection or slow intravenous injection/infusion, 4–6 mg/kg daily in 2 divided doses.

Tobramycin

- By intramuscular injection or slow intravenous injection/infusion, 3 mg/kg daily in 3 divided doses.

Once-daily gentamicin

- The rationale for pulse dosing of aminoglycosides is based on the following observations:
  - Aminoglycosides exhibit a significant post-antibiotic effect. An antibacterial effect is detectable beyond the time that the drug is detectable in the serum.
  - The bactericidal action of aminoglycosides is concentration dependent. The higher the ratio between the peak aminoglycoside concentration and minimum inhibitory concentration (MIC), the higher the kill rate. The multiple daily dosing regimen usually results in relatively low peak/MIC ratios (<5). When the same total daily dose is given as a single bolus (infused over 30-60 minutes), much higher ratios are obtained (>10).
  - Aminoglycoside uptake into renal tubule cells and the inner ear appears to be saturated at relatively low serum concentrations, suggesting that higher peaks do not necessarily result in a greater risk of toxicity.

Exclusion criteria for once-daily aminoglycoside dosing

- Pregnancy
- Severe liver disease (e.g. ascites)
- Neutropenia
- Extensive burns (>20% of body surface area)
- Patients with Gram-positive infection (when the aminoglycoside is used for synergy)
- Severe renal disease (creatinine clearance < 30 mL/min)
- Patients with enterococcal endocarditis

Dosage

- The *single dose* for gentamicin is 7 mg per kg body weight, unless the patient is more than 20% heavier than the ideal body weight. For obese patients, calculate a dosing weight:

Dosing weight = ideal body weight (in kg) + 0.4 x (actual body weight –ideal body weight)

- The calculated dose is diluted in 100 mL of isotonic saline and infused over 1 hour.
- Measure the serum concentration at 7–12 hours after the dose (take a careful note of the actual time).
- Use the nomogram (see diagram) to calculate the frequency of dosing.

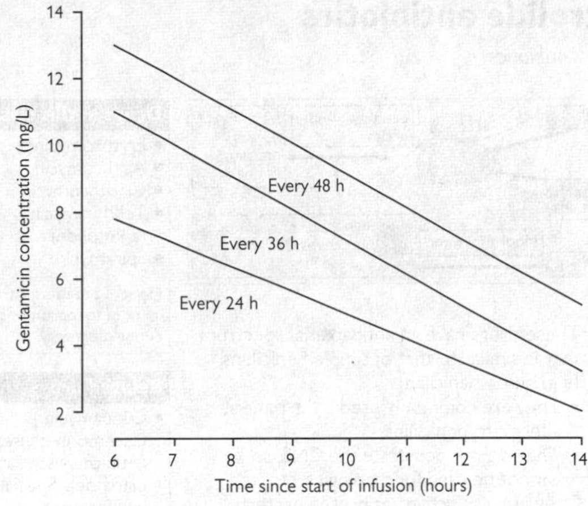

Hartford nomogram for calculating gentamicin dosing frequency

Macrolide antibiotics

Antibiotics

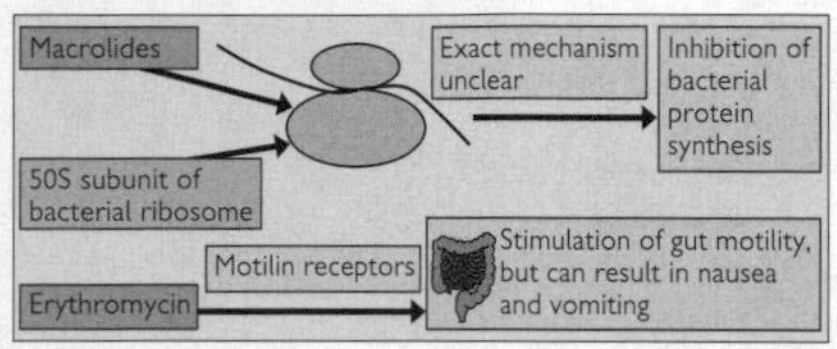

Drugs in this class
- Erythromycin
- Azithromycin
- Clarithromycin
- Telithromycin (a ketolide)
- Spiramycin*

*Specialized use, for treatment of toxoplasmosis during pregnancy.

Related drugs
- Clindamycin. Commonly causes antibiotic-associated diarrhoea. Specialist use for bone infection. Used in combination with other antibiotics.
- Steptogramins (Synercid®). See teaching point in glycopeptides, p. 335.

- These drugs have an antibacterial spectrum that is similar to that of simple penicillins (e.g. benzylpenicillin).
    - They are commonly used if the patient is allergic to penicillins.
    - They do not penetrate the CNS, so cannot be used for meningitis.
- They are also active against the bacteria that cause atypical pneumonias (e.g. *Mycoplasma, Chlamydia, Legionella*).
- Azithromycin has a slightly different spectrum from erythromycin:
    - It covers *Haemophilus influenzae.*
    - It can be given as single dose for treatment of chlamydial and non-gonococcal urethritis.
- Clarithromycin is commonly used as part of *Helicobacter pylori* eradication regimens (see proton pump inhibitors, p. 28).
- Erythromycin is used topically for the treatment of acne.
- Erythromycin stimulates motilin receptors in the gut. This increases gut motility and is used therapeutically on the ICU and in patients with diabetic autonomic neuropathy.

- Avoid macrolides in hepatic insufficiency; the risk of hepatotoxicity is increased.
    - They can also cause idiosyncratic heptatotoxicity.
    - Avoid macrolides if the patient has porphyria.
- Reduce the dose if the patient has renal insufficiency.
    - Halve the dose of clarithromycin in mild renal insufficiency.
    - Limit the total daily dose to 1.5 g of erythromycin in mild renal insufficiency.
- Macrolides are not known to be harmful in pregnancy, but the manufacturers advise that they should be avoided unless essential.
- Macrolides can prolong the QT interval; avoid them in patients with known cardiac conduction abnormalities.

- Always consider the likely causative organisms when treating infection empirically.
- Avoid using a broad-spectrum drug when one with a narrow spectrum will cover the causative organism.
- Using a broad-spectrum antibiotic increases the risk of antibiotic-associated diarrhoea (see cephalosporins, p. 331).
- Erythromycin commonly causes nausea and vomiting; this can be reduced by giving a lower dose (e.g. 250 mg qds).
  - The higher dose is required if *Legionella* could be the causative organism.
  - Clarithromycin and azithromycin cause less vomiting but are more expensive.
- Intravenous erythromycin can cause thrombophlebitis; only give it into a large vein via a free-flowing cannula.
- Erythromycin is used for the treatment of acne (see tetracyclines (p. 339) for more information).
  - Bacterial resistance is increasing, so limit its use to patients with moderate acne with an inflammatory component.
  - Use a non-antibiotic antimicrobial (e.g. benzoylperoxide) when possible.
  - Erythromycin can be given systemically for moderate to severe acne, but resistance is widespread. More commonly it is given topically for moderate acne.
  - Do not use different oral and topical antibiotics at the same time.

- Nausea and vomiting are the most common adverse effects of these drugs; see above for advice on how to mitigate this.
- Macrolides can cause a rash, which may be severe.
- Macrolides can prolong the QT interval; take care in patients who are cardiovascularly unstable.
- Macrolides can cause cholestatic jaundice.
- Eradication of the patient's normal flora can cause antibiotic-associated diarrhoea; see cephalosporins (p. 331) for guidance.

- Erythromycin and clarithromycin inhibit cytochrome P450 enzymes in the liver. This will reduce the metabolism of other drugs, increasing their effect. See teaching point below.
- Clarithromycin reduces the absorption of zidovudine.

Safety and efficacy

- Measures of clinical improvement are the most important, but inflammatory markers such as the CRP and ESR are often helpful.
- Whenever possible, take cultures before staring antibiotic treatment. Check the sensitivities of the causative organism. Discuss any unusual results with a microbiologist.
- Measure liver function tests, especially if long-term treatment is required (more than 7 days).
- Measure the QT interval on an ECG, especially if the patient is cardiovascularly unstable.

- Warn the patient of the risk of nausea and vomiting.
- Warn female patients that if they develop diarrhoea the oral contraceptive pill may be ineffective.

Prescribing information: **Macrolide antibiotics**

There are many formulations of these drugs. The following are given as examples. Dosages and duration of treatment will depend on the indication. Check your local antibiotics policy.

Erythromycin

Several salts of erythromycin are available; the estolate is the best absorbed when given by mouth and causes less nausea, vomiting, and anorexia.

- By mouth, 250–500 mg every 6 hours, or 0.5–1 g every 12 hours.
- By intravenous infusion, 50 mg/kg by continuous infusion, or in divided doses every 6 hours.

Azithromycin

- By mouth, 500 mg daily for 3 days.
  - Uncomplicated chlamydial infections and non-gonococcal urethritis, 1 g single dose.

Clarithromycin

Eradication of *H. pylori*; see proton pump inhibitors, p. 28)

- By mouth, 250 mg bd.
- By intravenous infusion, 500 mg bd.

Telithromycin

- By mouth, 800 mg daily.

TEACHING POINT Drugs that inhibit cytochrome P450 enzymes

- Drugs are metabolized in the liver by cytochrome P450 enzymes. The isoform called CYP 3A4 is responsible for the metabolism of many drugs. Erythromycin and clarithromycin (but not azithromycin) are inhibitors of CYP 3A4. They therefore slow down the metabolism of any other drugs that are metabolized by CYP 3A4. This can increase the effect of these other drugs.
- The interaction with warfarin is particularly important. The dose of warfarin may need to be reduced when these drugs are started. Remember also that the dose may need to be increased again when they are stopped.

Drugs that are metabolized by cytochrome 3A4.

These may be affected if they are co-administered with drugs that inhibit CYP 3A4 (see below).

Warfarin
HIV protease inhibitors
Antiepileptic drugs (phenytoin, carbamazepine)
Benzodiazepines
Clozapine
Sildenafil
Corticosteroids
Erythromycin, clarithromycin
Antihistamines
HMG CoA reductase inhibitors ('statins')
Immune modulators (ciclosporin, tacrolimus)
Calcium channel blockers
Theophylline
Ergotamine
Quinidine
St John's wort

Drugs that inhibit CYP 3A4

Erythromycin, clarithromycin
HIV protease inhibitors
Some SSRIs (fluoxetine, fluvoxamine)
Grapefruit juice
Amiodarone
Cimetidine
Some antifungal drugs (itraconazole, ketoconazole)

Sulfonamides and trimethoprim

Antimicrobials that act by interfering with bacterial folate metabolism

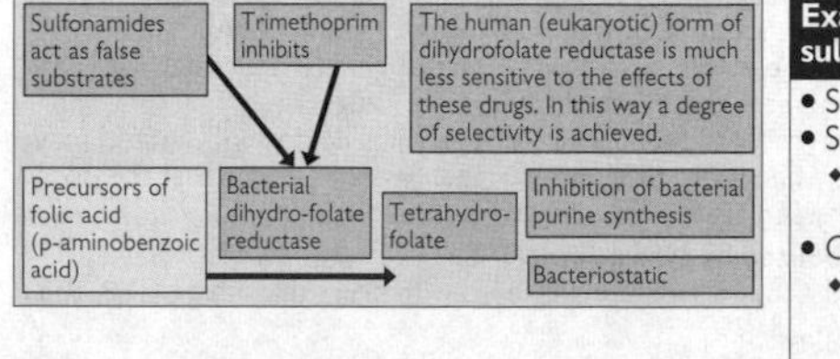

Examples of sulfonamides

- Sulfamethoxazole
- Sulfadiazine
  - Silver sulfadiazine (Flamazine®)
- Co-trimoxazole
  - Trimethoprim plus sulfamethoxazole (Septrin®)

- Trimethoprim is most commonly used for the treatment of urinary tract infections.
  - It can also be used for the treatment of prostatitis, shigellosis, and invasive *Salmonella* infections. Seek specialist advice.
- Co-trimoxazole is an effective antibiotic but is associated with rare, severe adverse effects. For this reason, its use should be restricted to the following indications.
  - Drug of choice for *Pneumocysitis jiroveci* pneumonia.
  - Also given for toxoplasmosis and nocardiasis (seek specialist advice).
- Sulfadiazine is used for the treatment of toxoplasmic encephalitis.
  - It is also used for the prevention of recurrence of rheumatic fever (specialized use).
  - Silver sulfadiazine is given topically for prevention of infection in wounds (commonly, burn wounds).

- Avoid all these drugs if the patient has severe hepatic or renal insufficiency.
- These drugs can cause crystalluria; ensure an adequate fluid intake in all patients, but especially those with any degree of renal insufficiency.
- Avoid all these drugs if the patient has an existing haematological disease; they can suppress the bone marrow.
- All these drugs should be avoided during the last trimester of pregnancy.
- Avoid all these drugs if the patient is folate deficient.
- Avoid sulfonamides if the patient has G6PD deficiency (see antimalarials, p. 387).
- See box below if the patient reports an allergy to sulfur.

Urinary tract infection

- Trimethoprim is commonly used empirically for urinary tract infections, but resistance is increasing and nitrofurantoin is an alternative. Check your local guidelines for empirical therapy.
- Always consider the likely causative organisms when treating infection empirically.
- Trimethoprim is sometimes given long-term. In this case special monitoring is required; see below.

Pneumocystis jiroveci (carinii)

- Treatment of toxoplasmic encephalitis and *Pneumocystis jiroveci* should be under the direction of a specialist. These infections are sometimes the first presentation of AIDS. Consider these diagnoses in patients at risk from HIV infection and AIDS.

- Co-trimoxazole is the drug of choice for prophylaxis and treatment of *Pneumocystis jiroveci* infection.
- Pneumocystis is an opportunistic pathogen and is usually only a cause of disease in immunocompromised patients; the largest group are those with AIDS.
  - Prophylaxis is usually given to those patients with a white cell CD4 count below 200 x 10^6/L.

Toxoplasmic encephalitis

- This serious infection occurs most commonly in patients with AIDS.
- Sulfadiazine is used in combination with pyramethamine (a folate antagonist), although it is unlicensed for this indication.
  - Alternatives include the combination of a macrolide antibiotic with pyramethamine (specialist use only).

Topical treatment

- Silver sulfadiazine is commonly used in the prophylaxis and treatment of infection in burn wounds. The care of extensive burns requires specialized nursing and medical supervision.
- Systemic absorption can be significant if this drug is applied over large areas. See adverse effects and interactions below.

- The adverse effects of trimethoprim are similar to those of co-trimoxazole, but are less common and usually less severe.
- The most serious adverse effects are:
  - Severe rash and Stevens–Johnson syndrome.
    - These are hypersensitivity phenomena.
    - Other hypersensitivity phenomena include anaphylaxis, serum sickness, systemic vasculitis, and pneumonitis.
  - Bone marrow depression (usually agranulocytosis).
    - An antifolate effect; see mechanism of action above.
  - The drug should be withdrawn immediately if these occur.
- Patients with G6PD deficiency or abnormal haemoglobins are at risk of haemolytic anaemia.
- Gastrointestinal disturbance, headache, and drowsiness tend to be dose-related.
- Crystalluria can occur, but urinary tract obstruction is uncommon.
- These drugs can cause antibiotic-associated diarrhoea (see cephalosporins, p. 331).

Co-trimoxazole

- Increased risk of ventricular arrhythmias with amiodarone; avoid concomitant use.
- Effect of warfarin increased.*
- Antifolate effect and plasma concentration of phenytoin increased.
- Increase risk of nephrotoxicity when given with ciclosporin.*
- Increased risk of toxicity when given with other drugs that have an antifolate action.*
  - Pyramethamine (includes Fansidar® and Maloprim®).*
  - Azathioprine and mercaptopurine.*
  - Methotrexate.*
  - Phenytoin.*

Trimethoprim

- The interactions marked * also apply to trimethoprim.

Safety and efficacy

- Measures of clinical improvement are the most important, but inflammatory markers such as the CRP and ESR are often helpful. Arterial blood gas measurements indicate the severity of *Pneumocystis carinii* infection.
- Whenever possible, take cultures before staring antibiotic treatment. Advise the laboratory if you suspect that the patient has HIV.
    - This is to protect the laboratory staff, and to ensure that special cultures for opportunistic organisms are set up.
    - Check the sensitivities of the causative organism. Discuss any unusual results with a microbiologist.
- No specific monitoring is required if trimethoprim is given in a short course for a urinary tract infection.
- If used for long-term treatment, patients should be advised how to recognize the symptoms and signs of bone marrow suppression (see below).
- Patients given sulfadiazine and pyramethamine should also be given folinic acid and should have a full blood count measured at least weekly.
- Patients given co-trimoxazole for long-term prophylaxis against *Pneumocystis jiroveci* should have a full blood count measured monthly.

- Advise patients how to recognize the symptoms and signs of bone marrow suppression (easy bruising, unexpected sore throat, bleeding). Advise them that they should seek immediate medical attention if these occur.
- Advise patients that they should seek immediate medical attention if they develop a rash.
- Warn female patients that if they develop diarrhoea, the oral contraceptive may be ineffective.

Prescribing information: **Sulfonamides and trimethoprim**

There are many formulations of these drugs. The following are given as examples. Dosages and duration of treatment will depend on the indication. Check your local antibiotics policy.

Trimethoprim

- For urinary tract infections
    - By mouth, 200 mg bd.

Co-trimoxazole

- Prophylaxis against *Pneumocystis jiroveci (carinii)* infection
    - By mouth, usually 960 mg daily.
- Treatment of *Pneumocystis jiroveci (carinii)* infection
    - By mouth or by intravenous infusion, usually 120 mg /kg daily in 2–4 divided doses over 14 days.

Sulfadiazine

- Treatment of toxoplasmic encephalitis, seek specialist advice.
- Prophylaxis and treatment of infection in burn wounds.
    - Cream 1%. Apply with sterile applicator. Note cautions above about applying to large areas.

TEACHING POINT Sulfur allergy

There are two distinct forms of 'sulfur' allergy:
- Allergy to sulfonamides.
- Allergy to sulfiting agents; these are present in foods, beverages, and some pharmaceutical formulations.

Drugs that contain sulfonamide groups	Drugs that are commonly formulated with sulfiting agents
• Sulfonamides • Sulfasalazine • Sulfanilamide • Sulfonylureas (allergy rare) • Thiazide diuretics (allergy rare) • Loop diuretics (allergy rare) • Acetazolamide (carbonic anhydrase inhibitor) • Celecoxib	• Amino acids • Aminoglycosides • Dexamethasone • Dopamine • Adrenaline • Isoprenaline • Phenylephrine
• The risk of cross-reactivity is relatively low. • Re-exposure to the causative drug after a period time will not cause a reaction in up to 50% of cases, especially if the initial reaction was a mild rash. • However, only reintroduce the drug if it is absolutely necessary and ensure that facilities to treat anaphylaxis are available. • Patients with an allergy to sulfonamides do not usually have an allergy to sulfiting agents.	• These patients commonly have a history of atopy and asthma. • The risk of cross-reactivity with sulphonamides is low.

Metronidazole and tinidazole

Nitroimidazole antibiotics

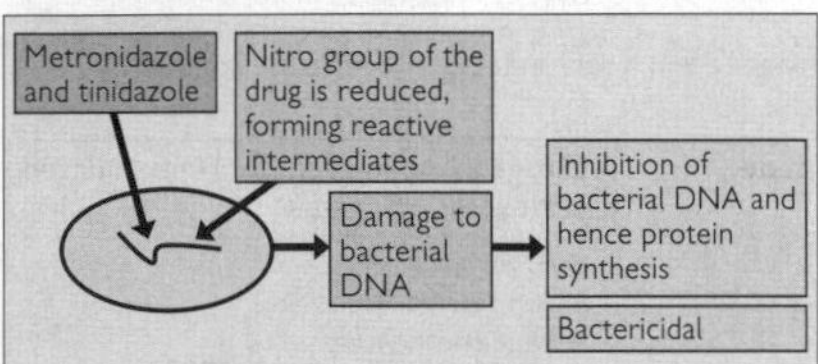

Drugs in this class

- Metronidazole
- Tinidazole
  - Similar spectrum of activity to metronidazole but has a longer duration of action

Drugs that are effective against anaerobic bacteria

- Metronidazole
- Tinidazole
- Tazocin
- Imipenem
- Clindamycin

- Treatment of infection by anaerobic (and microaerophilic) bacteria and protozoa.
  - Prophylaxis and treatment of infection from colonic anaerobes, especially *Bacteroides fragilis*.
    - Commonly used for prophylaxis during abdominal surgery.
    - Metronidazole is used for the treatment of antibiotic-associated diarrhoea (*Clostridium difficile*).
  - Treatment of amoebiasis (*Amoeba enterohepatica*) and amoebic abscesses.
  - Treatment of giardiasis (*Giardia lamblia*).
  - Treatment of tetanus (*Clostridium tetani*). Specialized use; seek expert advice.
  - Treatment of trichomonal vaginitis and bacterial vaginosis.
  - Metronidazole is a component of several regimens for the eradication of *Helicobacter pylori* (see proton pump inhibitors, p. 28).
  - Metronidazole can be used topically to reduce the odour from fungating tumours.

- No dosage adjustment is usually required in renal insufficiency.
- These drugs are metabolized by the liver; reduce the dose to one-third and give it once daily in severe hepatic insufficiency.
- The manufacturers of tinidazole recommend that it should be avoided during the first trimester of pregnancy.
- The manufacturers of metronidazole recommend that high dosages should be avoided during pregnancy.

- Always consider the likely causative organisms when treating infection empirically; is an anaerobic organism likely to be the cause?
- Advise the laboratory that you suspect an anaerobic infection, to ensure that the samples are cultured appropriately.
- If metronidazole is given for treatment of antibiotic-associated diarrhoea it should be given by mouth or rectum, even if the drug is also given intravenously for systemic infection.

⚠

- These drugs are usually well-tolerated.
- Gastrointestinal adverse effects are the most common: nausea and vomiting, unpleasant taste in the mouth.
- A rash can occur and can be severe. Anaphylactic reactions also occur rarely.

- Liver function test abnormalities occur occasionally.
- Prolonged treatment can cause a peripheral neuropathy.

Note on prophylactic antibiotic treatment

- The prophylactic use of antibiotics (commonly a cephalosporin plus metronidazole) has an important role in the prevention of postoperative infection. However, if the patient develops a postoperative infection, it is unlikely that the organism responsible will be sensitive to the antibiotics used for prophylaxis. Take appropriate cultures and discuss a change in antibiotic regimen with a microbiologist or specialist in infection.
- Do not continue prophylactic antibiotic treatment for inappropriately long periods.
- Guidelines on the use of prophylactic antibiotics during surgery are provided by the Scottish Intercollegiate Guidelines Network (*http://www.sign.ac.uk/guidelines*)

- Metronidazole enhances the effect of warfarin; take care to adjust the dose when starting or stopping a course of metronidazole.
- Metronidazole inhibits the metabolism of phenytoin and fluorouracil (5-FU), increasing the risk of toxicity.
- Both metronidazole and tinidazole can cause a disulfiram-like reaction (disulfiram = Antabuse®) if the patient also takes alcohol.

Safety and efficacy

- Measures of clinical improvement are the most important, but inflammatory markers such as the CRP and ESR are often helpful.
- Whenever possible, take cultures before staring antibiotic treatment. Check the sensitivities of the causative organism. Discuss any unusual results with a microbiologist.
- Measure liver function tests if long-term treatment is required (>10 days).

- Patients given antibiotics should be advised to avoid alcohol. This is particularly important with these drugs, since they can cause a disulfiram-like reaction, which is very unpleasant and potentially harmful.
- Warn female patients that if they develop diarrhoea, the oral contraceptive may be ineffective.

Prescribing information: **Metronidazole and tinidazole**

There are many formulations of these drugs. The following are given as examples. Dosages and duration of treatment will depend on the indication. Check your local antibiotics policy.

Metronidazole

- Treatment of anaerobic infections.
  - By mouth, either 800 mg initially then 400 mg tds, or 500 mg tds.
  - By rectum, 1 g tds.
  - By intravenous infusion, 500 mg tds.
- Surgical prophylaxis.
  - By mouth, 400–500 mg 3 hours before surgery. Up to 3 further doses can be given every 8 hours after high-risk procedures
  - By rectum, 1 g 2 hours before surgery. Up to 3 further doses can be given every 8 hours after high-risk procedures.
  - By intravenous infusion, 500 mg at induction. Up to 3 further doses can be given every 8 hours after high-risk procedures.

- Treatment of antibiotic-associated diarrhoea.
  - By mouth, 400 mg tds for 10 days (see also cephalosporins, p. 331).
  - By rectum, 1 g tds.

Tinidazole

- Treatment of anaerobic infections.
  - By mouth, either 2 g initially then 1 g daily, or 500 mg bd.

TEACHING POINT Treatment of tetanus

- Tetanus is an acute, often fatal, disease caused by a toxin of the bacillus *Clostridium tetani*. The bacterium is found in soil, street dust, and animal and human faeces. Infection results from an injury or puncture wound; however, these may be trivial or unnoticed cuts/abrasions. Less commonly, it can result from injection using contaminated needles.
- Symptoms occur within 3–21 days, usually 8 days, after exposure to tetanus spores. Most cases require hospitalization.

Immunization
- The outcome once the disease is established is often poor; prevention is therefore particularly important.
- In the UK, children are offered immunization with tetanus toxoid (as part of the DTP vaccine). This is a course of 3 injections every 4 weeks, starting at 2 months of age.
- This is then boosted before school entry (DTaP vaccine) and before leaving school.
- Adults should be given a booster injection every 10 years.
- Give a booster injection to any patient who presents with a potentially contaminated wound who does not have up-to-date tetanus immunization.

Clinical features
- Stiffness and contraction of muscles, especially those of the abdomen, back, and jaw. This can be painful. Death can result from asphyxiation.
- Symptoms of systemic infection, fever, tachycardia, sweating.

Treatment
- Seek specialist advice.
- Supportive:
  - Paralysis and mechanical ventilation
  - Diazepam for muscle spasm
- Specific:
  - Metronidazole
  - (Anti) tetanus immunoglobulin

Quinolone antibiotics

Antibiotics

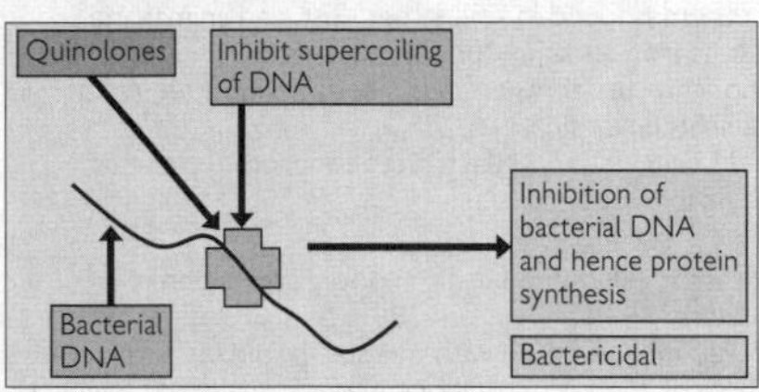

Drugs in this class

- Ciprofloxacin
- Levofloxacin
- Ofloxacin
- Nalidixic acid
- Norfloxacin
- Moxifloxacin

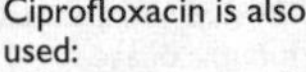

Ciprofloxacin is also used:

- For treatment and prophylaxis against anthrax.
- As a component of some regimens for the treatment of multi-resistant *Mycobacterium tuberculosis* (TB) and other atypical mycobacteria.
- As an alterative to rifampicin for meningococcal disease prophylaxis.

- Treatment of infection by both Gram-positive and Gram-negative organisms, especially:
  - Urinary tract sepsis.
  - Biliary tract sepsis.
  - Food poisoning due to *Campylobacter* (if antibiotics indicated), *Shigella*, and *Salmonella* species.
    - Food poisoning is a notifiable disease (see antituberculosis drugs, p. 361, for more information).
- Ciprofloxacin is the only drug currently available with good activity against *Pseudomonas aeruginosa* that can be given by mouth.
- Ciprofloxacin is not active against *Streptococcus pneumoniae*; levofloxacin gives better pneumococcal cover.
- All these drugs have relatively poor activity against staphylococci; they are therefore not ideal choices for the treatment of skin and soft-tissue infections.

- Quinolones are excreted by the kidney; halve the dose in renal insufficiency.
- Quinolones can cause hepatotoxicity; reduce the dose in hepatic insufficiency.
- Quinolones lower the seizure threshold; avoid them if possible in patients with epilepsy.
- Avoid quinolones during pregnancy; there is a theoretical risk of causing an arthropathy in the baby.
  - Animal studies suggest that children and adolescents are also at risk of arthropathy. Avoid these drugs if possible; but short-term use may be justified in some circumstances.
- Quinolones can cause tendon rupture; avoid them if the patient has tendonitis. The elderly and those taking corticosteroids are at increased risk.
- Avoid quinolones if the patient has G6PD deficiency. See teaching point in antimalarials (p. 387).

- Always consider the likely causative organisms when treating infection empirically.
- Avoid using a broad-spectrum drug when one with a narrow spectrum will cover the causative organism.
- Quinolones are very well absorbed when given by mouth. Intravenous administration is expensive and usually only justified if the patient cannot take drugs by mouth.
  - Ciprofloxacin is available as eye drops, for local application.

- Gastrointestinal adverse effects are common (8% of patients). These are usually nausea, vomiting, and abdominal pain.
- A photosensitive rash occurs in 1–2% of patients; it can be severe. Anaphylactic reactions also occur.
- Liver function test abnormalities occur in 5% of patients. In a small number this will progress to hepatitis.
- Quinolones can cause tendon rupture; the risk is greater if there is existing tendonitis, or if the patient is elderly or taking corticosteroids.
- Quinolones have effects on the CNS. These include convulsions, restlessness, confusion, and hallucinations. If any of these occur, the drug should be withdrawn.
- Rare adverse effects include haemolytic anaemia and hypoglycaemia.

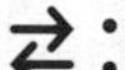

- Quinolones enhance the effect of warfarin.
- The risk of nephrotoxicity from ciclosporin is increased if it is given with quinolones.
- Quinolones increase the plasma theophylline concentration; a dose reduction may be required.
- There may be an increased risk of convulsions from quinolones if they are given with NSAIDs.
- Antacids significantly reduce the absorption of ciprofloxacin, levofloxacin, ofloxacin, and norfloxacin.

Safety and efficacy

- Measures of clinical improvement are the most important, but inflammatory markers such as the CRP and ESR are often helpful.
- Whenever possible, take cultures before staring antibiotic treatment. Check the sensitivities of the causative organism. Discuss any unusual results with a microbiologist.
- Measure liver function tests, especially if long-term treatment is required (more than 7 days).

- Warn the patient of the risk of rash and other hypersensitivity phenomena.
- Warn female patients that if they develop diarrhoea, the oral contraceptive may be ineffective.

Prescribing information: **Quinolones**

There are many formulations of these drugs. The following are given as examples. Dosages and duration of treatment will depend on the indication. Check your local antibiotics policy.

Ciprofloxacin

- By mouth, 250–750 mg twice daily.
- By intravenous infusion, 200–400 mg twice daily. Infuse over 60 minutes.

Levofloxacin

- By mouth, 250–500 mg once or twice daily.
- By intravenous infusion, 500 mg once or twice daily. Infuse over 60 minutes.

Nalidixic acid (for urinary tract infections only)

- By mouth, 1 g every 6 hours.

Norfloxacin

- By mouth, 400 mg twice daily.

Ofloxacin

- By mouth, 200–400 m once or twice daily.
- By intravenous infusion, 200–400 mg once or twice daily. Infuse over 30–60 minutes.

Antituberculosis drugs

A group of different anti-infective drugs that are effective against Mycobacterium tuberculosis

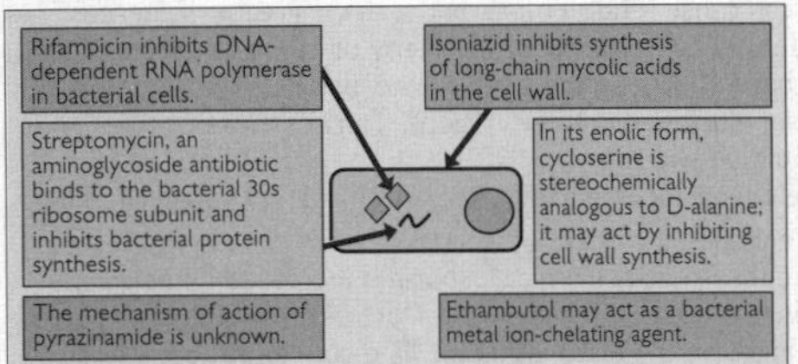

Drugs used in the treatment of tuberculosis

Fully-sensitive organisms
- Rifampicin
- Isoniazid
- Pyrazinamide
- (Ethambutol)
- (Streptomycin; specialist used only)

Multidrug-resistant organisms
- Streptomycin
- Capreomycin
- Cycloserine
- Rifabutin (for prophylaxis in patients with a low CD4 count)

- Many drugs are available for the treatment of *Mycobacterium tuberculosis* (TB).
- Treatment regimens are complex. Seek expert advice.
- If the patient is immunocompromised (e.g. HIV infection), infection may be due to atypical mycobacteria. Seek expert advice.
- Rifampicin is used to treat brucellosis and Legionnaires' disease.
  - Always in combination with other drugs.

- The standard treatment regimen can be given during pregnancy, but do not include streptomycin.
- Ethambutol and streptomycin are best avoided in renal insufficiency.
  - If their use is essential, measure plasma concentrations to guide the dosage regimen.
- These drugs can cause liver damage; take care in patients with hepatic insufficiency.

Bacille Calmette–Guérin (BCG)

Immunization is recommended for:
- Contacts of those with active respiratory TB
- Immigrants from areas of high prevalence
- Children aged 10–14
- Veterinary staff
- Prison/hostel workers
- Those staying for more than 1 month in an area of high prevalence

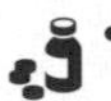

- Take care to protect yourself and other contacts if TB is suspected.
  - TB is a notifiable disease (see below).
- The principle of standard treatment is that of an initial killing phase (triple therapy) followed by a long continuation phase.
  - The challenge of treating TB is that the bacteria divide slowly, so the kill rate is low.
  - The initial phase is usually for 2 months (after which sensitivities should be available).
  - The continuation phase is usually for 4 months.
- Combination formulations are preferred for long-term treatment.
- Multidrug resistance is an increasing problem, especially in some Eastern European countries (e.g. Latvia), parts of China, and Iran. Seek expert advice immediately.

Prevention of reactivation of latent TB

In those given chemotherapy or who are immunosuppressed.

- Patients given steroids alone do not need prophylaxis.
- The usual treatment is isoniazid alone for 6 months, or in combination with rifampicin for 3 months.

Contact prophylaxis

- Give this to close contacts of those with established TB and to those who become tuberculin-positive on testing.
- See below for regimen.

Rifampicin

- Commonly causes a transient rise in transaminases.
- Can cause a number of other recognized syndromes; these are rare.
  - Flu-like syndrome, abdominal and respiratory symptoms, shock, renal insufficiency, and thrombocytopenic purpura.

Isoniazid

- Can cause a peripheral neuropathy.
  - This is more common in those with HIV infection, with chronic renal failure, who are malnourished, or who drink excess alcohol.
  - The incidence is reduced by giving pyridoxine 10 mg daily, which should be routine therapy with isoniazid.
- Can also cause optic atrophy, convulsions, and psychosis.
  - The incidence can be reduced by giving pyridoxine.
- Isoniazid can cause hepatitis; this is rare.

Pyrazinamide

- Can cause rare but serious liver toxicity.

Ethambutol

- This can damage visual acuity, especially if given in doses above 25 mg/kg/day, or if the patient has renal insufficiency.

- Rifampicin is a classic example of a drug that induces hepatic enzymes. It will induce its own metabolism and that of a large number of other drugs.
  - See carbamazepine (p. 246) for more information and a list.
  - Bacterial resistance to rifampicin develops very rapidly if it is given on its own. Rifampicin should only be given in combination with other anti-infective drugs for treatment of active infection.
- Isoniazid inhibits the metabolism of carbamazepine, phenytoin, diazepam, and theophylline. This will enhance their effect.

Safety and efficacy

- Measures of clinical improvement are the most important.
- Whenever possible, take cultures before staring antibiotic treatment. Sensitivities of the causative organism may take a month or more to be determined. Discuss your treatment strategy with an expert.
- Measure the patient's liver function tests weekly during the first 2 months of treatment, and then if there is any suggestion of liver toxicity.
- Measure the patient's visual acuity with a Snellen chart and colour vision using an Ishihara chart before starting treatment with ethambutol. Remeasure them if the patient complains of any visual symptoms.

- Close supervision of patients given antituberculosis therapy is essential. If you think that there is a risk that they will not take the medication as directed, consider directly observed therapy (DOTS) or admission to hospital.
- Plasma concentration for measurement is recommended for patients with renal insufficiency given ethambutol or streptomycin. These are specialist assays; liaise with your laboratory before sending samples.
  - Ethambutol target peak concentration 2–6 mg/L (7–22 micromol/L) 2–5 hours after the dose; trough <1 mg/L (4 micromol/L).
  - Streptomycin target peak concentration 15–40 mg/L one hour after the dose; trough <5 mg/L.

- Warn the patient that rifampicin will make their urine and tears orange (and will stain soft contact lenses).
- Warn female patients that rifampicin will reduce the effectiveness of the oral contraceptive. They should take additional precautions.
- Advise the patient how to recognize the symptoms and signs of liver toxicity: jaundice, vomiting, and malaise. They should seek medical attention if any of these develop.

Prescribing information: **Antituberculosis drugs**

There are many formulations and regimens of these drugs. The following are given as examples only. Dosages and duration of treatment will depend on the precise clinical circumstances. Seek expert advice and supervision.

Standard unsupervised treatment

- Initial 2 month phase
  - Rifampicin, isoniazid, and pyrazinamide, given as a combination tablet (e.g. Rifater®).
    - Rifampicin 600 mg daily.
    - Isoniazid 300 mg daily.
    - Pyrazinamide 2 g daily.
  - Ethambutol (if given) 15 mg/kg daily.
- Continuation phase (4 months)
  - Rifampicin and isoniazid in a combination tablet (e.g. Rifinah®).
    - Rifampicin 600 mg daily.
    - Isoniazid 300 mg daily.

Prevention of reactivation of latent TB or contact prophylaxis

- Isoniazid 300 mg daily for 6 months *or*
- Isoniazid 300 mg daily and rifampicin 600 mg daily for 3 months.

Supervised treatment (DOTS)

- This must be observed directly throughout.
- Patients are given isoniazid, rifampicin, pyrazinamide, and ethambutol (or streptomycin) 3 times a week for the first 2 months, followed by isoniazid and rifampicin 3 times a week for a further 4 months.
- Doses:
  - Rifampicin 600–900 mg 3 times a week.
  - Isoniazid 15 mg/kg 3 times a week.
  - Pyrazinamide 2.5 g 3 times a week.
  - Ethambutol 30 mg/kg 3 times a week.

TEACHING POINT Notifiable diseases

- Doctors in England and Wales have a statutory duty to notify a 'proper officer' of the local authority of suspected cases of certain infectious diseases. The proper officers are required every week to give the Communicable Disease Surveillance Centre (CDSC) details of each case of each disease that has been notified. The CDSC has responsibility for collating these weekly returns and publishing analyses of local and national trends. This is important, as it is a method of detecting, and so limiting, outbreaks.

List of notifiable diseases under the Public Health (Infectious Diseases) Regulations 1988: Some of the more common ones are highlighted in **bold**.

Acute encephalitis	**Meningitis**	Ophthalmia neonatorum	Typhoid fever
Acute poliomyelitis	*Meningococcal*	Paratyphoid fever	Typhus fever
Anthrax	*Pneumococcal*	Plague	Viral haemorrhagic fever
Cholera	*Haemophilus influenzae*	Rabies	Whooping cough
Diphtheria	*Viral*	Relapsing fever	**Viral hepatitis**
Dysentery	*Other specified*	Rubella	*Hepatitis A*
Food poisoning	*Unspecified*	Scarlet fever	*Hepatitis B*
Leptospirosis	Meningococcal septicaemia (without meningitis)	Smallpox	*Hepatitis C*
Malaria	Mumps	Tetanus	Other
Measles		**Tuberculosis**	Yellow fever

Antiviral guanine derivatives

Inhibit the replication of herpesviruses

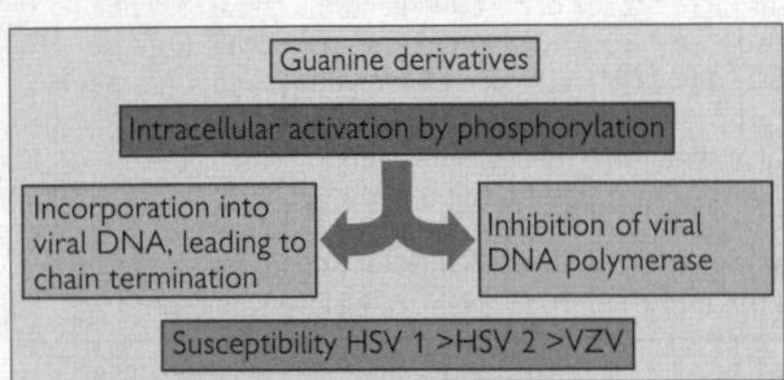

Drugs in this class

- Aciclovir
- Valaciclovir (prodrug of aciclovir)
- Penciclovir
- Famciclovir (prodrug of penciclovir)
- Ganciclovir is active against cytomegalovirus (CMV) (the other drugs are not) but is considerably more toxic. It is therefore reserved for the treatment of CMV infections.
- Valganciclovir (prodrug of ganciclovir)

- Treatment and prophylaxis against herpesvirus (HSV 1 and 2) infection.
- Ganciclovir only: treatment and prophylaxis against cytomegalovirus (CMV) infection.

- Avoid the combination of ganciclovir with zidovudine, as this can cause profound myelosuppression.
  - The combination of ganciclovir with didanosine is better tolerated.
- These drugs are given during pregnancy, but experience is limited. Seek expert advice.
- No dosage adjustment is usually required in hepatic insufficiency.
- Aciclovir is renally excreted. Reduce the dose in moderate to severe renal impairment.
  - Aciclovir can crystallize in the renal tubules if the patient is not adequately hydrated during treatment.
- Ganciclovir:
  - Pregnancy (ensure effective contraception during treatment and barrier contraception for men during and for at least 90 days after treatment).
  - Breastfeeding (until 72 hours after last dose).
  - Caution if the neutrophil or platelet count is low. See adverse effects below.

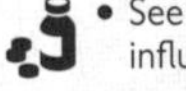

- See below for an approach to viral infections and the treatment of influenza.

Herpesvirus infection

- These drugs are effective against HSV, but they do not eradicate the virus and so are only really effective when used early.
- Valaciclovir is a prodrug of aciclovir. It is much better absorbed than aciclovir after oral administration.
- Famciclovir is a prodrug of penciclovir; it is 70% available after oral administration.
- The dosages of these drugs are different for each indication (see over for details) but they can be used for:
  - Treatment of:
    - Generalized/systemic HSV infection, including encephalitis.
    - Skin and mucous membrane infections, including shingles and genital infection.

    - Chickenpox in adults. (Not usually necessary in children, in whom the disease is milder.)
    - Keratitis and corneal ulcer. Ganciclovir eye drops are available for acute herpetic keratitis.
  - Prophylaxis against:
    - HSV infection in immunocompromised patients.
    - Recurrent HSV infection, especially genital infections.

CMV infection (ganciclovir only)

- CMV retinitis in patients with AIDS.
  - Initially, treatment is by intravenous infusion, followed by oral maintenance therapy.
  - Slow-release ocular implants containing ganciclovir can be inserted surgically to treat immediate sight-threatening CMV retinitis.
  - Local treatments do not protect against systemic infection or infection in the other eye.
- Oral prophylaxis in liver and renal transplant patients.
- Ganciclovir is considerably more toxic than the other guanine derivatives.
  - About one-third of patients need to have the drug withdrawn owing to adverse effects.
  - Neutropenia is the most frequent adverse effect; it is dose-dependent. Suppression of production of the other blood components is also seen. These effects are usually reversible on withdrawal of the drug.
    - Patients who develop neutropenia and require continuing treatment with ganciclovir may benefit from therapy with G-CSF (granulocyte colony-stimulating factor).
  - 5% of patients taking ganciclovir develop neurological adverse effects. These range from headache to confusion, hallucinations, and seizures.
- Treatment with the other guanine derivatives is usually associated with few adverse effects.
  - Aciclovir can cause severe local inflammation at the site of intravenous infusion.
  - Neurological reactions are rarely seen and are associated with high plasma drug concentrations.

- Topical formulations do not usually cause interactions.
- Ganciclovir is subject to more drug interactions than the other drugs in this class.
- Ganciclovir can cause myelosuppression; the risk of this is increased when it is given with other drugs that can cause myelosuppression (e.g. didanosine, zidovudine, lamivudine).
- Avoid these drugs with Primaxin® (imipenem with cilsastin); convulsions have been reported.

Safety

- Ensure that patients who receive guanine derivatives by intravenous infusion are adequately hydrated.
- Measure the full blood count (especially neutrophil and platelet counts) in patients receiving ganciclovir. The greatest risk is during intravenous treatment, but patients taking maintenance therapy should also have periodic checks.

Efficacy

- Review patients with HSV infection to ensure the episode has resolved.
  - Consider prophylaxis when the disease is recurrent.
- Arrange regular expert eye examinations for patients with CMV retinitis.

- Teach the patient taking long-term ganciclovir to recognize the signs of neutropenia (sore throat, skin infections) and thrombocytopenia (unexpected bruising or bleeding).

Prescribing information: **Guanine derivatives**

The following are given as examples.

Aciclovir

- Treatment by mouth
  - *Herpes simplex*, treatment, 200 mg (400 mg in the immunocompromised) 5 times daily, usually for 5 days.
  - *Herpes simplex*, prevention of recurrence, 200 mg 4 times daily *or* 400 mg twice daily, possibly reduced to 200 mg 2 or 3 times daily, and interrupted every 6–12 months.
  - *Herpes simplex*, prophylaxis in the immunocompromised, 200–400 mg 4 times daily.
  - *Varicella zoster*, treatment, 800 mg 5 times daily for 7 days.
- Treatment by intravenous infusion
  - Treatment of *Herpes simplex* in the immunocompromised, severe initial genital Herpes, and *Varicella zoster*: 5 mg/kg every 8 hours usually for 5 days, doubled to 10 mg/kg every 8 hours in *Varicella zoster* in the immunocompromised and in *Herpes simplex* encephalitis (usually given for 10 days in encephalitis).
  - Prophylaxis of *Herpes simplex* in the immunocompromised, 5 mg/kg every 8 hours.
- Treatment by topical application
  - Eye ointment, aciclovir 3%, apply 5 times daily (continue for at least 3 days after complete healing).
  - Skin *cream*, aciclovir 5%, apply to lesions every 4 hours (5 times daily) for 5–10 days, starting at the first sign of an attack.

Valaciclovir

- Oral administration
  - *Herpes zoster*, 1 g 3 times daily for 7 days.
  - *Herpes simplex*, first episode, 500 mg twice daily for 5 days (up to 10 days if severe); recurrent infection, 500 mg twice daily for 5 days.
  - *Herpes simplex*, suppression, 500 mg daily in 1–2 divided doses (in immunocompromised, 500 mg twice daily).

Ganciclovir

- Intravenous infusion
  - Initial (induction) treatment, 5 mg/kg every 12 hours for 14–21 days for treatment or for 7–14 days for prevention; maintenance (for patients at risk of relapse of retinitis) 6 mg/kg daily on 5 days per week *or* 5 mg/kg daily every day until adequate recovery of immunity; if retinitis progresses, initial induction treatment may be repeated.

- Oral administration
  - Maintenance treatment in AIDS patients when retinitis is stable (after at least 3 weeks of intravenous ganciclovir), use valganciclovir 900 mg daily with food.
  - Prevention of CMV disease in liver and kidney transplant patients, use valganciclovir 900 mg daily with food for 100 days.
- Topical application for acute herpetic keratitis
  - Ganciclovir 0.15% gel, apply 5 times daily until complete corneal re-epithelialization, then 3 times daily for 7 days (usual duration of treatment 21 days).

TEACHING POINT Treatment of influenza

- Patients often talk about 'having the flu', but this usually refers to infection with other viral causes of the common cold (e.g. adenovirus). Infection with influenza virus is potentially life-threatening.

Prevention

- Prevention is more effective than treatment.
- Influenza virus is antigenically unstable; the haemagglutinin and neuraminidase antigens on its surface change frequently. Large changes result in an epidemic as most people are not immune. The influenza vaccine available each year in the UK is different to provide cover for those strains that are considered most likely to be prevalent. For these reasons influenza vaccine cannot provide complete protection and will not control an epidemic. Immunization is only recommended for the following groups
  - Patients with
    - Chronic respiratory disease, including asthma.
    - Chronic heart disease.
    - Chronic renal failure.
    - Diabetes mellitus.
  - Patients who are immunosuppressed or who do not have a functioning spleen.
- Prophylaxis with amantadine is of limited efficacy and is only offered to
  - Unimmunized patients in the at-risk groups (see list above) during the 2 weeks that the vaccine takes to become effective.
  - At-risk patients who have a contraindication to immunization. Treatment should be limited to the duration of an outbreak.
  - Key healthcare workers during an epidemic.

Treatment

- Treatment of influenza infection is largely supportive.
- Zanamivir and oseltamivir are inhibitors of neuraminidase. If treatment with these drugs is started within 48 hours of the onset of symptoms, the duration of symptoms is shortened by one day. These drugs have not been shown convincingly to reduce morbidity or mortality. For this reason NICE has recommended that these drugs should not be prescribed in the NHS to otherwise healthy adults with influenza. Zanamivir can be given to patients in the high-risk groups (see list above) if treatment can be started within 48 hours of the onset of symptoms.

TEACHING POINT The treatment of viral infections

- Most anti-infective drugs exploit the differences between human and infective cells; the relative simplicity of viruses and the fact that they incorporate themselves into human cells makes them difficult to treat.
- For a long time treatment was entirely supportive, relying on the body's immune system to clear the infection. More recently a better understanding of the processes of viral replication and the enzymes involved has led to the identification of several novel drug targets. The emergence of HIV infection as a global health problem accelerated this process.
- Drugs used to treat are of several types:
  - Nucleoside analogues. These are incorporated into viral nuclear material and interfere with replication.
    - Zidovudine (and other nucleoside reverse transcriptase inhibitors).
    - Aciclovir.
    - Ribavirin.
  - Enzyme inhibitors. These exploit enzymes that are involved in viral replication only.
    - Non-nucleoside reverse transcriptase inhibitors.
    - Protease inhibitors.
  - Drugs that stimulate immune responses. These augment the body's own defence processes.
    - Interferon alfa for hepatitis B.
  - Monoclonal antibodies directed against viral antigens.
    - Palvizumab for respiratory syncitial virus.

Drugs used to treat human immunodeficiency virus (HIV) infection

Antiviral drugs

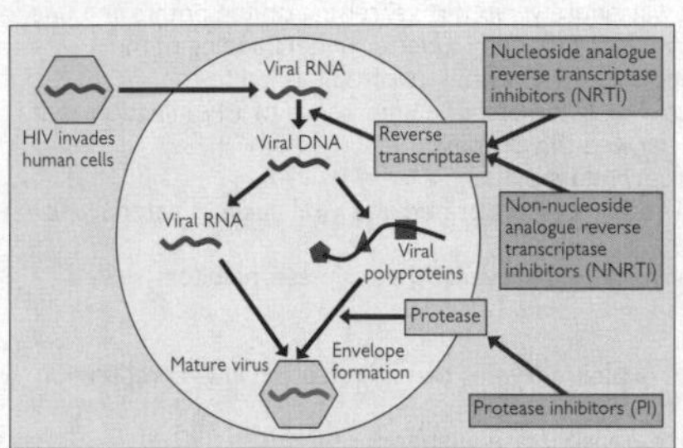

Groups of drugs

Nucleoside analogues (NRTI)
- Abacavir
- Didanosine
- Lamivudine
- Stavudine
- Tenofovir
- Zalcitabine
- Zidovudine

Non-nucleoside reverse transcriptase inhibitors (NNRTI)
- Efavirenz
- Nevirapine
- Delaviridine

Protease inhibitors (PI)
- Nelfinavir
- Indinavir
- Ritonavir
- Saquinavir
- Amprenavir
- Lopinavir plus ritonavir

- Treatment of infection with HIV.
  - Remember that these drugs suppress viral replication but do not effect a cure.
  - They are not a treatment for opportunistic organisms that cause infections in patients with AIDS.

- Hepatic insufficiency.
  - Avoid abacavir, ritonavir, saquinavir, nelfinavir, efavirenz, nevirapine, and zalcitabine.
  - Reduce the dose of indinavir from 800 mg tds to 600 mg tds.
  - Most of the nucleoside analogues can be used.
- Renal insufficiency.
  - Avoid abacavir, amprenavir, ritonavir, lopinavir.
  - Reduce the dose of the nucleoside analogues.
    - Stavudine, give half the dose in mild to moderate insufficiency. Give one quarter the dose if severe.
    - Zalcitabine, give two-thirds of the dose in mild insufficiency. Give one-third of the dose in moderate insufficiency.
    - Zidovudine, give half the dose in severe insufficiency.
    - Dose reduction may also be required for didanosine and lamivudine.
- Zidovudine is also known as AZT. Avoid this abbreviation, as it can be confused with azathioprine.
- These drugs are not recommended during pregnancy. However, they are sometimes given to pregnant women to reduce the risk of transmission of HIV to the baby. This is very a specialized area of practice; seek expert advice.

- Treatment of HIV is complex, and should be under the direction of a specialist. The following is offered as a general guide. It is based on the British HIV Association guidelines (*http://www.bhiva.org/guidelines.htm*).
- Acute seroconversion should usually be treated aggressively. The virus may be at its most vulnerable and least diverse at this point. However, treatment is unlikely to eradicate the virus.
- The decision when to treat established infection is not straightforward. On the one hand, HIV is an infectious disease and should be treated

hard and early. But in the asymptomatic patient this must be balanced against the toxicity of treatment, stringencies of the treatment regimen, and the current uncertainty as to whether early treatment will improve long-term outcome. Early treatment may just drive the emergence of resistant virus. See box for current suggested guidelines on when to treat.

- There are several highly active antiretroviral treatment regimens (HAART). None has been shown to be definitively better than any other. See box for guidance about choice of regimen.
- It is beyond our scope to discuss the strategy in the event of virological failure of treatment.
  - It is generally considered to be better to continue treatment even if there has been virological failure. Withdrawal of drug treatment causes a significant rebound in viral replication.
- The formulations of these drugs are not interchangeable.
- Many of these drugs have been developed and licensed on the basis of surrogate rather than clinical outcome data. See teaching point below for a discussion of this.

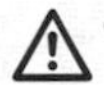

- Adverse effects of these drugs are very common.

Protease inhibitors

- As a group, these drugs are associated with metabolic abnormalities.
  - Abnormalities of lipid metabolism, characterized by raised cholesterol and triglycerides.
    - Consider switching to a non-protease inhibitor, or giving a statin or fibrate as appropriate.
  - Lipodystrophy. Characterized by atrophy and hypertrophy, and can be very distressing. The incidence of this is very variable between studies.

When to start treatment with antiretroviral drugs in HIV infection

Primary HIV infection
- Treat as soon as possible, ideally within 6 months.

Asymptomatic HIV infection
- CD4 count >350 x 10^6 cells/L: defer treatment.
- CD4 count 200–300 x 10^6 cells/L: offer treatment.
- CD4 count <200 x 10^6 cells/L: treatment recommended.

Symptomatic HIV infection
- Treat whatever the CD4 count or viral load.

Regimen	Advantages	Disadvantages
2NTRI + NNRTI (recommended)	Good surrogate outcome data. Simpler regimen.	Lack of clinical endpoint data.
2NRTI + PI	Long-term outcome data.	Toxicity common. Complex regimen. Drug interactions common.
2NTRI + 2PI	Good surrogate endpoint data. Simpler regimen.	Lack of clinical outcome data. Potential for drug interactions.
3NRTI	Few drug interactions. Simpler regimen.	May be less effective.

- Insulin resistance and worsening of diabetic control.
  - If treatment is required, metformin is preferred.
- If the patient is co-infected with hepatitis C virus there is an increased risk of liver abnormalities.
- Notes on specific drugs:
  - *Nelfinavir*, mild to moderate diarrhoea.
  - *Indinavir*, dose-related risk of renal stones and crystalluria, hyperbilirubinaemia.
  - *Ritonavir*, taste changes, nausea, diarrhoea, perioral tingling.
  - *Saquinavir*, nausea, diarrhoea, abdominal pain, and headache.
  - *Amprenavir*, nausea, diarrhoea, rash (usually in the first 2 weeks), perioral tingling.

Nucleoside analogues (NRTI)

- As a group these can cause:
  - Lactic acidosis. This can be fatal and is most associated with long-term treatment. It is difficult to predict those at greatest risk.
  - Hepatic steatosis.
- Notes on individual drugs:
  - *Abacavir*, life-threatening hypersensitivity, pancreatitis.
  - *Didanosine*, pancreatitis.
  - *Lamivudine*, hepatic steatosis, as above.
  - *Stavudine*, peripheral neuropathy.
  - *Tenofovir*, renal impairment and hypophosphataemia.
  - *Zalcitabine*, peripheral neuroathy, pancreatitis.
  - *Zidovudine*, hepatic impairment, anaemia.

Non-nucleoside reverse transcriptase inhibitors

- As a group, these drugs are better tolerated than the others.
  - Efavirenz
    - Can cause dysphoria.
    - Rash. Usually develops in the first 2 weeks and resolves after 1 month. Withdraw the drug if it is very severe.
    - Hypercholesterolaemia.
  - Nevirapine
    - Rash, can be severe (Stevens–Johnson syndrome).
    - Hepatitis (can be fulminant).

- Drug interactions are common, both with drugs for other indications and with other HIV drugs. This is not always detrimental. For example, ritonavir inhibits the metabolism of other protease inhibitors, increasing their effect.

Protease inhibitors

- The protease inhibitors are inhibitors of hepatic cytochrome 3A4 enzymes (see macrolides, p. 347, for more information).
- Ritonavir is a particularly potent inhibitor and will also increase the effects of opioids, tricyclic antidepressants, SSRIs, triptans, antifungal drugs, antipsychotic drugs, and amfebutamone (bupropion).
- Ritonavir and some of the other protease inhibitors increase the metabolism of the oral contraceptive. This may make it less effective. Warn women about this.

Nucleoside analogues (NRTI)

- Do not give with co-trimoxazole (increases lamivudine concentration).
- Do not give gancicolovir with zidovudine; this can cause bone marrow suppression.

Non-nucleoside reverse transcriptase inhibitors

- These drugs can interact with grapefruit juice; avoid this (see antihistamines, p. 610, for more information).
- Enzyme-inducing drugs (see carbamazepine, p. 246) reduce the concentrations of these drugs.
- These drugs can affect the metabolism of other anti-HIV drugs; use an established regimen.
- These drugs increase metabolism of the oral contraceptive. This may make it less effective. Warn women about this.

Safety

- Zidovudine — measure a full blood count every 2 weeks for the first 3 months of treatment, and monthly thereafter.
- Tenofovir — measure renal function and the serum phosphate concentration monthly.
- Nevirapine — measure liver function tests every 2 weeks for 2 months, and every 3–6 months thereafter.
- It has been suggested that patients taking long-term nucleoside analogues should have their anion gap, pyruvate, and lactate measured. However, it has not been established that this predicts the onset of lactic acidosis, so it is not routinely recommended.

Efficacy

- This is complex. In general, the patient's CD4 count is more predictive of the outcome in late disease, whereas the viral load (HIV-1 RNA copies/mL) is more predictive in early disease.
- Plasma drug concentration monitoring is still under development and is not routinely recommended. It may be useful, given that low plasma concentrations of drugs are associated with virological failure of treatment. At present, consider it for patients with liver insufficiency and those with dose-related adverse effects.

- Highly active antiretroviral treatment (HAART) regimens are complex and require considerable self-discipline to take correctly; these drugs will not be effective if taken randomly. Incorrect administration will promote viral resistance.
- These drugs can reduce the effectiveness of the oral contraceptive. Patients infected with HIV should use barrier methods of contraception to reduce the risk of transmission of HIV.
- Nelfinavir, saquinanvir, and lopinovir (with ritonavir) must be taken with food.
- Indinavir and didanosine must be taken on an empty stomach.
- Warn women about interactions with oral contraceptives.

Prescribing information: **Drugs used to treat HIV infection**

There are many regimens. Seek expert advice.

TEACHING POINT Surrogate markers in clinical trials

- It is often difficult to measure the therapeutic effect of a drug directly.
- For example, the effect of an antihypertensive drug on blood pressure may appear to be a simple outcome measure. However, it is not the blood pressure per se that we are most interested in, but rather the long-term reduction in risk of stroke or cardiovascular disease. These cannot be measured directly, and may not appear clinically for many years. Blood pressure is a useful surrogate because we know that lowering blood pressure lowers the risk of stroke.
- The situation in many other disease states is less clear. Many of the drugs used to treat HIV infection were granted licences quickly on the basis of effects on CD4 count and viral load rather than long-term clinical outcome. This may be appropriate when there are no effective treatments for a fatal disease, but it is essential that one tries to identify surrogates that are clinically relevant. Ideally, these should also include some measures of functional outcome, not just changes in biochemical markers.
- Another disadvantage of the surrogate approach is that it may not take into account the morbidity/mortality effect of late adverse effects of the drug. Drugs used to treat HIV carry a considerable risk of serious adverse effects. Always consider these along with the potential benefits.

TEACHING POINT Post-exposure HIV prophylaxis

- Based on the UK guidelines from the Department of Health (*http://www.doh.gov.uk/eaga*)
- Prevention is more important than post-exposure prophylaxis. HIV is not the only virus that can be transmitted (e.g. hepatitis B and C).
- Always follow guidelines when dealing with blood and other potentially contaminated material. Note that vomit, faeces, and urine are not considered high-risk unless they are blood-stained. Dispose of any sharps yourself. Do not expose others to risk by negligent behaviour.

Exposure is defined as:

- *Percutaneous injury* This carries the greatest risk, especially when there is frank contamination of the needle by blood. The risk of transmission is about 3 in 1000.
- *Exposure of broken skin* Eczema, abrasions.
- *Exposure of mucous membranes* (e.g. eye). The risk of transmission is about 1 in 1000.

Action

- Encourage any wound to bleed, but do not suck it. Wash with water. Irrigate mucous membranes with water. Do not use antiseptics.
- Contact the appropriate person (e.g. microbiologist, infectious diseases consultant, virologist) to discuss post-exposure drug treatment. This should include a discussion of the risk that the contaminated material poses. If the source is known, consider testing for HIV. This request should NOT be made by the person who has been exposed. Not all exposures are high-risk and drug treatment is not always necessary.
- If drug treatment is deemed appropriate it should be readily available. Ideally, this should start as soon as possible after exposure, but it is worth considering up to 2 weeks after exposure.
- A typical regimen consists of:
  - zidovudine 200 mg tds or 250 mg bd
  - plus lamivudine 150 mg
  - plus indinavir 800 mg tds.
- Make sure that the exposed individual has appropriate follow-up and support (e.g. with occupational health). Investigate the circumstance of the exposure and change practice if mistakes have been made.

Imidazole and triazole antifungal drugs

Inhibitors of fungal ergosterol synthesis

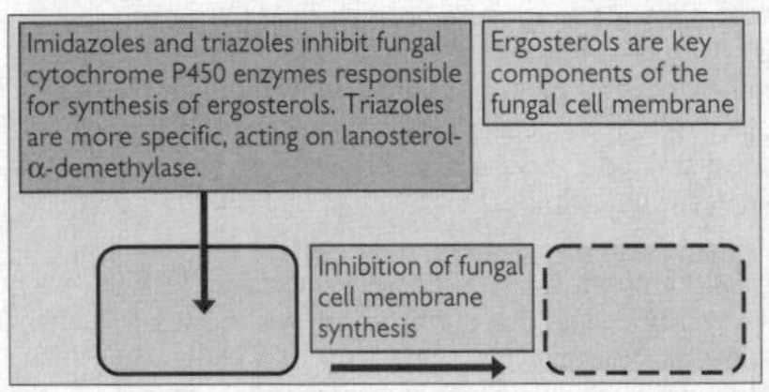

Drugs in this class

Triazoles
- Fluconazole
- Itraconazole
- Voriconazole

Imidazoles
- Ketoconazole
- Miconazole

Drugs used topically
- Clotrimazole
- Fenticonazole
- Sulconazole
- Tioconazole

Other antifungal drugs

- *Polyenes* (see p. 378).
- *Flucytosine*. Converted to fluouracil in fungal cells. Synergistic with amphotericin. Can cause bone marrow depression. Resistance is common.
- *Griseofulvin*. Largely replaced by newer drugs. Binds to keratin, making it more resistant to fungal infection.
- *Terbinafine* Used for fungal nail infections, and treatment of ringworm. Seek specialist advice.

- Treatment of infection by *Candida spp.*
  - Mucosal and skin infections commonly treated topically.
  - Invasive infections (fluconazole first-line).
    - Alternatively, give amphotericin with flucytosine.
- Cryptococcal infection
  - Treatment (e.g. meningitis).
  - Prevention in patients with AIDS (fluconazole).
    - Alternatively, give amphotericin with flucytosine.
- Aspergillus infection. Itraconazole is a second-line option.
- Histoplasmosis (rare in temperate climates).
  - Indolent infection (itraconazole or ketoconazole).
  - Severe infection. Can be life-threatening in patients with AIDS.
    - Itraconazole, given intravenously, is an option.
- Fungal skin and nail infections, treatment usually topical.
- Prevention of fungal disease in immunocompromised patients (fluconazole).

- Most of the following cautions apply to systemic rather than topical administration of these drugs.
  - Miconazole is given topically for oral infections, but is absorbed systemically and can cause drug interactions (see below).
- Ketoconazole and itraconazole carry a particular risk of liver damage.
  - The risk from fluconazole is much lower.
  - Itraconazole or ketoconazole should only be used when the potential benefits are significant (see above).
  - Avoid systemic administration of these drugs if there is any history of liver disease.
    - If treatment is essential use lower doses.

- If the patient has renal insufficiency, avoid giving itraconazole or ketoconazole.
  - Give the usual first dose of fluconazole, but halve subsequent doses if the patient has mild or moderate renal insufficiency.
- Long-term use of these drugs can cause congenital abnormalities if given during pregnancy.
- Antifungal drugs can precipitate heart failure. Avoid them in patients with cardiac disease, especially if they are taking drugs with negative inotropic actions (e.g. calcium channel blockers).

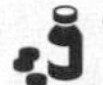

- Antifungal drugs are used for two types of clinical problem.
  - Non-invasive local infection. In this case, topical treatment is usually appropriate.
  - Invasive disease, often in vulnerable patients (e.g. those with AIDS). In this case, specialist advice and supervision is essential.
- Infection by fungi is commonly an indication of immunocompromise.
  - Investigate the underlying cause.
- Culture and identification of fungi is a specialized procedure.
  - Tell the laboratory if you suspect fungal infection and take advice about what sort of samples to send.

Topical treatment

- *Genital infection* (especially vaginal candidiasis). Topical treatment with a pessary, or fluconazole by mouth, are appropriate. Recurrence is more common in diabetes mellitus. If recurrent, consider the partner as a possible source.
- *Eyes.* Infection is uncommon but can occur after agricultural injuries. There are no licensed topical formulations for application to the eye. Seek specialist advice. Can also present with metastatic endophthalmitis.
- *Ears.* For treatment of fungal otitis externa.
- *Oropharynx.* The decision to treat topically or systemically will depend on the extent of the infection.
- *Skin.* Systemic treatment is usually necessary for scalp or nail infections. Seek specialist advice and take skin scrapings to confirm the diagnosis.

- The following adverse effects are usually associated with systemic administration.
  - Adverse effects from local administration are rare. The most common is local irritation.
- Antifungal drugs can cause a rash and other hypersensitivity phenomena.
  - The rash can be severe (including Stevens–Johnson syndrome) and is more common in patients with AIDS.
- Antifungal drugs commonly cause nausea, vomiting, and abdominal pain.
- Antifungal drugs can cause bone marrow suppression.
- Antifungal drugs can cause hepatotoxicity; this is characterized by cholestatic jaundice.
  - The risk is lower with fluconazole.
  - The risk is increased if treatment exceeds 1 month.
- Itraconazole can cause heart failure. This risk is increased if it is given in high doses for long periods.
- Long-term oral treatment with these drugs can cause hypokalaemia, oedema, and peripheral neuropathy.

- Antifungal drugs interact with many other drugs, the following refers to systemic administration.
  - Antifungal drugs inhibit cytochrome P450 enzymes (see macrolides, p. 347). This means that they increase the action of many other drugs.
- The absorption of ketoconazole depends on an acid environment in the stomach. Antacids will reduced its absorption.
- Ketoconazole can cause a disulfiram-like (Antabuse®) reaction if taken with alcohol.

Safety and efficacy

- No specific monitoring, other than appropriate clinical review, is usually required for topical treatment.
- Measures of clinical improvement are the most important, but inflammatory markers such as the CRP and ESR are often helpful.
- Whenever possible, take cultures before starting antifungal treatment. Check the sensitivities of the causative organism. Discuss any unusual results with a microbiologist.
- Long-term treatment with itraconazole or ketoconazole.
  - Measure liver function tests after 14 days' treatment and monthly thereafter.
  - Measure the full blood count and plasma electrolytes regularly if long-term systemic treatment is required.

- Advise the patient to seek urgent medial attention if they develop symptoms of:
  - Liver toxicity (jaundice, pale stools, dark urine).
  - Bone marrow suppression (easy bruising, bleeding).
- Topical vaginal formulations damage latex condoms and diaphragms.

Prescribing information: **Antifungal drugs**

The following are given as examples. Dosages and durations of treatment will depend on the indication. Check your local antibiotics policy.

Fluconazole

- By mouth for mucosal candidiasis, 50 mg daily for 7–14 days.
- By mouth or by intravenous infusion, for invasive candidal infections, initially 400 mg daily.
  - Long-term treatment usually 200 mg daily.
- By mouth, for prevention of fungal infections in the immunocompromised, 50–400 mg daily.

Itraconazole

- By mouth or intravenous infusion for systemic aspergillosis, 200 mg twice daily.
  - Reduced to 200 mg once-daily if responding.

Clotrimazole (Canesten®)

- 1% cream, spray, powder, and solution for topical application for skin infections.
- For vaginal candidiasis:
  - Pessary 500 mg, one daily.
  - Vaginal cream 10%.

Polyene antifungal drugs

Antifungal drugs

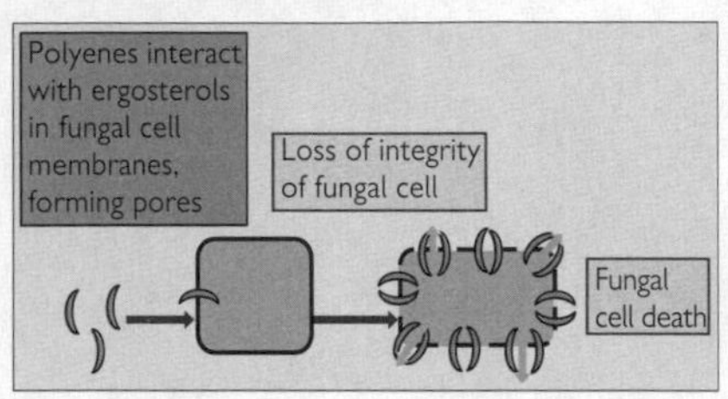

Drugs in this class

- Nystatin
- Amphotericin: standard and lipid formulations

Lipid and liposomal formulations of amphotericin

- Amphotericin in a lipid complex (Abelcet®)
- Amphotericin encapsulated in liposomes (AmBisome®)
- Amphotericin as a complex with sodium cholesteryl sulfate (Amphocil®)

- Nystatin is only given for superficial infection. Amphotericin is given for systemic infection.
- Treatment of infection by *Candida spp.*
  - Mucosal and skin infections commonly treated topically, nystatin and amphotericin.
  - Invasive infections, intravenous amphotericin with flucytosine.
- Cryptococcal infection.
  - Treatment of meningitis, intravenous amphotericin plus flucytosine.
  - Aspergillus infection, amphotericin first-line.
- Histoplasmosis (rare in temperate climates).
  - Severe infection. Can be life-threatening in patients with AIDS. Intravenous amphotericin, first-line.

- Most cautions apply to systemic rather than topical administration of these drugs.
  - Nystatin and amphotericin are not absorbed systemically when given by mouth.
- If the patient has renal insufficiency, only use if there is no alternative.
- These drugs are not known to be harmful during pregnancy, but use only when the potential benefits are clear.

- These drugs are used for two types of clinical problem.
  - Non-invasive local infection. In this case, topical treatment is usually appropriate.
  - Invasive disease, often in vulnerable patients (e.g. the immunosuppressed, patients in intensive care). In these cases, specialist advice and supervision is essential.
- Infection by fungi is commonly an indication of immunocompromise.
  - Investigate the underlying cause.
- Culture and identification of fungi is a specialized procedure.
  - Tell the laboratory if you suspect fungal infection and take advice about what sort of samples to send.

- Amphotericin penetrates tissues poorly; the doses required commonly cause nephrotoxicity.
  - Lipid formulations allow higher doses to be given without toxicity, but are considerably more expensive.
  - Keeping the patient well hydrated will reduce the risk of nephrotoxicity.

Topical treatment

- *Genital infection* (especially vaginal candidiasis). Topical treatment with a nystatin pessary or cream are appropriate. Recurrence is more common in diabetes mellitus. If recurrent, consider the partner as a possible source.
  - Treatment is usually for 14–28 days.
- *Oral and perioral infection.* The decision to treat topically or systemically (with an imidazole) will depend on the extent of the infection. Nystatin and amphotericin are available as pastilles and suspensions for local treatment.
- *Skin.* Seek specialist advice and take skin scrapings to confirm the diagnosis. Nystatin is effective for skin infections due to *Candida spp*, but not due to dermatophytes. See imidazoles (p. 374).

- Nystatin is too toxic to be given systemically, but adverse effects following topical administration are rare. The most common is local irritation.
- Adverse effects due to amphotericin given systemically are common.
  - Amphotericin can cause anaphylactic and anaphylactoid reactions (see acetylcysteine, p. 625).
    - Give a test dose before starting regular treatment (e.g. 1 mg in 10 mL of 5% glucose over 30 minutes).
  - Febrile reactions, nausea, and vomiting are common.
  - Amphotericin can cause a rash, which can be severe (including the Stevens–Johnson syndrome).
    - These reactions can be treated with hydrocortisone and antipyretics, which should be reserved for those with severe symptoms, as the steroid can exacerbate hypokalaemia due to amphotericin.
  - Rapid infusion of amphotericin can cause cardiac arrhythmias.
    - Give the dose over 2–4 hours.
  - Nephrotoxicity is almost universal and usually dose-limiting. It is due to renal vascular constriction and a direct toxic effect on the tubules.
    - Hypokalaemia and hypomagnesaemia can occur.
    - Lipid formulations are less nephrotoxic.
- Other adverse effects include convulsions, peripheral neuropathy, hearing loss, and hepatotoxicity. Amphotericin should be withdrawn if these occur.

The following refers to systemic administration of amphotericin.

- Avoid giving amphotericin with cytotoxic or other nephrotoxic drugs (e.g. ciclosporin); the risk of nephrotoxicity is very great.
- Amphotericin can cause hypokalaemia.
  - Corticosteroids can exacerbate this.
  - Avoid diuretics.
  - Hypokalaemia can cause digoxin toxicity.

Safety and efficacy

- No specific monitoring, other than appropriate clinical review, is usually required for topical treatment.
- Measures of clinical improvement are the most important, but inflammatory markers such as the CRP and ESR are often helpful in systemic infections.
- Whenever possible, take cultures before starting antifungal drug treatment. Check the sensitivities of the causative organism. Discuss any unusual results with a microbiologist.
- Treatment of a systemic fungal infection often requires a long course.
- Monitor renal function closely. The manufacturers advise that treatment should be suspended if the serum creatinine rises above 260 micromol/L.
  - This monitoring should include electrolytes; treat hypokalemia, which can be accompanied by hypomagnesaemia.
  - Measure a full blood count and liver function tests at least weekly. Withdraw amphotericin if liver function tests become abnormal.

- Topical vaginal creams, but not pessaries, damage latex condoms and diaphragms.
- Nystatin cream stains clothing yellow.

Prescribing information: **Polyene antifungal drugs**

The following are given as examples. Dosages and durations of treatment will depend on the indication. Check your local antibiotics policy.

Amphotericin

- Lozenge (10 mg) or oral suspension (10 mg/mL), for oral or perioral fungal infections, 10 mg 4 times daily after food.
- By intravenous infusion, for systemic fungal infections.
  - Initially 250 micrograms/kg daily.
  - May be increased to a maximum of 1.5 mg/kg daily in severe infections, if tolerated.
- Consider lipid formulations if nephrotoxicity is dose-limiting. Seek specialist advice.

Nystatin

- For vaginal candidiasis.
  - Cream 100 000 units/4 g, for topical vaginal application. Insert 4–8 g (supplied with applicator) at night for 14–28 nights.
  - Pessary 100 000 units, 1 or 2 daily for 14–28 nights.
- For skin infection due to *Candida spp.*
  - Cream or ointment 100 000 units/g, apply 2–4 times daily.
- For oral or perioral fungal infections.
  - Pastilles or oral suspension (100 000 units/mL), 100 000 units 4 times daily after food.

Antimalarial drugs

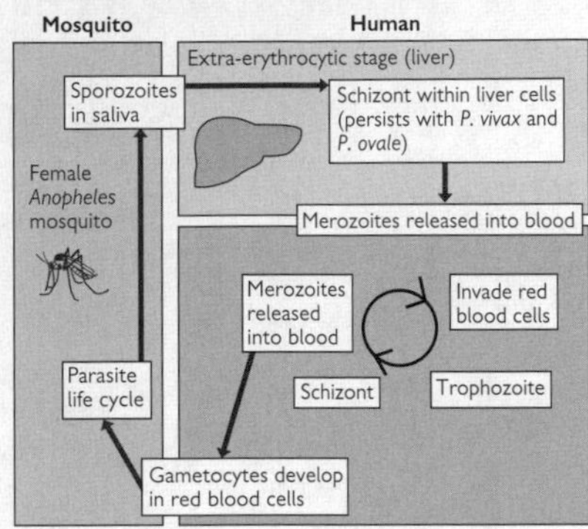

Drugs in this class

The drugs listed here are not interchangeable. The choice of drug should be directed by a specialist familiar with resistance patterns.

Drugs used for prophylaxis

(Note the importance of protection from bites)

- Chloroquine and proguanil
- Mefloquine (Lariam®)
- Proguanil with atovaquone (Malarone®)
- Doxycycline

Drugs used for treatment of malaria

'Benign' malarias *P. vivax, malariae*, and *ovale*

- Chloroquine followed by primaquine

Acute uncomplicated falciparum malaria

- Quinine (followed by pyrimethamine with sulfadoxine (Fansidar®) or doxycycline
- Artemether with lumefantrine
- Mefloquine
- Proguanil with atovaquone

Complicated falciparum malaria

- Intravenous quinine
- Intravenous artesunate (artemisinin derivative)
- Intramuscular artemether (artemisinin derivative)

- Treatment and prophylaxis of infection by:
  - *Plasmodium falciparum.*
  - *Plasmodium vivax, malariae*, and *ovale.*
- See pp. 336 and 570 for more information on chloroquine and doxycycline.

- The choice of drug for treatment or prophylaxis depends on the risk and resistance patterns for the area of proposed travel.
  - Patterns of resistance are constantly changing; seek up-to-date advice.
  - The risk of malaria varies widely, depending on the proposed area of travel. For example, the risk is often low in large cities. Take a detailed history of the proposed itinerary so that the risk can be evaluated fully.
- Pregnancy.
  - Quinine is preferred because there is considerable experience of its use.
  - Do not give doxycycline; it stains the baby's teeth.
  - Do not give primaquine during pregnancy; continue chloroquine until after delivery.
  - If proguanil is required, give it with folic acid 5 mg daily.
  - Avoid Maloprim® (pyrimethamine and dapsone) and Malarone®. Mefloquine may be safe.
- Epilepsy.
  - Avoid chloroquine and mefloquine.
  - Doxycycline interacts with some antiepileptic drugs.

- If Maloprim® is required, and the patient is taking phenytoin or phenobarbital, give folic acid 5 mg daily.
- Mefloquine lowers the seizure threshold.

- Renal insufficiency.
  - Proguanil is renally excreted; avoid it.
  - Avoid Malarone® and chloroquine in moderate to severe renal insufficiency.
  - Mefloquine and doxycycline are usually safe.
- G6PD deficiency
  - Take care with chloroquine, primaquine, pyrimethamine plus dapsone, and quinine. See teaching point below.
- Cardiac conduction defects
  - Avoid giving quinine or artemether plus lumefantrine; they can prolong the QT interval.

Malaria prophylaxis

- Always seek up-to-date specialist advice, as patterns of malarial resistance are constantly changing.
- Other measures, such as avoidance, bed nets, and repellent sprays (diethyltoluamide/DEET), are as important for the prophylaxis of malaria as drug treatment. You cannot catch malaria unless you are bitten.

Features of severe falciparum malaria

Clinical features

- Impaired consciousness, convulsions
- Respiratory distress
- Jaundice
- Bleeding
- Shock

Biochemical features

- Renal impairment (serum creatinine >265 micromol/L or urine output <400 mL/day)
- Acidosis (plasma bicarbonate <15 mmol/L)
- Hepatic impairment (transaminases >3 times normal)
- Hypoglycaemia (blood glucose <2.2 mmol/L)
- Hypoxia (pO_2 <8 kPa on room air)

Haematological features

- Parasitaemia >5%
- Haemoglobin <6 g/L or haematocrit <20%
- Evidence of disseminated intravascular coagulation (DIC)

Treatment of malaria

- Infection by *P. falciparum* can be fatal (see box on features of severe malaria). In most cases, patients suspected of having *P. falciparum* infection should be admitted to hospital for investigation and treatment.
- Symptoms and signs of malaria may present as early as 7 days after exposure (average 10–21 days). Longer incubation periods can occur in patients who have been taking chemoprophylaxis or selected antibiotics (e.g. co-trimoxazole, tetracycline, macrolides, chloramphenicol, and quinolones). Incubation periods for *P. falciparum* of 6–18 months are unusual, but are on record. Malaria due to infections with *P. vivax, P. ovale, or P. malariae* can take up to 12 months to the first manifestation.
- The presentation of *P. falciparum* malaria is very variable and it can mimic many other diseases.
  - Have a high index of suspicion in anyone who has returned from a malarious region.
- The diagnosis is usually made from examination of a blood smear.
  - A negative smear does not exclude the diagnosis.
- The box above indicates the suitable treatments, but seek expert advice in each case.

- These drugs commonly cause nausea, vomiting, and diarrhoea.
- Other rarer, but serious adverse effects are summarized in Table 5.1.
- See pp. 570 and 336 for chloroquine and doxycycline.

Table 5.1 Adverse effects of antimalarial drugs

	Drug						
	Quinine	**Mefloquine**	**Primaquine**	**Proguanil**	**Proguanil plus atovaquone**	**Pyrimethamine (commonly combined with other drugs e.g. dapsone, sulfadoxine)**	**Artemisinin derivatives**
Relatively common	'Cinchonism' (tinnitus, hot, flushed skin, abdominal pain, rash)	Sleep disorders (insomnia, abnormal dreams)		Mouth ulcers, stomatitis, hair loss	Mouth ulcers, stomatitis, hair loss Abnormal dreams and insomnia		Sleep disturbance Myalgia Rash
Rare but serious	Angio-oedema Temporary blindness and other visual disorders Thrombocytopenia (can cause disseminated intravascular coagulation (DIC))	Neurological symptoms (<1%) Sensory and motor neuropathy Tremor and ataxia Anxiety, depression, panic, and psychosis Convulsions Rash (urticaria most common but can cause Stevens–Johnson syndrome)	Methaemoglobinaemia Haemolytic anaemia Leukopenia	Urticaria and angio-oedema	Urticaria and angio-oedema Visual disturbance	Methaemoglobinaemia Thrombocytopenia Psychosis Jaundice Eosinophilic pulmonary infiltrates	

- Drugs that prolong the QT interval (quinine and artemether plus lumefantrine) should not be given with other drugs that prolong the QT interval: antiarrhythmic drugs, some antihistamines (e.g. terfenadine), macrolide and quinolone antibiotics, imidazole and triazole antifungal drugs, and antipsychotic drugs.
- Many of these drugs lower the seizure threshold (see above); this will reduce the efficacy of antiepileptic drugs.
- Quinine increases the plasma digoxin concentration and can cause digoxin toxicity.

Safety

- Measure the blood glucose concentration before and often during treatment. Treat hypoglycaemia.
- Measure the patient's core temperature, respiratory rate, blood pressure, level of consciousness.
- Laboratory measurements should include: regular measurement of haemoglobin, glucose, urea and creatinine, electrolytes, liver function, and acid-base status.
- Monitor fluid balance carefully. Avoid over- and underhydration. Fluid overload is dangerous; it can precipitate potentially fatal respiratory failure. However, hypovolaemia can potentiate renal failure, metabolic acidosis, and circulatory collapse. Accurate recording of fluid input and output is essential. Frequent central venous pressure (CVP) monitoring is recommended; maintain the CVP at 0–5 cm of water.
- Monitor urine output constantly and carefully observe for the appearance of haemoglobinuria.
- Reduce high body temperatures (>39°C) by vigorous tepid sponging and fanning. Antipyretics (paracetamol) can be given, but avoid aspirin-containing compounds and NSAIDs.

Efficacy

- Measure the parasite density at least daily.

- Malaria prophylaxis
  - Drug treatment alone is not sufficient. Do not forget to cover up and to use an impregnated bed net and repellent spray.
  - Report any feverish illness especially within 3 months of return; say if you have been to a malarious region.

Prescribing information: **Antimalarial drugs**

The following is offered as a general guide only, seek expert advice in all cases.

Quinine

- Treatment of malaria. By mouth, 600 mg tds for 7 days (usually followed by pyrimethamine plus sulfadoxine (Fansidar®)).
- Treatment by intravenous infusion for severe malaria.
  - Loading dose of 20 mg/kg over 4 hours.
  - Followed by 10 mg/kg every 8–12 hours (given over 4 hours), until able to take treatment by mouth (or for 7 days).
  - Usually followed by pyrimethamine plus sulfadoxine (Fansidar®).

Pyrimethamine plus sulfadoxine (Fansidar®)

- Treatment of malaria, following quinine. Tablets contain pyrimethamine 25 mg and sulfadoxine 500 mg. Give 3 tablets as a single dose.
- If resistant to Fansidar®, give doxycycline 200 mg for 7 days.

Mefloquine

- Chemoprophylaxis. By mouth, 250 mg once weekly. See notes above.
- Treatment of malaria. Daily dose 20–25 mg/kg given as 3 doses 8 hours apart.

Proguanil with atovaquone (Malarone®)

- Treatment of malaria. By mouth, 4 tablets once daily, for 4 days.
    - Tablets contain proguanil 100 mg with atovaquone 250 mg.

Proguanil

- Chemoprophylaxis. By mouth, 200 mg daily.
    - Given with chloroquine.

Primaquine

- Adjunct to treatment of *P. vivax* and *P. ovale* (eradication of liver stages). By mouth, 15 mg daily for 14–21 days, following chloroquine treatment.

Artemisinin derivatives

- Seek expert advice.

TEACHING POINT Glucose 6-phosphate dehydrogenase (G6PD) deficiency

- G6PD is an important component of the oxidative pathways within cells. Deficiency is common amongst people from most of Africa, most of Asia, Oceania, and Southern Europe (400 million people affected worldwide).
- These patients are liable to develop an acute haemolytic anaemia when given an acute oxidative stress. Severe illness is a cause, as are several drugs.
- Avoid the following drugs in patients with G6PD deficiency
  - Dapsone and other sulfones
  - Nitrofurantoin
  - Primaquine (low doses may be safe)
  - Quinolone antibiotics
  - Sulfonamides (including co-trimoxazole); some sulfonamides (e.g. sulfadiazine) have been tested and found not to be haemolytic in many G6PD-deficient individuals)
- The following drugs carry a possible risk:
  - Aspirin (acceptable up to a dose of at least 1 g daily in most G6PD-deficient individuals)
  - Chloroquine (acceptable in acute malaria)
  - Menadione, water-soluble derivatives (e.g. menadiol sodium phosphate)
  - Quinidine (acceptable in acute malaria)
  - Quinine (acceptable in acute malaria)
- *Note.* Mothballs containing naphthalene can cause haemolysis.

Chapter 6

Endocrine system; obstetrics and gynaecology

Contents

Insulin

Naturally occurring peptide hormone and its analogues

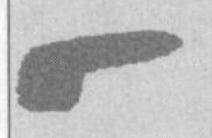

- Insulin is produced by the pancreatic beta cells in response to food and nutrients in the bloodstream.
- In Type I diabetes mellitus the islet cells are destroyed (this is usually immune-mediated). There is an absolute lack of insulin; without replacement insulin the patient will die.
- Type II diabetes mellitus is more complex. Insulin production may be low, medium, or high, but because there is peripheral resistance to insulin, it is relatively ineffective. Type II diabetes should be considered as a complex metabolic syndrome. Its features include:
- Hyperglycaemia with insulin resistance
- Hypertension
- Dyslipidaemia (raised LDL cholesterol, low HDL cholesterol, raised triglycerides)
- Obesity
- Renal impairment

Actions of insulin

- Promotes transport of glucose into cells and its utilization there
- Increases hepatic glycogen formation and inhibits gluconeogenesis
- Inhibits lipolysis
- Increases protein synthesis and decreases protein breakdown

Human Insulins

Short-acting
- Insulin lispro (analogue)
- Insulin aspart (analogue)
- Soluble insulin (clear): Actrapid®

Intermediate-acting
- Isophane insulin (cloudy)
  - Commonly mixed with soluble insulin
- Insulin zinc suspension

Long-acting
- Insulin zinc crystalline
- Insulin glargine (analogue)

Soluble, isophane, and zinc insulins all have the same insulin structure—that of endogenous insulin. Most patients use human insulin, but bovine and porcine forms are also still available. The kinetic differences between these forms of insulin arise from the different ways in which they are formulated, which alters the rate of absorption from the site of injection.

In contrast, insulin lispro, insulin aspart, and insulin glargine are analogues of endogenous insulin, in which two amino acids are different. These insulins have different rates of absorption and also different rates of onset of action.

- Treatment of hyperglycaemic states in diabetes mellitus.
- Essential treatment for Type I diabetes mellitus.
- Treatment of some patients with Type II diabetes mellitus.

- Insulin is essential for blood glucose control, but remember that dehydration is more likely to kill the patient with diabetic ketoacidosis first.

- Not all patients with Type II diabetes require insulin treatment. Most can be adequately managed using sulfonylurea drugs and metformin. However, pancreatic beta cell function usually deteriorates with time and patients become progressively resistant to the actions of sulfonylurea drugs. Once this has occurred, patients with Type II diabetes may require treatment with insulin.
- Insulin is anabolic (see box above). Treatment with insulin usually causes weight gain. Although the blood glucose control will be better, insulin can compound some of the other features of the metabolic syndrome in Type II diabetes.
- Oral hypoglycaemic drugs are contraindicated during pregnancy. Pregnant women should be treated with insulin under the close supervision of a specialist.

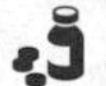

Treatment of diabetic ketoacidosis

- Establish the diagnosis first.
  - *Hyperglycaemia*. Ususally plasma glucose is greater than 11 mmol/L.
  - *Acidosis*. Arterial pH less than 7.3 and/or venous bicarbonate <15 mmol/L.
  - *Ketosis*. Measured in whole blood with a ketone meter ideally, but measure urine or serum ketones if this is not available.
- Fluid resuscitation is the first priority.
  - Give isotonic ('normal') saline initially. The following regimen is suggested but must be adusted to individual requirements.
  - Give 1 L over 30 mins, followed by 1 L over 1 hour, 1 L over 4 hours, 1 L over 6 hours, and then 1 L every 8 hours.
    - Once the plasma glucose is below 11 mmol/L, switch to 5% glucose (dextrose).
    - The aim is to replace the fluid deficit within 24 hours.
  - Measure the serum urea and electrolytes at baseline, 2 hours, 6 hours, and beyond as indicated. Use these to guide your fluid and potassium replacement regimen. See potassium, p. 552.
- The insulin regimen is aimed at reducing the blood glucose by 6 mmol/L per hour.
  - Very large doses are not usually required, even if the blood glucose is very high.
  - More insulin may be required if the patient is very acidotic, as this causes a degree of insulin resistance.
- Give an immediate dose of 10 units of soluble insulin intramuscularly.
- Set up an intravenous insulin sliding scale (see box on p. 397 for scale).
  - 50 units of soluble insulin (e.g. Actrapid®) in 50 mL isotonic ('normal') saline. Infuse according to the sliding scale (see box).
  - If intravenous access is impossible, insulin can be given intramuscularly, 10 units each hour.
    - Stop intramuscular insulin once the blood glucose falls below 15 mmol/L.
- Identify the underlying cause and identify strategies to avoid ketoacidosis in the future (see patient advice below).
- Switch to a subcutaneous regimen once the patient is clinically well, non-ketotic, non-acidotic, and normoglycaemic, and eating normally. Do not stop intravenous insulin until 1 hour after the first subcutaneous dose.

Treatment of non-ketotic hyperglycaemia, known as hyperosmolar non-ketotic coma (HONK)

- The clinical picture is usually one of insidious onset, unlike the acute presentation of ketoacidosis.
- The mortality from this condition is about 30%; seek help from specialists and intensive care.
- Establish the diagnosis:
  - Hyperglycaemia. The blood glucose is frequenly greater than 40 mmol/L.
  - Hyperosmolarity. Usually greater than 340 mosmol/L.
  - Exclude ketosis. Patients may have a lactic acidosis owing to sepsis.
- Excessively rapid rehydration can cause cerebral oedema owing to the intracellular hyperosmolarity. Rehydrate the patient with isotonic ('normal') saline (avoid hypotonic saline). Aim to replace the fluid deficit over about 48 hours.
  - Measure the serum urea and electrolytes at baseline, 2 hours, 6 hours, and beyond as indicated. Use these to guide your fluid and potassium replacement regimen. See potassium (p. 552).
- Set up an intravenous insulin sliding scale (see box below for scale)
  - These patients are usually very sensitive to insulin and require lower doses than patients with ketoacidosis.
  - Aim to reduce blood glucose by 3 mmol/h.
- Patients with non-ketotic hyperglycaemia are at risk of venous thromboembolism; anticoagulate the patient if there are no contraindications.
- Identify the underlying cause. Infection is the cause in more than 50% of cases; other causes include furosemide and phenytoin.
- Most patients presenting with non-ketotic hyperglycaemia will not require insulin in the long term.

Long-term insulin regimens

- Most patients are given recombinant human insulin. A dose reduction of 10% is usually required if a patient is switched from beef to human insulin; no dosage adjustment is usually required for pork insulin.
- All of these regimens are based on insulin given subcutaneously.
- Note that soluble insulin given subcutaneously takes 30 minutes to act, so it should be taken 30 minutes before a meal.
- The choice of insulin is often determined by the patient's preference for delivery device. There are many delivery systems available. Familiarize yourself with several of these, and involve a diabetes liaison nurse if you have access to one.
- The optimal regimen is one that takes account of the patient's lifestyle. The following are given as examples.

Basal-bolus regimen.

- A long-acting insulin is given at bedtime.
- A short-acting insulin is given 3 times daily with meals.
- This regimen has the advantage that it allows flexibility to take account of different meal times and meal sizes. It is commonly used for patients with Type I diabetes. However, it requires a high level of monitoring and understanding in order to adjust dosages safely.

Twice-daily biphasic insulin regimen

- This regimen is less flexible but may be suitable for patients who have predictable meal times.

- A biphasic insulin is given twice daily, once at breakfast and once with the evening meal.
- Biphasic insulins contain soluble insulin and intermediate (isophane) insulin in variable proportions. The number in the name refers to the proportion of soluble insulin (e.g. Humulin M3® and Mixtard 30® contain 30% soluble insulin and 70% isophane insulin.
- The major disadvantage of this regimen is that increasing the dose increases both the short- and intermediate-acting components.
- Patients using this regimen will often need to have snacks mid-morning and during the evening.
- The insulin dosage will always need to be adjusted to the patient's requirements. The following is offered as an initial calculation. Add up the daily requirement while the patient is on a sliding scale, and make sure that they are eating and drinking normally during this time. The average daily requirement is 0.5 units/kg. Use the two-thirds rule:
    - Use a biphasic insulin containing two-thirds isophane insulin (i.e. 30% soluble insulin).
    - Give two-thirds of the daily dose in the morning and one-third in the evening (e.g. in a 70 kg man requiring 36 units daily, give 24 units in the morning and 12 units in the evening).
    - See azathioprine (p. 515) for more information on giving drug dosages by body weight.

- The most common adverse effect is hypoglycaemia.
    - Tight control reduces microvascular complications of diabetes but increases the incidence of hypoglycaemia.
    - Patients who have been taking insulin for a long time, or who are taking beta-blocking drugs, may not develop the classical symptoms of hypoglycaemia. Beta-blockers do not block sweating, which can be the only sign of hypoglycaemia in a diabetic patient taking a beta-blocker.
    - Note that aggressive or disturbed behaviour can be a sign of hypoglycaemia.
    - Make sure that the patient and the patient's family/carers know how to recognize and treat hypoglycaemia (see also sulfonylureas, p. 403).
- Discomfort and local reactions around injection sites may be a sign of hypersensitivity. Generalized reactions are uncommon.
- Lipodystrophy (atrophy or hypertrophy) can occur around injection sites. This can be minimized by rotating injection sites. It is less common with recombinant human insulins.
- Insulin is anabolic; treatment with insulin commonly causes weight gain.

- Insulin and sulfonylurea drugs should not be combined.
    - Combinations with other antidiabetic drugs (e.g. metformin) may be beneficial.
- There has been concern that beta-blockers worsen diabetic control, but there is little objective evidence for this. The burden of cardiovascular disease is very great in these patients, so this potential disadvantage is usually outweighed by the cardiovascular benefits.
- The effect of insulin is reduced by the actions of corticosteroids and thiazide diuretics.

Safety and efficacy

- Teach patients how to measure their own blood glucose. Ideally, they should measure it 4 times daily. Teach the patient how to adjust their insulin on the basis of blood glucose measurements. Remember that a blood glucose measurement is affected by the previous dose of insulin, not the dose about to be taken.
- Review any episodes of hypoglycaemia to find the cause and develop a plan to prevent it in the future.
- Long-term control can be estimated by measurement of glycosylated haemoglobin (HbA_{1c}). Evidence suggests that the risk of microvascular complications is reduced if the HbA_{1c} is less than 7%.
- Remember to address the other components of the metabolic syndrome in Type II diabetes mellitus. Use an ACE inhibitor to protect renal function, whether or not the patient has hypertension or heart failure.

- Optimal control of diabetes mellitus requires a partnership between patient and healthcare professionals. There is a vast amount of information that a patient needs to assimilate, and education needs to be a continual process. Ensure that the patient has someone to contact for advice.
- Make sure the patient knows how to recognize and treat hypoglycaemia
- Make sure that the patient knows to continue taking insulin during an acute illness, although requirements may change. Drinking fluids is more important than eating. If they cannot drink any fluids, they should seek medical attention early.
- Many patients are expert at managing their disease. In hospital show them the insulin you are proposing to use, to allow them to check the formulation and dose.
- Patients using insulin or oral antidiabetic drugs are required by law to tell the DVLA about their medical status. They must also inform their insurers.
    - If the patient drives a heavy goods vehicle or a public service vehicle, they must inform the DVLA, even if they are treated by diet alone.

Prescribing information: **Insulin**

Table 6.1 gives information about the commonly used human insulins.

Table 6.1

	Type of insulin						
	Soluble insulin (clear)	**Insulin aspart or insulin lispro**	**Isophane insulin (cloudy)**	**Insulin zinc suspension (cloudy)**	**Insulin zinc crystalline (cloudy)**	**Insulin glargine**	**Biphasic insulin isophane/soluble (cloudy)**
Time to peak action (hours)	2–4	0.5–2	3–8	6–12	6–12	Slow release	Combined profile
Duration of action (hours)	6–12	4–6	12–20	16–30	24–36	24+	Combined profile
Examples	Actrapid®	Humalog®	Insuman basal® Insulatard®	Humulin lente® Monotard®	Ultratard®	Lantus®	Humulin® M2, M3, M4 Mixtard® 10, 20, 30, 40, 50

TEACHING POINT Management of diabetes mellitus during surgery

- Make sure that the surgical, nursing, and anaesthetic teams know that the patient has diabetes mellitus.
- Optimize control before elective surgery; delay if control is poor.
- Patients with diabetes should be on a morning list, and first on that list.

Patients with Type I or Type II diabetes treated with insulin

Minor surgery

- Give the patient's usual dose of insulin the evening before surgery.
- Fast from midnight.
- Do not give any insulin on the day of surgery.
- Give 5% dextrose by infusion at a maintenance rate (usually 125 mL/h); this should be continued until the patient is able to eat and drink satisfactorily.

After the procedure—

If the patient is able to eat and drink:

- If eating lunch, give 20% of the total daily dose as soluble insulin (e.g. Actrapid®).
- If eating tea/supper give 30% of the total daily dose of isophane insulin (e.g. Insulatard®).

Give the insulin after the meal to ensure that the patient has been able to eat.

If the patient is unable to eat and drink:

- Replace the maintenance fluids with a ***glucose-potassium-insulin infusion.*** To 1 litre of 10% (100 g/L) glucose (dextrose), add 16 units of **soluble** insulin and 10 mmol of potassium chloride.
    - Infuse this at the maintenance rate.
    - Measure the blood glucose hourly during the infusion.
- If the blood glucose is <4 mmol/L, only put 8 units of insulin in the next bag.
- If the blood glucose is 4–15 mmol/L, continue with 16 units of insulin in the next bag.
- If the blood glucose is 15–20 mmol/L, put 32 units of insulin in the next bag.
- Continue the infusion until 30 minutes after the patient has eaten and had their first dose of subcutaneous insulin.

Major surgery

- Give the patient's usual dose of insulin the evening before surgery.
- Fast from midnight.
- Do not give any insulin on the day of surgery.
- Give 5% dextrose containing 10 mmol/L potassium chloride by infusion at a maintenance rate (usually 125 mL/h).
- Set up a simplified intravenous insulin sliding scale (see below).
    - 50 units of soluble insulin (e.g. Actrapid®) in 50 mL isotonic ('normal') saline. Infuse as per the sliding scale.

Type II diabetes

Minor surgery

If the patient has good blood glucose control with oral antidiabetic drugs or diet

- Omit antidiabetic drugs on the morning of surgery.
- Restart when eating normally. Restart metformin only after renal function check (see metformin, p. 406).
- Avoid glucose-containing intravenous infusions.

Major surgery or unsatisfactory blood glucose control

- Omit antidiabetic drugs on the morning of surgery.
- Start a glucose-insulin-potassium infusion as shown opposite from 8.00 a.m. on the morning of surgery.
- Continue this until 30 minutes after the patient has eaten and had the first dose of antidiabetic drugs.
- Aim for blood glucose concentrations of 6.0–10.0 mmol/L (110–180 mg/dL).

An example of a sliding scale

Capillary glucose (mmol/L)	Soluble insulin infusion rate (Units/h) (Also mL/h if 50 units in 50 mL isotonic saline)
0–2.5	Treat for hypoglycaemia
2.6–4.0	0.5
4.1–7.0	1
7.1–11	2
11.1–14	3
14.1–17	4
17.1–20	5
>20	6

- Continue the infusion until 1 hour after the patient has eaten and had the first dose of subcutaneous insulin.

Glucagon

Naturally occuring peptide hormone

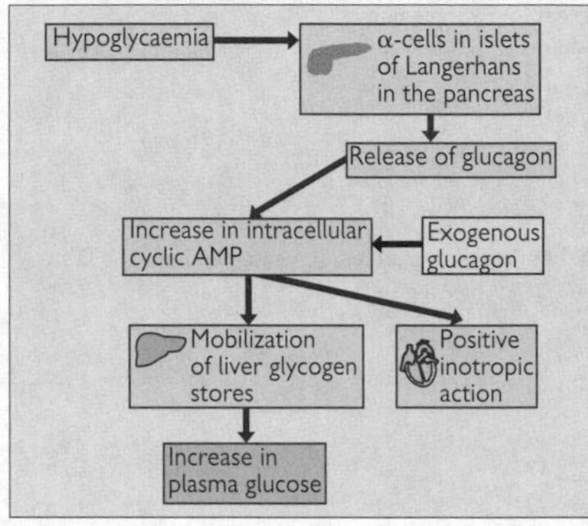

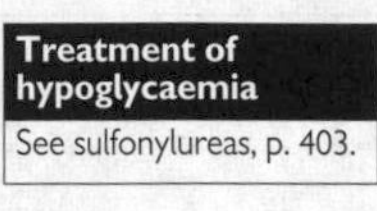

- Acute treatment of hypoglycaemia.
- Treatment of poisoning by beta-blocker drugs. Specialized, unlicensed use.

- Glucagon acts rapidly but only has a temporary effect.
- Glucagon will not work if there is no liver glycogen to mobilize (e.g. starvation, adrenal insufficiency).
- Glucagon is a peptide hormone and does not cross the placenta. Hypoglycaemia is a greater risk to the fetus.
- Avoid glucagon if the patient has a phaeochromocytoma; it can precipitate a crisis.
- No dosage adjustment is required if the patient has hepatic or renal insufficiency.

- Glucagon is a peptide and cannot be given by mouth; it must be given by injection, but any route (intravenous, intramuscular, subcutaneous) can be used.
- Glucagon is effective, but its action is temporary.
  - As soon as possible, give the patient something to eat (e.g. a slice of bread) or set up an intravenous glucose infusion, whichever is more appropriate.
  - Glucagon is not a suitable treatment for chronic hypoglycaemia (e.g. patients with an insulinoma).
- Sympathomimetic drugs (e.g. adrenaline) given to improve cardiac output can cause severe hypertension in patients poisoned by beta-blocker drugs, owing to unopposed α-adrenoceptor action. Glucagon increases intracellular cAMP and can have a positive inotropic effect. This is a specialized use.

- Adverse effects are uncommon, but glucagon can cause nausea and vomiting.
- Glucagon can cause hypokalaemia.

- Glucagon is not known to interact with other drugs.

Safety and efficacy

- Measure the blood or capillary glucose. Note that many meters are inaccurate in the lower range.
- Do not leave the patient alone until there is full recovery. Glucagon has only a short duration of action.

- Make sure that the patient knows how to avoid hypoglycaemia (e.g. by taking a mid-morning snack).
- If you prescribe a glucagon injection kit, make sure the patient and the patient's carers know how to use it in an emergency.
- Glucagon is supplied as a dry powder, which must be reconstituted before use.
- Make sure that the patient knows what to do after an attack of hypoglycaemia (see sulfonylurea, p. 403).

Prescribing information: **Glucagon**

- By intravenous, intramuscular, or subcutaneous injection, 1 mg.

Sulfonylureas

Oral hypoglycaemic drugs

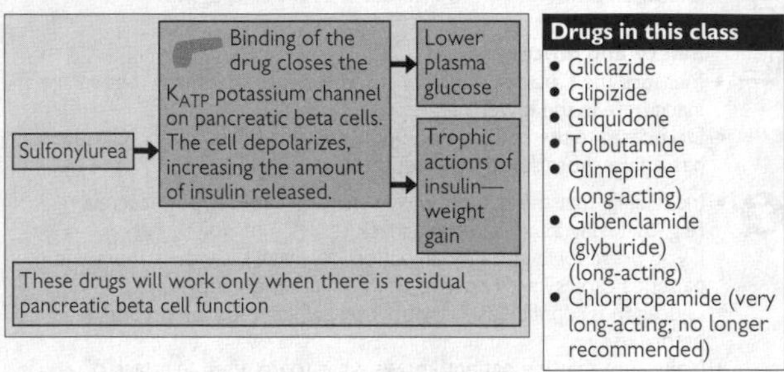

Drugs in this class

- Gliclazide
- Glipizide
- Gliquidone
- Tolbutamide
- Glimepiride (long-acting)
- Glibenclamide (glyburide) (long-acting)
- Chlorpropamide (very long-acting; no longer recommended)

- Treatment of Type II diabetes mellitus.
  - These drugs are not a treatment for Type I diabetes mellitus.

- Sulfonylureas will work only when there is adequate pancreatic beta cell function.
  - They will not work for patients with Type I diabetes mellitus.
  - Some patients with Type II diabetes mellitus no longer have any significant pancreatic beta cell function. These drugs will not work for them.
- Sulfonylureas are metabolized by the liver. Do not give them to patients with severe hepatic insufficiency.
- The risk of hypoglycaemia with chlorpropamide is increased if the patient has renal insufficiency. Chlorpropamide is no longer recommended.
- Avoid sulfonylureas in pregnancy. Pregnant women with diabetes, or who develop diabetes during pregnancy, should be treated with insulin.
- These drugs contain a sulfonamide group. Do not give them to patients with severe hypersensitivity to sulphonamides (see sulfonamides (p. 351) for more information).
- Insulin is almost always required for adequate, safe control of diabetes mellitus in medical or surgical emergencies.

- Sulfonylureas should be considered for patients who have not responded to a 3-month trial of diet and increased exercise. They should be used in addition to these measures, not instead of.
- Type II diabetes mellitus is a complex metabolic disease. Sulfonylurea drugs can help control hyperglycaemia, but the patient also needs a comprehensive assessment of the cardiovascular risks.
- Because sulfonylureas release insulin, they can cause hypoglycaemia; the risk is greatest with the long-acting drugs, chlorpropamide and glibenclamide. Hypoglycaemia can be particularly hazardous in elderly patients living alone. Use a short-acting sulfonylurea or an alternative drug for these patients.
- Release of insulin also causes weight gain, worsening insulin resistance. This reinforces the importance of diet and exercise in the treatment regimen.

- Pancreatic beta cell function usually deteriorates with time; patients become progressively resistant to the actions of sulfonylurea drugs. Once this has occurred, patients may require treatment with insulin.
- Patients with Type II diabetes require regular follow-up to ensure that blood glucose and the metabolic syndrome are managed optimally. See metformin (p. 409) for advice on the management of hypertension in patients with diabetes.

- Sulfonylureas can cause hypoglycaemia (also see notes above).
  - Titrate the dose upwards slowly.
  - Take particular care in the elderly and those with renal insufficiency.
- Sulfonylureas usually cause weight gain.
- Gastrointestinal adverse effects are common (nausea, vomiting, diarrhoea, constipation).
- Rare adverse effects include:
  - Hepatotoxicity: jaundice and increased transaminase activity.
  - Hypersensitivity: rash, can be severe; it may be related to the sulfur component. Avoid them in known sulfur allergy. See sulfonamides (p. 351) for a list of sulfur-containing drugs.
  - Blood dyscrasias, especially anaemia.

- There has been concern that beta-blockers worsen diabetic control, but there is little objective evidence of this. The burden of cardiovascular disease is very great in these patients, so this potential disadvantage is usually outweighed by the cardiovascular benefits.
- The effect of sulfonylureas is reduced by the actions of corticosteroids and thiazide diuretics.
- Alcohol can cause flushing and nausea in patients taking chlorpropamide.
- The metabolism of sulfonylurea drugs is inhibited by the antifungal drugs itraconazole and fluconazole. Avoid these combinations as they increase the risk of hypoglycaemia.

Efficacy

- Ensure that patients know how to monitor the blood glucose. Review the results with the patient and measure the glycated haemoglobin (HbA_{1c}). Aim for an HbA_{1c} concentration of less than 7%.
- Cardiovascular risk assessment and treatment is as important as blood glucose control. Also measure the patient's blood pressure, renal function, and lipid profile as part of your comprehensive assessment.

- Optimal control of Type II diabetes mellitus requires a partnership between patient and healthcare professionals. There is a vast amount of information that a patient needs to assimilate and education needs to be a continual process. Ensure that the patient has someone to contact for advice.
- Patients taking insulin or oral antidiabetic drugs are required by law to tell the DVLA about their medical status. They must also inform their insurers.
  - If the patient drives a heavy goods vehicle or public service vehicle, they must inform the DVLA, even if they are treated by diet alone.

Prescribing information: **Sulfonylureas**

There are many options; gliclazide and glibenclamide are given here as examples.

Gliclazide (short-acting)

- By mouth, initially 40–80 mg, with breakfast.
- The maximum daily dose is 320 mg. Doses above 160 mg should be divided.

Glibenclamide

- By mouth, 5 mg with breakfast.
- The maximum dose is 15 mg daily.
- Reduce the initial dose to 2.5 mg in the elderly.

TEACHING POINT Treatment of hypoglycaemia

- Hypoglycaemia is very frightening; many patients tolerate poor control in order to avoid the risk of hypoglycaemia.
- Prevention is important.
  - Teach the patient to recognize early symptoms.
  - Ensure that the patient and the patient's family/carers know what to look out for and what to do.
  - Regular meals and snacks can be important.
  - Do not increase dosages of sulfonylurea drugs too quickly.
  - Advise patients to avoid triggers (e.g. tiredness, certain foods).
- First-line treatment will depend on the circumstances.
  - If possible, give 10–20 g of sugar by mouth (this is two teaspoons of granulated sugar). Avoid very large amounts, which will cause hyperglycaemia. Then give the patient a longer-acting carbohydrate (e.g. a slice of bread).
  - If the patient is unconscious, this is an emergency; there are several options:
    - Give 50 mL of 20% glucose by intravenous injection.
    - Give 1 unit (1 mg) of glucagon by intramuscular, intravenous, or subcutaneous injection (Hypokit®).
      - This can be issued to patients and carers; make sure they know how to use it.
      - The action of glucagon is short; make sure that the patient receives glucose within 10 minutes
    - If there is no other option, glucose solution (e.g. honey or Hypostop® gel) rubbed into the buccal mucosa may help. Call for an ambulance or other help.
- Remember that the cause of the hypoglycaemia (e.g. long-acting insulin, sulfonylurea drugs) may act for longer than glucose. Continue to monitor the patient closely and treat with glucose as necessary. If the cause is a sulfonylurea drug, the patient should be admitted to hospital and may need an infusion of glucose.
- Once the patient has recovered, discuss why hypoglycaemia occurred, what can be done to prevent it in the future, and the action plan if hypoglycaemia should happen again.

Meglitinides

Oral hypoglycaemic drugs

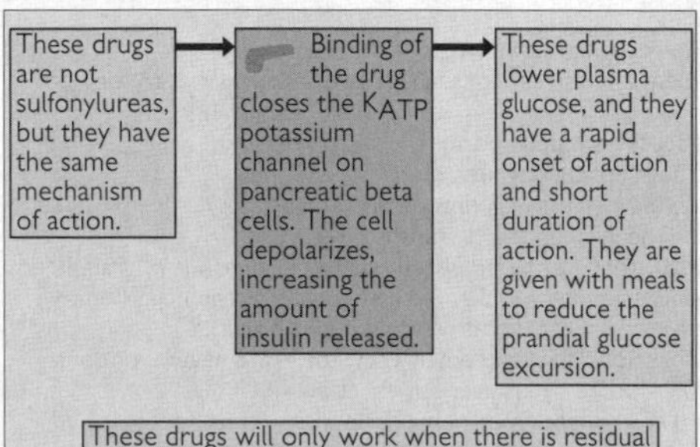

Drugs in this class

- Nateglinide
- Repaglinide

- Adjunct to the treatment of Type II diabetes mellitus.
  - These drugs are not a treatment for Type I diabetes mellitus.
  - Some patients with Type II diabetes mellitus no longer have any significant pancreatic beta cell function. These drugs will not work for them.
  - These drugs should usually be given in combination with metformin (see below).

- These drugs are metabolized by the liver. Do not give them to patients with severe hepatic insufficiency.
- Avoid these drugs in pregnancy. Pregnant women with diabetes, or who develop diabetes during pregnancy, should be treated with insulin.
- Stop these drugs if the patient suffers an intercurrent illness (e.g. infection, trauma, myocardial infarction), since there is a risk of hypoglycaemia. Insulin is almost always required for adequate, safe control of diabetes mellitus in medical or surgical emergencies.

- These drugs are not suitable for all patients with Type II diabetes mellitus.
  - They are most useful for those patients whose diabetes is generally well controlled with metformin, but in whom there is a considerable increase in blood glucose at around mealtimes.
  - They do not provide 24-hour control and should not be combined with sulfonylureas.
  - They are not an appropriate choice for patients who are debilitated or malnourished.
- Type II diabetes mellitus is a complex metabolic disease. These drugs can help control hyperglycaemia, but the patient also needs a comprehensive assessment of their cardiovascular risks. See metformin (p. 409) for advice on the management of hypertension in patients with diabetes.
- Because these drugs release insulin, they can cause hypoglycaemia. Hypoglycaemia can be particularly hazardous in elderly patients living alone.

- The release of insulin causes weight gain. Because these drugs act for a shorter time than sulfonylureas this effect is less marked. However, do not forget the importance of diet and exercise in the treatment regimen.
- Pancreatic beta cell function usually deteriorates with time, and patients become progressively resistant to the actions of these drugs. Once this has occurred, patients will require treatment with insulin.
- Patients with Type II diabetes require regular, formal follow-up to ensure that blood glucose and the metabolic syndrome are optimally managed.

- These drugs can cause hypoglycaemia (also see notes above).
  - Titrate the dose upwards slowly.
  - Take particular care in elderly people.
- These drugs can cause hypersensitivity. This is characterized by a rash and pruritus.
- Gastrointestinal adverse effects include nausea, vomiting, diarrhoea, and constipation.

- The effect of these drugs is reduced by the actions of corticosteroids and thiazide diuretics.

Efficacy

- Ensure that the patient knows how to monitor the blood glucose. Review the results with the patient and measure the glycated haemoglobin (HbA_{1c}). Aim for an HbA_{1c} concentration of less than 7%.
- Cardiovascular risk assessment and treatment is as important as blood glucose control. Also measure the patient's blood pressure, renal function, and lipid profile as part of your comprehensive assessment.

- Optimal control of Type II diabetes mellitus requires a partnership between patient and health-care professionals. There is a vast amount of information that a patient needs to assimilate and education needs to be a continual process. Ensure that the patient has someone to contact for advice.
- Patients taking insulin or oral antidiabetic drugs are required by law to tell the DVLA about their medical status. They must also inform their insurer.
  - If the patient drives a heavy goods vehicle or public service vehicle, they must inform the DVLA, even if they are treated by diet alone.

Prescribing information: **Nateglinide and repaglinide**

Nateglinide

- By mouth, initially 60 mg 3 times daily, with meals.
- The maximum daily dose is 180 mg 3 times daily.

Repaglinide

- By mouth, 500 micrograms 3 times daily, with meals.
- The maximum dose is 4 mg 3 times daily.

Biguanides (metformin)

Oral antidiabetic drug

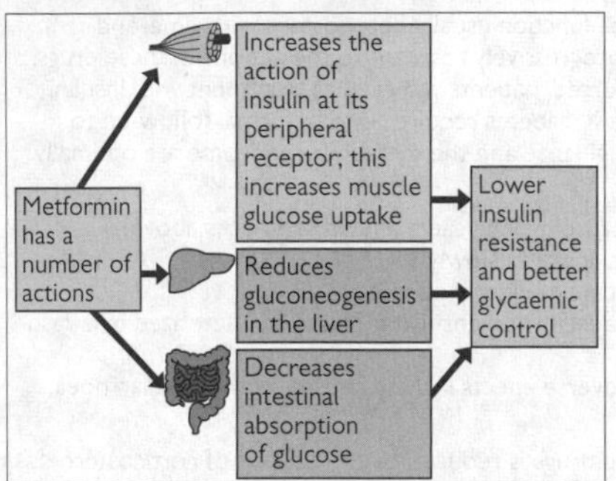

Drugs in this class

- Metformin
- Buformin and phenformin have been withdrawn because of adverse effects.

- Treatment of Type II diabetes mellitus.
  - Metformin is not a treatment for Type I diabetes mellitus.

- Metformin will work only when there is some pancreatic beta cell function.
  - It will not work for patients with Type I diabetes mellitus.
- Metformin is excreted by the kidney. Do not give it to patients with renal insufficiency; there is a risk of lactic acidosis.
- Avoid metformin in severe hepatic insufficiency.
- Avoid metformin in pregnancy. Pregnant women with diabetes, or who develop diabetes during pregnancy, should be treated with insulin.
- Insulin is almost always required for adequate, safe control of diabetes mellitus in medical or surgical emergencies.

Metformin and radiological examinations

- Metformin can cause lactic acidosis; this can be fatal. It is more common in patients with renal insufficiency. Intravenous radiological contrast agents in patients taking metformin can cause renal impairment and precipitate lactic acidosis.
- Measure the patient's renal function before any planned investigations involving intravenous contrast.
- Withdraw metformin on the day of examination, and for the following 48 hours.
- Do not delay emergency examinations, but ensure that the patient is well hydrated and that renal function is measured after the procedure.

- Metformin is not suitable for all patients with Type II diabetes mellitus.
  - It increases peripheral glucose sensitivity, but its effect on plasma glucose is less than other drugs (e.g. sulfonylureas, nateglinide, repaglinide).
  - Unlike sulfonylurea drugs, metformin does not cause weight gain, making it particularly useful in obese patients.
  - If the blood glucose is persistently high, metformin is often used in combination with other drugs.

- Type II diabetes mellitus is a complex metabolic disease. Metformin can help control the metabolic syndrome, but the patient also needs a comprehensive assessment of the cardiovascular risks. See below for advice on the management of hypertension in patients with diabetes.
- Patients with Type II diabetes require regular, formal follow-up to ensure that blood glucose and the metabolic syndrome are optimally managed.

- Metformin can cause lactic acidosis. This is due to increased glycolysis and inhibition of gluconeogensis from lactate in the liver.
  - The risk is very low but increases in renal insufficiency.
  - Follow the guidelines above for radiological procedures involving intravenous contrast media.
- Metformin alone rarely causes hypoglycaemia.
  - This can make it particularly useful in elderly people and those who live alone.
- Gastrointestinal adverse effects, including nausea, vomiting, diarrhoea, and constipation, are very common and may be intolerable. Giving the drug in divided doses can reduce this.
- Metformin can cause an unpleasant metallic taste.
- Metformin can reduce vitamin B_{12} absorption; this is rarely clinically important.

- There has been concern that beta-blockers worsen diabetic control, but there is little objective evidence for this. The burden of cardiovascular disease is very great in these patients, so this potential disadvantage is usually outweighed by the cardiovascular benefits.
- Avoid giving NSAIDs or any other drugs that can worsen reduced renal function in patients taking metformin; this can precipitate lactic acidosis.

Efficacy

- Ensure that the patient knows how to monitor the blood glucose. Review the results with the patient and measure the glycated haemoglobin (HbA_{1c}). Aim for an HbA_{1c} concentration of less than 7%.
- Cardiovascular risk assessment and treatment is as important as blood glucose control. Also measure the patient's blood pressure, renal function, and lipid profile as part of your comprehensive assessment.
- Pay particular attention to the patient's renal function. Withdraw the drug if there is significant impairment.

- Optimal control of Type II diabetes mellitus requires a partnership between patient and health-care professionals. There is a vast amount of information that a patient needs to assimilate and education needs to be a continual process. Ensure that the patient has someone to contact for advice.
- Patients taking insulin or oral antidiabetic drugs are required by law to tell the DVLA about their medical status. They must also inform their insurers.
  - If the patient drives a heavy goods vehicle or public service vehicle, they must inform the DVLA, even if they are treated by diet alone.

Prescribing information: **Metformin**

- By mouth, initially 500 mg with breakfast for at least 1 week.
- Increase to 500 mg 3 times daily.
- The usual maximum daily dose is 2 g in divided doses. In rare cases this can be increased to 3 g daily.

TEACHING POINT Management of hypertension in diabetics

- See also 'An approach to the treatment of hypertension.'
- For more information see British Hypertension Society Guidelines, *Br Med J*, 2004; **328**: 634–40.
- Type II diabetes is a complex metabolic syndrome, of which hyperglycaemia is only a part. 70% of patients with Type II diabetes have hypertension. By contrast, patients with Type I diabetes (without renal disease) have a risk of hypertension similar to that of the general population.
- Hypertension is an important contributor to the macrovascular and microvascular complications of diabetes.
- The threshold for treatment is lower than that for the general population: 140/90 mmHg.
- The target of treatment is a blood pressure below 140/80 mmHg. Most patients require two or more drugs to achieve this.

Type I or Type II diabetes without nephropathy

- There is evidence of benefit from treatment using ACE inhibitors, beta-blockers, low-dose thiazide diuretics, and dihydropyridine calcium channel blockers. The optimal choice of drug has not yet been established. Lowering blood pressure seems to be more important than the drug used.

Type I and Type II diabetes with nephropathy

- Blocking the actions of angiotensin using an ACE inhibitor or angiotensin receptor blocker reduces the rate of decline of renal function of patients with Type I and Type II diabetes. The differences in the evidence reflect the fact that ACE inhibitors were used for the Type I diabetes trials and angiotensin receptor blockers for the Type II diabetes trials. However, blocking the actions of angiotensin seems to be more important than the exact choice of drug.

Thiazolidinediones ('glitazones')

Oral antidiabetic drugs

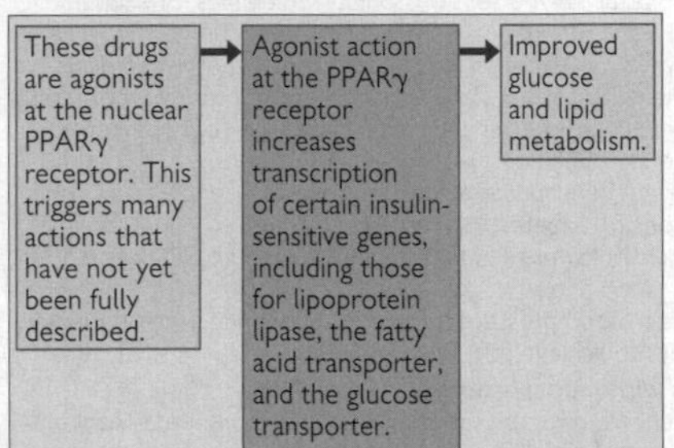

Drugs in this class

- Rosiglitazone
- Pioglitazone

Note

Troglitazone was withdrawn because of liver toxicity

- Adjunct to the treatment of Type II diabetes mellitus.
  - Thiazolidinediones are not a treatment for Type I diabetes mellitus.
  - NICE has recommended that thiazolidinediones may be used for patients:
    - Unable to tolerate the combination of metformin and a sulfonylurea.
    - Who have inadequate control with metformin and a sulfonylurea.

- The first of these drugs, troglitazone, was withdrawn because of rare, but severe, liver toxicity. Experience to date suggests that rosiglitazone and pioglitazone do not cause severe toxicity (but see notes below).
  - Nevertheless, avoid these drugs in patients with hepatic insufficiency.
  - Advise the patient to report symptoms of liver impairment (see below).
- Avoid thiazolidinediones in pregnancy. Pregnant women with diabetes, or who develop diabetes during pregnancy, should be treated with insulin.
- Insulin is almost always required for adequate, safe control of diabetes mellitus in medical or surgical emergencies.
- These drugs can cause fluid retention, which can precipitate heart failure. Avoid giving them to patients with a history of heart failure or severely impaired left ventricular function.

- Thiazolidinediones are not suitable for all patients with Type II diabetes mellitus.
  - They are most useful for those patients who are inadequately controlled by other oral treatments.
  - Treatment with these drugs can delay the time before insulin treatment is needed.
    - Treatment with a thiazolidinedione plus metformin is preferred over the combination with a sulfonylurea (NICE guidance).
  - Thiazolidinediones take several months to have their full effect. They are not a suitable choice for acute presentations.
  - Thiazolidinediones improve the body's handling of glucose but are not the most appropriate choice when the glucose is very high.
- Type II diabetes mellitus is a complex metabolic disease. Thiazolidinediones can help control hyperglycaemia, but the patient also needs a comprehensive assessment of the cardiovascular risks.

- Patients with Type II diabetes require regular, formal follow-up to ensure that blood glucose and the metabolic syndrome are optimally managed.

- Thiazolidinediones cause hypoglycaemia rarely; their major effect is to alter the handling of glucose.
- The major concern with these drug is liver toxicity (see notes above).
  - Experience to date suggests that rosiglitazone and pioglitazone do not cause severe toxicity.
  - Mild impairment can occur, usually between 2 and 12 months of treatment.
  - Withdraw the drug if the patient becomes jaundiced.
- Thiazolidinediones can cause fluid retention and oedema. Avoid them in patients at risk of heart failure.
- Thiazolidinediones can also cause anaemia, probably by haemodilution.
- Gastrointestinal adverse effects include nausea, vomiting, diarrhoea, and constipation.

- Few drug interactions with the thiazolidinediones have been identified, but they are relatively new, so be alert to possible interactions.

Efficacy and safety

- Measure liver function tests before treatment; avoid giving these drugs if they are abnormal. The manufacturers advise that liver function tests should be measured every 2 months during the first year of treatment.
- Ensure that the patient knows how to monitor the blood glucose. Review the results with the patient and measure the glycated haemoglobin (HbA_{1c}). Aim for an HbA_{1c} concentration of less than 7%.
- Treatment with thiazolidinediones can modestly improve lipid handling, but they are not considered adequate if cholesterol-lowering treatment is indicated. Consider a statin.
- Cardiovascular risk assessment and treatment is as important as blood glucose control. Measure the patient's blood pressure, renal function, and lipid profile as part of your comprehensive assessment.

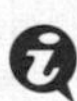

- Optimal control of Type II diabetes mellitus requires a partnership between patient and health-care professionals. There is a vast amount of information that a patient needs to assimilate and education needs to be a continual process. Ensure that the patient has someone to contact for advice.
- Advise the patient to report any symptoms of nausea, vomiting, fatigue, or dark urine. This could indicate liver toxicity.
- Patients taking insulin or oral antidiabetic drugs are required by law to tell the DVLA about their medical status. They must also inform their insurers.
  - If the patient drives a heavy goods vehicle or public service vehicle, they must inform the DVLA, even if they are treated by diet alone.

Prescribing information: **Thiazolidinediones ('glitazones')**

Pioglitazone

- By mouth, 15–45 mg daily.

Rosiglitazone

- By mouth, initially 4 mg daily.
- This may be increased to 8 mg daily (in single or divided doses) after 8 weeks' treatment if required.

Thyroid hormones

Naturally occurring hormones

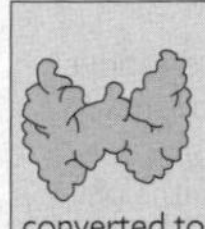

Thyroid hormones are essential co-factors in many cellular processes. Thyroxine (T4; levothyroxine) is secreted by the thyroid gland and is converted to the more active metabolite tri-iodothyronine (T3; liothyronine) in the tissues. They are either obtained from animal thyroid glands or prepared synthetically and are given as the sodium salts.

Causes of hypothyroidism

- Autoimmune thyroiditis.
- Ablative radio-iodine treatment.
- Surgical removal of the thyroid gland.
- Replacement of the thyroid gland by tumour (lymphoma).
- External radiation.
- Secondary to pituitary or hypothalamic disease.
- Drugs:
  - Interferon
  - Lithium
  - Amiodarone (can also cause hyperthyroidism)

- Treatment of hypothyroidism
  - The most common primary cause is autoimmune thyroiditis.
  - The most common secondary cause is ablative radio-iodine treatment for thyrotoxicosis.

- Pregnancy. Maternal hypoythyroidism can have adverse effects on the child's cognitive function.
  - Thyroid hormone requirements increase in pregnancy and the dose may need to be increased in women receiving replacement therapy.

Signs and symptoms of hypothyroidism

- Cold intolerance
- Coarse skin
- Alopecia
- Hoarseness
- Bradycardia
- Oedema
- Pericardial effusion
- Constipation
- Irregular or heavy menses
- Depression
- Mental impairment
- Weight gain
- Slow-relaxing reflexes

Signs and symptoms of hyperthyroidism

- Angina
- Cardiac arrhythmias
- Palpitation
- Tachycardia
- Skeletal muscle cramps
- Increased frequency of bowel movements
- Tremor
- Restlessness
- Flushing
- Sweating
- Insomnia
- Headache
- Flushing
- Fever

- Take great care when giving thyroid hormones to patients with ischaemic heart disease. Excessive doses can precipitate ischaemic events.
  - Note that hypothyroidism can cause changes in the ECG that mimic cardiac ischaemia.
- If the diagnosis is panhypopituitarism or includes adrenocortical insufficiency, the patient should be given a corticosteroid before thyroid hormone.
- Take care if the patient has diabetes mellitus; insulin or oral hypoglycaemic drug doses may need to be increased when thryoid hormone is given.
- Take care if the patient is elderly or has long-standing hypothyroidism; begin with a low dose and increase it gradually (see below).

- It is important to establish the cause of hypothyroidism. The most common cause is autoimmune thyroiditis, which can be diagnosed by the presence in the blood of autoantibodies to antithyroid peroxidase and antithyroglobulin.
  - Patients with autoimmue thyroiditis are at increased risk of other autoimmune diseases, such as vitiligo, Addison's disease, rheumatoid arthritis, diabetes mellitus, and pernicious anaemia.
  - Screen patients for these diseases, but be aware that they may develop many years in the future.

Levothyroxine sodium

- Levothyroxine (T4) is the treatment of choice for maintenance therapy of hypothyroidism.
- The mean replacement dosage of levothyroxine is 1.6 micrograms/kg/day. For an adult, this translates to a dosage of 100–200 micrograms/day.
  - The initial dosage should not exceed 100 micrograms/day.
  - Patients with ischaemic heart disease and the elderly should not be given more than 25 micrograms/day initially.
    - If required, the dosage may be increased by 25–50 micrograms/day at intervals of not less than 4 weeks.
- Levothyroxine replacement therapy should be given once daily, preferably before breakfast.

Liothyronine sodium

- Liothyronine (T3) has a similar action to levothyroxine but a more rapid onset (and offset) of action. It is principally given for the treatment of severe hypothyroidism when a rapid response is desired. Under these circumstances, it can be given by intravenous injection up to every 4 hours if required, but treatment should be under the direction of a specialist.
- Liothyronine 20 micrograms is approximately equivalent to levothyroxine 100 micrograms.
- Liothyronine acts within several hours, but the effect disappears after 24–48 hours.

- Excessive doses of thyroid hormone cause the symptoms and signs of hyperthyroidism (see above).
  - If the patient develops angina pectoris, withhold treatment for 1 or 2 days and reintroduce it at a lower dose. If ischaemic heart disease was not previously diagnosed, investigate this as a matter of urgency.
  - Many patients feel better while taking a dose of thyroid hormone in excess of their physiological requirements. However, do not over-treat patients; excessive dosages can have adverse cardiovascular effects in the long term.

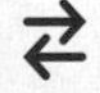

- Treatment of hyperthyroidism will alter the pharmacokinetics of drugs whose kinetics are changed by thyroid disease.

Efficacy and safety

- The best screening investigation for hypothyroidism is the serum thyroid stimulating hormone (TSH) concentration. This test can also be used to adjust the dosage of thyroid hormone replacement therapy. Aim for a TSH within the reference range. The reference range varies with age; check with your laboratory. Avoid over-treatment (see above).

- Other investigations, such as free thyroid hormone concentration and antithyroid antibodies, may also be required for adequate diagnosis of thyroid disease. See above and seek advice from a specialist.

- Advise the patient that replacement therapy for hypothyroidism is usually lifelong.

Prescribing information: **Thyroid hormones**

Levothyroxine

- By mouth, 50–100 micrograms/day initially, but see notes above.
- Usual maintenance dose 100–200 micrograms/day.

Liothyronine

- Usually reserved for treatment of severe hypothyroidism under specialist supervision.
- By intravenous injection, 5–20 micrograms given up to every 4 hours as required.

Carbimazole

Inhibitor of the formation of thyroid hormones

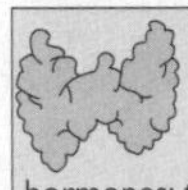

Carbimazole is metabolized to methimazole in the plasma. This inhibits the iodination of tyrosine, resulting in reduced production of the thyroid hormones: tri-iodothyronine (T3) and thyroxine (T4).

- First-line treatment for hyperthyroidism due to Graves' disease or toxic multinodular goitre.

- Pregnancy
  - Crosses the placenta and so may cause neonatal hypothyroidism.
  - Treatment in pregnancy is a risk/benefit decision.
  - Seek expert advice.
- Breastfeeding
  - Risk of neonatal goitre.
- No dosage adjustment is usually required in renal or hepatic insufficiency.

Hyperthyroidism

- Make a clear diagnosis before beginning treatment (beta-blocker therapy may be all that is required for thyroiditis).
- Treatment is usually for 1–2 years.
  - The relapse rate is 50% within 2–4 years of stopping carbimazole treatment. Patients who relapse should be considered for definitive ^{125}Iodine treatment.
- There are two common treatment regimens:
  - The first aims to render the patient euthyroid by treating with a relatively high dose first (15–40 mg daily). Ideally this will render the patient in euthyroid in 1–2 weeks, with a maximal effect at 4–8 weeks of treatment. Once the patient is euthyroid, the dose is reduced to a maintenance dose of 5–15 mg daily.
  - An alternative is a block and replace regimen. The patient is given a high dose (60 mg daily) for up to 18 months and given enough thyroxine (usually 100 micrograms daily) to keep them euthyroid.
- Thyroid ophthalmopathy does not always respond to carbimazole treatment. Severe cases may require steroid treatment and surgery.

- Gastrointestinal disturbance, headache, and rash are common (7% of patients); usually within the first 2 months of treatment. The rash is allergic in origin and the drug should be stopped. Hypersensitivity to carbimazole does not necessarily mean that the patient will be hypersensitive to propylthiouracil.

Practical treatment of hyperthyroidism due to Graves' disease or toxic multinodular goitre

Symptomatic relief
- Beta-blocker (e.g. propranolol)

Disease control
- Antithyroid drugs
  - Carbimazole (first-line)
  - Propylthiouracil
- ^{125}Iodine treatment (definitive)
- Surgery (especially if there is local compression).

Propylthiouracil

- This is an alternative for patients who are sensitive to carbimazole. It can cause hypersensitivity too, but not necessarily in the same patients.
- The daily dose is usually 200–400 mg, given until the patient is euthyroid. The maintenance dose is 50–150 mg daily.
- Halve the dose in moderate renal or hepatic insufficiency. Propylthiouracil can cause neonatal hypothyroidism if given to pregnant women.

- Carbimazole can cause agranulocytosis. The risk of this is low (<1%), but it can be severe, even fatal (see monitoring below). The risk of this diminishes with duration of treatment but is always present.
- Over-treatment will cause hypothyroidism (see thyroid hormones, p. 412).

Efficacy

- Carbimazole reduces the production of thyroid hormones; it does not have any effect on hormone already formed. Use a beta-blocker for rapid symptomatic relief. See the patient frequently (how frequently will depend on the severity of symptoms) when starting treatment to ensure adequate titration of the dose.
- TSH can remain suppressed for months. The free T4 concentration is usually the best measure of thyroid status.

Safety

- The risk of agranulocytosis is small; its onset is rapid and without warning. Prophylactic measurement of a full blood count is therefore unlikely to be helpful.

CSM advice

1. Patients should be asked to report symptoms and signs suggestive of infection, especially a sore throat.
2. A white blood cell count should be performed if there is any clinical evidence of infection.
3. Carbimazole should be stopped promptly if there is clinical or laboratory evidence of neutropenia.

- Advise the patient to seek medical advice immediately if they develop an unexpected sore throat, fever, mouth ulcers, or malaise.
- Warn patients with ophthalmopathy that the appearance of their eyes may not respond to this treatment.

Prescribing information: **Carbimazole**

Treatment of hyperthyroidism

- Initially 15–40 mg daily. Occasionally a larger dose (60 mg) may be required.
- This dose is continued until the patient becomes euthyroid, usually after 4–8 weeks.
- The dose is then gradually reduced to a maintenance dose of 5–15 mg.
- Therapy is usually given for 12–18 months.

An alternative block and replace regimen is sometimes used; see how to use section for details.

Efficacy

Safety

Carbimazole

Treatment of hyperthyroidism

TEACHING POINT Rare but potentially fatal adverse effects

- Carbimazole can cause agranulocytosis. This is rare (<1%, and may be as low as 1 in 1000).
- Agranulocytosis develops rapidly, and although it is more common early in treatment, it can occur at any time. The problem for the prescriber is how best to protect the patient. The rarity and rapid development of the adverse effect means that prophylactic measurement of a full blood count, even if done frequently, would be unlikely to detect impending neutropenia.
- The best protection is vigilance from both prescriber and patient (see CSM advice above) and a low threshold for measuring a full blood count.
- Rare, potentially fatal adverse effects are a major challenge. Before it is licensed, a new drug may have been given to a few thousand patients. If an adverse effect only occurs in 1 in 5000 patients it may never have been seen, much less associated with the drug, before a licence is granted.
- It is especially important for prescribers to be vigilant when using newly-licensed drugs (those marked with an inverted black triangle in the BNF). No matter how well the development of the drug was conducted, clinical experience before marketing is limited. Have a low threshold for making a report to the CSM ('yellow card') even if you cannot clearly associate the adverse effect with the drug. If the adverse effect is rare, it may require reports from several countries to detect a potential link.
- There have been several well publicized cases of drugs that have been withdrawn soon after launch because rare but serious adverse effects have been reported. Examples are:

Drug	**Adverse effect**
Troglitazone	Liver failure
Alosetron	Ischaemic colitis
Cerivastatin	Rhabdomyolysis

As an individual, you are most unlikely to see more than one case; send in a report even if you cannot attribute causality yourself.

Corticosteroids

Corticosteroids are primarily produced by the adrenal cortex and are essential for survival. The principal adrenal steroids are those with glucocorticoid and mineralocorticoid actions, but some sex steroids (particularly androgens) are also produced.

Glucocorticoids affect protein and carbohydrate metabolism (see below); the endogenous hormones are hydrocortisone and corticosterone. The mineralocorticoids, of which the endogenous hormone is aldosterone, affect fluid and electrolyte balance. The endogenous glucocorticoids have both glucocorticoid and mineralocorticoid actions. Synthetic molecules have been developed to provide clearer separation of these effects (see box below).

Potent mineralocorticoid action; little glucocorticoid action	Mixed mineralocorticoid and glucocorticoid actions	Principally glucocorticoid action	Potent glucocorticoid action; little mineralocorticoid action
Fludrocortisone	Cortisone (25 mg)	Prednisolone (5 mg)	Betamethasone (750 micrograms)
Aldosterone	Hydrocortisone (20 mg)	Methylprednisolone (4 mg)	Dexamethasone (750 micrograms)
		Triamcinolone (4 mg)	
		Beclomethasone (250 micrograms)	
		Deflazacort (6 mg)	

Approximate dose equivalents are given in brackets

Note on mineralocorticoids

The therapeutic use of these drugs is limited; see p. 178 (loop diuretics) for information on their use in postural hypotension and pp. 429 and 423 for information on their use in adrenocortical insufficiency.

TEACHING POINT Actions of glucocorticoids

- See p. 422 for clinical uses.
- The actions of corticosteroids are always a balance between desirable and undesirable effects.

Protein and carbohydrate metabolism

- Mobilization of glucose (including gluconeogenesis) and amino acids.
  - Weight gain.
  - Impaired glucose tolerance/diabetes mellitus.

Lipid metabolism

- Redistribution of fat.
- Weight gain.

Mineralocorticoid actions

- Hypokalaemia.
- Fluid retention.
  - Hypertension.
  - Worsening of heart failure.

Anti-inflammatory/immunosuppressant actions

- Acute reductions in the vascular response to injury (dilatation and permeability), cellular migrations, and actions of phagocytes.
- Chronic reductions in cellular proliferation and deposition of collagen.
  - Risk of infection (tuberculosis, oral candidiasis, chickenpox, and measles).
  - Skin changes (thinning, telangiectasia).
  - Masking of normal inflammatory responses (e.g. peptic ulcer more likely to present with bleeding or perforation).

Other adverse effects of glucocorticoids

- Over-treatment will result in Cushing's syndrome.
- Depression of the hypothalamic/pituitary/adrenal (HPA) axis can cause an Addisonian crisis after abrupt withdrawal of the drug.
  - Note that treatment of pregnant women will suppress the fetal HPA axis.
- Mental disturbance, including acute psychosis. Usually an acute effect associated with high doses.
- Glaucoma. This is determined by a recessive allele: 65% of patients have a small rise in intraocular pressure, 30% a moderate rise, and 5% a large rise.
- Cataract. 75% of patients who take more than 15 mg prednisolone equivalents per day for over 2 years develop cataracts, especially of the posterior subcapsular type.
- Osteoporosis. Bone protection is recommended when corticosteroid treatment (>7.5 mg prednisolone equivalents daily) is expected to exceed 3 months. Most bone loss is in the first 6–12 months.
- Ischaemic necrosis of the femoral head.

Glucocorticoids

Drugs in this class

Note that they are used for different indications (see below)
- Prednisolone
- Hydrocortisone
- Beclomethasone
- Betamethasone
- Methylprednisolone
- Dexamethasone
- Triamcinolone

- Replacement therapy in corticosteroid deficiency.
- Anti-inflammatory and immunosuppressant actions.
  - Systemic diseases (e.g. vasculitis, sarcoidosis, rheumatoid arthritis).
  - Lung disease (e.g. asthma).
  - Liver disease (e.g. chronic active hepatitis).
  - Renal disease (e.g. minimal change glomerulonephritis).
  - Bowel disease (e.g. ulcerative colitis).
  - Haematological disease (e.g. haemolytic anaemias).
  - Skin disease (e.g. psoriasis, pemphigus).
  - Eye inflammation (not infection).
  - Joint disease (e.g. intra-articular injections for gout — unlicensed use).
  - Malignant disease (e.g. acute lymphocytic leukaemia, Hodgkin's lymphoma, non-Hodgkin's lymphoma, hormone-sensitive breast cancer).
  - Infection and sepsis syndromes (e.g. meningococcal disease).
  - Anaphylaxis and transfusion reactions.
  - Prevention of transplant rejection.
  - Treatment of adrenal hyperplasia.
  - Treatment of hypercalcaemia due to sarcoidosis or vitamin D toxicity. For other treatments see bisphosphonates (p. 582).
  - Second-line treatment for certain forms of epilepsy (specialized use).

- Pregnancy
  - Glucocorticoids vary in their ability to cross the placenta. Betamethasone and dexamethasone cross the placenta well, while prednisolone does not. Seek expert advice if steroid treatment is required during pregnancy.
  - The CSM advises that there is no convincing evidence that glucocorticoids cause cleft lip or palate.
  - Intrauterine growth retardation is more common if treatment with glucocorticoids is prolonged, but is unlikely after short courses.
  - Treatment with glucocorticoids can suppress the fetal HPA axis, but this usually resolves rapidly after birth.
- Breastfeeding. Maternal dosages up to 10 mg prednisolone equivalents are unlikely to cause problems in children who are breastfed.
- Responses to live vaccines are reduced and may be inadequate in those taking moderate to large doses of glucocorticoids. A list of live vaccines is given on p. 486.

General advice

- Select the appropriate treatment by considering:
  - Glucocorticoid versus mineralocorticoid actions (see p. 420).
  - The route. Is systemic treatment required or can the drug be delivered to the site of action directly (e.g. topically, by inhalation, or by the intrarticular route)?
  - The dose. A high dose may be required initially to achieve control, but use the minimum effective dose.

    - The duration of treatment. Always consider how long you plan to continue treatment; this may change as the clinical problem develops, but avoid treatment for indefinite periods.
- Tell the patient to take the dose in the morning as this minimizes the disruption of the diurnal pattern of corticosteroid production. The regimen for replacement therapy is different; see below.
- Give the patient a steroid card if long-term treatment is required.
- Patients taking glucocorticoids who become unwell may need additional steroid treatment. See section below on steroids and surgery. Very high doses are sometimes given for sepsis syndromes (specialized use in ITU).

Tapering treatment
- Glucocorticoids can suppress the HPA axis; the CSM advises that treatment should be tapered if:
    - Treatment has been for more than 3 weeks.
    - The patient has received multiple short courses.
    - A short course has been given within 1 year of stopping long-term treatment.
    - The dose exceeds 40 mg prednisolone equivalents.
- Glucocorticoids can be stopped abruptly if given for less than 3 weeks (as is done commonly for exacerbations of asthma).

Suggested regimen for the withdrawal of prednisolone	
The disease has resolved and only a few weeks of treatment has been given	Reduce by 2.5 mg every 3 or 4 days down to 7.5 mg; then reduce more slowly (e.g. by 2.5 mg every week, fortnight, or month)
There is uncertainty about disease resolution and /or therapy has been given for many weeks	Reduce by 2.5 mg every fortnight or month down to 7.5 mg; then reduce by 1 mg every month
Symptoms of the disease are likely to recur on withdrawal of steroids (e.g. rheumatoid arthritis)	Reduce by 1 mg every month

Replacement therapy
- The dose required is not large; traditionally this has been 20 mg of hydrocortisone in the morning and 10 mg at lunch time, but this is more than many patients need. Tailor the dose to individual requirements by measuring an ACTH profile.
- Advise patients that they will need to increase the dose if they become unwell.
    - If an Addisonian crisis occurs give hydrocortisone 100 mg intravenously, 8-hourly.
- Mineralocorticoid replacement is usually also required (50–300 micrograms of fludrocortisone daily).

Inhaled glucocorticoids
- Glucocorticoids are central to the treatment of asthma, as they reduce the underlying inflammation.
- The British Thoracic Society guidelines for the treatment of asthma (*http://www.sign.ac.uk/guidelines*) advise that inhaled glucocorticoids should be added whenever inhaled β_2 agonist use exceeds once per day.

- Many patients with COPD do not have steroid-responsive disease. Give patients a formal 6-week trial of steroids and record whether there is improvement in symptoms or lung function. Reconsider glucocorticoid treatment if there is no improvement.
- Regular treatment is essential, and should be given via a large-volume spacer device. This increases delivery to the lungs and reduces systemic absorption.
- β_2 agonists should be taken (inhaled) first, as this increases delivery to the lungs, reduces the risk of paradoxical bronchospasm, and reduces coughing.
- Rinse the mouth after taking these drugs to reduce the risk of oral candidiasis.
- Avoid delivery by nebulizer if possible; the systemic dose delivered is large.
- Combination inhalers containing both a long-acting β_2 agonist and glucocorticoid are only suitable for patients who have stable disease and require both treatments regularly; they will still need a short-acting β_2 agonist for use as required.
- Advise patients that the new CFC-free inhalers may taste different from their previous ones, but that the dose delivered is the same.
- The steroids, budesonide and fluticasone, are subject to extensive first-pass metabolism in the liver. They may have fewer systemic adverse effects after inhalation, but because they are usually given to patients requiring high dosages this effect may not be apparent.

Allergic rhinitis (see antihistamines, p. 611, for general advice)

- Topical nasal formulations are useful for the treatment and prophylaxis of allergic rhinitis.
- An alternative is an oral antihistamine. Avoid decongestants.

Inflammatory conditions of the eye

- Never use topical steroids on the eye until an ulcer due to *Herpes simplex* virus has been excluded.
- Beware of the risk of glaucoma. Long-term treatment causes cataracts.
- Combination products with anti-infective drugs are rarely suitable and are not recommended.

Treatment of rheumatoid arthritis

- A Cochrane systematic review showed that low-dose oral corticosteroids, equivalent to prednisolone 15 mg daily or less, were more effective than NSAIDs within the first weeks of treatment.
- There is some evidence that a daily dose of prednisolone 7.5 mg reduces the rate of joint destruction, but this must be weighed against the long-term adverse effects of glucocorticoids.
- Glucocorticoids can be injected into joints to give pain relief, increase mobility, and reduce deformity. Triamcinolone is insoluble and so acts as a depot within the joint. Never inject a prosthetic joint or when there is the possibility of sepsis. Do not inject a single joint more than 3 times per year. Frequent injections into a joint can cause local osteoporosis and rupture of ligaments and tendons.
- Hydrocortisone can be injected into tendon sheaths for relief of compression neuropathies such as carpal tunnel syndrome. Do not inject the tendon itself and beware repeat injections, as this can cause wasting.

Inflammatory bowel disease

- Glucocorticoids are used to achieve disease control, but are not indicated for maintenance treatment.

- The usual treatment is prednisolone, but budesonide is also licensed for this indication. Budesonide is subject to extensive first-pass metabolism in the liver, so may have fewer systemic adverse effects.

Infections and sepsis syndromes

- Septic shock is associated with severe inflammation. High-dose intravenous glucocorticoids have been used in combination with anti-infective treatments, but the results have been variable. Lower doses of hydrocortisone (50 mg every 6 hours) and fludrocortisone (a mineralocorticoid, 50 micrograms daily by mouth) can be beneficial if the patient has adrenocortical insufficiency as a result of septic shock.

Cerebral oedema (see teaching point below)

- Glucocorticoids are effective in cerebral oedema resulting from intracranial malignancy. Use a pure glucocorticoid such as dexamethasone; a drug with mineralocorticoid actions will cause fluid retention.
- Do not use glucocorticoids for cerebral oedema that results from cerebral malaria; mortality is increased.

- Treatment with glucocorticoids is always a balance between desirable and adverse effects; see the corticosteroids (p. 421) for details.
- Adverse effects can be minimized by considering the following:
  - Use the smallest effective dose for the shortest possible time.
  - Consider the route of administration to limit systemic exposure (e.g. topical administration to eyes, nose, and skin).

Chickenpox (*Varicella zoster* infection) and measles

- Chickenpox and measles can be very severe in patients taking corticosteroids. The risk is lower with topical and inhaled steroids.
- If the patient has not had these infections in the past, the risk is high and the patient should be advised to avoid anyone with chickenpox or measles.
- **Chickenpox** If the patient is exposed to someone with chickenpox they should receive passive immunization with *Varicella zoster* IgG within 3 days (see immunoglobulins, p. 638).
  - If the patient develops chickenpox they should receive specialist care.
- **Measles** If the patient is exposed to someone with measles they should receive passive immunization with intramuscular, human, normal immunoglobulin.

- Steroids can mask the gastrointestinal adverse effects of NSAIDs (including aspirin). Avoid co-prescribing if possible and consider gastroprotection.
- Hypokalemia can cause digoxin toxicity.
- Hypokalaemia can be severe when glucocorticoids are given with other drugs that lower plasma potassium (e.g. loop and thiazide diuretics), amphotericin, acetazolamide, high-dose salbutamol.
- Drugs that induce liver enzymes (e.g. carbamazepine, phenytoin, barbiturates, rifampicin) accelerate the metabolism of glucocorticoids and can reduce their effects.
- Glucocorticoid treatment can affect anticoagulant control with warfarin; measure the INR more frequently.
- The effects of antihypertensive and oral hypoglycaemic drugs are antagonized by glucocorticoids.

Safety

- Minimize the impact of adverse effects by considering the following:
  - Measure the plasma potassium in patients with cardiac disease.
  - Measure the blood glucose; some patients may become glucose intolerant. Treatment with corticosteroids can worsen control of diabetes mellitus; be prepared to intensify treatment.
  - Osteoporosis. Bone protection is recommended when corticosteroid treatment (>7.5 mg prednisolone equivalents daily) is expected to exceed 3 months. Most bone loss is in the first 6–12 months.
  - Measure the intraocular pressure; glucocorticoids can cause glaucoma, especially when applied topically to the eye.
  - Examine the eyes for cataracts.

Efficacy

- The measure of efficacy will depend on the indication (e.g. PEFR for asthma, ESR for polymyalgia rheumatica, symptom scores in rheumatoid arthritis and inflammatory bowel disease).
  - For example, it is suggested that the dose of inhaled steroid given for asthma be reviewed every 3 months. If the dose can be reduced, this should be by 25–50%.
- It is very important that targets are set for treatment with glucocorticoids, so that effectiveness can be assessed. Do not commit patients to treatment for indefinite periods with poorly defined goals. The risks of treatment will almost certainly outweigh the benefits.

- Give the patient a steroid card if long-term treatment is required. Explain that they must not stop treatment abruptly after prolonged treatment.
- Patients are often aware of some of the adverse effects of glucocorticoids treatment, especially weight gain. Address their concerns directly to improve compliance with treatment. For example, a short course of glucocorticoids for an acute exacerbation of asthma will not cause weight gain.

TEACHING POINT Glucocorticoids and surgery

- Do not stop steroid treatment in patients admitted for surgery; their requirements may increase, especially if they are unwell.
- If the patient cannot take medication by mouth convert the oral dose to intravenous hydrocortisone. Note that intravenous hydrocortisone needs to be given 2 or 3 times daily.

The following advice is given for patients admitted for routine surgery.

- *Minor surgery under general anaesthesia.* Give the usual oral corticosteroid dose on the morning of surgery or hydrocortisone 25–50 mg (usually the sodium succinate) intravenously at induction. Restart the usual oral corticosteroid dose after surgery.
- *Moderate or major surgery. Give* the usual oral corticosteroid dose on the morning of surgery and hydrocortisone 25–50 mg intravenously at induction. Give hydrocortisone 25–50 mg 3 times a day by intravenous injection for 24 hours after moderate surgery (48–72 hours after major surgery), until the patient is eating. Start the usual pre-operative corticosteroid dose once the patient can take medication by mouth.

Prescribing information: **Glucocorticoids**

Hydrocortisone

- Replacement therapy. By mouth, 20 mg in the morning and 10 mg at lunch time, but titrate the dose to individual requirements (see note above).

Prednisolone

- By mouth, the dose will depend on the indication but will usually be in the range 20–60 mg.
- 7.5 mg daily is about twice endogenous glucocorticoid production.

Beclomethasone

- Metered-dose inhaler. The usual dose is 200 micrograms bd, but higher doses may be required (expert supervision advised).
- Note that metered-dose inhalers deliver 50–200 micrograms per actuation (puff). Check which strength is required (the most common is 100 micrograms per actuation).
- Give the patient a spacer device and demonstrate this.
- In addition to metered-dose inhalers, many proprietary delivery devices are available. These tend to be more expensive but may be more convenient for some patients. Seek expert advice locally if your patient cannot manage a metered-dose inhaler.

TEACHING POINT Treatment of rising intracranial pressure

Causes

- Vasogenic, due to increased capillary permeability (e.g. tumour, trauma, infection, stroke).
- Cell death due to hypoxia.
- Increased interstitial pressure (e.g. obstructive hydrocephalus).

Typical signs

- Irritability.
- Drowsiness.
- Coma.
- Irregular breathing.
- Cushing response (falling pulse with rising blood pressure).

Treatment

- This is an emergency; seek specialist advice.
- Maintain adequate cerebral oxygenation.
- An osmotic diuretic (e.g. mannitol 20% 5 mL/kg over 15 min) lowers intracranial pressure quickly, but the duration of effect is limited (a few hours).
- Dexamethasone has no mineralocorticoid actions and reduces vasogenic cerebral oedema. Give 4 mg every 8 hours by intravenous injection.
- Avoid fluid overload and nurse the patient with the head elevated at about 40 degrees.
- In the most severe cases, mechanical hyperventilation to maintain the partial pressure of CO_2 at 3.5 kPa reduces intracranial pressure. Anaesthetic drugs such as thiopental can also be effective.

Corticotrophins

Polypeptide hormones

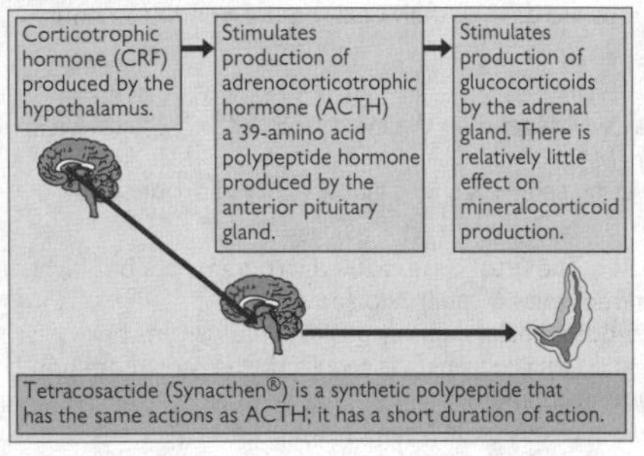

Drugs in this class

- Adrenocorticotrophic hormone (ACTH).
- Tetracosactide (Synacthen®)—synthetic derivative of ACTH with a short duration of action.

- Diagnosis of adrenocortical insufficiency (Addison's disease).
- Occasionally used as a short-term alternative to glucocorticoid treatment.

- The action of these drugs is short-lived and wanes with repeated administration. Long-term treatment should usually be with glucocorticoids.
- Do not use these drugs for the treatment of an Addisonian crisis; they will not work.

- Although ACTH can be used when glucocorticoid treatment is indicated, it produces a variable therapeutic response that rapidly wanes with time. Use a glucocorticoid instead (see glucocorticoids, p. 422).
- The principal use of these drugs is for the diagnosis of adrenocortical insufficiency (Addison's disease) by the 'short Synacthen® test'.
- There are some other uses in specialist endocrinological practice (e.g. the long Synacthen test to demonstrate adrenal suppression); seek specialist advice if these are required.

The short Synacthen® test

- Note that this test cannot be performed if the patient has received exogenous steroids.
- Give 250 micrograms of tetracosactide by either intramuscular or intravenous injection.
- Take blood samples for plasma cortisol (check locally to ensure that you collect these in the correct tube) at baseline, +30 minutes, and +60 minutes after the dose.

Interpretation

- If normal, the basal cortisol should be above 170 nmol/L.
- The plasma cortisol concentration at +30 minutes should be >580 nmol/L, and there should have been a rise of >190 nmol/L.

- Corticotrophins are polypeptides and so can cause anaphylaxis; this is very rare.
- Corticotrophins stimulate the production of glucocorticoids, so long-term treatment will cause the same adverse effects. Single doses do not usually produce any adverse effects.

- The Synacthen® test will be impossible to interpret if the patient has been given exogenous glucocorticoids.

Efficacy

- See box for interpretation of the Synacthen® test.

- Remember that steroid requirements increase when patients are acutely stressed (e.g. by infection, illness, or surgery).
- Advise patients with adrenocortical insufficiency to carry a Medicalert® bracelet.

Prescribing information: **Corticotrophins**

Diagnosis of adrenocortical insufficiency

- See box above.
- The use of ACTH for long-term treatment is not recommended.

Treatment of acute adrenocortical insufficiency

- The clinical features include hypotension, hyponatraemia (usually mild), hyperkalaemia, pigmentation, and hypoglycaemia.
- De novo presentation with an Addisonian crisis is rare. Remember that steroid requirements increase when patients are acutely stressed (e.g. by infection, illness, or surgery). Patients with hypopituitarism, adrenal insufficiency, or adrenal suppression (taking long-term steroids) may not be able to respond.
- Measure the blood glucose urgently (stick test). Give 50 mL of 50% glucose if it is less than 3.5 mmol/L.
- Give isotonic saline (e.g. 1 litre over 60 minutes). The patient may require several more litres over the next 24 hours. A central venous line may be required if the patient is cardiovascularly unstable.
- Give hydrocortisone 100 mg by intravenous injection.
  - If the patient is cardiovascularly unstable give 100 mg intramuscularly every 6 hours until they are stable.
  - If the patient is stable give hydrocortisone 20 mg every 8 hours.
- Mineralocorticoid replacement is rarely necessary in the acute phase, as glucocorticoids have some mineralocorticoid action.
- Once the crisis is over, consider why it occurred and how it can be avoided in the future. See box on corticosteroids and surgery.
- See glucocorticoid (p. 423) for notes on long-term replacement therapy in adrenocortical insufficiency.

Oestrogens and hormone replacement therapy (HRT)

Female sex hormones

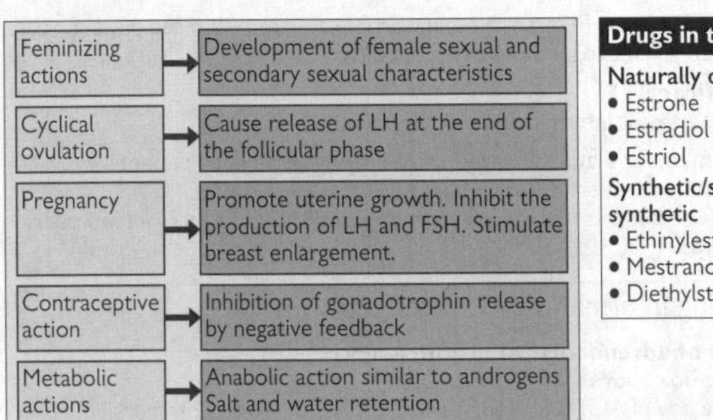

Drugs in this class

Naturally occurring
- Estrone (-1 ol)
- Estradiol (-2 ols)
- Estriol (-3 ols)

Synthetic/semi-synthetic
- Ethinylestradiol
- Mestranol
- Diethylstilbestrol

- Oestrogens alone.
  - Treatment of primary amenorrhoea.
  - Hormonal manipulation of carcinoma of the breast and prostate (specialized use).
  - Treatment of vaginal involution (topical).
- In combination with progestogens.
  - Replacement therapy in ovarian insufficiency.
  - Hormone replacement therapy (HRT).
  - Oral contraceptives (see p. 436).

- Do not give oestrogens during pregnancy (although there is little evidence of harm from oral contraceptives).
  - HRT is not a contraceptive.
- Do not give oestrogens if the patient has:
  - A history of venous thromboembolism.
  - A strong family history (e.g. antiphospholipid syndrome).
- Avoid oestrogens if the patient has endometrial or breast cancer (unless used specifically for treatment).

Risk factors for the development of osteoporosis

- Premature menopause (<40 years)
- Family history of osteoporosis
- Steroid treatment lasting >6 months
- Premenopausal amenorrhoea for >6 months
  - Due to low weight or exercise
- Liver, thyroid, or renal disease
- Excess alcohol intake
- Gonadotrophin-releasing analogue treatment for >6 months

Suggested diagnostic tests for patients at risk of osteoporosis

- ESR
- Serum calcium, phosphate, alkaline phosphatase, creatinine
- Serum and urine protein electrophoresis (if ESR raised and >50 years)
- TSH
- 9.00 a.m. testosterone in men (and LH/FSH)
- Plasma oestradiol and gondotrophins in amenorrhoeic premenopausal women
- Plasma prolactin (if hypogondal or suggestive features such as galactorrhoea)
- Endomysial antibodies in men and women with unexplained iron deficiency (coeliac disease)

- Avoid oestrogens in severe liver disease (they are metabolized by the liver).
  - Includes congenital syndromes such as Rotor and Dubin–Johnson.
- Do not give oestrogens if the patient has porphyria.
- Avoid oestrogens if the patient has fibroids; they may enlarge.
- Do not give oestrogens if the patient has endometriosis or undiagnosed vaginal bleeding.

Hormone replacement therapy

- The role of HRT has undergone a reassessment in the past few years.
- Relief of menopausal symptoms.
  - HRT is most effective for vasomotor and urogenital symptoms.
- Osteoporosis (see risk factors box).
  - Treat any underlying cause. See box for suggested diagnostic workup.
  - HRT reduces bone loss by 30–50% (similar to that from bisphosphonates).
  - Some would offer HRT to women with established osteoporosis or if they are at high risk; however, this is controversial and other drugs are available.
- Cardiovasular disease.
  - Do not offer HRT for prevention of cardiovascular disease or to those at high risk.
- Thromboembolic disease.
  - HRT increases the risk of thromboembolism to around 16–23 per 100 000 women per year. This is twice the baseline risk, but is still low.
- Breast cancer.
  - HRT increases the risk of breast cancer by 2.3% per year of treatment.
  - The risk becomes significant only after more than 5 years' treatment, and translates to 2 additional cases per 1000 women treated for more than 5 years.
- Other factors.
  - HRT may increase the risk of cervical cancer.
  - HRT increases the risk of endometrial cancer (those formulations that contain progestogen confer a lower risk).
  - HRT reduces the risk of colorectal cancer; the mechanism is not known.
  - The effect of HRT on the risk of ovarian cancer is inconsistent.
- See box for treatment suggestions for different groups of women
- If oestrogens are used topically, use the minimum effective amount. A systemic cyclical progestogen may need to be given if long-term treatment is required.
- It is recommended that HRT is suspended 1 month before major surgery.

Treatment of cancer (seek specialist advice)

- Diethylstilbestrol and fosfestrol are used to treat prostate cancer, but their use is limited by a high incidence of adverse effects.
- Ethinylestradiol is used in the treatment of some breast cancers.

Treatment suggestions	
Symptomatic perimenopausal women	Give continuous oestrogen with progestogen on the last 12–14 days of the cycle for 1–2 years.
Symptomatic postmenopausal women	There is probably a benefit. Include a progestogen if they have a uterus. Treatment is principally for symptoms.
Symptomatic women with premature menopause	Give long-term HRT.
Women with urogenital symptoms	Give local rather than systemic treatment.
Women with temporary ovarian failure (e.g. those given gonadorelin analogues for endometriosis or breast cancer)	If treatment is to be for more than 3 months, give HRT to reduce bone loss.
Do **not** give HRT to those with:	No symptoms. A low risk of osteoporosis. Breast cancer, cardiovascular disease, venous thromboembolic disease.

- Adverse effects are common and dose-related, they include:
  - Fluid retention and hypertension (affect 4% of women).
  - Painful breasts in women and gynaecomastia in men.
  - Endometrial bleeding.
    - Cyclical HRT causes a withdrawal bleed at the end of the progestogen-containing phase.
    - Initiation of continuous treatment (with oestrogen and progestogen) can cause irregular bleeding, but this should stop within 6 months.
  - Impaired glucose tolerance and diabetes mellitus.
  - Migraine.
- Rare but serious adverse effects include:
  - Thromboembolism. See box for risk. Treatment should be stopped, pending investigation, if this is suspected.
  - Endometrial carcinoma. The risk is increased 6-fold, but the overall incidence is low. Concomitant progestogens confer some protection.
- Oestogens given during pregnancy increase the risk of vaginal adenosis and increase the incidence of vaginal adenocarcinoma in female children.

- The effectiveness of oestrogens is reduced by drugs that are enzyme inducers (see carbamazepine, p. 246). Seek advice from a specialist if treatment with the following drugs is indicated: phenytoin, carbamazepine, St John's wort, rifampicin, griseofulvin, and some anti-HIV drugs.
- Drug interactions are unlikely with low-dose HRT.

Safety and efficacy

- Assess the patient's risk of venous thromboembolism (see progestogens, p. 434).
- Assess the patient's risk of osteoporosis (see box).
- Measure the blood pressure every 6 months.
- Women should have a cervical smear performed every 3 years.

- HRT should be stopped immediately, pending investigation, if any of the following occur:
  - Sudden chest pain suggestive of cardiac ischaemia.
  - Clinical features of venous thrombosis or pulmonary embolism.
  - New neurological symptoms, including headache and depression.
  - Hypertension (systolic BP >160 mmHg or diastolic BP >100 mmHg).

- Advise the patient of the risk of venous thromboembolism and breast cancer, but weigh this against the benefits (see above).
  - Advise the patient that it is particularly important to keep mobile and well-hydrated during long journeys.
  - Support stockings reduce the risk of venous thrombosis.
- Explain that HRT is most effective for menopausal vasomotor symptoms.

Prescribing information: **Oestrogens**

There are many formulations available. The following are offered as examples only.

Hormone replacement therapy

- See above for selection guidelines.
- Combination formulations (oestrogen plus progestogen) can be given continuously or with the progestogen given cyclically. Most products are available in both formats; specify which is required. See above for appropriate selection.
- **Conjugated oestrogens plus progestogen**
  - Conjugated equine oestrogens 625 micrograms plus medroxyprogesterone 5 mg (Premique®).
- **Estradiol with a progestogen**
  - Estradiol 2 mg plus norethisterone 700 micrograms (Climesse®).
- **Conjugated oestrogen only**
  - Conjugated equine oestrogens 625 micrograms (Premarin®).
- **Estradiol only**
  - Estradiol 1 mg (Progynova®).
- **Topical oestrogen**
  - Estradiol 0.1% (Ovestin®). Give 1 applicator dose daily for 2–3 weeks; then reduce to twice weekly.
  - Withdraw treatment every 2–3 months to assess the need for continued treatment.

Progestogens

Female sex hormones

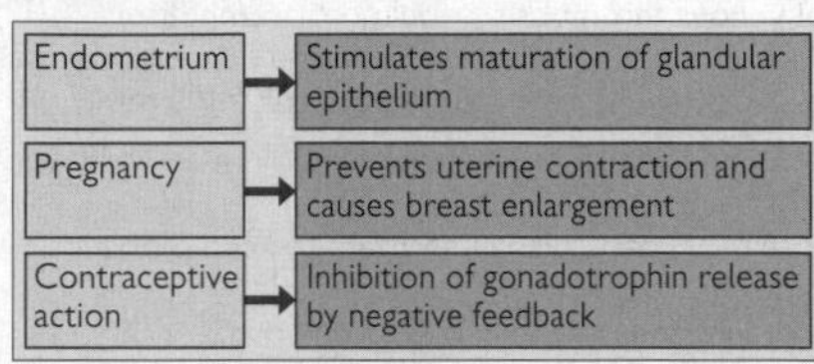

Drugs in this class

Naturally occurring
- Progesterone

Semi-synthetic steroids
- Norethisterone
- Levonorgestrel
- Ethynodiol
- Lynestrenol
- Norgestimate
- Medroxyprogesterone
- Etonorgestrel
- Third-generation drugs (fewer androgenic effects, but slightly increased risk of VTE)
  - Desogestrel
  - Gestodene
  - Drospirenone

Risk factors for VTE
- Family history (e.g. antiphospholipid syndrome, factor V Leiden)
- Obesity (body mass index >30 kg/m^2)
- Long-term immobilization
- Varicose veins

- Treatment of dysfunctional uterine bleeding.
  - Limited effect in menorrhagia (consider tranexamic acid instead).
- Treatment of endometriosis.
- Treatment of menstrual disturbance.
- Contraceptive (see p. 436).
- Have been used to prevent spontaneous abortion, but there is little evidence of their efficacy; not recommended.
- Treatment of cancer. Especially second-line or third-line for breast cancer, but also for endometrial cancer and renal cell cancer (specialized use).

- Do not give progestogens during pregnancy (although there is little evidence of harm from oral contraceptives).
- Do not give progestogens if the patient has a history of venous thromboembolism (VTE).
- Avoid progestogens if the patient has genital or breast cancer (unless used specifically for treatment).
- Avoid progestogens in severe liver disease (they are metabolized by the liver).
  - This includes a history of liver tumours or infective hepatitis.
- Do not give progestogens if the patient has porphyria.

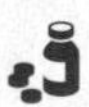

- The most common use of progestogens is for their contraceptive actions. See p. 436.

Endometriosis

- If this requires drug treatment, it may respond to a progestogen given continuously.
- Other drug treatments include danazol, gestrinone, and the gonadorelin analogues.

- Fluid retention is common and may worsen heart failure, hypertension, and renal insufficiency.
- Abdominal and lower back pain are also common.
- Breast tenderness is uncommon.
- Progestogens have specialized use in the treatment of breast cancer; in that case they can cause amenorrhoea and hypercalcaemia.
- Progestogens can cause virilization of the female fetus if given early in pregnancy.

- Long-term use can cause amenorrhoea (especially when given by depot injection for more than 7 years).

- The effect of warfarin is reduced by progestogens.
- The blood ciclosporin concentration is increased by progestogens.

Safety and efficacy
- Assess the patient's risk of venous thromboembolism (see risk factors box).
- Measure the blood pressure every 6 months.
- Women should have a cervical smear performed every 3 years.

- Advise the patient of the risk of venous thromboembolism.
    - Advise the patient that it is particularly important to keep mobile and well-hydrated during long journeys.

Prescribing information: **Progestogens**

There are many formulations available. The following is offered as an example.

Endometriosis
- By mouth, norethisterone 10–15 mg daily for 4–6 months (or longer).
    - Start on day 5 of the menstrual cycle.
    - If bleeding occurs, increase the dose to 20–25 mg daily. Reduce the dose once bleeding has stopped.

Oral contraceptives

Female sex hormones

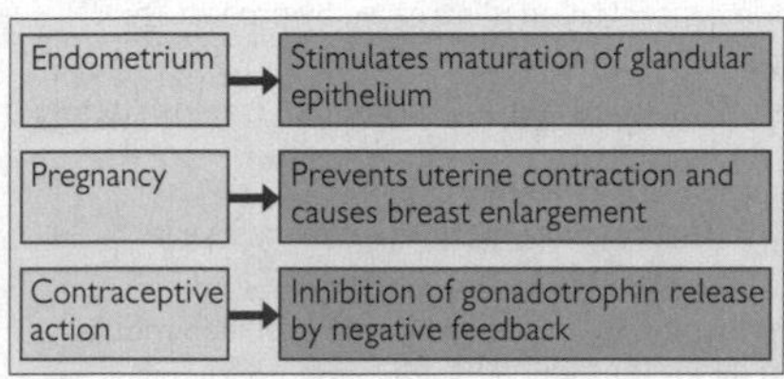

Relative contraindications to the use of combined oral contraceptives

- Strong family history of arterial disease (avoid if abnormal lipid profile)
- Diabetes mellitus (they worsen glucose tolerance)
- Hypertension (>140/100 mmHg)
- Smoking (avoid if >40/day)
- Age >35 years (avoid if >50 years)
- Obesity (avoid if body mass index >39 kg/m^2)
- Migraine (especially if with focal aura or if severe)

- Contraceptive.
  - Progestogen-only.
  - With an oestrogen–combined oral contraceptive.
  - Depot injections.
  - Intrauterine progestogen-only device.
  - Emergency contraception.
- See pp. 430 and 434 for other uses of oestrogens and progestogens.

- Do not give oral contraceptives if the woman is known to be pregnant, but there is little evidence of harm if they are given inadvertently.
- Avoid oral contraceptives if the patient has a history of venous thromboembolism.
- Avoid oral contraceptives if the patient has genital or breast cancer.
- Avoid oral contraceptives in severe liver disease (they are metabolized by the liver).
  - This includes a history of liver tumours or infective hepatitis.
- Do not give oral contraceptives if the patient has porphyria.
- The combined oral contraceptive is not suitable for all women; see cautions and contraindications box.

Oral contraception

- The combined oral contraceptive is the most effective contraceptive for general use. Progestogen-only contraceptives are suitable for older women, for heavy smokers, and for those with hypertension, valvular heart disease, diabetes mellitus, and migraine.
- Progestogen-only contraceptives are preferred over the combined oral contraceptive in women who are breast-feeding.
- Parenteral progestogen-only contraceptives are effective, but women should be carefully reviewed before they are administered, given their long duration of action.
  - The implants require specific training for insertion and removal.

Combined oral contraceptives

- If the amount of oestrogen and progestogen is fixed, the formulation is called monophasic. When the relative proportions change throughout the cycle, it is called biphasic or triphasic.

- Phased formulations are suitable for women who do not have withdrawal bleeding, or who have breakthrough bleeding with monophasic formulations.
- Use the lowest strength formulation that is effective.
  - For most women this will be one that contains 30–35 micrograms of oestrogen.
  - If the woman has risk factors for thromboembolism, and an oral contraceptive is still felt to be appropriate, consider giving a lower dose of oestrogen (20 micrograms).
- The third-generation progestogens are most suitable for women who have unacceptable androgenic adverse effects from other progestogens. However, note that the risk of thromboembolism is higher with these drugs (see box).
- Most formulations are taken for 21 days, followed by a 7-day break (during which a withdrawal bleed occurs). Some formulations contain inactive tablets for the last 7 days and are taken continuously.
- See below for advice to women who have missed a tablet or who require emergency contraception.

- The most common adverse effects of the combined oral contraceptive pill are:
  - Headache, vaginal discharge, depression, reduced libido, and urinary tract infection.
  - Uncommon adverse effects include thromboembolism (see box), benign liver tumours, and gallstones.
- Progestogen adverse effects; see p. 434.

Note on venous thromboembolism (VTE)

- The incidence of VTE
  - Is about 15 per 100 000 women per year of use in users of second-generation oral contraceptives.
  - Is about 25 per 100 000 women per year of use in users of third-generation oral contraceptives.
  - Is about 5 per 100 000 women per year if they are not taking an oral contraceptive.
  - Is about 60 per 100 000 pregnancies.
- This indicates a small excess risk for women using third-generation oral contraceptives. Note that the absolute risk of VTE in women taking third-generation combined oral contraceptives is very small, and is much less than the risk during pregnancy.

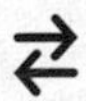

- The effectiveness of progestogen-only contraceptives and combined oral contraceptives is reduced by drugs that are enzyme inducers (see carbamazepine, p. 246). Seek advice from a family planning clinic if treatment with the following drugs is indicated: phenytoin, carbamazepine, St John's wort, rifampicin, griseofulvin, and some anti-HIV drugs.
- Drugs that can cause diarrhoea (e.g. broad-spectrum antibiotics) reduce the absorption of oral contraceptives.
  - Broad-spectrum antibiotics may also reduce their effect by altering the enterohepatic recirculation of oestrogens in the gut. The clinical importance of this effect has not been established.
  - Advise women to take additional precautions during and for 7 days after recovery from a diarrhoeal illness or a course of broad-spectrum antibiotics.

  - If the illness occurs during the last 7 days of a cycle of tablets, omit the next pill-free interval.
- The effect of warfarin is reduced by oral contraceptives.
- The blood ciclosporin concentration is increased by oral contraceptives.

Safety and efficacy

- Assess the patient's risk of venous thromboembolism (see risk factors in progestogens, p. 434).
- Measure the blood pressure every 6 months.
- Women should have a cervical smear performed every 3 years.
- Combined oral contraceptives should be stopped immediately, pending investigation, if any of the following occur:
  - Sudden chest pain suggestive of cardiac ischaemia.
  - Clinical features of venous thrombosis or pulmonary embolism.
  - New neurological symptoms, including headache and depression.
  - Hypertension (systolic BP >160 mmHg or diastolic BP >100 mmHg).

- Advise the patient of the risk of VTE, but weigh this against the risks of pregnancy (see above).
  - Advise the patient that it is particularly important to keep mobile and well-hydrated during long journeys.
- Warn the patient that a diarrhoeal illness or vomiting within 3 hours of taking the tablet may reduce absorption of the contraceptive.
- See advice below regarding 'missed pills'.

Prescribing information: **Progestogens**

Many formulations are available. The following are offered as examples.

Combined oral contraceptives

- Low strength
- Desogestrel 150 micrograms plus ethinylestradiol 20 micrograms daily (Mercilon®).
- Standard strength
- Levonorgestrel 250 micrograms plus ethinylestradiol 30 micrograms (Eugynon 30®).

Oral progestogen-only contraceptives

- Etynodiol diacetate 500 micrograms (Femulen®).

Parenteral progestogen-only contraceptives

- Medroxyprogesterone 150 mg by deep intramuscular injection every 12 weeks (Depo-Provera®).

Intrauterine progestogen-only system

- Releases levonorgestrel 20 microgams daily (Mirena®).

Emergency contraception

- Levonorgestrel 750 micrograms. Take 1 tablet as soon as possible (and not more than 72 hours) after unprotected intercourse. Take the second tablet 12 hours later (Levonelle-2®).

Endometriosis

- By mouth, norethisterone 10–15 mg daily for 4–6 months. Start the treatment on day 5 of the menstrual cycle.

Advice for women who have missed a dose of an oral contraceptive

- If less than 12 hours late, take the missed tablet immediately. Continue the pack as usual. There will be no extra risk of getting pregnant.
- If more than 12 hours late, take the last missed tablet immediately. Throw away any earlier missed tablets. Advise the patient to avoid sex for the next 7 days or to use condoms. If the packet is finished before the 7 days have passed, start another packet immediately (i.e. do not take a 7-day break).
  - If the patient is in the first week of the cycle, she may need to take emergency contraception before continuing the packet (unless she has not had sex in the previous week).*
  - If the patient starts the cycle of tablets later than she should, she may need to take emergency contraception before continuing treatment (unless she has not had sex in the previous week).*
  - If the patient misses 2 or more pills from the first 7 in the pack, she may need to take emergency contraception before continuing treatment (unless she has not had sex in the previous week).*

*In these cases the patient should be advised to seek urgent advice from her GP, family planning clinic, or sexual health clinic.

Emergency contraception

There are two main options for emergency contraception.

- High-dose progestogen ('morning-after pill'), which prevents implantation.
  - Levonorgestrel 750 micrograms taken up to 72 hours after unprotected intercourse. A second dose is taken 12 hours later. The patient should use barrier methods of contraception until the next period. Warn the patient that pregnancy can still occur despite emergency contraception.
  - Hormonal emergency contraception is widely available through GPs, family planning clinics, sexual health clinics, and A&E departments. It can also be purchased over the counter from pharmacies.
- Insertion of a intrauterine contraceptive device (IUCD or 'coil'). This is more effective than hormonal methods and can be inserted up to 120 hours after unprotected intercourse. Insertion should be covered by antibacterial prophylaxis (e.g. azithromycin 1 g by mouth). The patient should be offered testing for sexually transmitted diseases.

Gonadorelin analogues

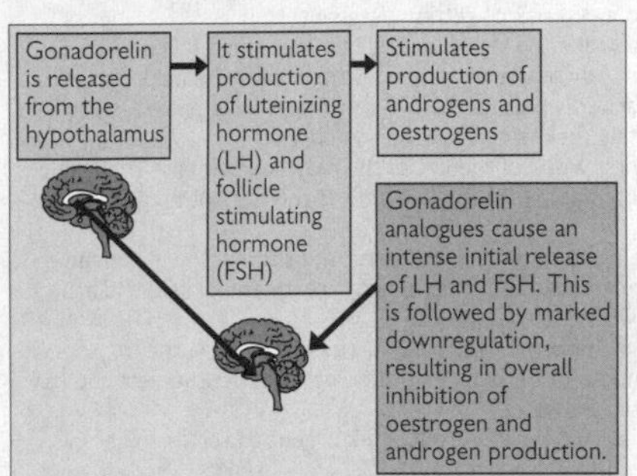

Drugs in this class

- Buserelin
- Goserelin
- Leuprorelin
- Nafarelin
- Triptorelin

Other drugs that inhibit pituitary gonadotrophins

(Not considered in further detail)

- Danazol
  - An inhibitor of pituitary gonadotrophins
  - Semi-synthetic steroid with androgenic actions
- Gestrinone
  - Similar actions to danazol
- Cestorelix and ganirelix
  - LH-releasing hormone antagonists

Analogues of naturally-occurring peptide hormones

- Most of the uses of these drugs are specialized.
  - Endometriosis.
  - Infertility. To cause desensitization before in vitro fertilization.
  - Treatment of anaemia due to uterine fibroids (plus iron).
  - To reduce uterine fibroid size before surgery.
  - Treatment of breast and prostate cancer.

- Women must use non-hormonal (barrier) methods of contraception while taking these drugs.
- Gonadorelin analogues are contraindicated during pregnancy. Pregnancy must be excluded before they are given.
- Gonadorelin analogues reduce bone mass; take care in those at risk of osteoporosis (see oestrogens (p. 430) for a list of risk factors).
- No dosage change is usually required in renal or hepatic insufficiency.
- Gonadorelin analogues should not be given to women with undiagnosed vaginal bleeding.
- Take care if the patient has polycystic ovaries; these drugs can cause them to increase in size.

Prostate cancer

- Treatment with one of the gonadorelin analogues is an alternative to orchidectomy.
- Some men are at risk of a tumour flare on starting these drugs; consider concomitant antiandrogen drug treatment (see antiandrogens, p. 444).
- The disease usually responds for between 12 and 18 months.
- There are no very satisfactory alternatives once the disease stops responding.

Breast cancer

- Gonadorelin analogues are indicated for:
  - Advanced breast cancer in postmenopausal and perimenopausal women as an alternative to chemotherapy (in those with oestrogen receptor positive tumours).
  - Early breast cancer in postmenopausal and perimenopausal women.

- The most common adverse effects of gonadorelin analogues are menopausal symptoms in women:
  - Vasomotor symptoms.
  - Reduced bone density.
  - Withdrawal bleeding.
  - The effect of these can be reduced by giving hormone replacement therapy (HRT).
- In men, gonadorelin analogues can cause a tumour flare (see above), sexual dysfunction, and gynaecomastia.
- Other adverse effects include:
  - Headache.
  - Palpitation.
  - Local irritation from the nasal spray formulations.
  - Rash and local irritation at injection sites.
- Less common adverse effects include:
  - Increase in the size of ovarian cysts (these can become very large).
  - Hypertension.
  - Hypersensitivity and anaphylaxis rarely.

- There are no important drug interactions.

Safety and efficacy

- It is recommended that treatment with gonadorelin analogues should not exceed 6 months, except for treatment of cancer.
- Consider bone protection if treatment with gonadorelin analogues is likely to exceed 3 months (see p. 582) for more information.

- Warn female patients that these drugs cause menopausal symptoms.
- Remember that smoking and excessive alcohol consumption will worsen bone loss.
- Avoid using nasal decongestant drugs if taking these drugs by nasal spray.

Prescribing information: **Gonadorelin analogues**

Goserelin

For breast or prostate cancer

- By subcutaneous injection into the anterior abdominal wall, 3.6 mg every 28 days (supplied with a special applicator).

Androgens and anabolic steroids

Male sex hormones

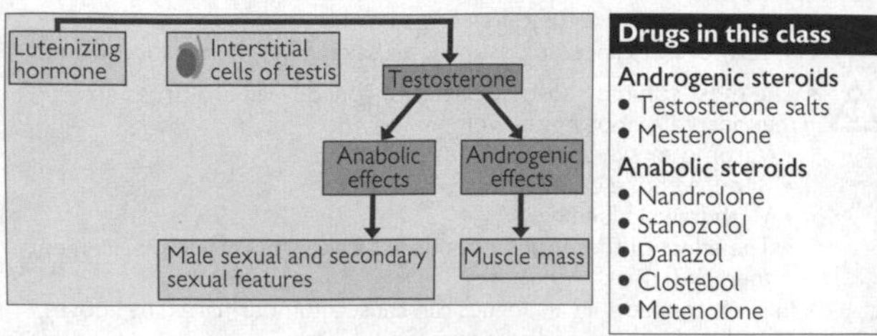

Drugs in this class

Androgenic steroids
- Testosterone salts
- Mesterolone

Anabolic steroids
- Nandrolone
- Stanozolol
- Danazol
- Clostebol
- Metenolone

- Replacement therapy (testosterone is the drug of choice).
  - Testicular or pituitary failure.
- To increase muscle bulk in wasting diseases (nandrolone or stanozolol).
- Nandrolone has been used for treatment of osteoporosis in postmenopausal women, but it is no longer recommended.
- Treatment of hereditary angio-oedema (specialized use): danazol, stanzolol.
- Sometimes used for treatment of aplastic anaemia, but this is controversial.
- Palliation of itching secondary to cholestatic jaundice in terminal care.

- Do not give androgens during pregnancy or breastfeeding; they cause virilization of female fetuses.
- Do not give androgens to men with prostate or breast carcinoma.
- If the patient has skeletal metastases these drugs can cause hypercalcaemia; take care.
- Androgens can cause fusion of the epiphyses; take care in children and young adults.
- Use androgens with caution in patients with cardiovascular disease, hypertension, or diabetes mellitus.
- Do not give stanozolol to patients with liver disease.

Replacement therapy

- Intramuscular depot formulations are the preferred method of delivery of testosterone for replacement.
  - Note that several depot injections contain peanut oil; check that the patient does not have a nut allergy.
- If the patient has pituitary insufficiency, continuous treatment will stimulate sexual development but may not restore fertility. Testosterone needs to be given in a pulsatile fashion if fertility is required.
- Hypogonadism is a risk factor for osteoporosis (see oestrogens (p. 430)) for more information.
- The other indications for androgens are specialized and are not considered further here.

- Adverse effects are common and result from the virilizing effects of these drugs.
  - Virilization effects in women may be unacceptable.
  - Acne is common.
- Androgens can cause fusion of the epiphyses causing short stature.
- Androgens cause sodium and water retention, and can cause hypertension.
  - They increase the risk of cardiovascular disease.
- Stanozolol can cause liver disease.
  - There may be an increased risk of liver tumours when androgens are given for long periods.

- Androgens can enhance the effect of warfarin.

Safety and efficacy

- Monitor growth in children given androgens.
- Measure the blood pressure regularly.
- Assess the patient's cardiovascular risk factors and treat appropriately.

- Advise the patient of the cardiovascular risks associated with inappropriate use of these drugs.

Prescribing information: **Androgens and anabolic steroids**

There are several formulations available. The following is offered as an example.

Sustanon 250® for replacement therapy

- By deep intramuscular injection, 1 mL monthly.
- Contains testosterone propionate 30 mg, testosterone phenylpropionate 60 mg, testosterone isocaproate 60 mg, and testosterone decanoate 100 mg.

Anti-androgens

A heterogeneous group, but all antagonize the actions of androgens (male sex hormones)

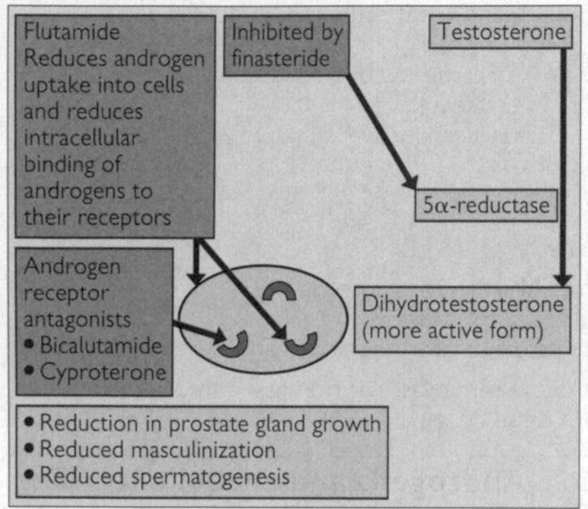

Drugs used for prostate cancer

First-line
- (Orchidectomy)
- Gonadorelin analogues
- (Diethylstilbestrol—poorly tolerated)

For prostate carcinoma refractory to gonadorelin analogues
- Anti-androgens
  - Bicalutamide
  - Cyproterone acetate
  - Flutamide

- Treatment of prostate carcinoma (see box above).
  - Inhibition of the tumour flare associated with initiation of gonadorelin analogue therapy.
  - Treatment of prostate carcinoma refractory to gonadorelin analogues.
- Treatment of benign prostatic hyperplasia (finasteride).
- Cytoproterone is occasionally used, in combination with ethinylestradiol, for the treatment of severe acne and hirsutism in women (specialized use).
- Cyproterone is occasionally used for the treatment of severe hypersexuality and sexual deviation (specialized use).

- These drugs are metabolized in the liver; their effects can be greatly enhanced if the patient has severe hepatic insufficiency. This is particularly true of cyproterone. Reduce the dose or consider another drug.
- These drugs are rarely given to women, but will cause feminization of a male fetus if given during pregnancy.
- No dosage adjustment is usually required in renal insufficiency.
- If cyproterone is to be used for hypersexuality, the following contraindications apply. They do not apply to the use of the drug for prostate cancer, when the risk/benefit equation is different.
  - Under 18 years old.
  - Severe diabetes mellitus.
  - History of thromboembolism.
  - Sickle cell disease.

Inhibition of the tumour flare associated with starting gonadorelin analogue therapy

- Gonadorelin analogues initially stimulate release of LH, followed by a prolonged fall. This initial release can induce a tumour flare; in rare cases this has led to spinal cord compression.

- Start the anti-androgen 3 days before the gonadorelin analogue and continue treatment for 3 weeks.

Treatment of prostate carcinoma refractory to gonadorelin analogues

- There are several therapeutic options in refractory prostate cancer. Specialist advice should be sought.

Treatment of benign prostatic hyperplasia (finasteride)

- See alpha-blockers (p. 474) for more information.
- Reduced testosterone metabolism reduces prostate size. This improves obstructive symptoms.
- It can take several months before the full effect of treatment is seen.
- An alternative drug treatment is an α_1-selective alpha-blocker (see p. 472), but finasteride may be a better choice if the prostate is very enlarged.

Treatment of severe acne and hirsutism in women (cyproterone)

- Cyproterone acetate is given in combination with ethinylestradiol in a cyclical manner. Treatment is usually for 21 days, followed by 7 days off.
- Once the acne has resolved, treatment should be stopped.

Treatment of severe hypersexuality (cyproterone)

- This is a specialized use and should only be undertaken by specialists.
- Cytoproterone reduces libido and fertility, but is not a male contraceptive.

- The anti-androgenic actions of these drugs will often cause the following symptoms in men:
  - Hot flushes.
  - Breast tenderness/gynaecomastia.
  - Reduced libido and erectile impotence.
- In addition, these drugs can cause gastrointestinal adverse effects: nausea, vomiting, anorexia, constipation, and diarrhoea.
- Hepatotoxicity
  - Cyproterone acetate. This is characterized by raised transaminases and can be severe. It is more common at higher dosages (200–300 mg daily) and usually develops 2–3 months after starting treatment. See monitoring section below.
  - Bicalutamide and flutamide can cause cholestasis.

- These drugs are subject to few drug interactions. The manufacturers of bicalutamide advise that terfenidine should not be given with bicalutamide.

Safety

- Cyproterone. Measure the liver transaminases before treatment starts, after 2–3 months, and 6-monthly thereafter.
- If cyproterone is to be used for hypersexuality it is recommended that a full blood count and spermatogram are performed before treatment starts.

Efficacy

- Assessment of treatment efficacy in prostate cancer is complex, but will usually include clinical assessment and measurement of the prostate-specific antigen (PSA).

- Note that finasteride can reduce markers such as the PSA and thus interfere with the diagnosis and monitoring of prostate cancer.

- Warn the patient of the risk of gynaecomastia and breast tenderness.
- Warn the patient about the possibility of erectile impotence.
- Warn the patient that these drugs can take some time to become fully effective.

Prescribing information: **Anti-androgens**

Bicalutamide

- With orchidectomy or gonadorelin therapy, by mouth, 50 mg daily (in gonadorelin therapy, started 3 days before; see notes above).
- For advanced prostate cancer, by mouth, 150 mg once daily.

Flutamide

- For prostate cancer, by mouth, 250 mg 3 times daily.

Finasteride

- For benign prostatic hyperplasia, by mouth, 5 mg daily.

Cytoproterone acetate

- Flare with initial gonadorelin therapy, 300 mg daily in 2 or 3 divided doses, reduced to 200 mg daily in 2 or 3 divided doses if necessary.
- Long-term palliative therapy when gonadorelin analogues or orchidectomy are contraindicated, or not tolerated, or when oral therapy is preferred, 200–300 mg daily in 2 or 3 divided doses.
- Hot flushes with gonadorelin therapy or after orchidectomy, initially 50 mg daily, adjusted according to response to 50–150 mg daily in 1–3 divided doses.
- Male hypersexuality, 50 mg twice daily after food.
- Hormone treatment for acne, co-cyprindiol 2000/35 (cyproterone acetate 2 mg, ethinylestradiol 35 micrograms).
  - 1 tablet daily for 21 days starting on day 1 of menstrual cycle and repeated after a 7-day interval. Usually given for several months.
  - Withdraw when acne or hirsutism has completely resolved (repeat courses can be given if they recur).

Tamoxifen

Antagonist of the effects of oestrogen on tissues; also a partial agonist

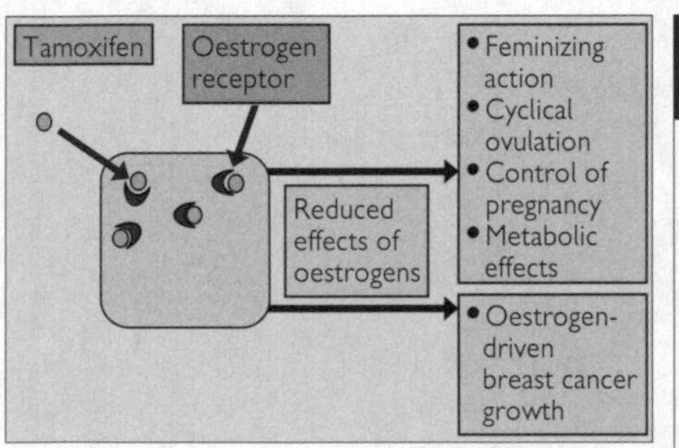

Additional treatments for breast cancer

- If a woman does not respond to treatment with tamoxifen, she is unlikely to respond to other hormonal treatments.
- If she does respond, consider the following in addition to tamoxifen.
- Premenopausal women
  - Ovarian ablation
  - Progestogen
- Postmenopausal women
  - Aromatase inhibitor*
  - Progestogen

*See notes below

- Adjuvant hormonal treatment of oestrogen receptor-positive breast cancer.
- Treatment of female infertility owing to oligomenorrhoea or secondary amenorrhoea (e.g. polycystic ovary syndrome); specialized use.
- Treatment of mastalgia when this is clearly cyclical and related to oestrogen production; unlicensed use.

- Tamoxifen is contraindicated in pregnancy. Ensure that premenopausal women taking tamoxifen use a non-hormonal form of contraception.
- There is an increased risk of thromboembolism when tamoxifen is given with cytotoxic drugs; take appropriate precautions.
- No dosage adjustment is usually required in renal or hepatic insufficiency.

Breast cancer

- Tamoxifen delays oestrogen-driven growth of tumours and metastases and prolongs life.
- If tolerated, it should be given for 5 years.
- About 60% of oestrogen receptor-positive cancers respond. Less than 10% of oestrogen receptor-negative cancers respond.
- No additional benefit has been demonstrated at daily doses above 20 mg.

Female infertility

- Tamoxifen reduces oestrogen feedback on the pituitary, increasing gonadotrophin release. This promotes effective ovulation.
- This is a specialized use and requires appropriate investigation and supervision.

Mastalgia

- Rule out serious causes of breast pain before considering treatment with tamoxifen.
- Consider simple analgesia first.
  - Gamolenic acid (derived from evening primrose oil) is no longer licensed for this indication because of lack of evidence of benefit.
- If tamoxifen is appropriate, give it on the days when symptoms are predicted.

- Adverse effects are related to inhibition of the effects of oestrogen.
- Tamoxifen causes endometrial changes and increases the risk of endometrial cancer.
  - Promptly investigate any menstrual irregularity, bleeding, discharge, or pelvic pain.
  - The CSM has advised that the risk of endometrial cancer is usually greatly outweighed by the benefits from treating breast cancer with tamoxifen.
- Tamoxifen can cause menopausal symptoms: hot flushes, vaginal bleeding, and discharge (note effects on the endometrium above).
- Tamoxifen increases the risk of thromboembolism. Take precautions and advise the patient to report swollen, painful legs or breathlessness promptly.
- Nausea and vomiting are common (10% of patients).
- Tamoxifen can cause oedema.
- Occasionally, tamoxifen causes a tumour flare with pain. It can also cause hypercalcaemia if bony metastases are extensive.
- There is a risk of multiple pregnancy when tamoxifen is used for infertility, but this is rarely more than twins.

- Tamoxifen potentiates the effect of warfarin.

Safety and efficacy

- Check the histology report to see if the patient is likely to benefit from treatment with tamoxifen (oestrogen receptor-positive).
- Ensure that the patient is well hydrated and measure the serum calcium if she has bony metastases and is starting to use tamoxifen.
- Look for signs of deep venous thrombosis or pulmonary embolism.

- Advise the patient to report menstrual irregularity or vaginal discharge/bleeding promptly.
- Warn the patient of the risk of VTE; advise her how to recognize the signs.
- Warn the patient of the risk of multiple pregnancy when tamoxifen is used for infertility.

Prescribing information: **Tamoxifen**

- Breast cancer, by mouth 20 mg daily.
- Infertility (specialized use), by mouth, 20 mg on days 2, 3, 4, and 5 of the cycle.

Note on aromatase inhibitors for breast cancer

Drugs in this class

- Anastrozole.
- Letrozole.
- Exemastane.
- (Aminoglutethimide and trilostane are poorly tolerated and may need corticosteroid replacement.)

Use

- There is increasing evidence of benefit from these drugs in the first-line adjuvant treatment of breast cancer.
- These drugs block the peripheral conversion of androgens to oestrogens.
- Take care if the patient has severe renal or hepatic insufficiency.
- They are contraindicated in pregnancy.
- None of these drugs is indicated in premenopausal women.
- Their adverse effects are similar to those of tamoxifen.
- They are usually well tolerated.
- These drugs should be given under the direction of a specialist.

Prostaglandins

Metabolites of arachidonic acid

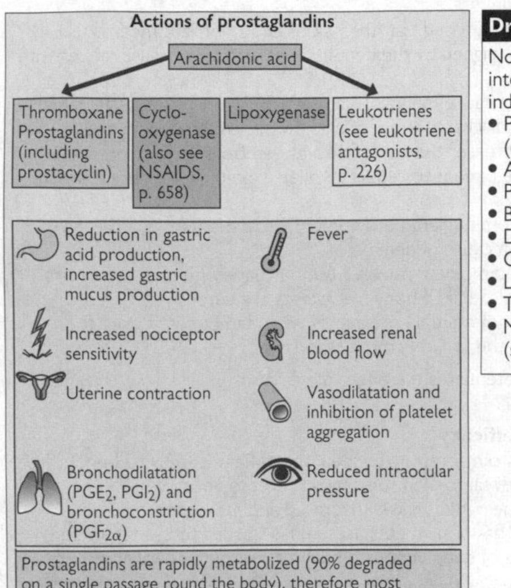

Drugs in this class

Note that they are not interchangeable (see indications section)

- Prostacyclin (epoprostenol)
- Alprostadil
- Prostaglandin E_1
- Bimatoprost
- Dinoprostone
- Gemeprost
- Latanoprost
- Travoprost
- Misoprostol (see p. 30)

- Prostaglandins and prostaglandin analogues have a wide range of clinical uses, but the drugs are not interchangeable.
- Prostacyclin (epoprostenol) is a potent vasodilator given by infusion for:
  - Inhibition of platelet aggregation during dialysis.
  - Primary pulmonary hypertension.
- Treatment of erectile dysfunction (alprostadil, prostaglandin E_1).
- Maintenance of patent ductus arteriosus in patients with congenital heart disease before surgery (prostaglandin E_1); specialized use.
- Treatment of glaucoma (latanoprost, travoprost, bimatoprost).
- Obstetric uses (gemeprost, dinoprostone, misoprostol).
  - Induction and augmentation of labour.
  - Second-line treatment of postpartum haemorrhage.
  - Induction of abortion.
- Misoprostol is used for treatment and prevention of benign gastric and duodenal ulcers (see misoprostol, p. 30).

- Consider all the potential actions of these drugs before giving them systemically.
- Systemic use of prostaglandins is contraindicated during pregnancy (unless used for obstetric purposes outlined above).
- Do not give prostaglandins to women with unexplained vaginal bleeding.

- Avoid giving prostaglandins for erectile dysfunction if the patient has a physical abnormality of the penis (e.g. cavernosal fibrosis). Refer the patient for a specialist opinion.
  - Take care if the patient is at risk of priapism (e.g. in sickle cell disease).

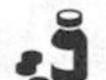

Treatment of glaucoma (see p. 605 for guidance)

- See also beta-blockers (p. 140).
- Until recently, beta-blockers were first-line therapy. Latanoprost is now an alternative first-line therapy.
- Latanoprost is more effective at lowering intraocular pressure than timolol (a beta-blocker). It causes fewer systemic unwanted effects and has fewer contraindications.
  - Latanoprost is given once daily.
  - It costs about four times as much as timolol.
- Many patients with glaucoma will require treatment with more than one drug in order to reduce their intraocular pressure sufficiently.

Obstetric uses

- The use of prostaglandins in obstetrics should be under the direction of a specialist. Prostaglandins are indicated for augmentation of uncomplicated labour. Seek further guidance if the pregnancy has been complicated in any way.
- Dinoprostone and gemeprost are given vaginally to ripen and soften the cervix.
- Misoprostol is then given systemically to augment uterine contraction.
  - See misoprostol (p. 30) for its other uses.
  - Oxytocin (Syntocinon®) is an alternative.
- NICE offers the following advice for the management of induction of labour;
  - Dinoprostone is preferred over oxytocin for induction in women with intact membranes.
  - Dinoprostone and oxytocin are equally effective, but dinoprostone is safer.
  - Wait 6 hours after a prostaglandin has been given before giving oxytocin.
- Carboprost is used as a second-line treatment in postpartum haemorrhage.
  - Ergometrine and oxytocin (Syntometrine®) are first-line drugs.

Erectile dysfunction

- See sildenafil (p. 205) for more information on the aetiology and investigation of erectile dysfunction.
- The Government has set limits on the prescribing of drugs in the NHS for erectile dysfunction in the UK. See sildenafil (p. 205) for details.
- Alprostadil is given by intracavernosal injection or intraurethral application.

Prostacyclin

- This is an effective treatment for primary pulmonary hypertension, but it has to be given by intravenous infusion as it has a short half-life (3 minutes). It is often given with an anticoagulant.

- Large doses of prostaglandins given during labour can cause uterine rupture.
- Other adverse effects from systemic prostaglandins include: nausea and vomiting, bronchospasm, flushing, hypertension, cardiovascular collapse.
    - The risk of severe effects is greatest with prostacyclin.
- Topical prostaglandins applied to the eye increase brown pigmentation of the iris and can cause local irritation.

- Prostaglandins are subject to few drug interactions.
    - Systemic prostaglandins can enhance the effects of other drugs that lower blood pressure.
    - Prostaglandins enhance the actions of oxytocic drugs.

- In patients taking a prostaglandin to prevent NSAID-induced blood loss, blood loss can nevertheless occur and can be occult and chronic. Have a low threshold for measuring a full blood count. Chronic diseases are often associated with an anaemia, but ensure that it is not due to iron deficiency through blood loss.

- Warn women that they should not take these drugs systemically if they are planning a pregnancy (topical formulations are safe).
- Warn patients that prostaglandin eye drops will increase brown pigmentation of the eye.

Prescribing information: **Prostaglandins**

The following is given as an example.

Glaucoma

- Latanoprost eye drops 50 micrograms/mL. Apply once daily, preferably in the evening.

The other indications are specialized; seek expert advice.

Oxytocin

An endogenous posterior pituitary hormone

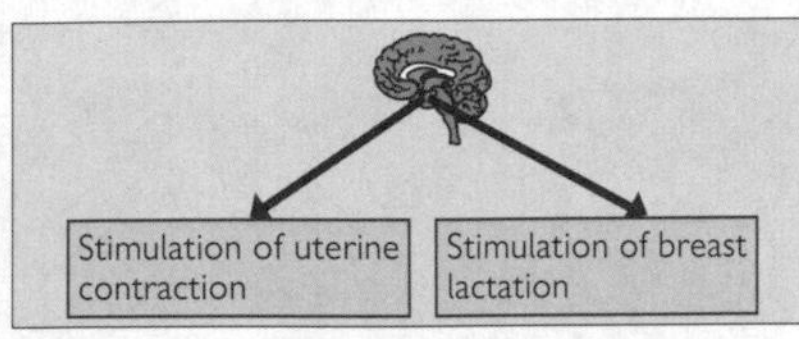

Formulations available

(Note the similar sounding names)
- Oxytocin alone (Syntocinon®)
- Oxytocin with ergometrine (Syntometrine®)

- To induce or augment labour.
  - Prostaglandins are preferred (see prostaglandins, p. 450).
- To treat and prevent postpartum haemorrhage.
  - Syntometrine® routinely used for the management of the third stage of labour.

- These drugs should never be used if there is a mechanical obstruction to labour.
- Induction and augmentation of labour should be under the direction of a specialist.

Obstetric uses

- These drugs are indicated for augmentation of uncomplicated labour. Seek further guidance if the pregnancy has been complicated.
- Oxytocin should usually only be given 6 hours after a prostaglandin has been given vaginally.
- Oxytocin is given by intravenous infusion. Start with a very low dose (see below) and gradually increase the dose as required. See below for more information.
- Take care — excessive doses can cause serious adverse effects.

Postpartum haemorrhage

- Give oxytocin by intravenous infusion at a rate to control uterine atony. Note that oxytocin will not constrict blood vessels directly.
- If the patient does not respond, consider giving a prostaglandin.

- Very rapid induction of labour can cause amniotic fluid embolism; increase the dose gradually.
- Large doses can cause fluid retention (water intoxication and hyponatraemia).
- Oxytocin can cause hypersensitivity reactions. The most common reaction is a rash, but it can also cause anaphylactoid reactions (see acetylcysteine, p. 625).

- These drugs are subject to few drug interactions.
  - They enhance the actions of prostaglandins given during labour.

- Measure the number of contractions in 10 minutes (aim for 3 or 4). Measure the fetal heart rate. Seek expert advice if labour is not progressing or there are signs of fetal distress.
- Follow the advice below on drug dilution, so that the concentration delivered is standardized.

- Warn women that uterine contractions will be painful and that oxytocin will make contractions more frequent and stronger.

Prescribing information: **Oxytocin**

Induction and augmentation of labour (NICE guidance)

- Oxytocin, 10 units in 500 mL of 5% glucose or 0.9% saline. A rate of 3 mL/h will deliver 0.001 units/min.
- Start the infusion at 0.001–0.002 units/min.
- Increase the rate at intervals of not less than 30 minutes.
- Aim for 3 or 4 contractions every 10 minutes.
- 0.012 units/min is usually adequate.
- The maximum rate is 0.032 units/min.

Prevention of postpartum haemorrhage

- Syntometrine® (oxytocin 5 units, ergometrine 500 micrograms); single intramuscular injection on delivery of the baby.

Treatment of postpartum haemorrhage

- Begin with oxytocin, 5–10 units by intravenous injection.
- If required, follow this with an infusion of 5–30 units in 500 mL, given at a rate to induce uterine contractions.

TEACHING POINT

Practical advice on the safe use of variable-rate intravenous infusions

- If drugs are given by variable-rate intravenous infusion (e.g. in intensive care), precision is essential; the potential for harm is great.

The following is offered as general advice.

- Maintain strict asepsis throughout. Change intravenous cannulas regularly (every 2 days). Remove any lines that show signs of infection.
- Ensure that you have secure, free-flowing venous access.
  - In many cases, central venous access is required (e.g. when giving noradrenaline).
- It is good practice to give each drug through a separate intravenous line.
  - Some drugs must not be mixed (e.g. calcium gluconate and sodium bicarbonate will form insoluble calcium carbonate if mixed). If two infusions must be given together, check the compatability with a pharmacist.
  - Stop the infusion if the solution becomes discoloured or cloudy.
- Check whether the solution needs special handling. For example:
  - To be shielded from light.
  - To be buffered to a certain pH before use.
- Control the rate of infusion with an infusion pump whenever possible. Relying on counting the drip rate in a standard giving set is unwise; the rate can change with the position of the infusion bag or position of the intravenous cannula.
- Use standard dilutions of drugs. It is usually better to alter the rate of the infusion rather than the amount of drug in the infusion.
  - Standard dilutions make calculations easier and are recognizable to other healthcare professionals, reducing the risk of administration errors.
  - For example, if one adds 50 units of soluble insulin to 50 mL isotonic saline, the rate (in mL/h) is clearly related to the dose delivered (in units/h). By contrast, an infusion containing 35 units soluble insulin in 50 mL of isotonic saline delivers 0.7 units/mL; this is likely to cause confusion and makes calculating the rate required much more difficult.

Somatostatin and analogues

Naturally occurring peptide hormone and its analogues

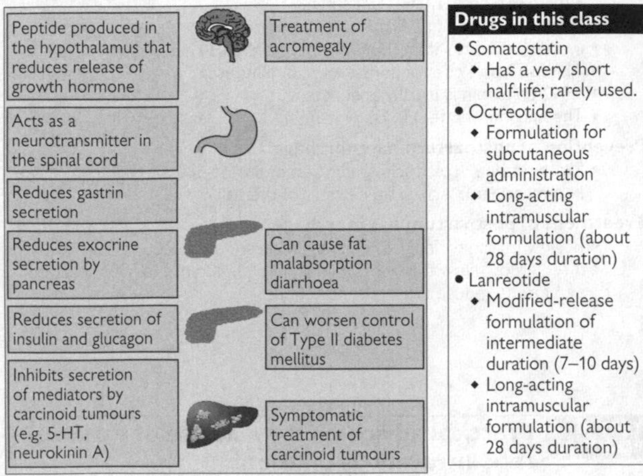

- Treatment of acromegaly.
- Relief of symptoms of neuroendocrine tumours (especially carcinoid tumours).
- Adjunctive treatment of bleeding oesophageal varices; specialized, unlicensed use.
- Prevention of complications following pancreatic surgery; specialized use.
- Treatment of nausea and vomiting in palliative care.

- No dosage reduction is usually required in renal or hepatic insufficiency.
- These drugs suppress fetal growth; avoid them during pregnancy if possible.

- Initiation and titration of treatment with these drugs should be by a specialist.

Treatment of acromegaly

- Somatostatin analogues are usually indicated in patients who are not cured by surgery or radiotherapy.
- The aim of treatment is to suppress the secretion of growth hormone (GH) and insulin-like growth factor (IGF-1).
  - Somatostatin analogues are effective in about 60% of patients.
  - Long-acting formulations usually give better control than short-acting ones.

Treatment of carcinoid tumours

- Somatostatin analogues are effective for the classical symptoms of the carcinoid syndrome (flushing, watery diarrhoea) but do not usually have any effect on the progression of the disease.

- Treatment usually begins with subcutaneous octreotide in order to stabilize the patient, after which a long-acting formulation can be used. These take several weeks to reach their maximum effect, so should be covered by subcutaneous octreotide at first.
  - Give the patient a supply of short-acting octreotide to use for breakthrough symptoms.
- Intravenous octreotide can be given perioperatively to stabilize patients with carcinoid tumours.
  - Similarly, it can be given to patients who are gravely ill owing to a carcinoid crisis.

Other uses

- Octreotide can be given as adjunctive treatment for bleeding oesophageal varices. Used alone, it is rarely sufficient; endoscopic intervention is usually the first-line treatment. Discuss the patient's management with a gastroenterologist. See also vasopressin (p. 476).
- See use of syringe drivers in palliative care section (p. 654) for treatment of nausea and vomiting.
- The use of these drugs after pancreatic surgery is very specialized; seek expert advice.

- Initiation of somatostatin analogue treatment for acromegaly can cause the pituitary to increase in size.
  - Monitor the patient very carefully during early treatment (see below).
- Local injection site reactions are common.
  - Rotate injection sites.
- Somatostatin analogues can cause fat malabsorption by reducing pancreatic exocrine function.
  - Consider giving pancreatin (Creon®).
- Somatostatin analogues reduce insulin release.
  - This can worsen symptoms if the patient has an insulinoma.
  - It can increase hypoglycaemic drug requirements in patients with Type II diabetes mellitus.
  - It can cause hyperglycaemia in a few patients.
- Somatostatin analogues can promote gallstone formation.
  - Avoid abrupt withdrawal; it can precipitate biliary colic and pancreatitis.
- Somatostatin analogues can cause hypothyroidism; this is rare.

- These drugs reduce the absorption of ciclosporin.
- These drugs affect insulin secretion, which can affect the treatment of Type II diabetes mellitus (see above).

Safety and efficacy

- Somatostatin analogue treatment for acromegaly can cause the pituitary to increase in size. Assess the patient's visual fields and ask about headache.
- Efficacy in acromegaly is assessed by measurement of the plasma concentration of growth hormone (GH) and insulin-like growth factor 1 (IGF-1). The usual target for GH is a plasma concentration below 5 mU/L.
- Efficacy in carcinoid syndrome is assessed in terms of symptom control. These drugs are effective for the classical symptoms of carcinoid syndrome, but remember to ask about others (e.g. pain).

- If long-term treatment is anticipated, measure thyroid function every 6 months.
- The manufacturers recommend that patients have an ultrasound scan to look for gallstones every 6 months.
    - The presence of gallstones would not necessarily lead to withdrawal of the drug.

- Advise patients with acromegaly to report any visual changes or headache (see above).
- Explain to patients with carcinoid tumours that these drugs may improve their symptoms but are unlikely to alter the progression of their disease.

Prescribing information: **Somatostatin analogues**

The initiation and supervision of these drugs should be under the direction of a specialist.

Octreotide

- By subcutaneous injection.
    - Usual initial dose 100 micrograms tds.
    - May be increased to 200 micrograms tds according to response.
- Depot modified-release formulation (Sandostatin LAR®).
    - Microsphere powder for resuspension and intramuscular injection, initially 20 mg monthly.
    - Can be increased to 30 mg monthly, or reduced to 10 mg monthly, as required.

Lanreotide

- Depot modified-release formulation (Somatuline LA®).
    - Microparticles for resuspension and intramuscular injection, initially 30 mg every 14 days.
    - Dose frequency can be increased to every 7–10 days if required.
- Depot modified-release formulation (Somatuline Autogel®).
    - Aqueous gel for intramuscular injection, dose range 60–120 mg monthly.

Chapter 7

Kidneys and the urinary tract

Contents

Renal insufficiency

Drugs are subjected to three processes in the kidneys:

- Glomerular filtration (GFR) of non-protein-bound drug.
- Active secretion.
- Passive reabsorption.

GFR is quantified by measuring the clearance of molecules such as creatinine and inulin. Creatinine clearance is calculated from a 24-hour urine collection:

$$\text{Creatinine clearance (mL/min)} = \frac{\text{Urine concentration of creatinine (micromol/L)} \times \text{urine volume (mL)}}{\text{Serum concentration of creatinine (micromol/L)} \times \text{time (min)}}$$

Creatinine clearance is higher than GFR owing to tubular excretion of creatinine. The difference between GFR and creatinine clearance is greater as renal function worsens. At around 10% of normal renal function (the level at which dialysis may be considered), creatinine clearance is around twice GFR (as tubular creatinine excretion is relatively preserved).

The serum creatinine concentration can be used as a surrogate of creatinine clearance, but is not ideal, as it is affected by the patient's age, sex, and weight. The Cockroft–Gault equation provides a reasonable estimate of creatinine clearance by taking these factors into account:

$$\text{Creatinine clearance (mL/min)} = \frac{[140 - \text{age (in years)}] \times \text{body weight in kg} \times F}{\text{Serum creatinine (micromol/L)}}$$

(F = 1.04 for women, 1.23 for men)

The definitions of mild, moderate, and severe renal impairment are as follows. These are used throughout this book and are the same as those stated in the BNF.

Severity of renal impairment	GFR (mL/min)	Approx. serum creatinine concentration (micromol/L)
Mild	20–50	150–300
Moderate	10–20	300–700
Severe	Less than 10	More than 700

The effects of age, weight, and sex on creatinine clearance estimated using the Cockroft–Gault equation

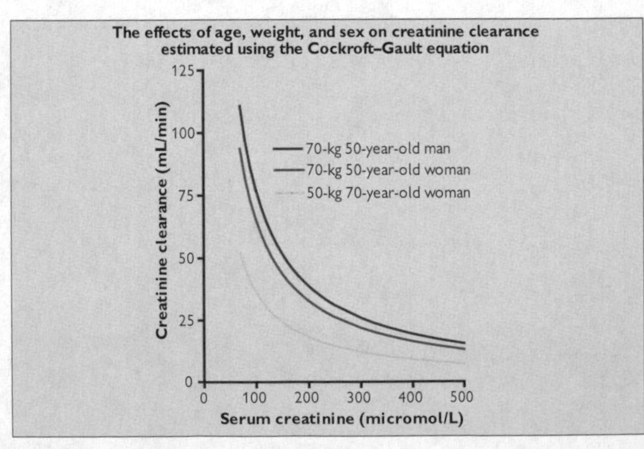

Drug-induced renal damage

Drugs can cause renal damage in a number of ways, including effects on:

- Renal blood flow
- The nephron
- The interstitial tissues

The lists given below are not exhaustive. See adverse effects sections of individual drugs for more information on renal toxicity.

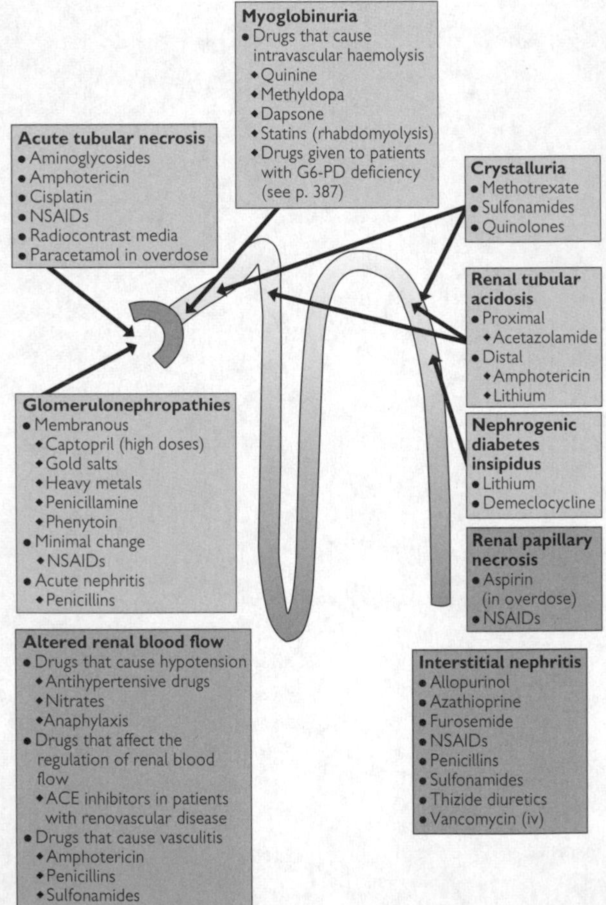

Drugs and renal stones

Symptomatic treatment of renal colic

- Relief of pain:
  - Give *either* an opioid (e.g. morphine 10 mg sc or im). (Pethidine is widely used, but is not recommended, as its metabolites accumulate in renal insufficiency and can cause seizures.)
  - *Or* an NSAID (e.g. diclofenac 75 mg im followed by a second dose 30 minutes later, or a single dose of 100 mg pr).
- Management of the renal stone itself should be under the direction of a specialist.

Prevention of renal stones

- In most cases, treatment of renal calculi should involve definitive treatment of the underlying cause (e.g. parathyroid adenoma), but in some conditions this is not possible, and drugs have a role in long-term prevention.
- In all cases a high fluid intake is important.
- Aim for a urine output of 2.5–3.0 L/day.

Calcium oxalate and apatite stones in patients with hypercalciuria

- Thiazide diuretics promote renal tubular calcium reabsorption (e.g. bendroflumethiazide 5 mg daily).
- Reducing calcium absorption from the gut reduces stone formation (e.g. sodium cellulose phosphate 12–15 g daily).
- If the patient also has high uric acid secretion, allopurinol can help.

Uric acid stones

- In most cases maintaining a high fluid intake and treatment with allopurinol is all that is required.
- An acidic urine promotes uric acid stone formation; consider urinary alkalinization with potassium citrate 10 mL tds.
  - Adjust the dose to keep the urinary pH at around 8.0; excessive alkalinization promotes calcium stone formation.

Cystinuria

- Alkalinize the urine with either potassium citrate 10 mL tds or sodium bicarbonate 12 g daily.
  - Adjust the dose to keep the urinary pH above 8.0.
- In the most severe cases, consider treatment with penicillamine. The usual dose is 250 mg tds, but this can be increased to 500 mg qds.

Drugs and renal replacement therapy (dialysis or filtration)

Drugs that are removed from the body in significant quantities by dialysis or filtration are listed in Table 7.1. Haemodialysis or filtration are important in several circumstances relating to drug therapy:

- During chronic haemodialysis.
  - Removal of drugs by dialysis can reduce the effectiveness of some drug treatments. Avoid taking these drugs just before dialysis. Discuss the treatment regimen with a renal physician.
  - Routine dialysis or filtration can cause changes in the body's physiology (e.g. changes in fluid and electrolyte balance) which may alter the response to the drug.
  - Drugs can alter the kinetics of dialysis or filtration. For example, vasodilators and vasoconstrictors can alter the rate of clearance of drugs by dialysis or filtration by altering the rate of blood flow.
- During emergency haemodialysis/haemofiltration.
  - Continuous filtration can remove significant amounts of drugs such as antibiotics, rendering them less effective. Seek expert advice from a medical microbiologist and renal physician.
- For severe cases of self poisoning.
  - Drugs for which dialysis is effective in poisoning are marked in Table 7.1 with an asterisk.

The extent to which a drug is removed from the body during renal replacement therapy (dialysis or haemofiltration) depends on the drug, characteristics of the patient, and the equipment.

- The drug
  - *Molecular weight* The larger the drug molecule the less quickly it is cleared by dialysis. For drugs of molecular weight below 500 Da the effective membrane surface area and the rate of flow of blood and dialysate are important. For drugs with molecular weights above 500 Da, only the membrane surface area is important.
  - *Water solubility* Poorly water-soluble drugs are poorly dialysed and filtered, since dialysis fluids are aqueous.
  - *Protein binding* Drugs that are highly protein-bound are poorly cleared by dialysis or filtration.
  - *Volume of distribution* If a drug is extensively bound in body tissues, even if it passes readily across dialysis or filter membranes, little of the total drug will be removed from the body.
  - *The usual route of drug clearance* If a drug is mostly eliminated by hepatic metabolism at a rate of clearance appreciably greater than the rate of dialysis or filtration clearance, dialysis or filtration will have little effect on total clearance.
- Characteristics of the patient
  - The total clearance of a drug is proportional to body weight, but dialysis or filtration clearance is constant for a given piece of equipment and a given flow rate. This means that the smaller the patient, the more dialysis will contribute to total body clearance.
- Characteristics of the equipment
  - *The membrane* The rate of clearance of a drug by dialysis or filtration varies with the type of membrane used.
  - *The rate of flow of fluid* The higher the rate of flow of dialysis or filtration fluid, the higher the rate of clearance.

Table 7.1

Drugs removed from the body in significant quantities by dialysis or filtration

ACE inhibitors	Diphenhydramine	Nitroprusside
Aciclovir	Ethambutol	Paracetamol
Allopurinol	Ethanol	Pentazocine
Aminoglycosides	Fluorides	Phenobarbital*
Amoxicillin	5-Fluorocytosine	Phenytoin*
Ampicillin	5-Fluorouracil	Prednisolone
Atenolol	Gallamine	Primidone
Azathioprine	Isoniazid	Procainamide
Bromides	Lithium*	Quinidine
Cephalosporins	Methanol	Quinine
Chloral hydrate derivatives*	Methotrexate	Ranitidine
	Methyldopa	Salicylates (aspirin)*
Cisplatin	Metoprolol	Sotalol
Co-trimoxazole	Metronidazole	Sulfonamides
Cyclophosphamide	Mushrooms, poisonous	Theophylline
Diazoxide	Nitrofurantoin	Trimethoprim

*Drugs for which dialysis is effective in poisoning

Drugs used in the management of chronic renal insufficiency

See individual articles for more information on the use of these drugs.

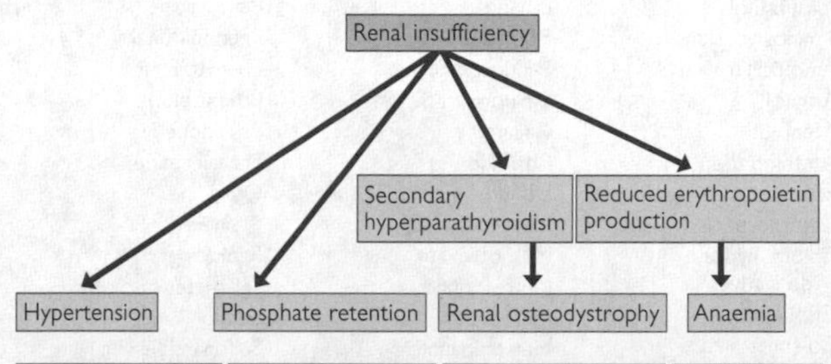

Hypertension

- Diuretics are not effective in severe renal insufficiency, as they act in the lumen of the tubule and require glomerular filtration.
- ACE inhibitors can be effective, but can cause further deterioration in renal function if the patient has renovascular disease.
- Avoid alpha$_1$-adrenoceptor antagonists in patients who are water- or sodium-depleted; they can cause severe hypotension.

Phosphate retention

- Calcium carbonate binds phosphate in the gut lumen and prevents its absorption.
  - The usual dose is 2.5–9.0 g/day taken with meals.
- Aluminium hydroxide also binds phosphate, but the aluminium causes encephalopathy with long-term use.

Renal osteodystrophy

Renal osteodystrophy is resistant to treatment with conventional forms of vitamin D because it requires 1-alfa-hydroxylation in the kidney to become active. Treatment is therefore with:

- 1-alfa-hydroxycholecalciferol (alfacalcidol).
- Or 1-alfa,25-dihydroxycholecalciferol (calcitriol).

Anaemia

Recombinant erythropoietin therapy.

Alpha-adrenoceptor antagonists (alpha-blockers)

Antagonists at alpha-adrenoceptors

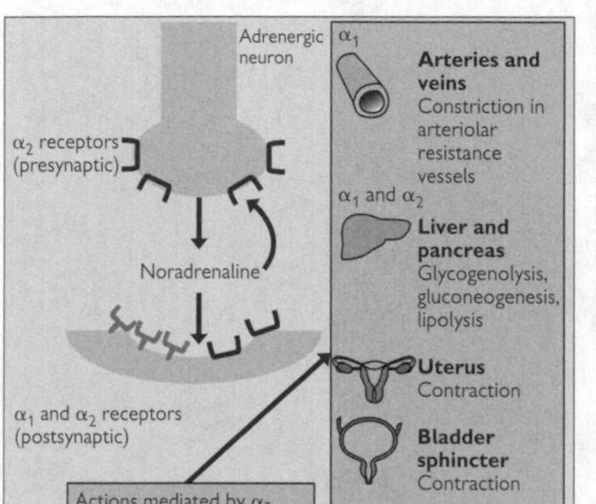

Drugs in this class

Non-selective drugs
- Phentolamine
- Phenoxybenzamine

α_1-selective drugs
- Prazosin
- Doxazosin
- Indoramin
- Terazosin
- Alfuzosin
- Tamsulosin

- The indications for non-selective α-blockers are specialized.
  - Treatment of hypertension due to a phaeochromocytoma.
  - Treatment of the hypertension due to drug interactions between amines and MAOIs.
  - Treatment of vasospasm (e.g. ergotism).
- The α_1-selective drugs are used for the treatment of:
  - Hypertension.
  - Benign prostatic hyperplasia (BPH).

- There is no evidence of toxicity from these drugs during pregnancy, but they should only be given when the indication is clear.
- The initial doses of these drugs may need to be reduced in renal or hepatic insufficiency.
- These drugs can precipitate or worsen heart failure.
- Do not give these drugs if the patient has micturition syncope (they can cause hypotension).

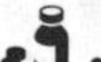

Hypertension (α_1-selective drugs)

- These drugs can cause the blood pressure to fall very rapidly as they have no presynaptic action (blocking α_2 receptors causes a tachycardia). This is particularly true for prazosin, terazosin, and alfuzosin.
- Start with a low dose and increase gradually.
- These drugs are most commonly used as add-on therapy in patients with hypertension that responds poorly to other drugs (e.g. in those with chronic renal insufficency).

Benign prostatic hyperplasia (BPH)

- See below for more information.
- These drugs should not be given to treat patients with acute retention, who should be catheterized.

- The treatment options for patients with BPH include:
  - Surgery.
  - An α_1-selective blocker.
  - Finasteride (see anti-androgens, p. 444).
- These drugs improve obstructive symptoms, but may not improve symptoms of bladder irritation.

Phaeochromocytoma

- Non-selective alpha-blockers are used short-term in combination with beta-blockers before and during surgery.
- The alpha-blocker is started before the beta-blocker (starting the beta-blocker first can cause severe hypertension).
- This is a specialized area of treatment.

- The most important adverse effect of these drugs is postural hypotension. This can be severe, especially after the first dose.
  - Advise the patient to take the drug in bed.
- These drugs can cause dry mouth, tachycardia, and headache.
- Occasionally they can cause erectile impotence and priapism.
- Indoramin can cause sedation.
- Hypersensitivity reactions are uncommon.

- The hypotensive action of these drugs is enhanced by diuretics and other drugs that lower blood pressure.
- Do not give indoramin with MAOIs or linezolid; this can cause a tyramine-like reaction (see MAOIs, p. 286).
  - Alcohol enhances the effect of indoramin.

Safety and efficacy

- Measure the blood pressure lying and standing before any dosage increments.
- Ask the patient about urinary outflow symptoms. Consider formal urodynamic studies.

- Warn the patient that indoramin can cause dizziness that can interfere with skilled motor tasks (e.g. driving).
- Warn the patient of the risk of postural hypotension and ways to minimize this (e.g. take the drug at night and stand up slowly).

Prescribing information: **Alpha-adrenoceptor antagonists**

The uses of phenoxybenzamine and phentolamine are specialized; detailed prescribing information is not given.

α_1-selective drugs

Several drugs and formulations are available (including modified-release formulations). The following are given as examples.

Doxazosin

- Hypertension. By mouth, 1 mg daily. Increased after 1–2 weeks to 2 mg daily.
  - Can be gradually increased to a maximum of 16 mg daily.

Indoramin

- For BPH. By mouth, 20 mg bd.
  - Can be increased by 20 mg every 2 weeks to a maximum of 100 mg daily in divided doses.

Alfuzosin

- For BPH. By mouth, 2.5 mg tds.

Benign prostatic hyperplasia

- This is very common and results in two groups of symptoms:
  - Obstructive symptoms (hesitancy, reduction in force of stream).
  - Irritative bladder symptoms (increased frequency, urgency, dysuria).
- Surgery is the treatment of choice, but is not suitable for all patients; if symptoms are mild, drug treatment is appropriate.
- All drug treatments are most effective for obstructive symptoms; irritative symptoms are difficult to treat.
- $Alpha_1$-selective receptor antagonists relax prostate smooth muscle.
- Growth of prostatic tissue is in part driven by testosterone; the other drug treatments for BPH antagonize the actions of testosterone.
  - Anti-androgen drugs (see p. 444).
  - Gonadorelin analogues (see p. 440).

Antidiuretic hormone (ADH, vasopressin) and analogues

Naturally occurring nonapeptide hormone

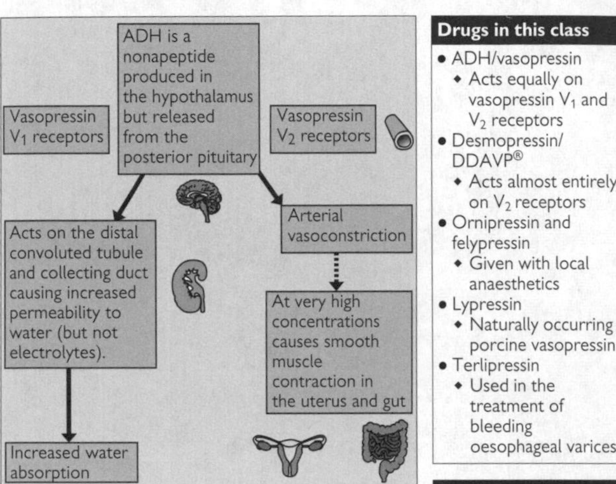

Drugs in this class

- ADH/vasopressin
  - Acts equally on vasopressin V_1 and V_2 receptors
- Desmopressin/DDAVP®
  - Acts almost entirely on V_2 receptors
- Ornipressin and felypressin
  - Given with local anaesthetics
- Lypressin
  - Naturally occurring porcine vasopressin
- Terlipressin
  - Used in the treatment of bleeding oesophageal varices

Syndrome of inappropriate secretion of ADH (SIADH)

See teaching point below.

- Treatment of cranial diabetes insipidus.
  - Long-term.
  - Short-term after trauma or pituitary surgery.
- Adjunctive treatment of bleeding oesophageal varices (terlipressin); specialized use.
- Treatment of nocturnal enuresis (desmopressin); specialized use.
- Given with local anaesthetics to delay systemic absorption (ornipressin, felypressin).
- To temporarily increase the circulating factor VIII concentration in mild/moderate haemophilia (desmopressin); specialized use.

- These drugs can cause coronary artery constriction; avoid them in patients with coronary artery disease.
  - Take care if the patient has a history of hypertension.
  - Take care if retention of water could cause problems (e.g. heart failure, raised intracranial pressure).
- These drugs increase the circulating blood volume; take care in elderly patients and those with impaired ventricular function.
- These drugs are excreted renally, but their effect is often reduced in renal disease, owing to their mechanism of action.
- Avoid these drugs in pregnancy; they have an oxytocic effect.

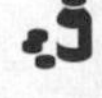

- Initiation and titration of treatment with these drugs should be by a specialist.
- Vasopressin can be given by intranasal spray or injection (sc, im, or iv). Desmopressin can be given by mouth.

- Terlipressin can be given as an adjunctive treatment for bleeding oesophageal varices. Used alone, it is rarely sufficient; endoscopic intervention is usually the first-line treatment. Discuss the patient's management with a gastroenterologist.

- These drugs are usually well tolerated; the most common adverse effects are abdominal cramp, nausea, and vomiting.
- Higher dosages can cause coronary artery constriction and cardiac ischaemia.
- Terlipressin is given in a high dose for oesophageal varices. It can cause uterine contraction, bowel evacuation, and abdominal cramps.
- Nasal sprays can cause nasal congestion and ulceration.
- Hypersensitivity to these drugs is rare.
- The most common serious adverse effect of these drugs is hyponatraemia, caused by fluid overload. See advice to patients (below) and avoid drugs that promote secretion of endogenous vasopressin.
- Some drugs stimulate the secretion of vasopressin; these may cause SIADH. They are listed below. Avoid giving these drugs with vasopressin and its analogues.

- Chlorpropamide and carbamazepine potentiate the effect of vasopressin. This action is sometimes used in the treatment of mild diabetes insipidus.

Safety and efficacy

- Assess the patient's intravascular volume clinically and by measurement of the serum sodium concentration. This is especially important while the optimal dose is being established, and if the patient's clinical condition changes in a way that might affect salt and water balance (e.g. diarrhoea, fever).

- Advise the patient to avoid water overload (drinking large volumes, swallowing a lot of water while swimming).
- Advise the patient to suspend treatment with a vasopressin analogue if they have diarrhoea or vomiting.

Prescribing information: **Vasopressin analogues**

Vasopressin

- By subcutaneous or intramuscular injection for cranial diabetes insipidus, 5–20 units every 4 hours.
- By intravenous infusion for initial treatment of bleeding oesophageal varices, 20 units over 15 minutes.

Desmopressin

- Diabetes insipidus.
  - By mouth, initially 100 micrograms tds. May be increased to a maximum of 400 micrograms tds.
  - By intranasal spray, 10–40 micrograms daily in 1 or 2 divided doses.
  - By subcutaneous, intramuscular, or intravenous injection, 1–4 micrograms daily.
- Treatment of haemophilia A (seek expert advice)
  - 0.3 micrograms/kg diluted in 50 mL of 0.9% saline and infused over 20 minutes.

Terlipressin

- By intravenous injection for bleeding oesophageal varices, 2 mg followed by 1–2 mg every 4–6 hours until bleeding is controlled. Maximum duration of treatment, 72 hours.

The syndrome of inappropriate ADH secretion (SIADH)

Diagnostic criteria

- Concentrated urine sodium (>20 mmol/L) in the presence of hyponatraemia (<125 mmol/L), or low plasma osmolality (<260 mmol/kg) in the absence of hypovolaemia.
- Caused by the inappropriate release of vasopressin or ectopic production.

Causes

- Malignancy, especially small cell lung cancer.
- CNS disorders (e.g. infection, haemorrhage, vasculitis).
- Chest disease (e.g. TB pneumonia, abscess).
- Metabolic disease (e.g. porphyria).
- Trauma, especially to the head.
- Drugs that stimulate secretion of vasopressin: chlorpropamide, clofibrate, cyclophosphamide, opioids, tricyclic antidepressants, SSRIs, vincristine.

Treatment

- Identify and treat the underlying cause whenever possible. For mild cases, fluid restriction may be all that is required.
- If the cause is chronic and cannot be removed, consider treatment with demeclocycline (demethylchlortetracycline). This causes nephrogenic diabetes insipidus (lithium also causes nephrogenic diabetes insipidus, but is not used therapeutically for this purpose).
- The drugs chlorpropamide and carbamazepine potentiate the effect of vasopressin; this action is sometimes used in the treatment of mild diabetes insipidus.
- Vasopressin receptor antagonists are in development.

Chapter 8

Malignant disease and immunosuppression

Contents

Drugs used to treat cancer

Most traditional cytotoxic drugs are designed to exploit the fact that malignant cells behave differently from normal cells in that they divide more rapidly. Cytotoxic drugs interfere with the processes of DNA replication and cell division. Their effects will be most readily seen in rapidly dividing cells. The target is the tumour, but other tissues that have rapid cell turnover rates are likely to be affected (e.g. gastrointestinal tract mucosa, hair follicles, bone marrow). This approach will always be limited by toxicity in these other organs, but for a long time it has not been possible to distinguish malignant from normal cells qualitatively. Molecular biology techniques are now dissecting the detailed phenotypes of malignant cells, and a new range of treatments (e.g. cytotoxic monoclonal antibodies) are starting to exploit the subtle differences.

As well as consisting of abnormal cells, tumours have an abnormal architecture. New treatments exploit the processes that promote this (e.g. angiogenesis, cell-cell interactions).

The last types of drug treatments target the external processes that drive and maintain malignant growth. The most recognizable of these are the glucocorticoids and drugs that block the actions of sex steroids (e.g. tamoxifen).

Drug treatments for cancer are depicted pictorially below.

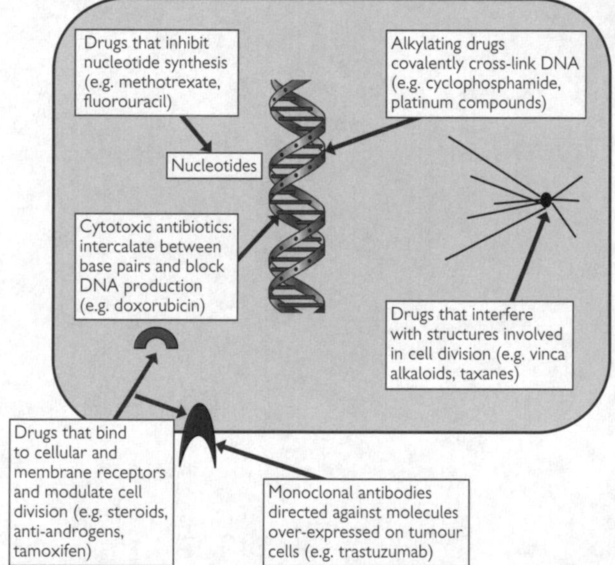

Note. Drugs used for cancer chemotherapy should only be prescribed by specialists. For this reason, detailed prescribing information is not given in this section.

Adverse effects of cytotoxic chemotherapy

Drugs used in cancer chemotherapy share adverse effects that arise from their cytotoxic actions. Drug-specific information is given in individual articles. This is intended as a general guide.

Remember that cytotoxic drugs are a hazardous to all who come into contact with them. Make sure that you are adequately protected.

- Follow your local protocol for reconstitution, storage, and administration of these drugs.
- There are special guidelines for intrathecal chemotherapy.

Local effects

Extravasation

- See cytotoxic antibiotics (p. 493) for information.

Effects that result from damage to rapidly dividing cells

Many cytotoxic drugs act on the cell cycle. They have their greatest effect on rapidly dividing cells. Cancer cells commonly divide rapidly and are destroyed. However, other cells that also divide rapidly are commonly subject to adverse effects of cytotoxic drugs.

Gastrointestinal tract

- Oral mucositis is common during treatment with fluorouracil, methotrexate, and anthracyclines.
  - Treatment is supportive.
  - Ensure good oral and dental hygiene; the mouth can be a portal for blood-borne infection.
- Diarrhoea is common.

Bone marrow

- All but bleomycin and vincristine are toxic to the bone marrow.
- The neutrophil cell line is most susceptible.
- The time course can be very variable. See individual articles for times of greatest risk.
- Colony stimulating factors are sometimes used to boost the neutrophil count (see colony stimulating factors (p. 536) for more information).
- Anaemia and thrombocytopenia are usually treated by transfusion of erythrocytes or platelets.
- Erythropoietin (see p. 532) increases erythrocyte production but is not widely used.

Hair follicles

- Alopecia is common.
- There are no effective pharmacological interventions for this.

Gonads

- Male sterility is most common when alkylating drugs are used.
- Women are less commonly affected (ova are already formed).
- Counsel patients about the risk of sterility before treatment starts. Consider sperm storage before treatment starts, in appropriate cases.

Fetus

- Almost all cytotoxic drugs are teratogenic.
- They should not be given during pregnancy; appropriate contraceptive measures should be taken.

Systemic effects

Nausea and vomiting

- See $5HT_3$ antagonists (p. 73) for more information.

Adverse effects that are specific to particular drugs

- Specific adverse effects (e.g. autonomic neuropathy due to vinca alkaloids, pulmonary fibrosis due to bleomycin) are listed in individual articles.

Chlorambucil

Alkylating cytotoxic drug

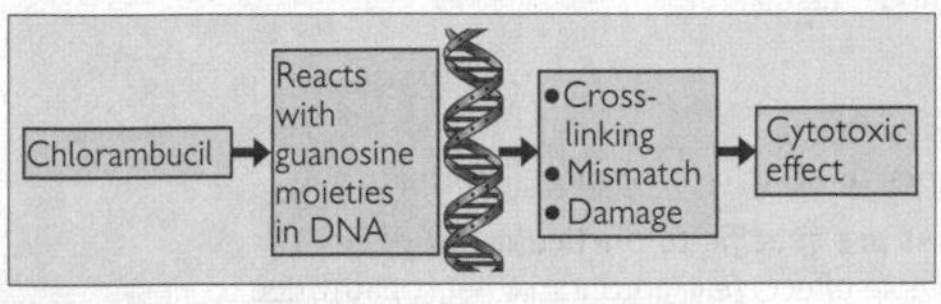

Examples of alkylating cytotoxic drugs

- Busulfan
- Carmustine
- Chlorambucil
- Chlormethine
- Cyclophosphamide
- Estramustine
- Ifosfamide
- Lomustine
- Melphalan
- Mitobronitol
- Thiotepa
- Treosulfan

- Treatment of:
  - Chronic lymphocytic leukaemia.
  - Indolent non-Hodgkin's lymphoma.
  - Hodgkin's lymphoma.
  - Ovarian carcinoma.
  - Primary (Waldenström's) macroglobulinaemia.

- Like all cytotoxic drugs, chlorambucil is potentially teratogenic; the greatest risk is during the first trimester of pregnancy.
- Chlorambucil enters breast milk; advise women not to breastfeed.
- Do not give chlorambucil if the patient has porphyria.
- No dosage adjustment is usually required in renal or hepatic insufficiency.

- Patient selection and choice of chemotherapeutic regimen is a specialist decision.
- Do not prescribe a cytotoxic drug unless you are familiar with it and certain about the regimen. Most hospitals restrict the prescribing of these drugs to specialists of registrar grade and above.
- The dose of a cytotoxic drug varies with indication, and is usually calculated on the basis of body surface area. It is good practice to check these calculations if you are asked to give a cytotoxic drug, even if you are not the prescriber.

- Bone marrow suppression is the most common adverse effect and is dose-related.
  - Chlorambucil causes leukopenia, and to a lesser extent anaemia and thrombocytopenia, at therapeutic doses. It is not necessary to withdraw the drug at the first sign of these, but the patient must be monitored closely.
  - Be aware that the neutrophil count can continue to fall for up to 10 days after the last dose of chlorambucil.
- Spermatogenesis is reduced; this is usually reversible, but can become progressive and irreversible.
- Rash is uncommon but can be severe (Stevens–Johnson syndrome). If the patient develops a rash, withdraw the chlorambucil and change to another drug, such as cyclophosphamide.

Examples of live vaccines			
BCG	Measles	Polio	Rubella
Influenza	Mumps	Rabies	Yellow fever

- Do not give live vaccines to patients taking cytotoxic drugs; there is a risk of overwhelming sepsis and severe local reactions.

Safety

- Measure the full blood count, including the differential white cell count. Neutropenia is the most common finding, but also look for anaemia and thrombocytopenia.
- If neutropenia develops, measure the blood count daily in case it is progressive.
- Do not forget that neutropenia can develop up to 10 days after the last dose of chlorambucil.
- Patients with renal insufficiency are at greater risk of bone marrow suppression.

- Warn patients about the effect on spermatogenesis before treatment begins.
- Make sure the patient knows the warning symptoms of neutropenia, what precautions to take, and what to do if they become feverish or unwell.
- If the patient is receiving chemotherapy as an outpatient, ensure that they know whom to contact out of hours.

Cyclophosphamide

Alkylating cytotoxic drug

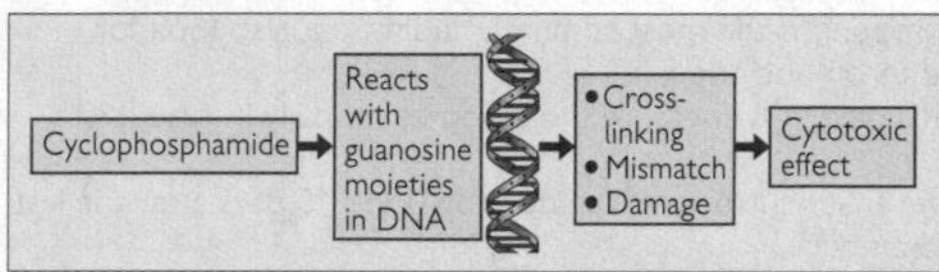

Examples of alkylating cytotoxic drugs

- Busulfan
- Carmustine
- Chlorambucil
- Chlormethine
- Cyclophosphamide
- Estramustine
- Ifosfamide
- Lomustine
- Melphalan
- Mitobronitol
- Thiotepa
- Treosulfan

- Cyclophosphamide should only be used by specialists.
- It can be used for the treatment of:
  - Chronic lymphocytic leukaemia.
  - Hodgkin's and non-Hodgkin's lymphoma.
  - Solid tumours.

- Successful use of cytotoxic drugs involves achieving a balance between the desired actions and toxicity.
- Cytotoxic chemotherapy is associated with a range of adverse effects, which are summarized separately (p. 484). The information given here is specific to cyclophosphamide.
- Dosage calculation for cytotoxic drugs is complex, and should be checked by an oncologist and a pharmacist. If you are asked to administer a cytotoxic drug, it is good practice to check that the correct dosage adjustments have been made.
  - Reduce the dose in hepatic insufficiency; cyclophosphamide requires metabolism to active metabolites.
  - Reduce the dose in renal insufficiency.
- Cytotoxic drugs should not be given to women who are pregnant; ensure that premenopausal women use adequate contraception.
- Do not give live vaccines to patients receiving cytotoxic chemotherapy. See chlorambucil (p. 486).

- Treatment with cyclophosphamide should always be under the supervision of a specialist familiar with the condition and the role of cytotoxic drugs in its treatment.
- Do not prescribe a cytotoxic drug unless you are familiar with it and certain about the regimen. Most hospitals restrict the prescribing of these drugs to specialists of registrar grade and above.
- The dose of a cytotoxic drug varies with indication. It is good practice to check these calculations if you are asked to give a cytotoxic drug, even if you are not the prescriber.

- Acrolein, a metabolite of cyclophosphamide, can cause haemorrhagic cystitis.
  - This can affect 10% of patients; the risk is greater if the patient has had previous radiotherapy to the bladder or around it, and if the drug is given intravenously.
  - The drug mesna binds to acrolein and reduces its toxicity.
  - Check whether routine treatment with mesna is required. Treatment with the related drug ifosfamide always includes mesna prophylaxis.

    - Mesna has a shorter half-life than cyclophosphamide; it needs to be given several times after a dose of cyclophosphamide.
    - Other prophylaxis measures include bladder irrigation and maintaining urine output above 100 mL/hour.
- Bone marrow suppression is the most common adverse effect and is dose-related.
    - Bone marrow toxicity can be severe, even after a single dose.
    - Recovery is usually complete by 21 days after a dose.
- High doses of cyclophosphamide can cause SIADH, leading to fluid retention and hyponatraemia.
- Spermatogenesis is reduced; this is usually reversible, but it can become progressive and irreversible. This is a particular problem with long-term treatment.
- Prolonged treatment, especially when combined with radiotherapy, increases the incidence of acute non-lymphocytic leukaemia.

- Do not give live vaccines to patients taking cytotoxic drugs; there is a risk of overwhelming sepsis and severe local reactions. See chlorambucil (p. 486).
- Cyclophosphamide inhibits pseudocholinesterase; do not give suxamethonium.
- Allopurinol potentiates the bone marrow toxicity due to cyclophosphamide.

Safety
- Measure a full blood count according to local protocol, taking into account the time when the patient is at greatest risk of bone marrow suppression.
- Measure the urine output and monitor for haemorrhagic cystitis.

- Warn patients about the effect on spermatogenesis before treatment begins.
- Make sure the patient knows the warning symptoms of neutropenia, what precautions to take, and what to do if they become feverish or unwell.
- If the patient is receiving chemotherapy as an outpatient, ensure that they know whom to contact out of hours.
- Advise the patient to report any blood in the urine immediately.

Cytotoxic antibiotics

Cytotoxic drugs

The mechanism of action of these drugs is not fully understood, but is related to their ability to intercalate into DNA. The mechanism is similar to that of radiotherapy and so they are not usually used in combination, as there is a risk of severe toxicity.

Drugs in this class

Anthracyclines
- Aclarubicin
- Daunorubicin
- Doxorubicin
- Epirubicin
- Idarubicin

Derivative of anthracycline
- Mitoxantrone

Others
- Bleomycin
- Dactinomycin (actinomycin D)
- Mitomycin

℞
- Cytotoxic antibiotics should only be used by specialists.
- Different drugs are not equivalent; the following list gives an indication of their different uses.
  - *Doxrubicin*. Widely used for leukaemias, lymphomas, and solid tumours.
  - *Epirubicin*. Breast cancer and bladder cancer by instillation.
  - *Aclarubicin*. Relapsed or refractory acute non-lymphocytic leukaemia.
  - *Idarubicin*. Second-line treatment for breast cancer and acute leukaemias.
  - *Daunorubicin*. Acute leukaemia and Kaposi's sarcoma in patients with AIDS.
  - *Mitoxantrone*. Breast cancer, non-Hodgkin's lymphoma, adult non-lymphocytic leukaemia.
  - *Bleomycin*. Lymphomas, solid tumours, squamous cell carinoma.
  - *Dactinomycin*. Paediatric cancers.
  - *Mitomycin*. Upper gastrointestinal and breast cancer, bladder tumours by instillation.

General notes
- Successful use of cytotoxic drugs involves achieving a balance between the desired actions and toxicity.
- Cytotoxic chemotherapy is associated with a range of adverse effects, which are summarized separately (p. 484). The information given here is specific to certain drugs.
- Dosage calculation for cytotoxic drugs is complex and should be checked by an oncologist and a pharmacist. If you are asked to administer a cytotoxic drug, it is good practice to check that the correct dosage adjustments have been made.
- Factors to consider are given below.
- The anthracyclines are all very irritant to tissues; see teaching point below for guidelines on avoiding extravasation of cytotoxic drugs.
- Most of these drugs are associated with cardiac toxicity. This is usually related to the cumulative dose. Serial ECG measurement, echocardiography, and radionuclide scans should be considered.
  - The risk is greater if the patient has heart disease or has received radiotherapy to the chest/heart: reduce the dose.
- Cytotoxic drugs should not be given to women who are pregnant; ensure that premenopausal women use adequate contraception.
- Do not give live vaccines to patients receiving cytotoxic chemotherapy. See chlorambucil (p. 486).

Notes on specific drugs

Doxorubicin

- Reduce the dose according to the bilirubin (the drug is excreted via the bile):
    - If the bilirubin is 22–50 micromol/L (1.2–3 mg/dL) reduce the dose by 50%.
    - If the bilirubin is greater than 50 micromol/L (3 mg/dL) reduce the dose by 75%.
- The cumulative dose is associated with a cardiomyopathy; restrict the total dose to 450 mg/m^2.
- Bone marrow suppression is maximal at 10–14 days after a dose and has usually recovered by 21 days.
- Doxorubicin is usually given by fast-running intravenous infusion. This can cause a supraventricular tachycardia in rare cases.
- Liposomal formulations are available. These are used when the risk of toxicity is very high (e.g. in patients with Kaposi's sarcoma with low CD4 counts).

Epirubicin

- Reduce the dose according to the bilirubin (the drug is excreted in the bile).
- Bone marrow suppression is greatest at 10–14 days after a dose and has usually recovered by day 21.
- The cumulative dose is associated with a cardiomyopathy; limit the total dose to 0.9–1 g/m^2.

Idarubicin

- Muscositis is common and occurs 2–10 days after a dose.
- Fever, chills, rash, and raised liver enzymes are experienced by 20–30% of patients.
- Reduce the dose according to the bilirubin (the drug is excreted in the bile).
- Reduce the dose in renal insufficiency.

Daunorubicin

- Bone marrow suppression is maximal at 10–14 days after a dose and has usually recovered by 3–4 weeks.
- The cumulative dose is associated with cardiomyopathy; limit it to 600 mg/m^2.
- Reduce the dose in renal insufficiency.
- Reduce the dose in hepatic insufficiency.

Mitoxantrone

- Mitoxantrone is generally well tolerated.
- Leukopenia is maximal at 10–14 days after a dose and has usually recovered by 21 days.
- Cardiac toxicity is seen at cumulative dosages above 160 mg/m^2.

Bleomycin

- Reduce the dose by 50% in mild to moderate renal insufficiency. Reduce further in severe renal insufficiency.
- This drug has little bone marrow toxicity, but skin toxicity is common (up to 38% of patients).
    - This is characterized by pigmentation of flexures and subcutaneous sclerotic plaques.
- Hypersensitivity phenomena, characterized by chills and fevers, manifest within a few hours of administration.
    - Give steroids prophylactically.

- Pulmonary fibrosis is the greatest long-term problem.
  - This is dose-related and is common at cumulative doses above 300 000 units.
  - The elderly are more susceptible.
  - Clinically it is characterized by basal lung crackles and infiltrates on the chest radiograph.
  - The manufacturer recommends weekly chest radiographs during treatment.
  - There is a risk of respiratory failure when patients receive a high FiO_2 (e.g. during anaesthesia). This is seen at cumulative dosages above 100 000 units. Warn the anaesthetist.

Dactinomycin
- Dactinomycin is not associated with cardiac toxicity.
- Bone marrow suppression is observed at 2–4 days after a dose; recovery is usually complete by 3 weeks.

Mitomycin
- Mitomycin is given at 6-week intervals because it causes delayed bone marrow toxicity.
  - The nadir is usually 4 weeks after a dose.
- Prolonged use can cause irreversible bone marrow suppression, lung fibrosis, and renal damage.
  - Limit the cumulative dose to 120 mg.

- Do not give anthracyclines with trastuzumab; there is a high risk of toxicity.
- Do not give live vaccines to patients taking cytotoxic drugs; there is a risk of overwhelming sepsis and severe local reactions. See chlorambucil (p. 486).

- Most of these drugs cause alopecia; warn the patient about this.
- Make sure that the patient knows when the greatest risk of bone marrow suppression occurs.
  - Tell the patient to seek urgent medical attention if they develop signs of myelosuppression: easy bruising, bleeding, infection.
- Some of these drugs (epirubicin, idarubicin) colour the urine red, and mitoxantrone colours the urine blue. Warn patients about this.

TEACHING POINT Treatment and prevention of extravasation of cytotoxic drugs

Prevention

- This is most important, as damage is almost certain once extravasation has occurred.
- If a patient requires a course of chemotherapy, they will often have a tunnelled central line inserted. This provides secure access to a large vein. Always check that the lumen is freely patent before using it. Remember to flush and 'lock' the line (with saline or heparinized saline) after use.
- If a peripheral cannula is to be used, use a large vein. If the only available vein is rather small, place a glyceryl-trinitrate patch distal to the cannula; this may help to maintain patency. Ensure that it is freely patent before use. Do not use peripheral cannulae for cytotoxic chemotherapy more than a couple of times before re-siting. Never force an injection if you encounter resistance to flow; re-site the cannula.
- Advise the patient to report any burning or stinging around the site immediately.

Treatment of extravasation

- Stop the drug infusion immediately.
- Leave the cannula in place and try to aspirate any fluid back. This is rarely successful.
- Local application of corticosteriods may reduce inflammation.
- Beyond this, there are two courses of treatment, but neither is entirely satisfactory. One approach is to localize the drug and try to administer an antidote. The other involves spreading and diluting the drug. Seek expert advice from a plastic surgeon. These methods should only be attempted by specialists, as they are potentially hazardous.

Antimetabolite drugs

Cytotoxic drugs

This is a large and diverse group of drugs. Their exact mechanisms of action are not known, but seem to involve at least two processes:

They are incorporated into new nuclear material and interfere with the process of mitosis. For example, 5–FU blocks the methylation reaction of deoxyuridylic acid to thymidylic acid, thereby interfering with the synthesis of deoxyribonucleic acid (DNA).	They bind to enzymes and other molecules involved in the normal process of mitosis. For example, cytarabine interferes with pyrimidine synthesis.

Drugs in this class

- Fluorouracil (5-FU)
- Capecitabine
- Gemcitabine
- Cytarabine
- Fludarabine
- Cladribine
- Raltitrexed
- Tegafur plus uracil
- Tioguanine
- Mercaptopurine*
- Azathioprine*
- Methotrexate*

*See separate articles

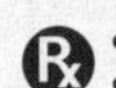

- These drugs should only be used by specialists.
- The different drugs are not equivalent; the following list gives an indication of their different uses.
  - Fluorouracil (5-FU). Treatment of solid tumours. Used topically for skin cancers.
  - Capecitabine. Colorectal cancer.
  - Cytarabine. Maintenance of remission of acute myeloid leukaemia.
  - Fludarabine. NICE recommends its use as a second-line drug for B-cell chronic lymphocytic leukaemia in patients who have failed treatment with an alkylating drug.
  - Cladribine. Treatment of hairy cell leukaemia.
  - Gemcitabine. NICE recommends its use:
    - First-line for advanced/metastatic pancreatic cancer in patients with a good level of function.
    - First-line for advanced non-small cell lung cancer (with platinum).
  - Raltitrexed. Palliation of advanced colorectal cancer.
  - Tioguanine. Induction of remission in acute myeloid leukaemia.

- Successful use of cytotoxic drugs involves achieving a balance between the desired actions and toxicity.
- Cytotoxic chemotherapy is associated with a range of adverse effects which are summarized separately (p. 484). The information given here is specific to certain drugs.
- Dosage calculation for cytotoxic drugs is complex and should be checked by an oncologist and pharmacist. If you are asked to administer a cytotoxic drug, it is good practice to check that the correct dosage adjustments have been made. Factors to consider are given below.
- Cytotoxic drugs should not be given to women who are pregnant; ensure that premenopausal women use adequate contraception.
- Do not give live vaccines to patients receiving cytotoxic chemotherapy. See chlorambucil (p. 486).

- Treatment with these drugs should always be under the supervision of a specialist familiar with the condition and the role of the drugs in treatment.

Adverse effects and monitoring: notes on specific drugs

Fluorouracil (5-FU)

- Absorption of fluorouracil is unpredictable when given by mouth; it is given intravenously.
- If used topically for skin cancer ensure that it is under an occlusive dressing, that other areas do not become exposed, and that others are not exposed to it.
- Fluorouracil is usually well tolerated but can cause:
  - Myelosupression.
  - Mucositis (hand/foot desquamative syndrome; see capecitabine below).
  - A cerebellar syndrome.
  - Myocardial ischaemia with ST segment elevation.
- Note that the effect of warfarin can be enhanced by 5-FU (mechanism not known).

Capecitabine

- Capecitabine is metabolized to 5-FU by an enzyme that is more prevalent in malignant tissue. It can therefore achieve a degree of selectivity. Capecitabine can be given by mouth.
- Reduce the dose by 25% in moderate renal insufficiency; avoid using it in severe hepatic or renal impairment.
- Diarrhoea is the most common adverse effect. It affects half the patients treated and can be severe in 13%. Withdraw the drug if severe. For less severe cases, give loperamide for symptomatic relief.
- Capecitabine also commonly causes a hand/foot syndrome. This is characterized by numbness, dysaesthesia/paraesthesia, tingling, painless swelling, or erythema of the hands and/or feet.

Cytarabine

- Cytarabine is a potent myelosuppressant. Toxicity can occur as early as 7 days but can occur up to 64 days after starting treatment. It is used for maintenance of remission.
- A cytarabine syndrome has been described. It is characterized by fever, myalgia, bone pain, occasionally chest pain, maculopapular rash, conjunctivitis, and malaise. It usually occurs 6–12 hours after administration. Corticosteroids are effective for treatment and prevention of this syndrome.

Fludarabine

- Avoid using fludarabine in severe renal insufficiency.
- Fludarabine is usually well tolerated but can cause:
  - Myelosuppression.
  - Immunosuppression; consider co-trimoxazole prophylaxis against *Pneumocystis carinii.*
  - Immune-mediated haemolytic anaemia; this is rare.
- Do not use fludarabine with pentostatin; there have been cases of fatal toxicity.

Gemcitabine

- Gemcitabine causes myelosuppression, but less commonly than other drugs. Reduce or delay the next dose if there is suppression of the granulocyte or platelet counts.
- A rash occurs in 25% of patients; it is pruritic in 10%.

Raltitrexed

- Avoid using raltitrexed in severe hepatic or renal insufficiency.

- Make sure that the patient knows when the greatest risk of bone marrow suppression occurs.
  - Tell the patient to seek urgent medical attention if they develop signs of myelosuppression: easy bruising, bleeding, infection.

Methotrexate

Methotrexate

Antimetabolite drug

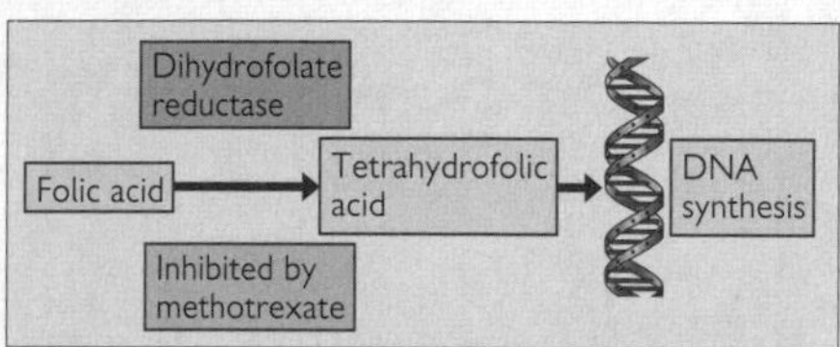

Drugs in this class
- Methotrexate
- Azathioprine
- Mercaptopurine
- See p. 494 for a further list of antimetabolite drugs

- Methotrexate should only be used by specialists.
- It is used as a cytotoxic drug for:
  - Maintenance treatment of acute lymphocytic leukaemia.
  - Treatment of choriocarcinoma, non-Hodgkin's lymphoma, and solid tumours.
- It is used for severe, treatment-resistant psoriasis.
- Methotrexate is a useful disease-modifying drug (DMARD) in rheumatoid arthritis.

- Avoid if the patient has severe renal impairment; it is excreted renally.
- Avoid if the patient has moderate or severe hepatic insufficiency; it can be hepatotoxic.
- Avoid if the patient has a large volume of ascites or pleural effusions. The drug can accumulate in these fluids and be released later, causing toxicity.
- Should not be given to women who are pregnant; ensure that premenopausal women use adequate contraception. Advise men and women to avoid conception for 6 months after stopping methotrexate treatment.

- Treatment with methotrexate should always be under the supervision of a specialist familiar with the condition and the role of the drug in treatment.

Chemotherapy
- Consult your local protocol for the treatment regimen.
- A course of methotrexate is usually followed by 'rescue' treatment with folinic acid. This reduces the severity of myelosuppression and mucositis.

Psoriasis
- Methotrexate should only be used when there is severe disease, resistant to other treatments.
- There are several regimens available; check your local protocol.

Rheumatoid arthritis
- Methotrexate is given once a week for this indication.
- Patients have died as a result of incorrect prescribing. Make sure that the patient understands the regimen.
- If you are giving the drug in hospital, strike out the other days of the week on the drug chart to avoid administration errors.
- Give folic acid 5 mg 3 days after each dose of methotrexate. This reduces the haematological, gastrointestinal, and mucosal adverse effects.

- Bone marrow toxicity (usually neutropenia) is dose-related and can be abrupt.
  - It can occur even if the drug is used correctly, and at low doses.
  - If bone marrow suppression occurs, stop the drug and give folinic acid (120 mg daily in divided doses).
    - Follow local guidelines for the care of neutropenic patients and seek expert advice.
    - Consider giving granulocyte colony stimulating factor if neutopenia persists.
- Can cause pulmonary toxicity. This is more common in patients with rheumatoid arthritis.
- Long-term treatment with methotrexate can cause liver fibrosis and even cirrhosis.

- Do not co-prescribe with aspirin and NSAIDs. These reduce methotrexate excretion and increase toxicity.
- Do not co-prescribe with antifolate antibiotics (trimethoprim, co-trimoxazole) and triamterene; there is a risk of severe toxicity.
- The antifolate action of methotrexate is enhanced by pyrimethamine.
- Penicillins (and probenecid) reduce the excretion of methotrexate; take care and be prepared to reduce the dose.
- There is an increased risk of toxicity from leflunomide (another DMARD), retinoids, and ciclosporin when they are co-prescribed with methotrexate. Avoid these combinations whenever possible.
- The following drugs increase the risk of bone marrow suppression when they are given with methotrexate: chloramphenicol, cisplatin, corticosteroids, kanamycin, nitrous oxide, omeprazole, phenytoin, tetracycline.

Safety

- When using methotrexate for psoriasis or rheumatoid arthritis, measure the full blood count, liver function tests, and renal function fortnightly until 6 weeks after the last dose increase.
- Thereafter measure the full blood count monthly and renal function every 6–12 months.
- Suspend treatment if any of the following occur:
  - White blood cell count below 4.0 x 10^9/L or neutrophil count below 2.0 x 10^9/L.
  - Platelet count is below 150,000 /mm^3 or if there are clinical signs of thrombocytopenia.
  - A greater than two-fold rise in aspartate aminotransferase, alanine aminotransferase, or alkaline phosphatase.
  - Ask about rash, oral ulceration, new or increasing dyspnoea, and cough.
- National guidelines for the monitoring of second-line drugs, British Society for Rheumatology, July 2000. *https://www.msecportal.org/portal/editorial/PublicPages/bsr/536883013/3.doc.*
- The monitoring regimen when methotrexate is used for chemotherapy is more intense; follow your local protocol.
- Obtain a baseline chest radiograph to allow comparison if the patient develops evidence of pulmonary toxicity.

- Advise the patient to avoid over-the-counter aspirin and NSAIDs.
- Advise the patient to report any dyspnoea or cough; these may be symptoms of pulmonary toxicity.

- Tell the patient to seek urgent medical attention if they develop signs of myelosuppression: easy bruising, bleeding, or infection.
- Make sure that patients with rheumatoid arthritis know to take the treatment only once a week and to take folic acid as well.

Prescribing information: **Methotrexate**

Psoriasis and tumours

- Methotrexate should only be prescribed by specialists, usually of registrar grade or above.

Rheumatoid arthritis

- The usual dose is 7.5 mg once weekly; this can be increased by 2.5 mg every 6 weeks, to a maximum of 20 mg weekly.

Vinca alkaloids

Cytotoxic drugs

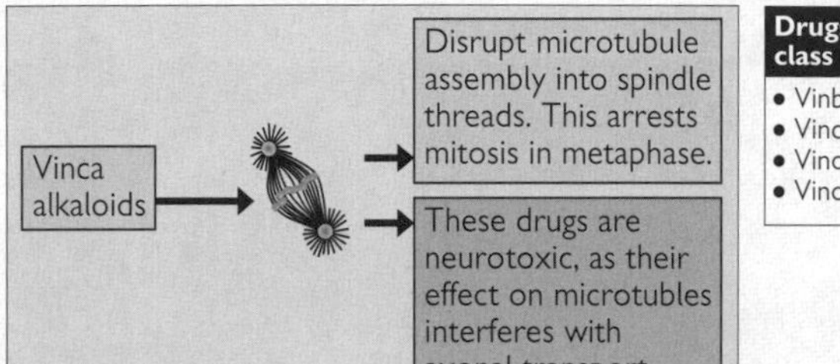

Drugs in this class

- Vinblastine
- Vincristine
- Vindesine
- Vinorelbine

- Vinca alkaloids should only be used by specialists.
- Different drugs are not equivalent; the following list gives an indication of their different uses.
  - *Vinblastine, vincristine, and vindesine* For acute leukaemias, lymphomas, and some solid tumours.
  - *Vinorelbine* First-line treatment for non-small cell lung cancer, and second-line for advanced breast cancer.

- Successful use of cytotoxic drugs involves achieving a balance between the desired actions and toxicity.
- Cytotoxic chemotherapy is associated with a range of adverse effects, which are summarized separately (p. 484). The information given here is specific to these drugs.
- Dosage calculation for cytotoxic drugs is complex and should be checked by an oncologist and a pharmacist. If you are asked to administer a cytotoxic drug, it is good practice to check that the correct dosage adjustments have been made.
  - Reduce the dose in hepatic insufficiency.
- Cytotoxic drugs should not be given to women who are pregnant; ensure that premenopausal women use adequate contraception.
- Do not give live vaccines to patients receiving cytotoxic chemotherapy. See chlorambucil (p. 486).
- Treatment with vinca alkaloids should always be under the supervision of a specialist familiar with the condition and the roles of the drugs in treatment.

Never give vinca alkaloids intrathecally

- Vinca alkaloids are not absorbed when given by mouth; all are given intravenously.
- There have been fatal incidents when vinca alkaloids have been given intrathecally. It is good practice to give vinca alkaloids on a different day from any intrathecal chemotherapy.

- The principal toxic effect is dose-related neurotoxicity; it is most severe with vincristine.
  - It is characterized by paraesthesia, loss of deep tendon reflexes, abdominal pain, and constipation. If these occur, reduce the dose.
  - If motor weakness develops, withdraw the drug.
- Bone marrow toxicity is also dose-related.
  - Vincristine causes very little myelosuppression.

- Bone marrow toxicity is greatest 7–10 days after a dose and has usually recovered by 21 days.
- Vinca alkaloids cause reversible alopecia.
- Vinca alkaloids are irritant to tissues; see teaching point under cytotoxic antibiotics (p. 493) for guidelines on the avoidance of extravasation of cytotoxic drugs.

- The antifungal drug, itraconazole, inhibits vincristine metabolism and so increases the risk of neurotoxicity. Avoid giving them together.

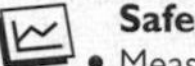

Safety

- Measure a full blood count according to local protocol, taking into account the time when the patient is at greatest risk of bone marrow suppression.
- Perform regular neurological examinations and reduce the dose if there is evidence of neurotoxicity.

- Warn the patient that these drugs cause alopecia (usually reversible).
- Tell the patient to seek urgent medical attention if they develop signs of myelosuppression: easy bruising, bleeding, infection.

Platinum compounds

Cytotoxic drugs

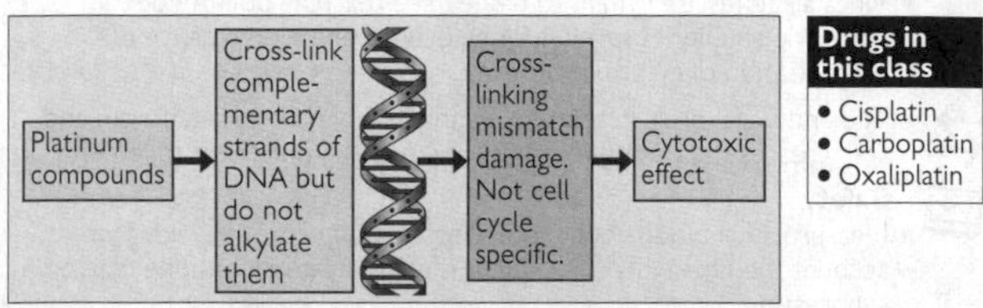

Drugs in this class

- Cisplatin
- Carboplatin
- Oxaliplatin

- Platinum compounds should only be used by specialists.
- The different drugs are not equivalent; the following list gives an indication of their different uses.
  - *Carboplatin.* Advanced ovarian cancer and small cell lung cancer.
  - *Cisplatin.* Germ cell tumours (seminoma, teratoma); bladder, lung, upper gastrointestinal, and ovarian cancers.
  - *Oxaliplatin.* Metastatic colorectal cancer.

- Successful use of cytotoxic drugs involves achieving a balance between the desired actions and toxicity.
- Cytotoxic chemotherapy is associated with a range of adverse effects which are summarized separately (p. 484). The information given here is specific to these drugs.
- Dosage calculation for cytotoxic drugs is complex, and should be checked by an oncologist and a pharmacist. If you are asked to administer a cytotoxic drug, it is good practice to check that the correct dosage adjustments have been made.
  - Reduce the dose in renal insufficiency.
- Cytotoxic drugs should not be given to women who are pregnant; ensure that premenopausal women use adequate contraception.
- Do not give live vaccines to patients receiving cytotoxic chemotherapy. See chlorambucil (p. 486).

- Treatment with platinum compounds should always be under the supervision of a specialist familiar with the condition and the roles of the drugs in treatment.
- Platinum compounds are not absorbed when given by mouth; all are given intravenously.
- Prehydrate the patient with 1–2 litres of intravenous saline before treatment. Ensure that the patient takes 2–3 litres of fluid daily during treatment.
- These drugs are highly emetogenic; premedicate before starting treatment (see teaching point in 5-HT_3 receptor antagonists, p. 73). If the patient is vomiting, give intravenous fluids to ensure adequate intake.

Cisplatin

- The principal toxic effect is dose-related nephrotoxicity. Cisplatin is excreted renally, so this adverse effect can be self-perpetuating.
  - The nephrotoxic effect is cumulative.
  - The maximal effect on renal function occurs at 2 weeks after a dose.
- These drugs are highly emetogenic. Nausea develops within 1–2 hours of starting treatment and can last a week (see teaching box below).

- Bone marrow toxicity is also dose-related.
  - Bone marrow suppression is greatest at 6–21 days after a dose and has usually recovered by day 45.
- Cisplatin is ototoxic; this manifests as tinnitus and deafness and is common (24% for cisplatin).
- When used in high doses, cisplatin can cause a peripheral neuropathy.
- Cisplatin can cause hypomagnesaemia; consider replacement if the patient is at a high risk of cardiac arrhythmias.

Carboplatin

- The pattern of toxic effects is similar. Carboplatin usually causes less nephrotoxicity and neurotoxicity, but more bone marrow suppression.

Oxaliplatin

- The pattern of toxic effects is similar. Oxaliplatin is dose-limited by neurotoxicity.

- Avoid giving with other drugs that are nephrotoxic (e.g. NSAIDs).
- Avoid giving with other drugs that are ototoxic (e.g. furosemide, aminoglycoside antibiotics).

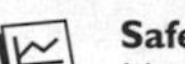

Safety

- Measure a full blood count according to local protocol, taking into account the time when the patient is at greatest risk of bone marrow suppression.
- Measure renal function regularly. Note that nephrotoxicity may not manifest until 2 weeks after a dose. Delay treatment or reduce the dose according to renal function.
- Perform audiometry before and after treatment. Cisplatin causes a 15 decibel loss in threshold in 25% of patients.

- Tell the patient to seek urgent medical attention if they develop signs of myelosuppression: easy bruising, bleeding, infection.

Taxanes

Cytotoxic drugs

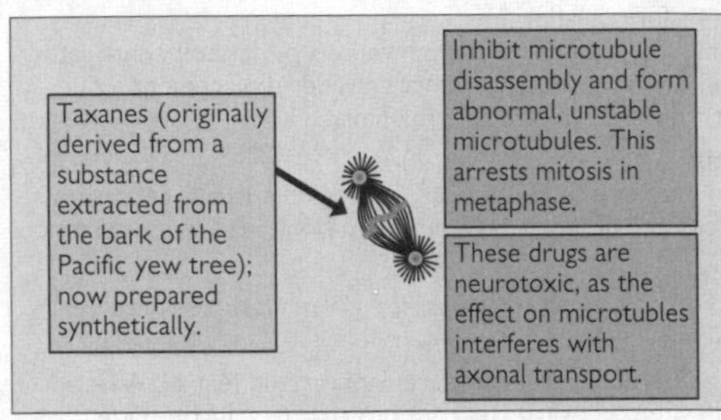

Drugs in this class

- Docetaxel
- Paclitaxel

- Taxanes should only be used by specialists.
- The different drugs are not equivalent; the following list gives an indication of their different uses.
- NICE has recommended that these drugs should be used for:
  - The treatment of advanced breast cancer when initial treatments have failed; adjuvant treatment should be restricted to clinical trials.
  - The first-line treatment of non-small cell cancer when curative treatment is not possible.
- In addition, NICE has recommended that:
  - *Paclitaxel* (in combination with platinum drugs) should be the standard initial treatment of ovarian cancer after surgery; use as a second-line drug should be restricted to women who have not already received it.
  - *Docetaxel* can be used for the treatment of non-small cell lung cancer that has relapsed with other treatments.

- Successful use of cytotoxic drugs involves achieving a balance between the desired actions and toxicity.
- Cytotoxic chemotherapy is associated with a range of adverse effects which are summarized separately (p. 484). The information given here is specific to the taxanes.
- Dosage calculation for cytotoxic drugs is complex and should be checked by an oncologist and a pharmacist. If you are asked to administer a cytotoxic drug, it is good practice to check that the correct dosage adjustments have been made.
- Cytotoxic drugs should not be given to women who are pregnant; ensure that premenopausal women use adequate contraception.
- Do not give live vaccines to patients receiving cytotoxic chemotherapy. See chlorambucil (p. 486).

- Treatment with taxanes should always be under the supervision of a specialist familiar with the condition and the role of the drugs in treatment.
- These drugs are not absorbed when given by mouth; both are given intravenously.

- The principal adverse effect is hypersensitivity.
  - This is common; it is severe in 8% of patients.
  - Premedicate the patient with a corticosteroid (e.g. dexamethasone 3 mg), an antihistamine (H_1 receptor antagonist e.g. chlorphenamine), and an H_2 receptor antagonist (e.g. ranitidine).
- Docetaxel causes fluid retention and peripheral oedema.
  - This can be reduced if steroid (dexamethasone) treatment is continued for 5 days.
- Bone marrow toxicity is also dose-related.
- Taxanes can cause a peripheral neuropathy, especially when used in high doses.
  - They can cause cardiac conduction defects; these are usually asymptomatic.
- Taxanes cause reversible alopecia.
- Arthralgia and myalgia are common; they can be severe in 12% of patients.
- Nausea and vomiting due to taxanes is usually mild.

- Ciclosporin, erythromycin, and ketoconazole inhibit the metabolism of taxanes. This may enhance their actions, but also increases the risk of adverse effects.

Safety
- Measure a full blood count according to local protocol, taking into account the time when the patient is at greatest risk of bone marrow suppression.
- Measure liver function tests during treatment; reduce the dose if there is evidence of toxicity.
- Perform regular neurological examinations and reduce the dose if there is evidence of neurotoxicity.

- Warn the patient that these drugs cause alopecia (usually reversible).
- Tell the patient to seek urgent medical attention if they develop signs of myelosuppression: easy bruising, bleeding, or infection.

Cytotoxic monoclonal antibodies

Trastuzumab is given here as an example of this new type of cytotoxic treatment

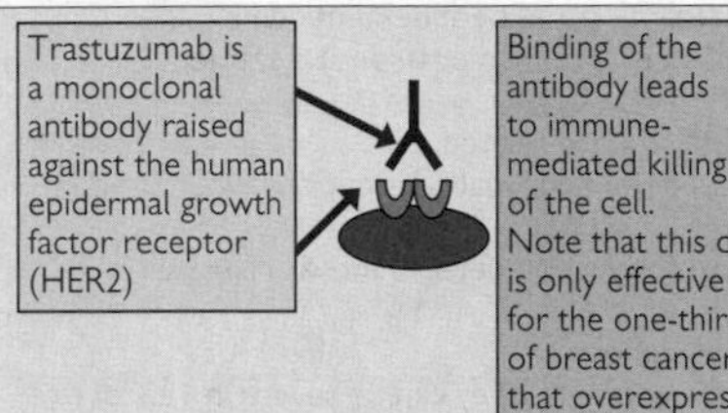

Note

This is a new type of treatment for cancer. It is likely that a number of similar drugs will become available in the near future.

- Monoclonal antibodies should only be used by specialists
- They have the potential to be powerful and specific anticancer drugs.
- Ideally, one would want to identify a molecule that is only expressed on malignant cells. In most cases, however, expression is not limited to malignant cells; rather, they overexpress a molecule that is expressed in a smaller amount by other cells.
- It is therefore very important to understand the biology of the target tumour when considering treatment with this type of drug.
  - For example, trastuzumab is only effective for breast cancer tumours that overexpress the HER2 receptor. This is only about one-third of cases. The other two-thirds have nothing to gain and so should be considered for alternatives.

- Although drugs of this type have the potential to be very specific, they bind to biologically active molecules. Often we do not fully understand the full extent of the actions of these molecules. Adverse effects may therefore be difficult to predict.
  - For example, trastuzumab can cause cardiotoxicity, the mechanism of which is not immediately obvious.
  - Avoid giving trastuzumab to patients with a history of coronary artery disease, heart failure, or hypertension.
- Drugs of this type can interact with other types of cytotoxic chemotherapy.
  - For example, there is a particular risk of cardiac toxicity if trastuzumab is given with anthracycline drugs.
  - Delay treatment with trastuzumab for 22 weeks after treatment with anthracycline drugs.
- Cytotoxic drugs should not be given to women who are pregnant; ensure that premenopausal women use adequate contraception.
- Do not give live vaccines to patients receiving cytotoxic chemotherapy. See chlorambucil (p. 486).

- Treatment with these drugs should always be under the supervision of a specialist familiar with the condition and the roles of the drugs in treatment.
- These drugs are not absorbed when given by mouth; all are given parenterally.

- The principal adverse effect is hypersensitivity.
  - This risk is particularly high with monoclonal antibody drugs.
  - It can range from fevers and chills to angio-oedema and anaphylaxis.
  - Monoclonal antibody drugs should only be given when adequate resuscitation facilities are immediately available.
- Trastuzumab can cause cardiac toxicity; see notes above.
- Other adverse effects of trastuzumab include gastrointestinal disturbance.

- There is a particular risk of cardiac toxicity if trastuzumab is given with anthracycline drugs; avoid this combination.

Safety

- Monoclonal antibody drugs have the potential to be less toxic than conventional cytotoxic drugs. The monitoring required will depend on the precise actions of the drug; follow the manufacturers' advice.

- New treatments are often hailed in the media as a 'breakthrough'. Drugs such as trastuzumab have an important role in the treatment of certain cancers, but they are not a panacea. Patients with cancer are often very well-informed; take time to explain why a treatment may not be suitable for them.

TEACHING POINT Reporting suspected adverse events

- This class of drugs is new. As with any new treatment, rare adverse effects may not have been identified.
  - See carbimazole (p. 419) for more information on rare but potentially fatal adverse effects.
- Recently-introduced drugs are identified in the BNF by an inverted black triangle ▼.
- Report any suspected adverse effects of new drugs to your local regulatory agency; for example:
  - To the Committee on Safety of Medicines in the UK, using a yellow card. These are available from pharmacists and are in the back of the BNF. The yellow card scheme in the UK invites reports from doctors, dentists, coroners, pharmacists, and nurses. In the future, patients may also be allowed to use this route. Meanwhile, patients who suspect they have suffered an adverse reaction to their medicines should report these to their doctor, pharmacist, or nurse who may then report it to the Scheme.
  - In the USA, the MedWatch scheme allows healthcare professionals and consumers to report to the Food and Drug Administration serious problems that they suspect are associated with drugs and medical devices they prescribe, dispense, or use.
  - The World Health Organization provides a forum for WHO member states to collaborate in monitoring drug safety. This is organized by the co-ordinating centre in Uppsala, Sweden.
- Regulatory agencies are also interested to hear about a suspected serious adverse effect due to an established drug, even if the effect is well-recognized. This information helps to build up a picture of how common an adverse effect is.
  - A serious adverse effect is defined as one that:
    - Is fatal.
    - Is disabling or incapacitating.
    - Prolongs hospitalization.
- Do not be deterred from making a report if you are not certain whether the drug was responsible; it can be difficult to ascribe causality, especially with new drugs.
- Regulatory authorities are particularly interested to hear about suspected adverse effects that:
  - Are delayed; these may not have been identified in early clinical trials.
  - Occur in elderly people; this group are more susceptible to the adverse effects of some drugs.
  - Result in a congenital abnormality.
  - Occur in children; clinical trial information on the use of drugs in children is often very sparse.

Azathioprine and mercaptopurine

Inhibitors of DNA synthesis

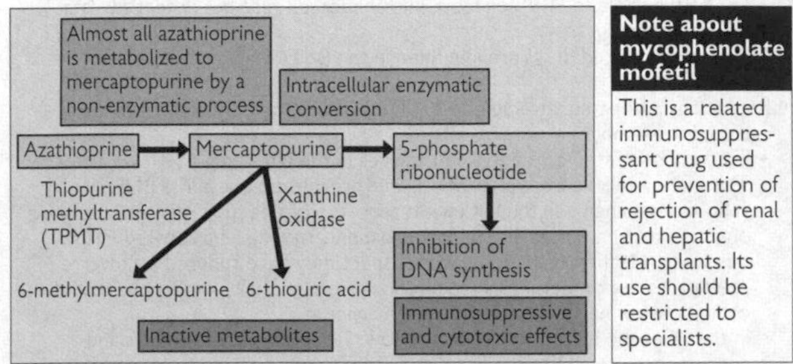

Note about mycophenolate mofetil

This is a related immunosuppressant drug used for prevention of rejection of renal and hepatic transplants. Its use should be restricted to specialists.

- Antiproliferative immunosuppression.
  - Transplant rejection.
  - Vasculitis: systemic lupus erthematosus, polyarteritis nodosa, dermatomyositis, Wegener's granulomatosis.
  - Rheumatoid arthritis.
  - Inflammatory bowel disease (unlicensed indication).
  - Myasthenia gravis.
- Cytotoxic maintenance therapy for acute leukaemias.

- Do not initiate treatment during pregnancy, although current treatment can be continued after a thorough assessment of the risks.
- Reduce the dose in patients with severe renal or hepatic insufficiency.

- Treatment with these drugs should always be under the supervision of a specialist familiar with the condition and the roles of the drugs in treatment.
- These drugs can be given on their own, but are usually combined with other immunosuppressants, such as corticosteroids or calcineurin inhibitors (ciclosporin, tacrolimus).
- The exact dose and treatment regimen will depend on the indication; details are not given here.
- The intravenous formulation of azathioprine is very irritant; use it only when treatment by mouth is not possible. Ensure that the cannula is patent and flush with 50 mL of saline after the drug has been infused.
- Do not give live vaccines to patients receiving immunosuppressant drugs. See chlorambucil (p. 486).
  - Passive immunization with *Varicella zoster* immunoglobulin should be given to non-immune patients exposed to chickenpox or shingles.
  - Pneumovax and an annual flu vaccine should be given.

- The principal toxic effect is dose-related myelosuppression; 5% of patients require a dose reduction or withdrawal of the drug for this reason.

- Hepatic toxicity can present with raised transaminases or cholestatic jaundice.
  - Whenever possible, it is advisable to start these drugs at a low dose and build up to the maintenance dose. In this way toxic effects can be identified early.
- Hypersusceptibility phenomena, such as fever, rigors, rash, and interstitial nephritis, are relatively common (2% of patients)
- Be aware that the patient is at greater risk of infection, owing to immunosuppression and leukopenia.
- Long-term treatment is associated with an increased risk of tumours (especially lymphomas). Regularly review the need for treatment.

- Allopurinol markedly inhibits the metabolism of these drugs. Reduce the dose by 75% when the patient is also taking allopurinol.
- There is an increased risk of myelosuppression when these drugs are co-prescribed with antibiotics that inhibit folic acid metabolism (trimethoprim and co-trimoxazole).

Safety

- Measure a full blood count (looking for myelosuppression), renal function, electrolytes, and liver function tests weekly for the first 6 weeks of treatment.
  - Also measure 2 and 4 weeks after each dose increase and monthly thereafter.
  - Suspend treatment if any of the following occur:
    - White blood cell count below 4.0×10^9/L or neutrophil count below 2.0×10^9/L.
    - Platelet count below 150×10^9/L or if there are clinical signs of thrombocytopenia.
    - A greater than two-fold rise in aspartate aminotransferase, alanine aminotransferase, or alkaline phosphatase.
- The frequency of monitoring blood tests should be increased if the patient has renal or hepatic insufficiency.
- A few patients are homozygous slow metabolizers of azathioprine (by thiopurine methyltransferase). They are at particular risk of myelosuppression. You should be able to identify them by close monitoring of the blood count and careful titration of the dose.

Efficacy

- The precise measures of efficacy will depend on the indication, but will usually include clinical assessment of symptoms and measurement of inflammatory markers. When using potentially hazardous drugs such as these it is especially important to set outcome targets, so that progress can be assessed properly. It is unwise to start treatments without a clear idea of your goals.

- Tell the patient to seek urgent medical attention if they develop signs of myelosuppression: easy bruising, bleeding, infection.

Prescribing information: **Azathioprine and mercaptopurine**

Azathioprine

- The dose will depend on the indication. Seek expert advice.
- The usual maintenance dose is in the range 2.0–2.5 mg/kg.

Mercaptopurine

- The dose will depend on the indication. Seek expert advice.
- The usual maintenance dose is in the range 1.0–1.5 mg/kg.

TEACHING POINT Giving drug dosages according to body weight

Some drugs are given in fixed doses to all patients across a stated dosage range. However, in some cases the dose should be calculated according to the weight of the patient (e.g. drugs that have a low therapeutic index, or toxic to therapeutic ratio). This index or ratio indicates the margin between the toxic dose and the therapeutic dose. The bigger it is, the better. For example, in the absence of penicillin hypersensitivity, penicillins have a high therapeutic index, or a high toxic to therapeutic ratio, since very high doses (much higher than are needed for therapeutic efficacy) are safe. The following classes of drugs have a low therapeutic index, and examples are given of weight-related doses:

- *Aminoglycoside antibiotics* When gentamicin is given once a day, the initial intravenous dose is 7 mg/kg.
- *Antiarrhythmic drugs* The intravenous maintenance dose of disopyramide is 400 micrograms/kg/h. However, recommendations for most antiarrhythmic drugs are not weight-corrected.
- *Anticoagulants* The total daily dose of subcutaneous dalteparin for deep venous thrombosis is 200 units/kg.
- *Cardiac glycosides* The usual loading dose of digoxin is 15 micrograms/kg and the usual oral maintenance dose is 5 micrograms/kg/day; in someone with renal impairment, adjust the maintenance dose according to the degree of renal insufficiency (p . 95); in severe renal insufficiency also reduce the loading dose to 10 micrograms/kg.
- *Cytotoxic and immunosuppressive drugs* The oral maintenance dose of azathioprine is 1–3 mg/kg/day.
- *Hypoglycaemic drugs* The usual total daily dose of insulin is 0.5 units/kg, although requirements vary greatly.

Although it is a good rule to give drugs with a low therapeutic index in weight-related doses, this is not always done. For example, the anticoagulant, warfarin, is given in doses that are not weight-corrected; however, in that case careful monitoring is necessary to titrate the dose to an individual's requirements.

Ciclosporin, tacrolimus, and sirolimus

Immunosuppressant drugs

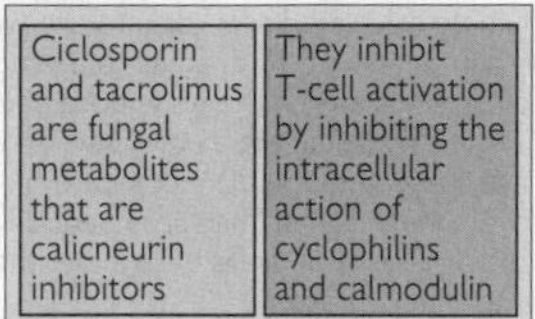

Immunosuppressant drugs

- Corticosteroids
- Azathioprine and mercaptopurine
- Ciclosporin, tacrolimus, and sirolimus
- Mycophenolate mofetil

Less commonly used

- Cyclophosphamide and chlorambucil

- Immunosuppressant.
  - After organ transplantation.
  - Treatment and prevention of graft versus host disease (GVHD).
  - Autoimmune disease (e.g. rheumatoid arthritis, psoriasis, atopic dermatitis, uveitis, Behçet's disease, Crohn's disease).

- Do not use these drugs in patients with uncontrolled hypertension; they are nephrotoxic and can worsen control.
- Do not use immunosupressant drugs in patients with uncontrolled infection or malignancy.
- Avoid using these drugs in women who are pregnant. There is evidence of toxicity in animal studies.
- Careful dosage adjustment is required in renal and hepatic insufficiency; see monitoring section below.

- These drugs should only be given by a specialist familiar with them and their roles in treatment.
- Dosage regimens are complex and should be checked by a senior member of staff and a pharmacist.
- Treatment is always a balance between beneficial and adverse effects. The target concentration ranges are wide because patient responses are very variable.
- Clinical outcome measures need to be taken into account along with the blood drug concentration.
- These drugs should be prescribed by brand name, as each formulation differs in its kinetics.

- These drugs are nephrotoxic; this can occur at therapeutic doses. See below for details of ciclosporin monitoring.
- These drugs can also cause hepatotoxicity and neurotoxicity.
- The intravenous formulations of these drugs contain polyethoxylated castor oil (Cremophor EL); this can cause anaphylactoid reactions. See teaching point in acetylcysteine (p. 625).
- These drugs can cause hypertension, abnormalities of liver function tests, and weakness.
- They can cause the haemolytic uraemic syndrome in bone marrow transplant patients.
- Long-term treatment can cause hirsutism and gum hyperplasia.

- Long-term treatment is associated with an increased risk of secondary lymphomas, especially those caused by Epstein–Barr virus (EBV). Patients will require long-term follow-up for this.

Note on tacrolimus

- The CSM has advised that tacrolimus carries an increased risk of neurotoxicity and nephrotoxicity.
- In addition, it can cause hypertrophic cardiomyopathy and disturbances of glucose metabolism (hyperglycaemia).

- These drugs are subject to a large number of metabolic drug interactions. Always check before starting or stopping a drug.

Examples of drugs that lower plasma ciclosporin concentrations	Examples of drugs that increase plasma ciclosporin concentrations
• Carbamazepine, phenytoin, barbiturates, St John's wort, rifampicin (enzyme inducers).	• Choloroquine, bile acids (increase absorption). • Calcium channel blockers, macrolide antibiotics. • **Corticosteroids** (important as these are often given together), oestrogens. • **Grapefruit juice** (inhibits CYP 3A4).

- These drugs increase the metabolism of the oral contraceptive; advise patients that they will also need to use non-hormonal methods.
- Avoid co-prescribing with other drugs that are potentially nephrotoxic (e.g. aminoglycoside antibiotics, antifungal drugs, and NSAIDs).
- Take care when co-prescribing with other drugs can than cause hyperkalemia (a consequence of nephrotoxicity) (e.g. ACE inhibitors, angiotensin receptor blockers, potassium-sparing diuretics).

Blood concentration measurement of ciclosporin

- Seek expert advice for tacrolimus and sirolimus.
  - Several methods are available and these yield slightly different results.
  - Ciclosporin concentrations are usually measured in whole blood.
  - Take the sample immediately before the next dose.
  - It takes 2 days to reach a new steady state after a dosage change.
  - The target plasma concentration range varies from individual to individual, and with indication.
  - For example, the risk of rejection increases if the trough concentration is below 200 nmol/L, but the risk of nephrotoxcity increases once the blood concentration is above 70 nmol/L.
  - Remember that stopping as well as starting a drug that interacts with these drugs will alter the blood concentration.
- Measure the following before treatment starts:
  - Full blood count, renal function, electrolytes, lipids, blood pressure.
- The following monitoring regimen is suggested.
  - Measure the serum creatinine and blood pressure fortnightly until the dosage has been stable for 3 months, and then monthly.
  - Measure the full blood count and liver function tests monthly until the dosage has been stable for 3 months, and then every 3 months.
  - Measure the serum lipids every 6 months.

- Make sure that the patient understands the importance of taking these drugs regularly.
- Avoid a high potassium diet.
- Avoid grapefruit juice. The oral solution formulations of these drugs can be taken with orange juice or apple juice.
- These drugs can affect the performance of skilled motor tasks (driving).
- Advise the patient to use a sunblock. This may reduce the risk of secondary skin malignancies.

Prescribing information: **Ciclosporin, tacrolimus, and sirolimus**

- Use of these drugs is specialized. Use your local protocol.

Chapter 9

Nutrition and blood

Contents

Drugs and anaemia

Drugs are used to treat anaemia, but can also be responsible for it. The following is offered as a general guide. See individual articles for more information.

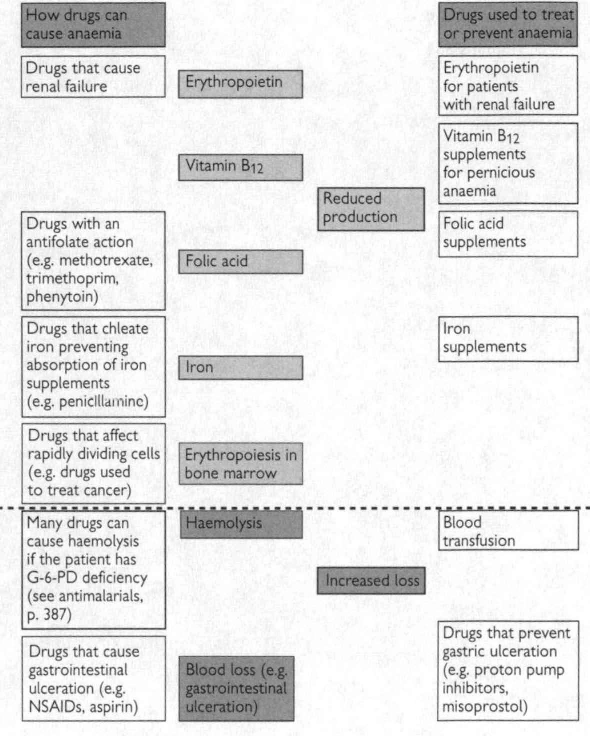

Blood transfusion

Blood group	Antigen on erythrocytes	Antibodies in plasma
O	None	Anti-A and anti-B
A	A	Anti-B
B	B	Anti-A
AB	AB	None

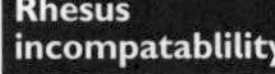

Rhesus incompatablility

See immunoglobulins (p. 639) for information on prevention of rhesus disease of the newborn.

- Treatment of blood loss and severe anaemia.

- Do not use blood indiscriminately. It should not be given for mild or asymptomatic anaemia, or to 'normalize the numbers'.
- There are several ways in which the need for blood can be reduced.
  - Checking for and correcting anaemia before elective surgery.
  - Careful use of anticoagulant drugs in the perisurgical period (see warfarin (p. 115) for guidance).
  - Sometimes stimulating erythropoiesis with erythropoietin is more appropriate than blood transfusion.
- Blood can affect the body's immunological response to a renal transplant; only give blood when it is essential, and having consulted an expert.
- Patients with haematological malignancies have special requirements for blood and blood products (e.g. leukocyte depleted, CMV-negative); always seek haematological advice before giving a transfusion to such patients.
- In the UK, blood is screened for HIV and Hepatitis B and C, but the presence of other, as yet unidentified viruses cannot be excluded.

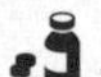

Practical considerations

- For more information consult the 'Handbook of Transfusion Medicine' (*www.transfusionguidelines.org.uk*).
- Record the reason for the transfusion in the notes. Obtain the patient's consent for transfusion. It may be prudent to record this formally using a consent form.
- Prescribe the blood on the infusion section of the drug chart. Do not use a circle with a dot inside to indicate a unit; this can be confused with a zero.

Crossmatching

- Samples for crossmatching blood require special handling.
  - To avoid mixing samples, only take blood for crossmatch from one patient at a time.
  - Write the patient's details on the tube by hand (do not use addressograph labels).
  - Many hospitals require an additional method of linking the patient to the sample (e.g. red label system).
  - Take time to complete the crossmatch form as completely as possible.
    - It is very important to advise the laboratory if any atypical antibodies have been identified, as this will complicate the crossmatch procedure.

- Telephone the laboratory if the sample is urgent. If the blood is required at a specific time (e.g. for a surgical procedure), ensure that this is clearly stated, especially if it is not for several days.
  - Make sure that you request a suitable amount of blood; check your local protocol for elective surgical cases.

Transfusion

- Identify the patient. Use the wristband, but if the patient can speak also check with them.
- Confirm that the name, date of birth, hospital number, and sex are correct on the blood unit.
- Check that the blood compatability information (ABO and rhesus groups) and unique blood unit donation number are correct on the blood unit and the form sent with the blood.
  - On some occasions the blood group may not be the same as the patient's group; check that it is still compatible (e.g. A group blood for an AB patient). If you are at all unsure, speak to the blood bank.
- Check that the blood matches any special requirements (e.g. gamma-irradiated, CMV-seronegative).
- Perform all these checks at the bedside, and put up the infusion immediately.
- Check the physical state of the unit of blood; do not infuse it if it looks damaged or abnormal in any way.
- Blood should be infused though a dedicated (large bore) cannula.
  - Do not add anything to, or infuse anything through, the same cannula as blood; this includes drugs, which should not be added to blood infusion bags.
- A unit of blood should be completely infused within 4 hours.

Acute, severe reactions

- These are most common within the first 15 minutes of the infusion. Four main types are recognized:
  - Acute haemolytic transfusion reactions. These should be avoided if the procedures above are followed.
  - Infusion of a bacterially contaminated unit.
  - Transfusion-associated lung injury. This is usually the result of an interaction between donor plasma antibodies and recipient leukocytes.
  - Severe allergic reactions or anaphylaxis. These are more common when products containing large volumes of plasma are given.
- Treatment of severe reactions is supportive. Stop the infusion. Treat anaphylaxis (see adrenoceptor agonists, p. 194). Summon senior help and notify the blood bank.

Febrile and non-haemolytic transfusion reactions

- These occur in about 1–2% of patients and are probably due to donor leukocytes. They tend to occur towards the end of the transfusion.
- Fever and rigors are the cardinal signs; this may represent a severe reaction, so monitor the patient closely, but in most cases it will not progress. The symptoms can be relieved by:
  - Slowing the rate of infusion.
  - Paracetamol for the fever.
  - Chlorphenamine (an antihistamine) for urticaria.
  - Intravenous steroids are not usually necessary; seek expert advice if the patient has a history of febrile reactions to transfusion.

Fluid overload

- Patients with chronic anaemia and cardiac disease are usually euvolaemic or hypervolaemic, and blood transfusion can precipitate pulmonary oedema. If blood transfusion is essential, the risk of fluid overload can be reduced by:
  - Only giving 1 unit in each 12-hour period (over 4 hours during that period).
  - Giving 20 mg furosemide (by intravenous injection) before each unit.

Delayed reactions

- These are rare, but can be life-threatening; seek expert advice.
- Delayed haemolysis due to red cell antibodies other than ABO.
- Transfusion graft versus host disease.
- Iron overload after repeated transfusions (see deferoxamine, p. 546).
- Post-transfusion purpura (thrombocytopenia).

- Blood is incompatible with almost all other drugs and infusion solutions. Give blood via a dedicated cannula and do not add drugs to units of blood.

Safety and efficacy

- Ensure that you have a sound indication for blood transfusion.
- Severe reactions are most common within 15 minutes of the start of the infusion.
  - Before starting transfusion, record blood pressure, pulse, and temperature.
  - Check the pulse and temperature 15 minutes after starting the transfusion.
  - Observe the patient throughout the transfusion.
  - Repeat the blood pressure, pulse, and temperature when the transfusion is completed.
  - If the patient is conscious, further recordings are only needed if the patient becomes unwell or has symptoms and signs of a reaction.
  - An unconscious patient should have their pulse and temperature measured at intervals during the transfusion.

- Objection to blood transfusion is not restricted to patients who are Jehovah's Witnesses. Always obtain consent for blood transfusion.
- Warn patients that a transfusion may be required if you are assessing them before major surgery.

Prescribing information: **Blood transfusion**

- Prescribe blood on the dedicated blood products section or infusion section of the drug chart.

Factor VIII and related products

Clotting factor

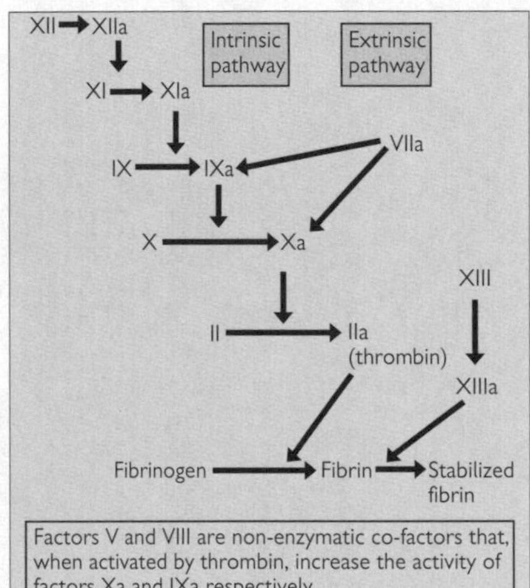

Related products

- Antithrombin III concentrate: used for congenital deficiency of antithrombin III
- Factor VIIa: recombinant product for patients with inhibitors of factors VIII and IX
- Factor VIII inhibitor bypassing fraction: for patients with inhibitors of factor VIII
- Factor IX: used for patients with haemophilia B
- Factor XIII: used for congenital deficiency of factor XIII
- Protein C concentrate: for patients with protein C deficiency

- Treatment and prophylaxis of bleeding in patients with haemophilia A.

- These blood products are used for the treatment of specific coagulation disorders only. If the patient has severe bleeding, consider whether there is a failure of coagulation or of platelet function. See below and heparins (p. 109) for guidance on the treatment of bleeding.
- These peptide coagulation factors can induce the formation of inhibitory antibodies. These can render clotting factors ineffective.

- The treatment of haemophilia should be under the direction of a specialist.
- Guidance from the United Kingdom Haemophilia Centre Directors Organisation Executive Committee is available at *http://www.medicine.ox.ac.uk/ohc/index.htm*.
- The dose and frequency of administration of factor VIII varies greatly between individuals. Always seek expert advice if a patient with haemophilia is admitted under your care.
- The following is offered as a guide only.

- The dose can be calculated using the following formula:
  - Required IU = body weight (kg) × desired factor VIII rise (% of normal) × 0.5

Degree of haemorrhage/ type of surgical procedure	Factor VIII level required (%) (IU/dl)	Example dose for a 70-kg patient (units)	Frequency of doses (hours)/duration of therapy (days)
Haemorrhage			
Early haemarthrosis, muscle bleed, or oral bleed.	20-40	1000	Repeat every 12–24 hours. Give for at least 1 day or until the bleeding episode has resolved.
More extensive haemarthrosis, muscle bleed or haematoma.	30-60	1500	Repeat infusion every 12–24 hours for 3–4 days or more until pain and disability have resolved.
Life threatening bleeds, e.g. intracranial or abdominal.	60-100	2800	Repeat infusion every 8 to 24 hours until the threat is resolved.
Surgery			
Minor, including tooth extraction.	30-60	1500	Repeat every 24 hours. Give for at least 1 day or until the bleeding episode has resolved.
Major.	80-100	3000	Repeat infusion every 8-24 hours until adequate.

- Patients with haemophilia should be immunized against hepatitis A and B.
- Recombinant factor VIII is very expensive and may not be available to all those who may benefit from it.
  - If the patient has mild disease consider treatment with desmopressin (see vasopressin, p. 476).
- Do not give patients with haemophilia intramuscular injections because of the risk of haematoma.

- These factors are peptides; they can cause allergic reactions (including anaphylaxis).
- Haemolysis has been associated with the administration of large doses of these drugs to patients with blood groups A, B, and AB.
- Less pure fractions contain fibrinogen, which can build up. This is less of a problem with recombinant products.

- These patients should not normally be given drugs that increase their risk of bleeding: warfarin, antiplatelet drugs, corticosteroids.

Safety and efficacy

- Measure the factor VIII concentration. Liaise with your laboratory about the practicalities of doing this before you send the sample.

- Patients with haemophilia need to be taught how to identify and avoid injury (especially to joints).

Prescribing information

This is a specialized area of practice. Liaise with your local haemophilia centre.

Drugs and blood products used in the treatment of bleeding

Identify whether the bleeding is the result of:
- Deficient clotting
  - Specific deficiency (e.g. haemophilia A).
  - Consumption (e.g. disseminated intravascular coagulation).
  - Depletion/dilution (e.g. massive transfusion and severe haemorrhage).
  - Anticoagulant or fibrinolytic drugs (see heparin and warfarin, pp. 109 and 115, for more information).
- Platelet factors
  - Specific deficiency (rare).
  - Consumption (e.g. disseminated intravascular coagulation and severe haemorrhage).
  - Antiplatelet drugs.
- Treat the underlying cause whenever possible.
- Treat the bleeding locally whenever possible (e.g. endoscopic intervention).

Fresh frozen plasma contains clotting factors and can be used if clotting factors are deficient. You will need to know the patient's blood group.

Remember to include the volume of any blood products in your calculations of fluid balance.

The following drugs are used in special circumstances.

Tranexamic acid

This is an inhibitor of the activation of plasminogen to plasmin. It is used short-term for haemorrhage or if there is a risk of haemorrhage in increased fibrinolysis or fibrinogenolysis. Local fibrinolysis occurs in the following conditions:
- Prostatectomy and bladder surgery.
- Menorrhagia.
- Epistaxis.
- Conization of the cervix.
- Traumatic hyphaema.
- Hereditary angio-oedema (danazol or stanozolol are preferred).
- Management of dental extraction in patients with haemophilia.

Tranexamic acid is renally excreted; halve the dose in moderate renal insufficiency and give one-quarter of the usual dose in severe renal insufficiency. Do not give during pregnancy. Tranexamic acid can cause thromboembolism, but this is rare.

Aprotinin

This is an inhibitor of plasmin that is used in open-heart surgery when optimal blood conservation is essential. It is also given to patients with some forms of acute promyelocytic leukaemia that produce large quantities of plasmin.

Etamsylate

This corrects abnormal platelet adhesion (with a normal number of platelets) and is used occasionally for menorrhagia and periventricular haemorrhage in neonates.

Erythropoietin (epoetin) and analogues

Recombinant analogues of the peptide erythropoietin

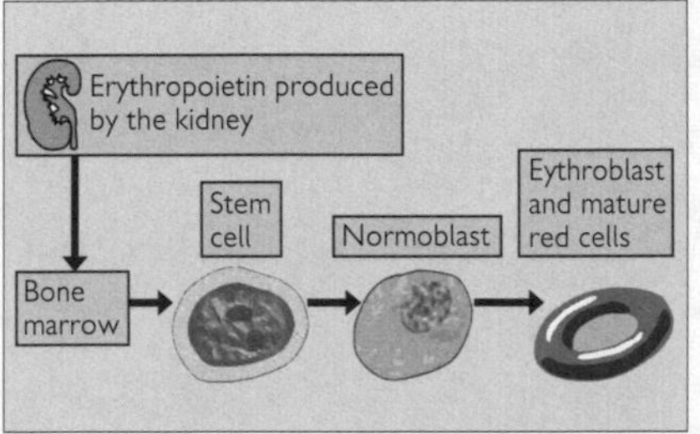

Drugs in this class

Erythropoietin is the endogenous hormone. Epoetin is recombinant human erythropoietin.

- Epoetin alpha
- Epoetin beta
  - These drugs are clinically indistinguishable.
- Darbepoetin
  - This drug has a longer half-life than epoetin.

- When stimulation of erythropoiesis is required.
  - Treatment of the anaemia associated with chronic renal insufficiency.
  - To reduce the duration of the period of anaemia following treatment with platinum-based chemotherapy.
  - To increase the yield of autologous blood from healthy donors in a predonation programme.

- These drugs increase the haematocrit; this can precipitate or worsen heart failure.
  - Avoid giving them to patients who have recently had a myocardial infarction.
  - Avoid them in patients with severe or uncontrolled hypertension.
- There is no evidence of harm from epoetin during pregnancy, but use it only when the benefits are clear.
- No dosage adjustment is usually required in hepatic insufficiency.
- Chronic renal insufficiency is one of the major indications for the use of these drugs.
- See notes below on actions in the case of pure red cell aplasia.

Chronic renal insufficiency

- Patients with chronic renal insufficiency may be anaemic for several reasons, only one of which is inadequate erythropoietin production.
  - Always exclude anaemia due to iron, folate, or vitamin B_{12} deficiency before giving epoetin.
  - Aluminium toxicity will reduce the efficacy of epoetin treatment (see deferoxamine, p. 546).
- Do not give epoetin by subcutaneous injection for long-term use; give it by intravenous injection.
- The target haemoglobin concentration is 10–12 g/dL.
  - Adjust the dose and frequency of administration to achieve this.
  - Darbepoetin has a longer duration of action; it can be given once weekly.

Chemotherapy

- Treatment with epoetin forms part of some regimens. It can shorten the period of anaemia but has not been shown to affect overall outcome.

- This is an expensive treatment and the benefit needs to weighed against the cost.
- Epoetin can be given by the subcutaneous route for this indication.

Predonation programmes

- Patients can donate blood before an operation during which it is expected that blood transfusion will be required. Epoetin treatment can increase the yield.
- Pay particular attention to the cautions above when assessing whether the patient will benefit. This procedure is not widespread in the UK; seek specialist guidance.

- Epoetin is usually well tolerated.
- Epoetin causes a dose-dependent increase in blood pressure; if not properly monitored it can cause hypertensive encephalopathy.
- Epoetin can also increase the platelet count, although thrombocytosis is uncommon.
- Epoetin can, very rarely, cause pure red cell aplasia.
  - The CSM has advised that, if this occurs, epoetin should be withdrawn and that patients should **not** be switched to another member of the class.

- The antihypertensive action of ACE inhibitors and angiotensin receptor blockers is antagonized by these drugs. This is important, because patients with chronic renal insufficiency are commonly given these drugs.
  - The risk of hyperkalaemia is increased when ACE inhibitors or angiotensin receptor blockers are given concomitantly with epoetin.

Efficacy

- The target haemoglobin concentration is 10–12 g/dL. If it rises above 13 g/dL, suspend treatment. If the haemoglobin has not risen by at least 1 g/dL after 8 weeks treatment, withhold the drug.

Safety

- Measure the blood pressure frequently; this should form part of the routine follow-up of patients with chronic renal insufficiency.

- Explain that this treatment may make the patient feel better, but that it will not have any effect on the long-term outcome of their disease (renal failure or tumour).

Prescribing information: **Epoetin analogues**

Dosage regimens are complex and require adjustment according to the indication and individual requirements. Use your local protocol. The following is given as an example. Epoetin alfa and epoetin beta are indistinguishable in effect, but you must specify in the prescription which one you want to be used, since the doses are slightly different.

Epoetin alfa

Chronic renal insufficiency

- By intravenous injection, 50 units/kg 3 times weekly.
- Can be increased by 25 units/kg 3 times weekly every 4 weeks to achieve the desired haemoglobin concentration.
  - Usual dose 25–100 units/kg 3 times weekly.

Cancer chemotherapy

- By subcutaneous injection, 150 units/kg 3 times weekly.
- Can be increased to 300 units/kg 3 times weekly if required.

Epoetin beta

Chronic renal insufficiency

- By intravenous injection, 40 units/kg 3 times weekly.
- Can be increased by 20 units/kg 3 times weekly every 4 weeks to achieve the desired haemoglobin concentration.

Colony stimulating factors

Recombinant analogues of the peptide colony stimulating factors

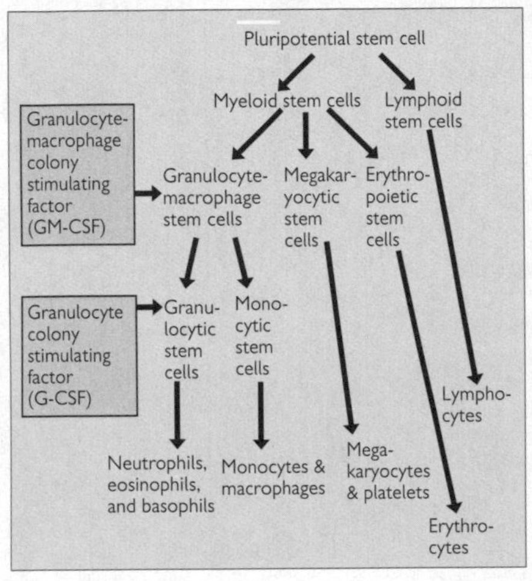

Drugs in this class

- Recombinant human granulocyte colony stimulating factor (rG-CSF); filgrastim
- Glycosylated recombinant human granulocyte colony stimulating factor (rHuG-CSF); lenograstim
- Recombinant granulocyte-macrophage colony stimulating factor (GM-CSF); molgramostim*

* Molgramostim stimulates a wider range of cell lines and is associated with a higher incidence of adverse effects.

- When stimulation of neutrophil production is required.
  - To reduce the duration of the period of neutropenia due to cytotoxic chemotherapy.
  - To increase the yield of autologous stem and progenitor cells for autologous or allogenic donation.
  - Treatment of congenital/cyclic/idiopathic neutropenia.
    - Note that molgramostim is ineffective in congenital neutropenia.
  - Treatment of persistent neutropenia in patients with HIV infection.

- Take care if the patient has abnormalities of the myeloid line.
  - For example, molgramostim is contraindicated in myeloid malignancy.
  - G-CSF can cause myelodysplastic syndromes in patients with severe congenital neutropenia.
- Also avoid these drugs if the patient has Kostmann's syndrome (reduced neutrophils with abnormal cytogenetics).
- There is evidence of harm from these drugs during pregnancy, but use only when essential.
- No dosage adjustment is usually required in hepatic or renal insufficiency.
- Do not give these drugs 24 hours before, or 24 hours after, a dose of chemotherapy.

Note on amifostine

- This drug, which is not a colony stimulating factor, can be used to reduce the neutropenia caused by treatment with cyclophosphamide or platinum compounds.
- It is thought to act by selectively protecting normal tissues from the actions of cytotoxic drugs. Its place in chemotherapy regimens is not yet fully established.

- Colony stimulating factors should only be used by specialists.
- They will reduce the duration of neutropenia after bone marrow transplant or cytotoxic chemotherapy, but have not been shown to affect overall survival.
  - They have not been shown to reduce the incidence of fever or infection.
- Colony stimulating factors are very expensive; the potential benefits (e.g. earlier discharge from hospital) must be weighed against this. Follow your local guidance.
- Always ensure that you know why the patient is neutropenic. Seek specialist help with investigation if the cause is not clear.

- The most common adverse effect is bone pain.
  - This occurs in about 13% of patients given G-CSF and 45% of patients given GM-CSF.
- Colony stimulating factors can cause a leukocytosis, but this is rare. Stop the drug if it occurs.
- Colony stimulating factors can cause thrombocytopenia. Measure the platelet count frequently and withdraw the drug if it becomes severe.
- Colony stimulating factors can cause splenic enlargement, especially in patients with sickle cell disease.
- Hypersensitivity reactions are more common after intravenous infusion.
- These drugs can cause a rash; it is more common with molgramostim.

- There are a few reports that filgrastim reduces the efficacy of fluorouracil.

Safety and efficacy

- Patients with neutropenia should have frequent blood counts (usually daily). Neutropenia is usually defined as a neurophil count less than 0.5×10^9/L. The target neutrophil count varies with indication; seek specialist advice.
- Chemotherapeutic regimens vary in the time when the neutrophil count is lowest; ensure that your treatment regimen covers this period.
- Make sure that you also look at the other elements of the blood count, in particular the lymphocyte and platelet counts.
- While the neutropenia persists, measure the patient's temperature 4 times daily and ask about symptoms of infection.

- Explain that this treatment may allow the patient to go home earlier, but that it will not have any effect on the long-term outcome of the disease.
- Advise the patient to report any symptoms of fever immediately.

Prescribing information: **Colony stimulating factors**

Dosage regimens are complex and require adjustment according to the indication and individual requirements. Use your local protocol. The following is given as an example.

Filgrastim

Cytotoxic drug–induced neutropenia

- By intravenous or subcutaneous injection, 500 000 units/kg daily.
- Do not start within 24 hours of administration of a cytotoxic drug.
- The duration of treatment is usually 14 days, but it may be up to 38 days in acute myeloid leukaemia. Follow your local protocol.

Iron salts

Essential element

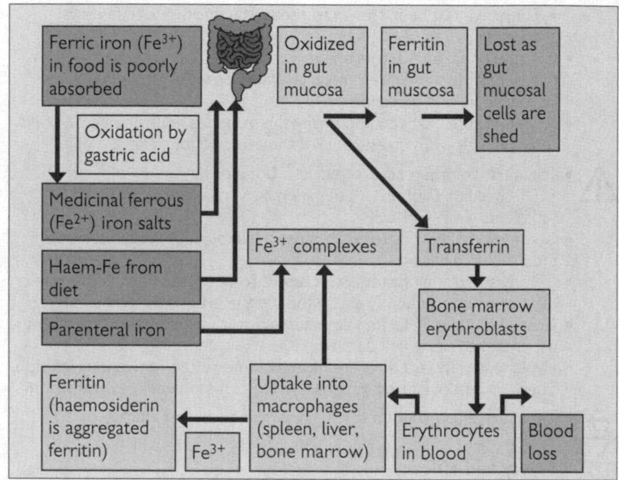

- Treatment and prevention of iron deficiency.

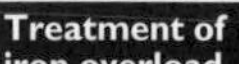

See deferoxamine (p. 546).

- Iron salts, given by mouth, can worsen inflammatory bowel disease.
- Avoid oral iron therapy in patients with strictures and diverticula.
- Parenteral iron therapy is rarely justified (see below) and should not be given to patients with severe hepatic or renal insufficiency.
- Allergic reactions to parenteral iron are common; avoid this route if the patient has a history of coeliac disease, asthma, or hypersensitivity to any drugs.
- Routine iron supplementation during pregnancy is not justified.
  - Consider it for women with identified deficiency or risk factors (poor diet and after subtotal or total gastrectomy).

Treatment of poisoning by iron

See teaching point below.

- Administration of iron by the parenteral route is only justified if the patient has:
  - Failed oral therapy owing to poor adherence.
  - Severe gastrointestinal adverse effects (see below for ways to minimize these).
  - Continuing severe blood loss.
  - Malabsorption.
  - Renal failure and is receiving haemodialysis (or in some cases peritoneal dialysis).

- Administration of iron by the parenteral route significantly improves the rate of increase of haemoglobin. However, if the patient needs a very rapid increase in haemoglobin, consider a blood transfusion.
- Ascorbic acid (vitamin C) increases the absorption of oral iron, but has not been shown to improve the overall clinical response. Combination tablets containing ascorbic acid are more expensive.
- Modified-release formulations are better tolerated, but the iron is released beyond the first part of the duodenum, so absorption may be reduced. They are not recommended.
- There is no justification for iron therapy in combination with multivitamins. Combination formulations of iron and folic acid may be useful for pregnant women, if both are required.
- You should aim to give the patient the equivalent of 100–200 mg of elemental iron daily. The amount of elemental iron varies with different formulations and salts. A table is provided in the prescribing section, as a guide.
- Treat the cause of the iron deficiency whenever possible (blood loss, poor diet).

- Nausea and vomiting are common and dose-related.
- Constipation is common (diarrhoea can also occur), but is less clearly dose-related.
- Elemental iron is thought to be responsible for these effects; no iron salt is less irritant than another (at equivalent dosages).
- Iron salts make the faeces black. This can be mistaken for melaena, but it smells different and is negative on testing for occult blood.
- Parenteral iron can cause severe allergic reactions, a metallic taste in the mouth, hypotension, bradycardia, abdominal pain, lymph node enlargement, and arthralgia.
- Hypotension is common (5% of patients) with intravenous iron.
- Intravenous iron can cause thrombophlebitis. Intramuscular injection of iron can stain the skin. The fear that intramuscular iron can cause muscle sarcoma has not been substantiated.

- Iron salts form chelates with some other drugs. This reduces the absorption of these drugs. Those most affected include: tetracyclines, quinolones, penicillamine, and levodopa.
- Magnesium trisilicate, an antacid, reduces the absorption of oral iron.

Safety and efficacy

- The haemoglobin should rise by 1–2 g over 3–4 weeks. Look for causes if it does not (e.g. poor compliance due to adverse effects, continuing blood loss).
- Continue iron therapy for 3 months after the haemoglobin is normal, to replace the body's stores.
- Atrophic glossitis and koilonychia improve, but can take a long time.

- Make sure that the patient knows that iron therapy takes time to increase the haemoglobin; improvement will be gradual.
- Warn the patient that iron salts turn the faeces black.
- Keep iron tablets away from children. Iron poisoning in children can be fatal.

Prescribing information: **Iron salts**

Oral iron

- Modified-release formulations and those containing ascorbic acid are not recommended (see above).
- The usual oral dose of elemental iron for treating iron deficiency is 100–200 mg daily.
  - The dose can be halved for prophylactic treatment (prophylaxis is justified in only a few patients).
  - The dose may need to be increased by 50% for patients with chronic renal insufficiency.
- The usual iron salt used is dried ferrous sulfate. The table below gives the suggested daily dosages for this and the other commonly prescribed iron salts.

Parenteral iron

- Giving iron by a parenteral route is rarely justified (see above).
- Calculate the total body iron deficit as follows:

Iron deficit (mg) = body weight (kg) × haemoglobin deficit (g/dL) × 2.21 + iron for stores (usually 500 mg)

Example: a 50-kg woman with a haemoglobin of 8 g/dL (normal 14 g/dL) has a deficit of 50 × (14 – 8) × 2.21 = 663 mg. She will require this and 500 mg (for stores).

Iron salt	Amount of iron salt per tablet	Content of elemental iron per tablet	Usual daily dose for treatment of iron deficiency
Dried ferrous sulfate	200 mg	65 mg	200 mg tds
Ferrous gluconate	300 mg	35 mg	4-6 tablets daily, in divided doses, with food
Ferrous fumarate (Fersaday®)	322 mg	100 mg	1 tablet bd
Ferrous fumarate (Fersamal®)	210 mg	68 mg	1 or 2 tablets tds
Ferrous fumarate	305 mg	100 mg	1 capsule bd

By intravenous infusion

- Give a test dose first.
- Iron dextran contains iron 50 mg/mL. Maximum daily dose 20 mg/kg. Test dose 25 mg.
- Iron sucrose contains iron 20 mg/mL. Test dose 50 mg. Usual dosage regimen for haemodialysis patients:
  - 100 mg 1–3 times per week, over sequential dialysis sessions, to a cumulative dose of 1000 mg.
  - Can be repeated if required.

By intramuscular injection

- Iron sorbitol contains iron 50 mg/mL. Maximum daily dose 100 mg.
- Give by deep intramuscular injection into the buttock (5-cm needle).
- To reduce staining of the skin, pull the skin of the buttock down before injection. When the needle is removed the track will form a zig-zag.

Treatment of iron poisoning

Likely toxicity	Ingested dose (mg/kg body weight)	Serum iron concentration at 4 hours
Mild	<20	3 mg/L (55 micromol/L)
Moderate	>20	3–5 mg/L (55–90 micromol/L)
Severe	150–300	>5 mg/L (90 micromol/L)

- Poisoning with iron is most common in children and is usually accidental.
- The most common symptoms are nausea, vomiting, abdominal pain, and diarrhoea.
- Stools and vomit are grey/black.
- Laboratory findings include a polymorphonuclear leukocytosis and hyperglycaemia.
- More severe findings include haematemesis and rectal bleeding (due to GI corrosion), drowsiness, convulsions, and metabolic acidosis.
- Treatment is supportive. Activated charcoal does not adsorb iron.
- If the poisoning is severe, take blood for urgent measurement of the serum iron concentration.
- Give deferoxamine intravenously without waiting for the serum iron result. The dose is 15 mg/kg/hour. The maximum dose advised is 80 mg/kg in 24 hours.
- Discuss the case with the National Poisons Information Service.
- If the poisoning is mild or moderate, measure the serum iron at 4 hours. If the patient is symptomatic, consider treatment with deferoxamine. Discuss the case with the National Poisons Information Service.
- (See also deferoxamine, p. 546).

Folic acid and folinic acid

Essential nutrients

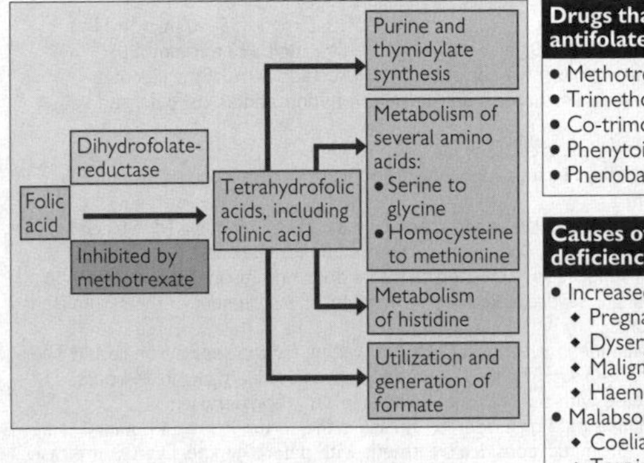

Drugs that have antifolate effects

- Methotrexate
- Trimethoprim
- Co-trimoxazole
- Phenytoin
- Phenobarbital

Causes of folate deficiency

- Increased demand
  - Pregnancy
  - Dyserythropoiesis
  - Malignancy
  - Haemodialysis
- Malabsorption
  - Coeliac disease
  - Tropical sprue
- Drugs (see above)

℞
- Prevention and treatment of folate deficiency.
- 'Rescue' therapy to reduce bone marrow toxicity during treatment with methotrexate.
- Prevention of neural tube defects during pregnancy.
- Prevention of cardiovascular disease.

- Folinic acid is not used for prevention and treatment of folate deficiency.
- Folic acid must be converted to folinic acid in order to act; this is inhibited by methotrexate.
  - Folic acid will not therefore be effective for the prevention of methotrexate-induced bone marrow toxicity during continuous administration of methotrexate; however, it is effective during intermittent administration.

- Whenever you suspect folic acid deficiency, find out if the patient has vitamin B_{12} deficiency as well. Do not give folic acid alone if there is a mixed deficiency (see below).

Pregnancy

- The daily requirement for folic acid is usually 50 micrograms, but this rises to 200 micrograms during pregnancy.
- Advise the patient to take folic acid throughout the period they are trying to conceive, and for the first 3 months of the pregnancy.
- A supraphysiological dose is recommended if the woman has had a previous child with a neural tube defect or is taking some antiepileptic drugs (phenytoin, sodium valproate, carbamazepine).
  - Counsel women about this; seek specialist advice in women considering pregnancy; and ensure folic acid supplementation (5 mg/day).

During treatment with methotrexate

- Give folinic acid 'rescue' therapy on a different day from the methotrexate (usually the day after).
- It is available in both oral and intravenous formulations.

Folate deficiency
- The initial dose is much higher than the maintenance dose (see below).
- Long-term treatment is rarely necessary; folic acid is obtained from food, so ensure that the patient has an adequate diet.

Primary prevention of ischaemic heart disease and stroke
- Meta-analysis of randomized controlled trials suggests that folic acid 0.8 mg/day reduces the risk of ischaemic heart disease by 16% and of stroke by 24% in those aged over 55 years. It is thought to do this by lowering the plasma homocysteine concentration.

- Adverse effects are very rare; hypersensitivity is occasionally observed during intravenous infusion.
- It is generally said that giving folic acid alone to a patient who is also vitamin B_{12} deficient can precipitate subacute combined degeneration of the spinal cord, although there is scant evidence that this is so. However, it is wise to give B_{12} first.

- The efficacy of treatment with fluorouracil (5-FU) for metastatic colorectal cancer is increased when the patient is also given folinic acid.

Efficacy
- In suspected deficiency, measure the red cell folate or plasma folate concentration. Also measure the plasma B_{12} concentration.

- Advise women who are considering becoming pregnant to take folic acid; this reduces the risk of fetal neural tube defects.

Prescribing information: **Folic acid and folinic acid**

Folic acid

Pregnancy
- Previous history of a neural tube defect, 5 mg daily.
- No previous history, 400 micrograms daily. This is available over the counter.

Folic acid deficiency
- Initially, 10–20 mg daily.
- Long-term treatment is rarely necessary.

During intermittent treatment with methotrexate for rheumatoid arthritis
- Give folic acid 5 mg 3 days after each dose of methotrexate. This can reduce the haematological, gastrointestinal, and mucosal adverse effects.

Primary prevention of ischaemic heart disease and stroke
- 0.8 mg daily.

Folinic acid (given as calcium folinate)

During treatment with methotrexate
- Initially 120 mg in divided doses over 12–24 hours
- Followed by 15 mg every 6–8 hours by mouth for 2–8 doses
- Usually given 24 hours after a dose of methotrexate.

Vitamin B_{12}

Essential vitamin

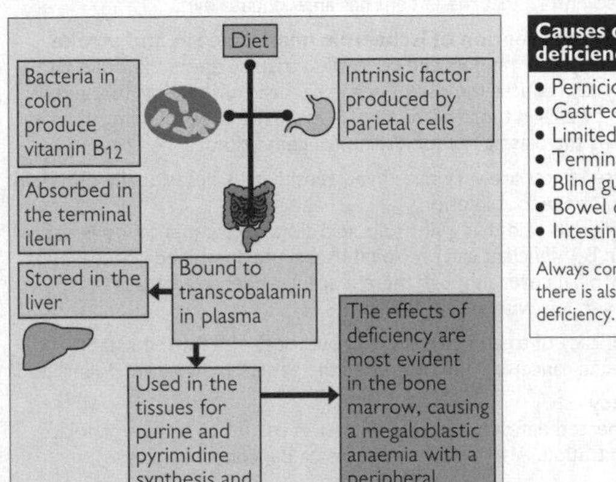

Causes of B_{12} deficiency

- Pernicious anaemia
- Gastrectomy
- Limited diet (vegans)
- Terminal ileal disease
- Blind gut loops
- Bowel diverticula
- Intestinal worms

Always consider whether there is also folate deficiency.

- Treatment and prevention of vitamin B_{12} deficiency
  - Given prophylactically after total gastrectomy (partial gastrectomy in some patients) and total ileal resection.

- Hydroxocobalamin has largely replaced cyanocobalamin, as it has preferable kinetic properties.
- If the patient has severe, undiagnosed megaloblastic anaemia, always give both vitamin B_{12} and folate; giving either alone can reportedly precipitate neuropathy, although the evidence supporting that is old and anecdotal.
- In other circumstances, determine whether there is vitamin B_{12} deficiency before giving treatment.

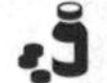

- The dose and route of administration will depend on the cause of the deficiency.
  - For example, if the cause is pernicious anaemia, B_{12} cannot be absorbed from the gut and must be given parenterally.
- If the patient has established deficiency, an initial period of loading will be needed in order to replenish body stores. This is not necessary if it is given prophylactically.

- Adverse effects are rare.
- Hypersensitivity to hydroxocobalamin is rare.

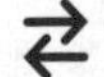

- There are no established drug interactions with vitamin B_{12}.

Safety and efficacy

- Measure the serum B_{12}. Usually B_{12} assay is a microbiological assay, which can give false low results if the patient is taking antibiotics.
- Measure a full blood count and folate (preferably red cell folate).

- Advise the patient that treatment will usually need to be lifelong.

Prescribing information: **Vitamin B_{12}**

Hydroxocobalamin

By intramuscular injection

- Pernicious anaemia without neurological involvement, initially 1 mg 3 times a week for 2 weeks, then 1 mg every 3 months.
- Pernicious anaemia with neurological involvement, initially 1 mg on alternate days, until no further clinical improvement, then 1 mg every 2 months.
- Prophylaxis, 1 mg every 2–3 months.

Cyanocobalamin

- Available for administration by mouth for the few patients for whom this route is appropriate. Not recommended for routine use. Seek specialist advice.

Deferoxamine (desferrioxamine)

Iron chelating drug

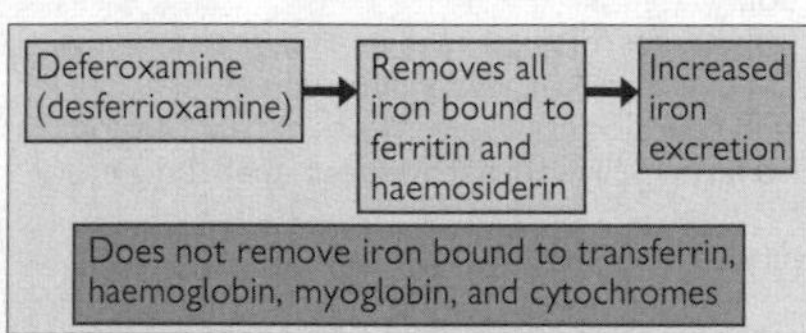

Note on deferiprone

- Deferiprone can be given by mouth for patients who cannot tolerate deferoxamine.
- However, it can cause neutropenia and liver damage, so it is not used first-line.

- Treatment of acute iron poisoning.
- Chronic iron overload:
  - Secondary to repeated transfusions.
  - Haemochromatosis. Note that venesection is usually preferred for this indication.
- Deferoxamine can also be used for chronic aluminium overload in renal dialysis patients.

- Deferoxamine is teratogenic in animals; avoid giving it long-term to women who are pregnant. However, if it is used for acute iron poisoning, the benefit is likely to outweigh the risk.

Iron poisoning *(see also p. 541)*

- Poisoning by iron is most common in childhood and is usually accidental.
- Remove iron from the stomach by lavage if the patient presents within 1 hour of the overdose.
  - Charcoal does not adsorb iron.
- Treat with intravenous deferoxamine according to the serum iron concentration measured 4 hours after the overdose.
  - Mild poisoning: <3 mg/L (<55 micromol/L). Treatment not usually necessary.
  - Moderate poisoning: 3–5 mg/L (55–90 micromol/L). Treat.
  - Severe poisoning: >5 mg/L (>90 micromol/L). Treat.
- If the dose is large (>20 mg iron/kg) treat immediately.

Chronic iron overload

- Deferoxamine is usually given subcutaneously 3–7 times per week over an 8–12 hour period (overnight).
- Deferoxamine can be given intramuscularly, but this can be painful.
- Deferoxamine can be given intravenously when the patient is receiving a blood transfusion as part of long-term treatment (e.g. in thalassaemia).
  - This can be via the same cannula, but do not add deferoxamine to the blood bag or use the same line.
  - Give up to 2 g of deferoxamine per unit of blood.

- Intravenous infusion can cause histamine release from mast cells; this in turn can cause hypotension, erythema, and pruritus.
- Local reactions around subcutaneous infusion sites are common.
  - If this is a problem, add hydrocortisone 2 mg to the infusion bag.
- Follow-up studies show that the changes in iron metabolism that result from long-term treatment increase the risk of infection due to *Yersinia* spp., *Pneumocystis carinii*, and *Staphylococcus aureus*.

- Long-term treatment can cause lens opacities, retinopathy, and hearing disturbances.

- Vitamin C (100–200 mg orally) can increase the effect of deferoxamine, but only if given separately from food.
- Avoid co-prescribing prochlorperazine and levomepromazine with deferoxamine; they can cause loss of consciousness.

Safety and efficacy

Long-term treatment

- Measure visual acuity and perform a hearing check before long-term treatment starts and every 3 months thereafter.
- Measure the serum iron and other markers of iron metabolism to tailor the dose correctly.

- Warn patients that deferoxamine can turn the urine brown.
- Advise patients to report any changes in vision or hearing.

Prescribing information: **Deferoxamine**

Acute poisoning

- The usual dose is 15 mg/kg/h, given intravenously, up to a maximum of 80 mg/kg.

Chronic overload

- In established overload the usual dose is 30–50 mg/kg daily.
- Once the overload has been treated the dose should not exceed 30 mg/kg daily.
- Measure the serum iron and markers of iron metabolism to tailor the dosage regimen.

Aluminium overload (specialist use)

- 100 mg of deferoxamine will bind 4.1 mg of aluminium.

Calcium salts

Essential ion

Calcium is an essential component of excitation–contraction coupling in muscle cells.

Corrected calcium concentration

- Clinical features are due to the ionized calcium concentration; the laboratory measures total calcium. Most calcium is bound to albumin.
- Adjust the calcium according to the plasma albumin.
- Add 0.02 mmol/L to the measured calcium concentration for every 1 g the albumin is below 40 g/L.
- And vice versa if the albumin is above 40 g/L.
- For example, measured calcium concentration 2.25 mmol/L, albumin 35 g/L; corrected calcium concentration = 2.25 + [(40 – 35) x 0.02] = 2.35 mmol/L.

Note

- Calcium salts are included in some antacid formulations.
- Excessive doses can cause the milk-alkali syndrome, characterized by hypercalaemia and alkalosis.

- Treatment of hypocalcaemia.
- Treatment of hyperkalaemia.
- Prevention of osteoporosis (with vitamin D).

- Collection of a blood sample in a tube containing EDTA, citrate, or oxalate will give a spuriously low result.

Treatment of hypocalcaemia

- Identify the underlying cause.
- See below for an intravenous regimen if emergency treatment is required.

Treatment of hyperkalaemia

- Calcium gluconate, given by intravenous injection over 3–5 minutes stabilizes cardiac membranes.
  - This has no effect on the serum potassium concentration.
  - See potassium (p. 552) for more information.

Prevention of osteoporosis

- Calcium and vitamin D supplements are recommended for patients at risk of osteoporosis over 65 years old.
- See bisphosphonates (p. 582) for more information on the treatment of osteoporosis.

Hypocalcaemia

Causes
- Chronic renal insufficiency (deficient vitamin D production)
- Hypoparathyroidism
- Vitamin D deficiency
- Malabsorption
- Hypomagnesaemia and hypokalaemia
- Rhabdomyolysis

Clinical features
- Tingling
- Tetany
- Mental changes

Hypercalcaemia

- Polyuria, polydipsia
- Anorexia, nausea, vomiting
- Constipation
- Muscle weakness
- Confusion, lethargy, and depression

Late findings
- Nephrolithiasis
- Bone pain
- Pathological fractures

Causes
- Parathyroid-associated
- Malignancy-associated (breast, bronchus, bone marrow, kidney)
- Vitamin D-related
- High bone turnover (hyperthyroidism, immobilization)
- Related to renal insufficiency (severe secondary hyperparathyroidism, aluminium intoxication)
- Drugs (thiazide diuretics)

- Adverse effects are uncommon.
  - Excessive doses can cause hypercalcaemia (see box).
  - See bisphosphonates (p. 585) for information on the treatment of hypercalcaemia.
  - Rapid infusion can precipitate cardiac arrhythmias.

- Take care when giving intravenous calcium to patients taking digoxin, whose actions it will enhance.

Safety and efficacy

- Measure the serum calcium concentration and monitor clinically for hypercalcaemia.
- The serum calcium concentration is not normally reduced in osteoporosis. Consider bone densitometry if this will change your treatment.

- If calcium is given for prevention of osteoporosis, make sure that the patient addresses the other risk factors for osteoporosis (e.g. smoking).

Prescribing information: **Calcium salts**

Emergency treatment of hyperkalaemia

- By intravenous injection, 10 mL of 10% calcium gluconate over 3–5 minutes.
- This has no effect on the serum potassium concentration.

Emergency treatment of hypocalcaemia

- By intravenous injection, 10 mL of 10% calcium gluconate over 3–5 minutes.
- Followed by a continuous infusion of 40 mL over 24 hours.

Prevention of osteoporosis (with vitamin D)

- By mouth, ergocalciferol (vitamin D_2) 800 IU (20 mg) and calcium gluconate 800–1500 mg daily.

Magnesium sulfate

Essential ion

Magnesium is an essential ion that is an important co-factor in many enzyme systems. Body magnesium stores often mirror body potassium stores.

Note

- Magnesium is not well absorbed when taken by mouth.
- It is commonly used as an osmotic laxative. This indication is not considered further here.
- See section on treatment of constipation for more information.

- Treatment of hypomagnesaemia.
- Treatment of some cardiac arrhythmias (e.g. torsade de pointes).
- Treatment of eclampsia and pre-eclampsia.
- Adjunctive role in the treatment of acute, severe asthma.

- Avoid giving magnesium if the patient has severe hepatic insufficiency.
- Magnesium can accumulate if the patient has severe renal insufficiency, but this is rare.
- Excessive doses given during labour can cause neonatal respiratory depression.

Treatment of hypomagnesaemia

- Body magnesium concentrations may be low when body potassium concentrations are low.
  - Excretion of magnesium is increased by diuretic drugs.
  - Potassium-sparing diuretics are also magnesium-sparing.
- Patients in ICUs are often given maintenance doses of 24 mmol daily.

Treatment of arrhythmias

- Intravenous magnesium is effective for certain ventricular arrhythmias, in particular torsade de pointes.
  - This arrhythmia can be precipitated by drugs that prolong the QT interval (see antihistamines, p. 610).

Eclampsia and pre-eclampsia

- Magnesium sulfate reduces the incidence of seizures in women with eclampsia.
- This is a potentially fatal condition and should be managed by an expert.

Asthma

- A single dose of intravenous magnesium sulfate is an effective adjunct in the treatment of acute severe asthma.
- Seek expert advice before giving magnesium.

- Adverse effects are uncommon.
  - Hypermagnesaemia is characterized by:
    - Muscle weakness and reduced tendon reflexes.
    - Nausea and flushing.
    - Double vision and slurred speech.
  - Calcium gluconate can be used to treat toxicity.

- The combination of large doses of magnesium and calcium channel blockers in eclampsia can cause profound hypotension.
- Magnesium potentiates the action of non-depolarizing muscle blockers.

Safety and efficacy

- Measure the serum magnesium concentration and monitor clinically for hypermagnesaemia.

- This drug is usually given in an emergency.

Prescribing information: **Magnesium sulfate**

Arrhythmias

- By intravenous infusion, 8 mmol over 10–15 minutes.

Eclampsia

- By intravenous infusion, 16 mmol over 5–10 minutes, followed by 4 mmol/h for 24 hours.

Note Magnesium sulfate 1g approximately equivalent to Mg^{2+} 4 mmol.

Potassium chloride

Essential ion

- Potassium is an essential ion involved in creating and maintaining electrochemical gradients in both excitable and non-excitable tissues.
- Total body potassium is about 3500 mmol, of which 90% is intracellular.
- Total body potassium may be low even in the presence of a high serum concentration (e.g. in diabetic ketoacidosis).
- The serum potassium concentration is tightly regulated; small changes can have important clinical effects, especially on cardiac tissues.
- A raised serum potassium concentration stabilizes excitable membranes and can cause asystole.
- A low serum concentration depolarizes membranes and can cause cardiac arrhythmias.

Serum potassium concentration reference range 3.5–5.0 mmol/L

Note on potassium chloride

Potassium chloride is the salt of choice in treating or preventing potassium depletion, since retention of potassium will not occur unless the concomitant chloride depletion is also corrected.

- Treatment and prevention of potassium depletion from any cause (e.g. patients taking diuretic drugs or corticosteroids).

- Do not give potassium supplements unless you know the serum potassium concentration.
  - Do not give supplements if the serum potassium is above 5 mmol/L.
- Patients with renal insufficiency are at particular risk of hyperkalaemia.
- Never give undiluted potassium by intravenous injection or infusion.
- Hypokalaemia can cause digoxin toxicity, even if the plasma digoxin concentration is in or even below the usual target range. Withhold digoxin and replace potassium urgently.

- Patients should not normally require potassium supplements. If the serum potassium concentration is low, always consider the likely cause.
  - Diuretics are a common cause. Regularly review the need for these drugs and the dose. Long-term prevention of hypokalaemia is best achieved with a potassium-sparing diuretic rather than potassium supplements. Combination formulation of diuretics and potassium supplements are not recommended. See potassium-sparing diuretics (p. 184) for more information.
  - Corticosteroids lower the serum potassium concentration. Remember that treatment with corticosteroids should be with the lowest effective dose for the shortest possible time.
  - Patients with heavy gastrointestinal loss (e.g. high-output ileostomy) may lose a lot of potassium (5–15 mmol/day). Provide supplements and consider whether losses can be reduced.
  - Extensive surgical (especially abdominal) procedures can result in significant potassium loss. Monitor the serum potassium closely and be prepared to give supplements.
- Patients with cardiac disease are at particular risk of arrhythmias if the serum potassium concentration is low. The target concentration is usually higher in these patients.

Suggested target serum potassium concentration in patients with cardiac disease is 4–5 mmol/L

- Oral potassium supplements are suitable for short-term mild potassium depletion. Review the need for supplements daily, and especially before discharge from hospital.
  - Enteric-coated formulations can cause intestinal ulceration and are no longer recommended.
  - Modified-release formulations can cause oesophageal ulceration in those with oesophageal obstruction (e.g. left atrial enlargement due to mitral stenosis). They also have a delayed onset of action. Their use is not recommended. Instead use effervescent formulations.

Parenteral infusion		
Peripheral	**Central**	**General notes**
• 40 mmol/L is the usual maximum recommended concentration that can be administered via a peripheral line. • Higher concentrations (60–80 mmol/L) can be given via a large peripheral vein in severe depletion, or during strict fluid restriction. • Usual maximum daily dose, 3 mmol/kg. • Usual maximum rate of infusion, 10–20 mmol/h.	• 20 mmol/100 mL is the usual recommended maximum concentration to be administered via a central line. • The usual maximum daily dose is 3 mmol/kg, although this can be increased to 6 mmol/kg in severe cases. • The usual maximum rate of infusion is 30 mmol/h.	• Use ready-mixed potassium infusion bags whenever possible. • Adding strong potassium chloride to bags can cause layering if it is not mixed properly. • The rate of replacement of potassium is limited by the rate of transfer of potassium from the extracellular to intracellular compartments. • Use an infusion pump if the concentration of potassium in the intravenous fluid is above 40 mmol/L.

- Cardiac toxicity. Because the rate of replacement of potassium is limited by the rate of transfer of potassium from the extracellular to the intracellular compartment, the plasma concentration can rise rapidly (within a few hours). Follow the monitoring guidelines outlined below.
- Pain and phlebitis are more likely when high concentrations of potassium are given intravenously.
  - Extravasation causes tissue necrosis.
- Oral potassium supplements commonly cause nausea and vomiting.

- There is a particular risk of hyperkalaemia when potassium supplements are co-prescribed with:
  - Potassium-sparing diuretics (e.g. amiloride, triamterene, spironolactone).
  - ACE inhibitors or angiotensin receptor antagonists; this can be severe.
  - Ciclosporin and tacrolimus.
  - NSAIDs, especially indometacin, which can worsen renal function and so cause hyperkalaemia.

Safety and efficacy

- Measure the plasma potassium concentration before giving potassium supplements.
- The continued need for oral supplements should be reviewed daily. They should not be required in the long term.
- If potassium is given parenterally:
  - Continuous ECG monitoring is recommended if the infusion rate exceeds 20 mmol/h.
  - Stop the infusion if peaking of the T waves occurs; measure the serum concentration urgently.
  - Measure the serum potassium concentration at least daily (more often if given via a central vein).
  - Patients with renal insufficiency are at particular risk of hyperkalaemia.

- Advise the patient at risk of hypokalaemia to maintain a good oral intake of potassium.
  - The recommended dietary intake is 3.5 g daily.
  - A banana contains 0.5 g and a baked potato 0.75 g.
- Similarly, warn patients with renal insufficiency to avoid food rich in potassium.
- Explain the importance of regular measurement of serum potassium concentrations.

Prescribing information: **Potassium**

Oral potassium

- The following are examples:
- Sando K® tablets, 12 mmol potassium per tablet. Usual dose 2 tablets tds.
- Kay-Cee-L® liquid, 1 mmol/mL. Usual dose 20 mL tds.

Parenteral potassium

- Follow the guidance on dose and administration given above.

TEACHING POINT Treatment of hyperkalaemia

Reduce intake and increase elimination

- Withhold oral potassium supplements and any drugs that conserve potassium (see interactions section above).
- Increase gastrointestinal potassium loss. Give a polystyrene sulfonate resin (e.g. Calcium Resonium®) by mouth.
- These take time to act and are only suitable if hyperkalaemia is mild and the patient is at a low risk of arrhythmias.

If hyperkalaemia is severe or if the patient has ECG changes

- The patient should have continuous cardiac monitoring and resuscitation facilities should be immediately available.
- Stabilize cardiac membranes with 10 mL of 10% calcium gluconate given by intravenous injection over 3–5 minutes. This has no effect on the serum potassium concentration.
    - Take care when giving this drug to patients taking digoxin; it potentiates the effect of digoxin and can cause arrhythmias.
- Drive potassium into cells (lowering the serum potassium concentration).
    - Give 10 units of soluble insulin with 50 mL of glucose (to prevent hypoglycaemia) by intravenous infusion over several minutes.
- Alternatives include:
    - Salbutamol (β_2 adrenoceptor agonist), 5–10 mg by nebulized solution.
    - Sodium bicarbonate, 50 mL of an 8.4% solution by intravenous infusion over several minutes into a central vein.
        - Note, do not give through the same lumen as calcium gluconate; insoluble calcium carbonate will precipitate.
- The most severe cases will require dialysis.
- Most of these measures move potassium rather eliminating it; urgently investigate the cause of the hyperkalaemia.

ECG features of hyperkalaemia

- Peaked T waves
- Flat P waves
- Prolonged PR interval
- Widened QRS complex

Vitamin D analogues

A complex group of metabolites and synthetic analogues of vitamin D

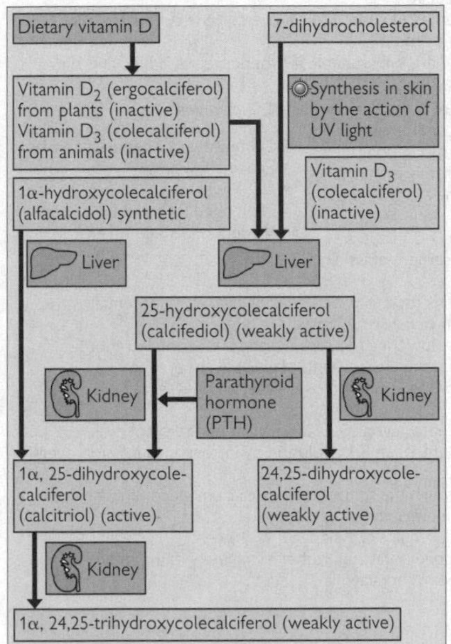

Causes of vitamin D deficiency

- Inadequate dietary sources
- Malabsorption
- Repeated pregnancy
- Drugs (e.g colestyramine reduces the absorption of fat-soluble vitamins)
  - Anticonvulsants

- Treatment of vitamin D deficiency (usually oral colecalciferol or ergocalciferol).
  - Prevention of osteoporosis (with calcium).
- Treatment of hypoparathyroidism (alfacalcidol).
- Treatment of renal osteodystrophy (alfacalcidol).
- Treatment of anticonvulsant-induced osteomalacia.
- Treatment of congenital rickets.
- Topical treatment of plaque psoriasis.

- Avoid these drugs if the patient has hypercalcaemia or metastatic calcification.
- No dosage reduction is usually required in renal or hepatic insufficiency.
  - The hydroxylated derivatives, alfacalcidol and calcitriol, should be used if the patient has renal insufficiency.
- High systemic doses of vitamin D are teratogenic in animals; therapeutic doses are unlikely to cause adverse effects.
- Vitamin D enters breast milk in significant quantities.

Vitamin D deficiency

- The elderly and those who do not take vitamin D in the diet are at risk of vitamin D deficiency.
  - This was classically described in Asian immigrants to the UK eating unleavened bread containing large amounts of phytate, but vitamin D deficiency is now uncommon in this group.
  - Vitamin D and calcium supplementation reduces the incidence of osteoporosis in the elderly, even in the absence of frank deficiency.
- Once the deficiency has been treated, long-term treatment is rarely necessary, unless the cause is persistent.
  - The most common persistent cause is malabsorption, in which very large oral doses may be required.

Prevention of osteoporosis

- Calcium and vitamin D supplementation is recommended in those aged over 65 years at risk of osteoporosis.
  - See below for dose. See bisphosphonates (p. 582) for more information on osteoporosis.
  - See oestrogens (p. 430) for a list of risk factors and suggested diagnostic workup.

Hypoparathyroidism

- Hypoparathyroidism can result de novo or can follow parathyroid or thyroid surgery.
- Post-surgical patients should be monitored for hypoparathyroidism.

Renal osteodystrophy

- Renal insufficiency leads to reduced plasma calcium and raised plasma phosphate concentrations. This stimulates parathyroid hormone (PTH) production and can lead to metastatic calcification.
- The initial treatment of renal osteodystrophy is a phosphate-binding drug. Once the phosphate concentration has fallen, give alfacalcidol with calcium supplements to reduce metastatic calcification.

Anticonvulsant-induced osteomalacia

- The anticonvulsants phenytoin and phenobarbital can cause osteomalacia during long-term use.
- The mechanism is not fully understood, but is probably the result of enhanced metabolism of colecalciferol.

Psoriasis

- Topical vitamin D analogues, calcipotriol and tacalcitol, and topical calcitriol, are used for the treatment of plaque psoriasis.
- They induce the differentiation of keratinocytes, reducing their proliferation.
- Used topically, these drugs do not affect systemic calcium metabolism.

- The adverse effects of vitamin D analogues are related to their effects on calcium metabolism.
  - The most common important adverse effect is hypercalaemia. This is dose-related.
  - The symptoms of hypercalcaemia include nausea, vomiting, anorexia, thirst, and lassitude.
  - Alfacalcidol and calcitriol have short half-lives. This makes it easier to titrate them to the correct dose than some of the long-acting alternatives.

- See bisphosphonates (p. 585) for guidance on the treatment of hypercalaemia.
  - Withdrawal of the drug or a dosage reduction may be all that is required for mild symptoms.
- Vitamin D analogues used topically for psoriasis can cause local itching, erythema, dermatitis, and burning.

- Drug interactions are uncommon.
- Thiazide diuretics reduce the excretion of vitamin D analogues; there is an increased risk of hypercalcaemia if they are given together.
- Phenobarbital and phenytoin increase the metabolism of vitamin D analogues (see above). The dose of vitamin D may need to be increased.

Safety and efficacy

- Measure the plasma calcium concentration at least weekly during the start of treatment.
- If long-term treatment is required, measure the plasma calcium concentration every few months.
- Measure the plasma calcium concentration if the patient has any symptoms of hypercalcaemia.

- Advise the patient to report nausea, vomiting, polyuria, polydipsia, or other symptoms that might suggest hypercalcaemia.
- Advise patients using vitamin D analogues topically to wash their hands thoroughly after use.
- There is evidence of diurnal variation in response to vitamin D; advise the patient to take the dose at the same time each day.

Prescribing information: **Vitamin D analogues**

There are many formulations of these drugs; the following are given as examples. See notes above to select the most apporiate for the proposed indication.

Treatment and prevention of vitamin D deficiency and osteoporosis

- Only available in combination with calcium.
  - Ergocalciferol 400 IU (10 micrograms) with a variable amount of calcium (depends on the formulation).
  - If used to prevent osteoporosis give ergocalciferol 800 IU (20 micrograms) and 800–1500 mg calcium gluconate daily.

Vitamin D deficiency due to malabsorption or chronic liver disease

- Calciferol by mouth, up to 40 000 units (1 mg) daily.

Hypoparathyroidism

- Calciferol by mouth, up to 100 000 units (2.5 mg) daily.

Renal osteodystrophy

- Alfacalcidol, by mouth, initially 1 microgram daily.
  - Usual maintenance dose 0.25–1 microgram daily.
- Calcitriol by mouth, initially 250 nanograms daily.
  - Usual maintenance dose 500–1000 nanograms daily.
  - Available by injection for patients receiving haemodialysis; usual maintenance dose 500–3000 nanograms 3 times a week.

Vitamin K_1

Essential fat-soluble vitamin

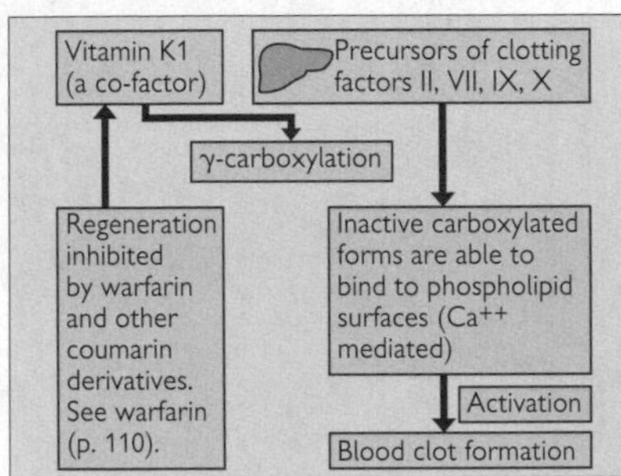

Drugs in this class

- Phytomenadione
  - Lipid-soluble
- Menadiol
  - Synthetic analogue
  - Water-soluble
  - Do not give to neonates

- Treatment of clotting disorders that result from vitamin K deficiency.
  - Reduced synthesis (e.g. hepatic cirrhosis).
  - Drugs (e.g. warfarin and other coumarin anticoagulants). Colestyramine given for primary biliary cirrhosis reduces absorption of fat-soluble vitamins.
  - Nutritional deficiency.
    - Neonates are relatively deficient in vitamin K. This can cause haemorrhagic disease of the newborn. Vitamin K is given to prevent this. This risk is increased if the mother is taking anticonvulsant drugs.
    - Malabsorption of fat-soluble vitamins (A, D, E_1, K) (e.g. in biliary obstruction).
    - Lack of enteric bacteria.

- Vitamin K can be used to correct a clotting disorder, but is rarely sufficient on its own for treatment of haemorrhage.
- Do not give menadiol (a synthetic analogue of vitamin K) to neonates; there is a risk of haemolysis.
- Do not give by intramuscular injection if the patient has abnormal clotting.
- Anticoagulation using warfarin or other coumarin anticoagulants will be very difficult for several weeks after a large dose of vitamin K. See how to use section.

- The Chief Medical Officer in the UK has recommended that all newborn babies should be offered vitamin K to reduce the risk of haemorrhagic disease of the newborn.
  - This can be given as a single intramuscular injection of 1 mg at birth; or 2 mg orally at birth, after 1 week, and after 1 month. Bottle-fed babies can omit the last dose, as formula feeds contain vitamin K.
- Some intravenous formulations of phytomenadione contain polyethoxylated castor oil (Cremophor EL) which can cause anaphylactoid reactions when given by rapid intravenous injection (see acetylcysteine, p. 625). Give slowly (1 mg/min) by intravenous infusion.
- If the patient has fat-soluble vitamin malabsorption give menadione, as this is water-soluble.

- Vitamin K can be given to reverse anticoagulation due to warfarin and other coumarin analogues (see warfarin, p. 115).
    - A dose of 10 mg of vitamin K will fully reverse the action of warfarin. Blood clotting may not return to normal immediately, as new clotting factors will have to be synthesized.
    - If the patient is bleeding, see teaching point in heparin (p. 109) for guidance.
    - Partial reversal of the effect of warfarin can be achieved by giving small doses of vitamin K (e.g. 0.5–2.0 mg by intravenous injection). This will require close monitoring and dose titration.

- Adverse effects are rare.
    - Note the advice about intravenous adminstration of phytomenadione.
    - Intramuscular injection can cause a haematoma if the patient has abnormal clotting.

- Vitamin K antagonizes the action of warfarin and other coumarin anticoagulants.

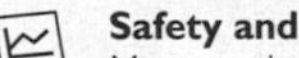

Safety and efficacy

- Measure the prothrombin time (or INR — see warfarin, p. 110) to assess the requirement for treatment.
- Ensure that the patient is closely observed if there is a risk of bleeding.

- Discuss the recommendation that the baby be given vitamin K with women and their partners before they go into labour; record the parents' preference in the notes.

Prescribing information: **Vitamin K_1**

Menadiol

- By mouth for prevention of vitamin K deficiency in fat malabsorption syndromes, 10 mg daily.

Phytomenadione

- By mouth for prevention of haemorrhagic disease of the newborn, 2 mg at birth and on days 7 and 30.
- By intramuscular injection for prevention of haemorrhagic disease of the newborn, 1 mg at birth.
- By slow intravenous injection/infusion for treatment of abnormal clotting, 0.5–10 mg; see notes above.

Chapter 10

Musculoskeletal and joints

Contents

Colchicine

Inhibitor of cellular microtubule function

The mechanism by which colchicine has its effect is not completely understood, but it seems to be related to inhibition of microtubule function in leukocytes. This reduces migration of phagocytes into gouty tissues. In turn, this reduces the deposition of urate and breaks the vicious cycle of inflammation and further urate deposition.

Drugs used for hyperuricaemia

Acute gout
- NSAIDs
- Colchicine

Long-term prophylaxis
- Allopurinol (reduced uric acid production)
- Sulfinpyrazone (uricosuric, increased excretion)
- Probenecid (increased excretion); rarely used

Cytotoxic drug-induced hyperuricaemia
- Allopurinol
- Rasburicase

- Treatment of acute gout.
- Prophylaxis against allopurinol-induced gout.
- Prophylaxis against attacks of familial Mediterranean fever (recurrent polyserositis); unlicensed indication.

- Colchicine is mainly metabolized by the liver, but the proportion excreted by the kidney increases in hepatic insufficiency. Reduce the dose by half in severe liver or renal impairment.
- Colchicine is teratogenic in animals; it is therefore contraindicated in pregnancy. The manufacturers advise that it should not be given to mothers who are breastfeeding.

Acute gout
- Colchicine can produce an analgesic effect within a few hours.
- Colchicine is not a treatment for causes of secondary gout (see box above).
- Unlike NSAIDs, colchicine does not cause fluid retention, making it a suitable choice for patients with heart failure.
- The first few days of treatment with allopurinol are associated with an increased risk of an acute attack of gout. Colchicine can be used as prophylaxis during this period. Most doctors wait until an acute attack has fully settled (usually after 1 month) before starting allopurinol.
- Colchicine has a narrow therapeutic range, and adverse effects are common. Start with a low dose and titrate to optimal symptomatic relief.
- Long-term treatment is associated with the risk of several serious adverse effects and is rarely indicated.

- Gastrointestinal adverse effects are very common at therapeutic doses. The most common adverse effect is diarrhoea; in severe cases (usually associated with overdose) this can be a cholera-like enteritis.
- Colchicine can cause bone marrow suppression. Leukopenia and thrombocytopenia are sometimes seen with long-term treatment.
- Long-term treatment can cause steatorrhoea, a myopathy, and a peripheral neuropathy. These are more common in patients with renal impairment.

- Colchicine interacts with ciclosporin; the plasma ciclosporin concentration is increased and there is an increased risk of nephrotoxicity.

- Low doses of aspirin and other salicylates reduce uric acid excretion; it may be necessary to avoid these drugs in patients with gout.
- Diuretics (especially thiazides) increase the risk of gout. Ask the patient about previous attacks of gout before starting these drugs.
- Colchicine, unlike NSAIDs, does not interact with warfarin.

Safety and efficacy

- Clinical improvement and reduction in pain are the measures of efficacy.
- Although colchicine can cause leukopenia, routine measurement is unlikely to be helpful.
- If long-term treatment is required, measure the creatinine clearance and use the lowest effective dose (less than 0.6 mg/day). Measure the serum creatinine kinase if there is evidence of myopathy.

- Advise the patient how to avoid acute attacks of gout.
  - Certain meats, seafood, dried peas, and beans are particularly high in purines.
  - Alcoholic beverages, especially beer, can precipitate attacks of gout.
  - Ensure adequate daily fluid intake (2–3 litres per day).

Prescribing information: **Colchicine**

Treatment of gout

- By mouth, 1 mg initially, followed by 500 micrograms every 2–3 hours until relief of pain is obtained or vomiting or diarrhoea occurs, or until a total dose of 6 mg has been reached. The course should not be repeated within 3 days.

Prevention of gout

- During initial treatment with allopurinol or uricosuric drugs, 500 micrograms 2 or 3 times daily.

Allopurinol

Inhibitor of the enzyme xanthine oxidase

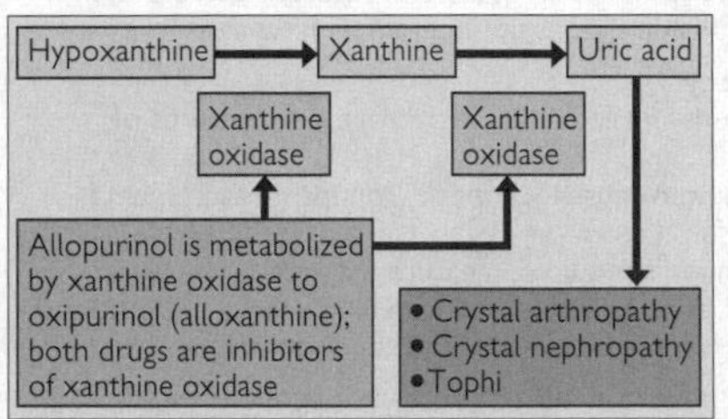

Drugs used for hyperuricaemia

Acute gout
- NSAIDs
- Colchicine

Long-term prophylaxis
- Allopurinol (reduced uric acid production)
- Sulfinpyrazone (uricosuric, increased excretion)
- Probenecid (increased excretion); rarely used

Cytotoxic drug-induced hyperuricaemia
- Allopurinol
- Rasburicase

- Treatment of chronic hyperuricaemia and its complications:
  - Gout.
  - Uric acid nephropathy.
  - Tophi.
- Treatment of hyperuricaemia associated with chemotherapy.
- Treatment of certain rare enzyme deficiencies associated with hyperuricaemia (specialized use).

- Do not start allopurinol during an acute attack of gout (see below).
- The safety of allopurinol in pregnancy has not been formally assessed, but it has been used for many years without apparent adverse effects.
- Limit the daily dose to 100 mg or less in moderate to severe renal insufficiency (see prescribing information).
- Reduce the dose in severe hepatic insufficiency.

Chronic hyperuricaemia
- Allopurinol is not a treatment for acute gout, nor is it an analgesic; use NSAIDs or colchicine.
- The first few days of treatment with allopurinol are associated with an increased risk of an acute attack of gout. Colchicine can be used as prophylaxis during this period. Most prescribers wait until an acute attack has fully settled (usually after 1 month) before starting allopurinol.
- If an acute attack of gout occurs while the patient is taking allopurinol, continue the allopurinol and treat the acute attack.

Hyperuricaemia associated with chemotherapy
- Chemotherapy that results in rapid tumour lysis can cause hyperuricaemia. This is particularly associated with treatment of leukaemia and non-Hodgkin's lymphoma.
- The metabolism of mercaptopurine and azathioprine is significantly reduced by allopurinol. The dosage requirements are reduced by 75% when allopurinol is co-administered. Check that this has been taken into account.
- Allopurinol should be started at least 24 hours before chemotherapy in order to be effective.
- Adequate hydration is as important as allopurinol in reducing the risk of nephropathy. Ensure that the patient takes 2–3 litres of fluid daily.

- Rash and hypersensitivity are common with allopurinol.
  - Rash affects about 2% of patients.
  - The rash may rarely be severe (Stevens–Johnson syndrome).
- Other manifestations include:
  - Renal failure (interstitial nephritis).
  - Hepatitis.
  - Eosinophilia.

- The metabolism of azathioprine and mercaptopurine are significantly reduced by allopurinol. Reduce the dose by 75% if allopurinol is co-administered.
- The toxic effects of cyclophosphamide on the bone marrow are increased when allopurinol is co-administered.
- The risk of toxicity of ACE inhibitors and angiotensin receptor antagonists is increased when they are co-administered with allopurinol, especially when the patient has renal impairment.
- Low doses of aspirin and other salicylates reduce uric acid excretion; it may be necessary to avoid these drugs in patients with gout.
- Diuretics (especially thiazides) increase the risk of gout. Ask the patient about previous attacks of gout before starting these drugs and consider allopurinol prophylaxis.

Safety and efficacy

- Measure renal function to ensure both adequate hydration and that the drug is effective. This is especially important when using allopurinol during chemotherapy.
- Measuring the serum uric acid concentration is fraught with difficulties of interpretation. There is no absolute correlation between the uric acid concentration and symptoms and no consensus about the target uric acid concentration.
  - The manufacturers suggest that if facilities are available to monitor plasma concentrations of the active metabolite oxipurinol, the dose of allopurinol should be adjusted to maintain plasma oxipurinol concentrations below 100 micromol/L (15.2 mg/L). However, this is rarely available.
  - Treat the clinical presentation rather than the uric acid concentration.

- Advise the patient how to avoid acute attacks of gout.
  - Certain meats, seafood, dried peas, and beans are particularly high in purines.
  - Alcoholic beverages, especially beer, can precipitate attacks of gout.
  - Ensure an adequate daily fluid intake (2–3 litres per day).

Prescribing information: **Allopurinol**

Prophylaxis against gout

- Initially 100 mg daily, preferably after food.
- Usual maintenance dose 100–200 mg/day. Severe disease may require doses up to 900 mg daily.
- Doses above 300 mg/day should be divided (e.g. 200 mg bd).
- Reduce the initial dose to 100 mg daily in moderate renal insufficiency.
- Reduce the initial dose to 100 mg on alternate days in severe renal insufficiency.

Hyperuricaemia associated with chemotherapy

- Follow local protocols according to chemotherapy regimen.

Rheumatoid arthritis (disease-modifying drugs)

Note on the treatment of rheumatoid arthritis

Rheumatoid arthritis is a complex systemic disease that should ideally be managed by a multidisciplinary team. It is not our purpose in this section to provide a treatment guide, but to provide information on the drugs used. Rheumatoid arthritis is common and the drugs used to treat it commonly cause adverse effects.

See also:
NSAIDs p. 658
Penicillamine p. 630
Methotrexate p. 498
Sulfasalazine p. 42

Drugs used to treat rheumatoid arthritis

- Analgesics

Disease-modifying drugs

- Sulfasalazine
- Antimalarial drugs
- Methotrexate
- Gold salts
- Penicillamine

Second-line drugs

- Azathioprine
- Cyclophosphamide
- Chlorambucil
- Leflunomide
- Etanercept
- Infliximab

Chloroquine and hydroxychloroquine

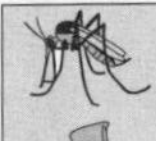

The antimalarial actions of these drugs are based on their ability to interfere with plasmodial DNA replication.
See also antimalarials, p. 382.

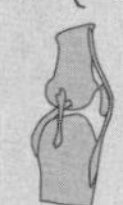

These drugs can also be used as disease modifying agents (DMARDs) in the treatment of rheumatoid arthritis. The mechanism of action is not known but may be related to stabilization of lysosomes.

- Treatment and prophylaxis against chloroquine-sensitive *Plasmodium* infection.
  - Resistance to chloroquine is very common and it is no longer recommended for the treatment of *Plasmodium falciparum* malaria. It can still be used for *P. ovale*, *P. malariae*, and *P. vivax* infections.
- As a disease-modifying drug in the long-term control of rheumatoid arthritis.
- Occasionally used for the treatment of systemic and discoid lupus erythematosus and psoriasis (specialized uses).

- Reduce the dose in patients with renal or hepatic insufficiency. The doses used for prophylaxis do not usually need to be reduced.
- Do not give these drugs to patients with G6PD deficiency.
- Avoid using these drugs for prolonged periods in women who are pregnant; there is a risk of fetal ototoxicity. If used short-term for the treatment of acute malaria, the benefit will usually outweigh the risk.
- Do not use in patients with epilepsy; these drugs lower the seizure threshold.
- Although occasionally used for the treatment of psoriasis, these drugs more commonly precipitate psoriasis. Avoid using them if possible in patients with psoriasis.

Malaria prophylaxis

- Patterns of malarial resistance are constantly changing; seek up-to-date specialist advice.
- When using these drugs for prophylaxis, aim to establish a routine and tolerability by starting them 2 weeks before travel. Continue treatment for 4 weeks after returning.
- Other measures, such as avoidance, bed nets, and repellent sprays (diethyltoluamide/DEET), are as important as drug treatment for the prophylaxis of malaria. You cannot catch malaria unless you are bitten.
- Choloroquine can be used for up to 5 years for long-term prophylaxis.
- Choloroquine alone will eradicate *P. malariae* but if used for *P. ovale* or *P. vivax* infection the liver stage will need to be treated by another drug (e.g. primaquine).

Rheumatoid arthritis

- The choice of a DMARD should be taken by the supervising specialist.
- These drugs are generally better tolerated than gold or penicillamine.
- The dose should be calculated on lean body mass; do not exceed 4 mg/kg in obese patients.
- The effect will take 4–6 months to develop.

- These drugs can form deposits in the cornea and retina. The risk is higher (seen at daily doses of 250 mg) with chloroquine than with

hydroxychloroquine (seen at daily doses of 400 mg). See monitoring section below.
- Hypersensitivity phenomena are common and can be severe, ranging from a rash to angio-oedema.
- Gastrointestinal disturbance and headache are common adverse effects.
- These drugs can cause thrombocytopenia and ototoxicity.
- These drugs are very dangerous in overdose, owing to cardiac toxicity. Doses above 8 g are usually fatal.
- Long-term treatment can cause a bluish pigmentation of the skin and bleaching of the hair.
- These drugs have very long half-lives (~45 days); it takes several months before they reach a steady state (see teaching point in amiodarone, p. 103).

- Do not prescribe these drugs with amiodarone; there is a risk of ventricular tachycardia.
- Avoid prescribing these drugs with other drugs that can cause severe rash (e.g. gold, phenylbutazone, pyramethamine/sulfadoxine); the risk is greatly increased.
- These drugs lower the seizure threshold; take care if the patient is taking another drug that lowers the threshold.
- These drugs can increase plasma digoxin and ciclosporin concentrations, causing toxicity.

Safety
- Before long-term treatment
  - Measure visual acuity and record the result. Measure renal and liver function, a lower dose is required if there is impairment.
- During long-term treatment
  - Measure acuity annually. If the patient reports any blurred vision or reduction in acuity, refer them for an expert opinion.

- Malaria prophylaxis
  - Drug treatment alone is not sufficient. Do not forget to cover up, and to use an impregnated bed net and repellent spray.
  - Report any feverish illness especially within 3 months of return; say that you have been to a malarious region.
- Report any deterioration in vision immediately during long-term treatment.

Prescribing information: **Chloroquine and hydroxychloroquine**

Chloroquine for malaria

- Note: chloroquine dosages are calculated on the basis of the amount of chloroquine base.
- Chloroquine base 150 mg ≡ chloroquine sulphate 200 mg ≡ chloroquine phosphate 250 mg (approximately).
- Prophylaxis
  - Seek expert advice for the proposed area of travel.
  - When cholorquine is appropriate, the dosage is usually chloroquine base 300 mg taken once weekly.
- Treatment
  - Chloroquine is not recommended for the treatment of *P. falciparum* malaria.

- When appropriate, the usual regimen is:
  - Initial dose of 600 mg (of base) *then*
  - A single dose of 300 mg after 6–8 hours *then*
  - A single dose of 300 mg daily for 2 days

DMARDs for rheumatoid arthritis

- This is a specialized use and should be initiated and supervised under expert guidance.
- Chloroquine
  - Chloroquine (base) 150 mg daily. Can be increased to a maximum of 2.5 mg/kg daily.
- Hydroxychloroquine
  - Initially 400 mg daily in divided doses.
  - The maintenance dosage is usually 200–400 mg daily.
  - Can be increased to a maximum of 6.5 mg/kg daily (but not exceeding 400 mg daily).

Gold salts

Disease-modifying antirheumatic drug

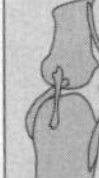

These drugs are used as disease modifying agents (DMARDs) in the treatment of rheumatoid arthritis. Their mechanism of action is not fully understood, but they suppress inflammatory and immune responses. This may be due to reduced lysosomal enzyme activity and phagocytosis.

Drugs in this class

- Sodium aurothiomaleate (intramuscular)
- Auranofin (oral)

- As a disease-modifying agent (DMARD) in rheumatoid arthritis.
  - Also given for juvenile arthritis.

- Avoid giving gold salts to patients with severe renal or hepatic insufficiency, or those with a history of blood disorders.
- Avoid gold salts in patients with a history of systemic lupus erythematosus, inflammatory bowel disease, porphyria, or pulmonary fibrosis.
- Gold salts are contraindicated during pregnancy and breastfeeding.

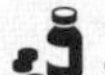

Rheumatoid arthritis

- The choice of a DMARD should be made by the supervising specialist.
- Sulfasalazine, methotrexate, gold, and penicillamine are of similar efficacy, but sulfasalazine and methotrexate tend to be used first, as they are better tolerated.
- Intramuscular gold is more effective than oral gold.
- If a gold salt is given by the intramuscular route, a test dose of 10 mg should be given first.
  - The patient should then be given 50 mg weekly. A beneficial effect is not usually seen until a total of 300–500 mg has been given.
  - Stop the treatment if there has been no response after a total of 1 g has been given.
  - Once the patient has responded, gradually increase the interval between injections, up to a maximum of 4 weeks.
  - Treatment can be continued for up to 5 years.
- If gold is given by mouth, it should be stopped if there has been no response after 6 months.

- Adverse effects from gold are very common (40% of patients) and are serious in 10% of patients.
  - Severe reactions can be treated with corticosteroids.
- A rash affects 25% of patients. This is most common after 2–6 months and can lead to irreversible pigmentation of sun-exposed areas.
- Gold salts can cause blood disorders; thrombocytopenia, agranulocytosis, and aplastic anaemia are the most common.
- Proteinuria is common. If this is only a trace amount treatment can continue, but if it becomes heavier treatment should be stopped. Gold can cause the nephrotic syndrome (membranous glomerulonephritis).
- Gastrointestinal adverse effects are common.
  - Nausea and vomiting are the most common, but gold can also cause stomatitis.
  - Diarrhoea is common; this may improve with bulking agents such as bran.

- Rare serious adverse effects include neuritis, pulmonary fibrosis, and hepatotoxicity with cholestatic jaundice.

- Do not give gold with chloroquine; there is risk of severe exfoliative dermatitis.

Safety and efficacy

- Perform the following investigations monthly if gold is given by mouth, and before each injection if it is given intramuscularly.
- Full blood count and urine dipstick for protein.
  - Suspend treatment if the platelet count is below 150 x 10^9/L or if there are clinical signs of thrombocytopenia.
  - Suspend treatment if the total white blood cell count is less than 4.0 x 10^9/L or the neutrophil count is below 2.0 x 10^9/L.
  - A trace of proteinuria is common; stop treatment if it becomes more severe.
  - Ask about rash and oral ulceration.
  - National guidelines for the monitoring of second-line drugs, British Society for Rheumatology, July 2000 (*https://www.msecportal.org/portal/editorial/PublicPages/bsr/536883013/3.doc*)
- Set clear targets against which the success of treatment can be judged. Ideally, these should include functional outcomes.

- Explain that this drug affects the disease process but does not provide rapid pain relief.
- Advise the patient to report symptoms of bone marrow suppression immediately (e.g. easy bruising, bleeding).

Prescribing information: **Gold salts**

Sodium aurothiomaleate

- By intramuscular injection, give an inital test dose of 10 mg. Subsequent dose 50 mg. See above for suggested regimen.

Auranofin

- By mouth, usual dose 3 mg bd. Can be increased to 3 mg tds after 3 months.

Leflunomide

Inhibitor of pyrimidine synthesis

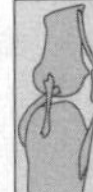

- Leflunomide is an inhibitor of pyrimidine synthesis and affects T cell proliferation; this is thought to be its mechanism of action in rheumatoid arthritis.
- This action accounts for its major adverse effect, bone marrow suppression.

- As a disease-modifying agent (DMARD) in rheumatoid arthritis.
  - Usually given second-line.

- Avoid leflunomide if the patient has moderate or severe renal insufficiency.
- Leflunomide can accumulate in hepatic insufficiency; avoid it.
- Leflunomide is teratogenic; it must not be used during pregnancy.
  - Women should be advised not to become pregnant for 2 years after stopping this drug (contraception is essential). See also monitoring section.
  - Men should not attempt to father a child while taking this drug and for 3 months after stopping it. See also monitoring section.
- Do not give leflunomide to patients with:
  - A history of tuberculosis.
  - Impaired bone marrow function.

Rheumatoid arthritis

- The choice of a DMARD should be made by the supervising specialist.
- Sulfasalazine, methotrexate, gold, and penicillamine are of similar efficacy, but sulfsalazine and methotrexate tend to be used first, as they are better tolerated.
- Leflunomide is more toxic than these drugs and is reserved for patients who are unresponsive to these first-line drugs.
- A clinical effect is usually seen after 4 weeks of treatment and increases over the next 4–6 weeks.

- Gastrointestinal adverse effects are common.
  - Nausea and vomiting are the most common, but leflunomide can cause oral ulcers and anorexia.
- Leflunomide can cause bone marrow suppression; this is characterized by falls in platelet and white cell counts.
- Treatment with leflunomide increases the risk of serious infection and malignancy.
  - Do not give leflunomide if the patient has a chronic infection or a history of tuberculosis.
- Leflunomide can cause hypertension.
- Hepatotoxicity is uncommon but can be severe. It usually occurs in the first 6 weeks of treatment. If hepatotoxicity occurs, carry out the washout procedure outlined below.
- Rashes can be severe (including the Stevens–Johnson syndrome). If severe, consider the washout procedure outlined below.

Washout procedure
Leflunomide persists in the body for a long time because it undergoes enterohepatic recirculation (see activated charcoal (p. 620) for more information); if severe toxicity occurs, it may be necessary to carry out the washout procedure: • Stop leflunomide. • Give colestyramine 8 g tds or activated charcoal 50 g qds for 11 days. • Repeat this 14 days later.

- Do not give leflunomide with other drugs that can suppress the bone marrow (e.g. cytotoxic drugs) or impair hepatic function.
- Colestyramine increases the elimination of leflunomide, which may be a desired action (see above).

Safety and efficacy

- Perform a full blood count every 2 weeks for the first 6 weeks of treatment, then every 8 weeks.
  - Suspend treatment if the platelet count is below 150 000/mm^3 or if there are clinical signs of thrombocytopenia.
  - Suspend treatment if the white blood cell count is less than 4.0×10^9/L or the neutrophil count is below 2.0×10^9/L.
- Perform liver function tests every month for the first 6 months, then every 2 months.
  - Suspend treatment if there is a greater than two-fold rise in aspartate aminotransferase or alanine aminotransferase.
- Measure the blood pressure every month for the first 6 months, then every 2 months.
  - From National guidelines for the monitoring of second-line drugs, British Society for Rheumatology, July 2000 (*https://www.msecportal.org/portal/editorial/PublicPages/bsr/536883013/3.doc*).
- Set clear targets against which the success of treatment can be judged. Ideally, these should include functional outcomes.

- Explain that leflunomide affects the disease process but does not provide rapid pain relief.
- Advise the patient to report symptoms of bone marrow suppression immediately (e.g. easy bruising, bleeding).

Prescribing information: **Leflunomide**

Rheumatoid arthritis

- By mouth, 100 mg daily for 3 days, then
- Maintenance dose of 10–20 mg daily.

Tumour necrosis factor (TNF) blocking drugs

Inhibitors of the actions of TNF

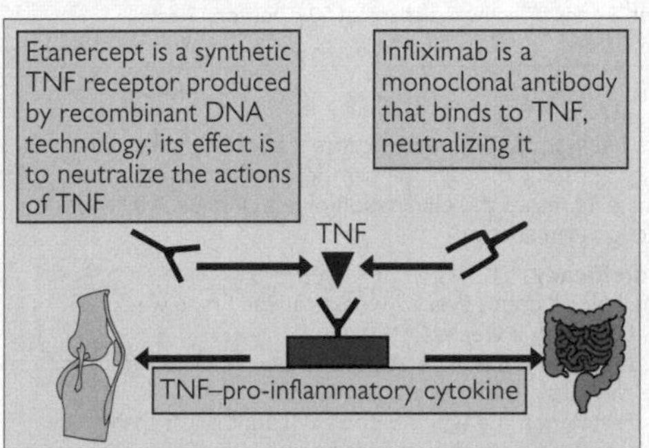

Note

An increasing number of therapeutic monoclonal antibodies is available. See trastuzumab (p. 508) for more information about this type of drug.

- These drugs should only be used by specialists.
- NICE has recommended that these drugs be considered for adult patients with highly active rheumatoid arthritis who are refractory to treatment with at least two other disease modifying drugs (DMARDS). One of these drugs should usually have been methotrexate.
- Infliximab is also licensed for the treatment of severe active Crohn's disease refractory to corticosteroids and immunosuppressants.

- The British Society for Rheumatology Working Party has recommended that patients with the following should not be given TNF blocking drugs.
  - Chronic leg ulcers.
  - Previous tuberculosis. (Note: patients with previous TB may be eligible if they have completed a full course of modern antituberculosis therapy, but measures should be taken to prevent the reactivation of tuberculosis and the risk/benefit for the patient should be considered before starting treatment.)
  - Sepsis of a prosthetic joint within the last 12 months, or indefinitely if the joint remains in situ.
  - Septic arthritis of a native joint within the last 12 months.
  - Persistent or recurrent chest infection.
  - Indwelling urinary catheter.
  - Multiple sclerosis.
  - Malignancy or premalignancy states, excluding:
    - Basal cell carcinoma.
    - Malignancies diagnosed and treated more than 10 years before (when the probability of total cure is very high).
- These drugs can exacerbate heart failure; do not give them to patients with unstable or severe heart failure (NYHA classes III or IV).
- These drugs should not be given to women who are pregnant. Women should also avoid becoming pregnant for 6 months after stopping these drugs.
- No dosage adjustment is usually required in hepatic or renal insufficiency.

- Treatment with these drugs should always be under the supervision of a specialist familiar with the condition and the role of the drug in treatment.
- These drugs are not absorbed when given by mouth; they are given parenterally.
- The British Society for Rheumatology Working Party has suggested that patients with a 28 joint disease activity score (DAS 28) of greater than 5.1 have severe active disease and should be considered for these drugs.
- Infliximab should usually be given in combination with methotrexate, as this reduces the incidence of antibody formation.
- Stop treatment with these drugs if there has been no response after 3 months (see below for criteria).

- The principal adverse effect is hypersensitivity.
  - This can manifest as anaphylaxis. Ensure that adequate resuscitation facilities are available when these drugs are given.
  - Delayed hypersensitivity can also occur.
- These drugs reduce inflammation; this may be useful in inflammatory disease but it is also part of the normal response to infection.
  - Hence, patients given these drugs are at greater risk of opportunistic infection, especially by *M. tuberculosis*.
- These drugs can exacerbate heart failure.
- These drugs can cause CNS demyelination. Clinically this is similar to multiple sclerosis.
- Long-term effects on the risks of malignancies are not yet known.

- To date, no important drug interactions have been identified. However, these are relatively new drugs and experience is limited.

Safety

- Exclude tuberculosis before beginning treatment with these drugs.
  - As a minimum, this will usually involve a tuberculin skin test and a chest X-ray.
- Neutralizing antibodies to etancercept have been reported to interfere with assays that involve monoclonal antibodies (e.g. serum troponin was raised in one study).

Efficacy

- The British Society for Rheumatology Working Party suggests that response is defined as improvement in the DAS 28 score by more than 1.2, or the achievement of a DAS 28 score of less than 3.2.

- These drugs can offer important benefits to patients with severe disease; however, they are associated with significant risks. Some of the long-term effects of these drugs may not have been identified yet.

Prescribing information: **Tumour necrosis factor (TNF) blocking drugs**

- These drugs should only be prescribed by specialists.

Calcitonin

Naturally occurring peptide hormone produced by the parathyroid gland

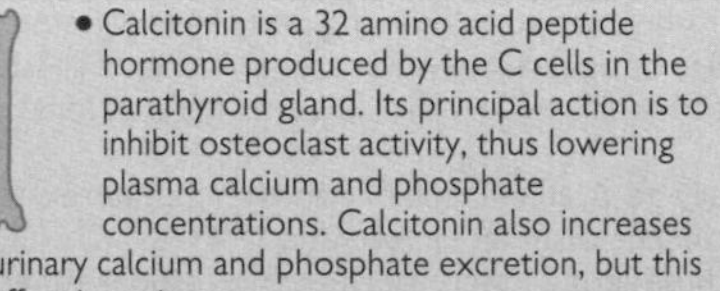

- Calcitonin is a 32 amino acid peptide hormone produced by the C cells in the parathyroid gland. Its principal action is to inhibit osteoclast activity, thus lowering plasma calcium and phosphate concentrations. Calcitonin also increases urinary calcium and phosphate excretion, but this effect is a minor one.
- The commercially available drug is salmon calcitonin (both natural and recombinant), as this is more potent than the endogenous form.

Treatment and prevention of osteoporosis

- See also bisphosphonates (p. 582)

Royal College of Physicians guidelines (http://www.rcplondon.ac.uk/pubs/wp_osteo_update.htm):

Bisphosphonates

- First-line
  - Alendronate
  - Risedronate
- Second-line
  - Etidronate

Other treatments

- Calcium and vitamin D
- Hormone replacement therapy (HRT)
- Calcitonin
- Raloxifene

- Treatment and prevention of postmenopausal osteoporosis.
- Treatment of Paget's disease of bone.
- Treatment of hypercalcaemia of malignancy.

- Do not give during pregnancy and breast-feeding; there is evidence of reduced birth weight and inhibition of lactation in animals.
- Patients with a history of atopy/allergic conditions should receive a test injection of one-hundredth of the usual dose before starting regular treatment.
- No dosage reduction is usually required if the patient has renal or hepatic insufficiency.

- Calcitonin is a polypeptide, so cannot be given by mouth; it is available for administration intravenously, subcutaneously, intramuscularly, and intranasally.
- Calcitonin is less effective than bisphosphonates for the prevention of osteoporosis and treatment of hypercalaemia of malignancy (see treatment of hypercalcaemia in bisphosphonates, p. 585).
  - Hypercalcaemia is a poor prognostic feature.
- Calcitonin is particularly effective for pain from osteoporotic fractures. It can be used up to 3 months after a fracture and is worth considering if other simple analgesia is ineffective. The mechanism of action may involve endogenous opioids.
- If calcitonin is to be used for the prevention of osteoporosis, the patient should also be given calcium and vitamin D supplements (calcium 0.5–1.0 g and vitamin D 800 IU daily).
  - See oestrogens (p. 430) for list of risk factors and suggested diagnostic workup.

- The most common adverse effects are nausea, vomiting, and flushing (20% of patients). These may abate with continued treatment.
- A few patients complain of an unpleasant taste and tingling of the hands.

- Local irritation around injection sites is common. Hypersensitivity phenomena, including rashes, can occur with all routes of administration. These drugs are polypeptides and so can cause anaphylaxis; this is very rare.
- Neutralizing antibodies can form during long-term treatment; these can reduce the effectiveness of treatment.

- Calcitonin treatment increases lithium clearance, and so the serum lithium concentration may fall. Measure the serum lithium concentration after 1 week of treatment to ensure that the dosage is still adequate.

Safety

- Measure the serum calcium daily. An effect can be seen within 3 hours, but it lasts only 2–3 days.

Efficacy

- Serum calcium is the efficacy measure when these drugs are used for the treatment of hypercalcaemia.
  - See calcium (p. 548) for calculation of the corrected serum calcium concentration.
- Dual energy X-ray absorptiometry (DXA) measurement of bone mineral density can be used to monitor the effectiveness of treatment. Bone mineral density correlates with the risk of fracture but does not tell you whether that individual will have a fracture. DXA should be restricted to patients in whom you are considering additional interventions.

- Remind patients that lifestyle adjustments (smoking, alcohol intake, and exercise) are also important in the maintenance of bone density. Drug therapy should be in addition to, not instead of, these interventions.

Prescribing information: **Calcitonin (Salmon)**

Treatment of hypercalcaemia

- *By subcutaneous or intramuscular injection,* the dose ranges from 5–10 units/kg daily (in 1 or 2 divided doses), up to 400 units every 6–8 hours. Adjust the dose according to clinical and biochemical response. There is no additional benefit over 8 units/kg every 6 hours.
- *By slow intravenous infusion (Forcaltonin® and Miacalcic® ampoules* only), 5–10 units/kg over at least 6 hours.

Paget's disease of bone

- *By subcutaneous or intramuscular injection,* the dose ranges from 50 units 3 times weekly to 100 units daily (in single or divided doses).

Bone pain in neoplastic disease

- *By subcutaneous or intramuscular injection,* 200 units every 6 hours or 400 units every 12 hours for 48 hours. These doses may be repeated at the discretion of the physician.

Postmenopausal osteoporosis

- *By subcutaneous or intramuscular injection,* 100 units daily with dietary calcium and vitamin D supplements.
- *Intranasally,* 200 units (1 spray) into one nostril daily, with dietary calcium and vitamin D supplements.

Bisphosphonates

Structurally similar to endogenous pyrophosphate

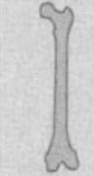

These drugs mimic endogenous pyrophosphate; as a result they are incorporated into bone. Unlike pyrophosphate, they are resistant to enzymatic degradation; they therefore inhibit precipitation and dissolution of bone minerals. They also inhibit osteoclast action.

Drugs used for the treatment of hypercalcaemia and pain from lytic bone metastases

- Pamidronate
- Clodronate
- Zolendronic acid
- Ibandronic acid

Treatment and prevention of osteoporosis

Royal College of Physicians guidelines http://www.rcplondon.ac.uk/pubs/wp_osteo_update.htm:

- Treat secondary causes
- Optimize lifestyle factors (smoking, diet exercise)
- Minimize falls; consider hip protectors
- Drug treatment

Bisphosphonates

- First-line: alendronate, risedronate
- Second-line: etidronate

Other drug treatments

- Calcium and vitamin D
- Hormone replacement therapy (HRT)
- Calcitonin
- Raloxifene

- Treatment and prevention of osteoporosis.
  - Postmenopausal.
  - Corticosteroid-induced.
- Treatment of Paget's disease of bone.
- Treatment of hypercalcaemia of malignancy.
- Treatment of pain from lytic bone metastases.

- There is insufficient evidence that bisphosphonates are safe in pregnancy and/or during breastfeeding.
- Bisphosphonates can cause gastric or oesophageal erosions; avoid using them in patients with delayed gastric or oesophageal emptying (e.g. achalasia).
- Bisphosphonates can cause hypocalcaemia; do not use them in those who are already hypocalcaemic.
- Bisphosphonates are excreted via the kidney; most manufacturers advise avoiding them if the patient has moderate or severe renal impairment.

Treatment and prevention of osteoporosis

- Protect bones early. Bisphosphonates reduce the risk of further fractures once one has occurred, but in many ways this is too late. Remember that those over 65 years are at greater risk.
- See oestrogens (p. 430) for a list of risk factors and suggested diagnostic workup.
- The principal action of bisphosphonates is to protect existing bone; there may be some building of new bone, but whether this is structurally sound is controversial. Long-term outcome data are not yet available.
- Other treatments are important:
  - Promote regular, non-impact exercise.

- Ensure adequate calcium and vitamin D intake. Most people do not have an adequate intake, so give a supplement. Suggested dosages: calcium 0.5–1.0 g and vitamin D 800 IU daily.
- Consider whether HRT is appropriate.

- Bone protection is recommended when corticosteroid treatment (>7.5 mg prednisolone equivalent daily) is expected to exceed 3 months.
  - Most bone loss is in the first 6–12 months.

Pain and hypercalcaemia due to malignancy (see also below)

- Treatment is usually by a single intravenous infusion, although clodronate can be given by mouth for pain.
- Before starting treatment with a bisphosphonate, ensure that the patient is adequately hydrated. This may be all that is required for mild hypercalaemia; it will also reduce the toxicity of the bisphosphonate.
- The dose of bisphosphonate should be adjusted according to the initial serum calcium. The dosage table for pamidronate is given below. The effect lasts 3–4 weeks.
- Bisphosphonate treatment can be scheduled (e.g. every 4 weeks) to coincide with chemotherapy for cancers that cause lytic bone lesions.
- Remember that radiotherapy is an effective treatment for pain from lytic bone lesions.

Treatment of Paget's disease

- Intermittent treatment is advised, as long-term treatment can cause hypocalaemia and defective bone mineralization.
- Calcium and vitamin D supplements may be required if these drugs are given in high doses.

- Gastrointestinal disturbance, especially pain, is the most common adverse effect. These drugs can cause gastric and oesophageal ulceration. The risk of this can be minimized by following the administration advice given below.
- Intravenous pamidronate is associated with pyrexia, 24–72 hours after administration. This occurs in about one-third of patients.
- Bisphosphonates can cause renal toxicity, especially when given intravenously. Reduce the risk of this by ensuring that the patient is adequately hydrated.

- Do not give bisphosphonates with calcium salts (including milk), as they bind them and prevent their absorption.
- Avoid co-prescribing these drugs with NSAIDs, as they can also cause gastric ulceration and renal impairment.

Safety

- These drugs have unusual pharmacokinetics — there is no clear relation between the plasma kinetics and their action (see teaching point below).
- Measure the serum calcium daily for the first 7 days when bisphosphonates are given intravenously. In those who respond, the maximum effect is usually seen at between 4 and 7 days.
  - Oral treatments (for osteoporosis) do not usually cause hypocalcaemia as long as calcium and vitamin D intake is adequate.

Efficacy

- Serum calcium is the efficacy measure when bisphosphonates are used for the treatment of hypercalcaemia.
- Dual energy X-ray absorptiometry (DXA) measurement of bone mineral density can be used to monitor the effectiveness of treatment. Bone mineral density correlates with the risk of fracture, but does not tell you whether that individual will have a fracture. DXA should be restricted to patients in whom you are considering additional interventions.

- Take bisphosphonates on an empty stomach (30 minutes before food) but do not take before going to bed.
- Take bisphosphonates with plenty of water (a full cup).
- Report any gastrointestinal symptoms before they become severe.
- Avoid NSAID painkillers such as ibuprofen (Brufen®, Nurofen®).

Prescribing information: **Bisphosphonates**

Alendronic acid

- Treatment of postmenopausal osteoporosis and osteoporosis in men, 10 mg daily by mouth or (in postmenopausal osteoporosis) 70 mg once weekly.
- Prevention of postmenopausal osteoporosis, 5 mg daily by mouth.
- Prevention and treatment of corticosteroid-induced osteoporosis, 5 mg daily (postmenopausal women not taking hormone replacement therapy, 10 mg daily).

Risedronate

- Treatment and prevention of osteoporosis (including corticosteroid-induced osteoporosis) in postmenopausal women, 5 mg daily by mouth.
- Paget's disease of bone, 30 mg daily for 2 months; may be repeated, if necessary, after at least 2 months.

Etidronate

- Treatment and prevention of osteoporosis. Given cyclically with calcium carbonate under the trade name of Didronel PMO®.

Pamidronate

- Hypercalcaemia of malignancy, according to serum calcium concentration (see below) as a single infusion, or in divided doses over 2–4 days. Do not exceed 90 mg per treatment course.

Initial serum calcium (mmol/L)	Recommended total dose (mg)
Up to 3.0	15–30
3.0–3.5	30–60
3.5–4.0	60–90
>4.0	90

- Osteolytic lesions and bone pain in bone metastases associated with breast cancer or multiple myeloma, 90 mg every 4 weeks (or every 3 weeks to coincide with chemotherapy in breast cancer).
- Paget's disease of bone, 30 mg once a week for 6 weeks (total dose 180 mg) or 30 mg in first week then 60 mg every other week (total dose 210 mg). Maximum total 360 mg (in divided doses of 60 mg) per treatment course. May be repeated every 6 months.

Clodronate

- Osteolytic lesions, hypercalcaemia, and bone pain associated with skeletal metastases in patients with breast cancer or multiple myeloma, by mouth, 1.6 g daily in single or 2 divided doses, increased if necessary to a maximum of 3.2 g daily.
- Hypercalcaemia of malignancy, by slow intravenous infusion, 300 mg daily for a maximum of 7–10 days or by a single-dose infusion of 1.5 g.

TEACHING POINT Treatment of hypercalcaemia of malignancy

- See calcium salts (p. 548) for other causes.
- Certain tumours are more likely to cause hypercalcaemia:
  - Breast cancer.
  - Squamous cell lung cancer.
  - Myeloma.
  - Genitourinary tract tumours (kidney, cervix, uterus, ovary).
- Hypercalcaemia is a poor prognostic feature.
- The severity of symptoms does not always correlate with the serum calcium concentration.
  - See calcium (p. 548) for calculation of the corrected serum calcium.
- Many of the symptoms of hypercalcaemia (e.g. fatigue, lethargy, weakness, constipation, anorexia) are common in patients with malignancy anyway. Have a high index of suspicion and measure the serum calcium concentration.

Rehydration

- Most appropriate for mild symptoms and a corrected calcium of 2.6–2.8 mmol/L.
  - Give 6–8 L of 0.9% saline ('normal saline') over 48 hours.
  - Give potassium supplementation.
  - Can be oral or intravenous.
- The calcium is lowered by sodium-linked calcium diuresis, usually by about 0.2–0.4 mmol/L.

Bisphosphonates and calcitonin

- If the patient has more severe symptoms or a serum calcium concentration above 2.8 mmol/L, consider treatment with a bisphosphonate or calcitonin.
  - Bisphosphonates take several days to act. Their effect is maximal at 5–7 days but the effect lasts 3–4 weeks.
  - Calcitonin has a rapid effect (2–3 hours) but a short duration of action (2–3 days). It is most useful in conjunction with a bisphosphonate for control of pain.

TEACHING POINT Drugs with unusual kinetic properties

- The bisphosphonates are polar molecules and are poorly absorbed from the gut into the body; hence the complex administration instructions.
- Less than 10% of the orally administered dose is absorbed.
- Once in the body, these molecules are avidly taken up by metabolically active bone. They are incorporated into bone and have their action there.
- The drug in the plasma is excreted by the kidney; this is a relatively rapid process, measured in hours. The drug will no longer be measurable in plasma after a few days, but some of the drug has been incorporated into bone and will only be released as that bone is turned over; this takes place over months and years.
- In other words, the apparent half-life in the plasma is short, but the half-life in bone is very long.
- Measuring the plasma kinetics of drugs like the bisphophonates tells one little about their therapeutic properties. These unusual kinetics can have implications for dosage regimens. For example, when alendronate is given as a single large dose once a week, the effect on bone mineral density is the same as giving a smaller dose daily.
- Aminoglycoside antibiotics are another class of drugs with unusual kinetic properties. They have a relatively short half-life in plasma but their antibacterial effect lasts for much longer. This is called a 'hit and run' effect.
    - In this case, the peak plasma concentration correlates with bactericidal action, but not with duration of action. The trough plasma concentration is of greater use; it correlates with the risk of ototoxicity. See aminoglycosides, p. 342, for more information.
- The plasma half-life of a drug often gives you useful information about the likely duration of the drug, but always ask whether it is relevant to the drug you are using.

Baclofen

Presynaptic GABA receptor antagonist

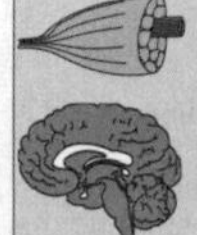

Baclofen probably acts as an antagonist at presynaptic GABA receptors; this has the effect of increasing GABA neurotransmission in the spinal cord by reducing feedback inhibition of synaptic GABA release. Since GABA is an inhibitory neurotransmitter, this results in muscle relaxation. This effect is not limited to the spinal cord; baclofen can also cause marked sedation.

- To alleviate muscle spasm.
  - Multiple sclerosis.
  - Spinal cord tumours.
  - Transverse myelitis.
  - Stroke.

- Baclofen is not an appropriate treatment for muscle spasm associated with an acute injury.
- Baclofen is contraindicated in peptic ulceration. This is based on the effects of GABA on gastric acid secretion rather than on clinical events.
- Baclofen can cause unpredicatable psychiatric reactions; avoid it in patients with a history of psychiatric disorders.
- The elderly are more sensitive to the CNS effects of baclofen; halve the starting dose.
- Baclofen is renally excreted; halve the dose in renal impairment.
- Avoid baclofen in pregnancy whenever possible; there is evidence of toxicity in animal studies.

- The underlying cause of the spasticity should be identified and treated whenever possible. Aggravating factors, such as local infection and pressure sores, should also be treated.
- The muscle relaxant effect of baclofen can lead to loss of the splinting action of muscles in a spastic limb. This can adversely affect mobility. Consider carefully which is the greater problem, spasticity or mobility.
- Baclofen is available as an intrathecal injection; this should only be used under specialist supervision. The dose needs to be slowly titrated at daily intervals.
  - A test dose must be given before beginning to titrate to the maintenance dose.
- Abrupt withdrawal of baclofen can cause hallucinations and hyperspasticity. Withdraw it over a 1–2 week period.
- Discontinue baclofen if there has not been a response after 6 weeks.

- CNS adverse effects are common, especially in the elderly. These include drowsiness, confusion, and fatigue. The incidence of these can be minimized by starting with a low dose, then carefully increasing it.

Skeletal muscle relaxants

- Dantrolene
  - Acts directly on skeletal muscle and so has fewer CNS effects. Drug of choice.
- Baclofen
  - Can cause marked sedation.
- Benzodiazepines
  - Muscle relaxant dosages are similar to anxiolytic dosages. Cause sedation.
- Tizanidine
  - Recently introduced alpha-2 adrenoceptor antagonist. Its place in therapy is yet to be established.

- Baclofen can cause convulsions.
- Generalized hypotonia is common at doses above 60 mg daily.
- Gastrointestinal adverse effects, such as nausea and vomiting, can be minimized by taking baclofen with meals.
- Baclofen can cause the blood pressure to fall.

- Baclofen potentiates the effect of antihypertensive drugs.

Safety and efficacy

- Patients starting baclofen need to be reviewed frequently during the dose titration phase to assess the balance between desired and adverse effects. If there has been no response after 6 weeks, withhold the drug.
- Measure the blood pressure on each visit to ensure that the patient is not hypotensive.
- Warn the patient about the risk of drowsiness, particularly with regard to driving.

Prescribing information: **Baclofen**

Treatment by mouth

- 5 mg three times daily, preferably with or after food. Gradually increased to a maximum of 100 mg daily.
- Halve the initial dose in the elderly and those with renal insufficiency.

Treatment by intrathecal injection

- Specialist use only.

Dantrolene

Muscle relaxant

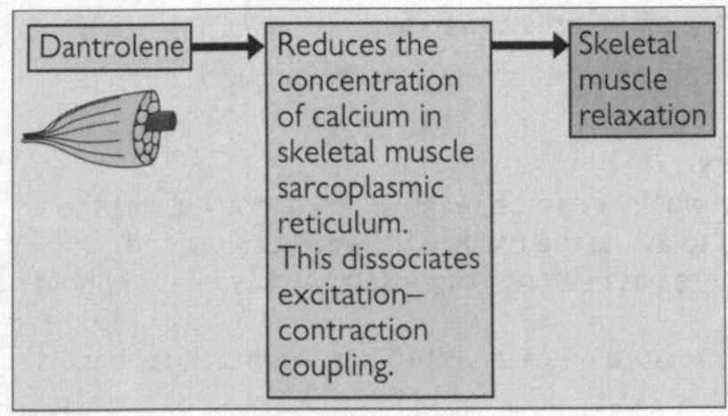

Skeletal muscle relaxants

- Dantrolene
  - Acts directly on the muscle and so has fewer CNS effects. Drug of choice.
- Baclofen
  - Can cause marked sedation.
- Benzodiazepines
  - Muscle relaxant dosages are similar to anxiolytic dosages. Cause sedation.
- Tizanidine
  - Recently introduced alpha-2 adrenoceptor antagonist. Its place in therapy is yet to be established.

- Treatment of chronic muscle spasm.
  - Multiple sclerosis.
  - Spinal cord injury.
  - Cerebral palsy.
- Treatment of malignant hyperpyrexia.
- Treatment of the neuroleptic malignant syndrome.

- Dantrolene is not an appropriate treatment for muscle spasm associated with an acute injury.
- Do not use dantrolene in patients with liver disease. It can cause severe liver toxicity.
- *Pregnancy*. The safety of dantrolene has not been established; avoid giving it unless essential.
- Take care to avoid extravasation; dantrolene can cause severe local tissue damage (see cytotoxic antibiotics (p. 493) for advice on the management of extravasation).

Malignant hyperpyrexia

- Predisposition to this syndrome is inherited in an autosomal dominant manner. It affects 1 in 20 000 patients.
  - The syndrome is characterized by hyperpyrexia (>40°C), stiffness, tachycardia and raised plasma creatine kinase (CK) activity.
  - The most common triggers are halothane, methoxyflurane, and suxamethonium (succinylcholine).
  - Ask about a family history of problems with anaesthetics when preparing a patient for surgery.
- Dantrolene can also be used to treat neuroleptic malignant syndrome; this shares many of the same clinical features.
  - Dantrolene is given by intravenous infusion for this indication.
- Do not forget to stop the causative drug and to institute other measures, such as cooling and intravenous fluids.

Chronic muscle spasm

- This is a specialized area of practice; seek expert advice. Dantrolene is not first-line treatment for this indication.
- Dantrolene is given by mouth for this indication.
- Begin with a low dose and gradually increase at weekly intervals to the desired effect (see below).

- Assess the patient after 4–6 weeks of treatment with the target dose. Stop the drug if there has not been a satisfactory result.

- Adverse effects from short-term intravenous use are rare.
- The principal problem with long-term use is in achieving a satisfactory balance between relief of spasm and muscle weakness and hypotonia.
- Dantrolene can cause drowsiness, vertigo, and dizziness during long-term use.
- Long-term treatment can cause liver damage. This is rare, but the risk is increased if the patient is taking oestrogens.

- See note above about liver toxicity.

Safety and efficacy

- Long-term treatment
  - Measurement of liver function tests is recommended during long-term treatment. There is little guidance about how often this should be done.
  - Do not continue long-term treatment if it has not been effective after 4–6 weeks.

- Warn patients that the muscle relaxant effect can interfere with skilled motor tasks, especially driving.

Prescribing information: **Dantrolene**

Malignant hyperpyrexia

- The usual dose is 1 mg/kg, given intravenously.
- This can be repeated according to the response, up to a cumulative maximum of 10 mg/kg.

Chronic muscle spasm

- Begin with a low dose of 25 mg bd by mouth.
  This can be increased by 25 mg bd at weekly intervals to a maximum of 100 mg qds.

Neuromuscular blocking drugs

Blockers of the effects of acetylcholine at the neuromuscular junction

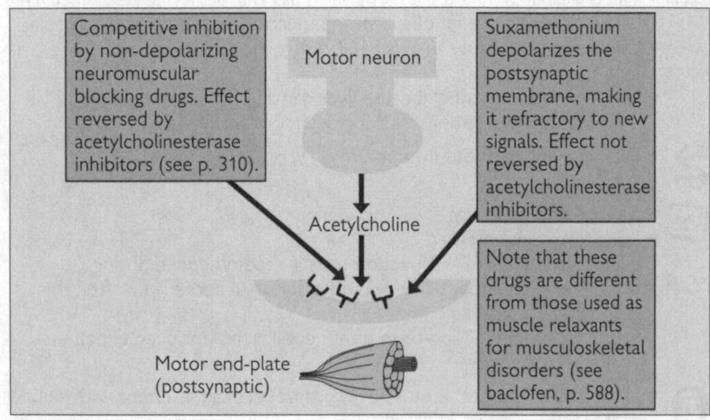

Drugs in this class and their approximate durations of action

Non-depolarizing blockers

• Mivacurium	15–20 mins
• Tubocurarine	20–30 mins
• Atracurium	30–40 mins
• Vecuronium	30–40 mins
• Rocuronium	30–40 mins
• Pancuronium	60–120 mins

- Gallamine is used rarely, as it has vagolytic and sympathomimetic actions
- Rapacuronium has been withdrawn because of adverse effects

Depolarizing blocker

• Suxamethonium	3–5 mins

- Whenever generalized muscle paralysis is required, for example:
  - In anaesthesia to aid intubation.
  - Major surgery (abdominal).
  - In ICUs.
- Suxamethonium is commonly used to induce muscle paralysis because it has a rapid onset of action. Other drugs are then used if prolonged muscle paralysis is required.

Note on botulinum toxin

Botulinum toxin is a potent, long-lasting inhibitor of neuromuscular transmission. It lasts too long to be given systemically (see p. 596).

- There is no evidence of toxicity from these drugs during pregnancy, but they should only be given when the indication is clear.
- These drugs have no anaesthetic or analgesic actions, but render patients unable to respond to noxious stimuli. Ensure that the patient has adequate anaesthesia and analgesia.
  - Also ensure that resuscitation facilities are immediately available.

Never give a neuromuscular blocking drug without the facilities and skills to ventilate the patient mechanically.

- Suxamethonium
  - Patients with pseudocholinesterase deficiency cannot metabolize suxamethonium in the usual way; this results in prolonged paralysis. Ask about a family history of prolonged paralysis after anaesthesia.
  - Suxamethonium increases intraocular pressure (muscarinic action); it should not be used for ocular operations or in people with glaucoma.
  - Suxamethonium can cause hyperkalaemia; avoid it in patients with hyperkalaemia or severe crush injuries.
- Renal insufficiency prolongs the actions of pancuronium, vecuronium, and rocuronium.
  - Atracurium does not depend on the liver or kidney for its elimination. It is a good choice in renal or hepatic insufficiency.

Suxamethonium (depolarizing drug)

- When given by bolus intravenous injection, suxamethonium acts within 30 seconds and lasts for 3–5 minutes.
- It also has muscarinic actions (see adverse effects below).

Non-depolarizing drugs

- All of these drugs take time to act (several minutes).
  - Rocuronium has the fastest onset of action and mivacurium the shortest duration of action.
- Some of these drugs cause histamine release to greater or lesser extent.
  - This can cause bronchospasm and hypotension.
  - Give them into a large vein and separately from other drugs.
  - Pancuronium, vecuronium, and rocuronium do not cause histamine release.

Suxamethonium

- Suxamethonium has muscarinic actions; this can cause salivation, an increase in intraocular pressure, increased gastric motility, and increased bronchial secretions.
- Because of its mechanism of action, suxamethonium causes muscle fasciculation; this can cause postoperative muscle pain.
  - Fasciculation will also release potassium and can result in hyperkalaemia (see cautions above).
- Pseudocholinesterase deficiency will result in prolonged apnoea.
- Rarely, suxamethonium can cause malignant hyperthermia when given with some inhalational anaesthetics.
- Repeated administration can cause dual block (depolarizing and non-depolarizing block); edrophonium can be used to reverse this.

Non-depolarizing drugs

- Some of these drugs release histamine (see above).
- Vecuronium can cause bradycardia because it does not act on sympathetic ganglia.

- Inhalational anaesthetics potentiate the action of non-depolarizing drugs.
- The following drugs potentiate the action of both depolarizing and non-depolarizing drugs: aminoglycosides, polymixins, clindamycin, colistin, quinine, quinidine, and magnesium salts.

- Drugs that inhibit pseudocholinesterase potentiate the action of suxamethonium; these include: MAOIs, cyclophosphamide, chlorpromazine, trimethoprim, glucocorticoids.
- Suxamethonium can potentiate the action of cardiac glycosides (e.g. digoxin).

Safety and efficacy

- Measure the respiratory rate and effort as a measure of the effectiveness of neuromuscular blockade.
- Neuromuscular stimulators placed over a muscle group can be used to monitor prolonged neuromuscular blockade (e.g. during a long operation).
- Whenever possible, measure the plasma potassium concentration and renal function before using these drugs.

- Patients may be concerned about being awake and in pain while paralysed. Take time to explain that they will also receive anaesthetic and analgesic drugs.

Prescribing information: **Neuromuscular blocking drugs**

- Several are available; the following are given as examples.
- Never give a neuromuscular blocking drug without the facilities and skills to ventilate the patient mechanically.

Suxamethonium

- By intravenous injection, usually 1 mg/kg.

Atracurium

- By intravenous injection, initially 300–600 micrograms/kg.
- Then by intravenous infusion, 300–600 micrograms/kg/h.

Pancuronium

- In ICUs, by intravenous injection, 60 micrograms/kg every 60–90 minutes.

Botulinum toxin

Inhibitor of neuromuscular transmission

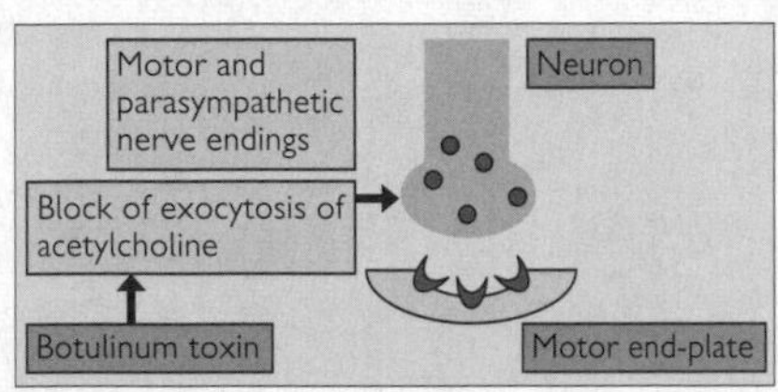

Drugs in this class
- Botulinum toxin A-haemagglutinin complex
- Botulinum toxin B

- Relief of muscle spasticity.
  - Continuous spasm (e.g. dynamic equinus foot deformity, cerebral palsy).
  - Intermittent spasm (e.g. blepharospasm, hemifacial spasm, torticollis).
- Treatment of severe hyperhidrosis.
- Widespread unlicensed use for cosmetic purposes (Botox®).
- Numerous other potential indications under investigation (currently unlicensed).

- Botulinum toxin should only be given by a specialist.
- Do not give botulinum toxin to patients with myasthenia gravis.
- The manufacturers advise that botulinum toxin should not be used during pregnancy.
- No dosage adjustment is usually required if the patient has renal or hepatic insufficiency.
- Avoid botulinum toxin in patients with bleeding disorders; administration requires repeated injections.

- Botulinum toxin is given by direct injection into the site. This requires technical skill and adequate training.
- Take care to avoid inadvertent intravenous injection.
- The dose required is determined by the indication and requires adjustment in the individual.
- The effect of botulinum toxin is temporary. The duration of action varies between individuals but is usually of the order of 4–6 weeks.

- Adverse effects result from muscle weakness and are determined by the site of injection.
  - *Face.* Ptosis, and diplopia. Reduced blinking can cause corneal ulcers.
  - *Neck.* Dysphagia (if persistent can cause aspiration) and pooling of saliva.
  - *Leg.* Leg weakness and urinary incontinence.
- Local bruising at the site of injection.
- Can also cause fever and lethargy.

- The effect of these drugs is enhanced by aminoglycoside antibiotics; avoid giving them together.
- Similarly, their effect is enhanced by non-depolarizing muscle blocking drugs.

Safety and efficacy

- Initial treatment should be with a low dose. The dose and exact site of injection can then be adjusted to give the best symptomatic relief for that patient.
- This requires regular clinical review in the early stages; once a regimen has been established review can be less frequent.
- At present, there is relatively little information regarding long-term use of these drugs.

- Warn patients of the possible adverse effects, depending on the site of injection.
- Advise patients that the effect is only temporary and that they will require repeated treatment.

Prescribing information: **Botulinum toxin**

- The dose, site of injection, and frequency of administration require specialist supervision.
- Consult the specific product literature for each indication; the formulations are not interchangeable.
- Detailed prescribing information is not given here.

Chapter 11

Eye

Contents

Acetylcholine receptor agonists

Agonists at muscarinic acetylcholine receptors

These drugs have the same effects as stimulation of the parasympathetic nervous system. A degree of specificity can be achieved by local administration (e.g. eye drops).

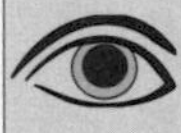

Pilocarpine causes contraction of the iris (small pupil); this opens the trabeculae, lowering intraocular pressure.

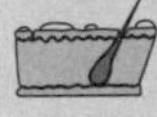

Muscarinic agonists increase bronchial and salivary secretions.

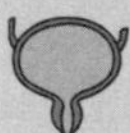

Parasympathomimetics increase detrusor muscle (bladder) contraction and can relieve acute urinary retention.

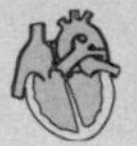

Muscarinic agonists mimic the effect of the vagus nerve on the heart, producing bradycardia.

Drugs in this class
- Pilocarpine
- Carbachol
- Bethanechol (now rarely used)

- Treatment of glaucoma.
  - Treatment of open-angle and closed-angle glaucoma.
  - To induce pupillary constriction preoperatively for surgery for glaucoma.
- For xerostomia (dry mouth) following radiotherapy to the head and neck or due to Sjögren's syndrome.
- Previously used to relieve postoperative acute urinary retention. This requires intravenous administration, which can be hazardous; it has been superseded by catheterization.

- Glaucoma due to inflammation (acute iritis, anterior uveitis).
- Avoid systemic treatment (tablets) in pregnancy and breastfeeding, asthma/COPD (increased secretions and bronchospasm), and cardiovascular disease (bradycardia and hypotension).
- Reduce the dose if these drugs are given systemically to patients with severe renal or hepatic insufficiency.

Glaucoma *(see p. 605 for guidance)*
- Available as eye drops, ocular inserts, and gel.
  - The eye drops work for only 2 hours, so require administration 3 times daily.
- Patients with a darkly pigmented iris may require a higher dose.

Dry mouth
- These drugs only work when there is residual salivary gland function. Stop the drug if ineffective.

- Headache and browache are the most commonly reported adverse effects. They are most common in young patients who have recently started treatment.

- Transient blurred vision, local stinging, and painful ciliary spasm are relatively common.
- Systemic parasympathetic adverse effects (nausea, diarrhoea, sweating, pallor, and bronchoconstriction) are rare with local ocular treatment.
  - Systemic exposure can be minimized by pressing on the medial canthus for 1 minute during administration.
- Retinal detachment has occurred during treatment with these drugs; ensure that the fundus has been examined before starting these drugs.

- Because they are usually given topically, these drugs do not usually cause drug interactions.

Efficacy

- Ensure that patients with glaucoma have regular follow-up, including measurement of intraocular pressure and visual fields.

- Warn about the possibility of stinging, pain, and transiently blurred vision with eye drops.
- Warn patients that they may have difficulty performing skilled visual tasks. This is especially true of driving at night.
- The preservative used in the eye drops will form deposits on soft (hydrophilic) contact lenses. After instilling the eye drops, wait for 15 minutes before putting in soft contact lenses.

Prescribing information: **Acetylcholine receptor agonists**

Glaucoma

- Pilocarpine eye drops (concentrations range from 0.5 to 4% — check which is required). Apply up to 4 times daily.
- Carbachol eye drops 3%. Apply up to 4 times daily.

Dry mouth

- Pilocarpine tablets 5 mg 4 times daily (with meals and at bedtime). May be increased to 30 mg daily.
- Discontinue if no response after 3 months.

Acute urinary retention

- These drugs are not recommended for this indication.

Carbonic anhydrase inhibitors

Inhibitors of the enzyme carbonic anhydrase

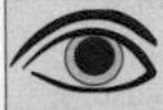

Inhibition of carbonic anhydrase results in reduced formation of aqueous humour.

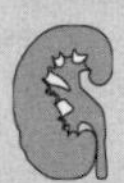

Inhibition of carbonic anhydrase inhibits bicarbonate reabsorption. This causes a diuresis of alkaline urine and an initial kaliuresis. The resulting acidosis prevents further potassium loss after a week or two.

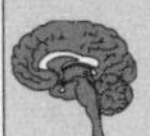

Inhibition of carbonic anhydrase causes resetting of the central pH set point.

Drugs in this class

- Acetazolamide (oral)
- Brinzolamide (eye drops)
- Dorzolamide (eye drops)
  - This is also available as a combination product with a beta-blocker

- Treatment of glaucoma.
  - Licensed for use in patients who are beta-blocker resistant or in whom a beta-blocker is contraindicated.
- Unlicensed use as prophylaxis against mountain sickness (acetazolamide).
- Occasionally used as a second-line treatment for atypical absent, atonic, and tonic seizures (specialized use).
- No longer used for their diuretic action.
- There is evidence of toxicity due to systemic acetazolamide during pregnancy. There is no evidence to determine whether these drugs given as eye drops are safe or not. Only use if essential.

- Acetazolamide is a sulfonamide derivative; do not use in people with a history of severe allergy to sulfonamides (see sulfonamides (p. 351) for more information).
- Do not use acetazolamide for long-term treatment; it carries a high risk of metabolic adverse effects.
- These drugs are excreted via the kidney. Avoid them in severe renal impairment, as they accumulate.
- Do not use a carbonic anhydrase inhibitor for chronic congestive closed-angle glaucoma.
- Avoid these drugs in pregnancy; there is no evidence that they are safe. The greatest risk is likely to be associated with systemic administration.

Glaucoma *(see p. 605 for guidance)*

- These drugs reduce intraocular pressure in open-angle glaucoma and secondary glaucoma. They are also used perioperatively in closed-angle glaucoma.
  - Beta-blockers or a prostaglandin analogue are first-line treatments (see pp. 140 and 450).
  - If these drugs are used, dorzolamide (eye drops) is preferred.
  - Carbonic anhydrase inhibitors can be given alone if a beta-blocker is contraindicated. More commonly, they are added in patients who have an inadequate response to a beta-blocker.
  - Acetazolamide is available as tablets and an intravenous injection. Avoid intramuscular administration, as this is painful.

Prophylaxis against mountain sickness (unlicensed indication)

- Suggested dose is acetazolamide 125 mg twice daily.
- Suggested regimen is to start treatment 24 hours before ascending to altitude (>8000 feet, 2500 meters), and to continue treatment for at least 5 days once at altitude.
- Acetazolamide is not a treatment for mountain sickness; if symptoms develop, the individual should descend.
- Seek expert local advice before prescribing acetazolamide for this indication.

- Carbonic anhydrase inhibitors (especially acetazolamide) can cause severe hypokalaemia and acidosis. Hypokalaemia is most common in the first weeks of treatment and tolerance then occurs because of the acidosis.
  - The acidosis can be corrected by giving potassium bicarbonate as effervescent tablets.
- Paraesthesia, especially of the lips, is relatively common.
- Other common adverse effects include drowsiness and fatigue, headache, flushing, and gastrointestinal upset.
- Acetazolamide is a sulfonamide derivative. It can cause sulfonamide-like adverse effects (see sulfonamides, p. 348).
  - Stevens–Johnson syndrome is a rare adverse effect.

- The hypokalaemia caused by these drugs can result in digoxin toxicity.
- Co-administration with aspirin can worsen the acidosis.
- The excretion of flecainide, mexiletine, and quinidine is reduced in alkaline urine. Reduce the dose.
- The excretion of lithium is enhanced by treatment with carbonic anhydrase inhibitors. Measure the serum lithium concentration 1–2 weeks after starting treatment. Note that the sample should be taken exactly 12 hours after the previous dose of lithium.
- Ensure that the patient has been instructed about the correct use of the eye drops and that they know which eye requires treatment, if only one is affected.

Safety

- The metabolic effects of carbonic anhydrase inhibitors are most marked during the first 2 weeks of treatment. The frequency with which you should measure the patient's electrolytes will depend on the clinical problem and concomitant medications (see above).
- Measure the arterial pH if the patient becomes unwell and you suspect acidosis.

Efficacy

- Ensure that patients with glaucoma have regular follow-up, including measurement of intraocular pressure.

- Glaucoma. Make sure the patient knows which eye requires treatment if only one eye is affected, or to treat both, and for how long.
- Altitude sickness. Ensure that the patient knows that this is a prophylactic treatment, not a treatment for established altitude sickness.

Prescribing information: **Carbonic anhydrase inhibitors**

Glaucoma

- Acetazolamide 0.25–1.0 g daily in divided doses, by mouth or intravenous infusion.
  - Tablets contain 250 mg of acetazolamide.
- Brinzolamide eye drops (10 mg/mL). Apply twice daily; increased to 3 times daily if necessary.
- Dorzolamide eye drops (2%). Apply 3 times daily if used alone. Apply twice daily if used in combination with a beta-blocker.

Epilepsy (specialized use)

- Acetazolamide 0.25–1.0 g daily in divided doses.

Altitude sickness

- Unlicensed use. See how to use section for suggested regimen.

TEACHING POINT Treatment of glaucoma

Simple glaucoma, also called open-angle glaucoma, although asymptomatic, can lead to severe visual field impairment and eventually blindness. The cause is obstruction in the trabecular network, resulting in raised intraocular pressure. In turn this causes a gradual reduction in the blood supply to the optic nerve head. Reducing intraocular pressure prevents the progression of glaucoma. Most clinicians begin with medical therapy, proceed to laser therapy if necessary, and finally perform surgery if control remains inadequate.

Drug treatments for open-angle glaucoma act by reducing aqueous humour production or by increasing aqueous humour outflow. They are given topically as eye drops, providing good efficacy with a low incidence of systemic adverse effects.

Drugs used for the chronic treatment of simple (open-angle) glaucoma

Mechanism of action	Drug class	Examples
Reduced aqueous humour production	Beta-blockers	Betaxolol, carteolol, levobunolol, metipranolol, timolol
	Alpha-adrenoceptor agonists	Brimonidine, dipivefrine
	Carbonic anhydrase inhibitors	Acetazolamide (oral), brinzolamide, dorzolamide
Increased aqueous humour outflow	Prostaglandin derivatives	Bimatoprost, latanoprost, travoprost
	Alpha-adrenoceptor agonists	Brimonidine, dipivefrine
	Acetylcholine receptor agonists	Carbachol, pilocarpine

See individual topics for more information.

The choice of treatment is determined by several factors: efficacy, relative frequency or severity of local or systemic adverse effects, and cost. Beta-blockers and prostaglandin analogues are considered first-line treatments; they are effective and have a low incidence of local and systemic adverse effects. Prostaglandin derivatives are more effective than beta-blockers, but are considerably more expensive.

The other drug treatments are usually added to first-line treatment for patients who have an inadequate response. They are not considered first-line treatments because of limited efficacy (carbonic anhydrase inhibitors) or a high incidence of local adverse effects (acetylcholine receptor antagonists, alpha-adrenoceptor agonists). The goal of therapy is usually to reduce the intraocular pressure below 21 mmHg.

Acute closed-angle glaucoma results from complete blockage of flow of aqueous humour into the anterior chamber of the eye; it is a medical emergency (seek specialist advice). Osmotic agents (e.g. mannitol, glycerine, urea), which act by shrinking vitreous humour volume and are given systemically, are sometimes used for short periods for acute closed-angle glaucoma, or before incisional surgery.

Chapter 12

Skin

Contents

Antihistamines

Antagonists at H_1 histamine receptors

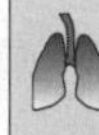

A structurally diverse group of drugs sharing the ability to block the H_1 histamine receptor. Histamine causes bronchoconstriction, increases bowel peristalsis, is a vasodilator, and increases vascular permeability. These are all features of allergic reactions and the major use for these drugs is in the symptomatic relief of allergic conditions. These drugs also have antagonist properties at muscarinic and dopaminergic receptors. These properties may well be responsible for their decongestant and antiemetic actions.

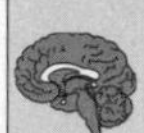

Antihistamines that do not penetrate the CNS, such as loratadine and acrivastine, are less sedative than those that do.

Antihistamines

Sedative
Azatidine
Brompheniramine
Chlorphenamine
Clemastine
Cyproheptadine
Diphenhydramine
Hydroxyzine
Promethazine
Trimeprazine

Less sedative
Acrivastine
Cetirizine/levocetirizine
Fexofenadine
Loratadine/desloratadine
Mizolastine
Terfenadine

Astemizole is no longer available

- Symptomatic treatment of allergic conditions (hay fever, urticaria)
- Treatment of anaphylaxis and angio-oedema.
- Prophylaxis against motion sickness.
- Symptom relief for vertigo and Menière's disease (see teaching point in prochlorperazine, p. 67).
- Cinnarizine has been used as a treatment for peripheral vascular disease because of its calcium channel blocking properties, but it is not recommended for this use.

- Antihistamines have antimuscarinic actions; avoid using them in patients with prostatic hyperplasia, closed-angle glaucoma, or pyloroduodenal obstruction.
- These drugs are probably safe in pregnancy, but their routine use is not recommended.
- Avoid antihistamines in patients with severe hepatic insufficiency; the sedative action may precipitate coma.
- Most of these drugs do not require dosage reduction in renal insufficiency, but halve the dose of cetirizine.

Allergy
- See below for advice on treatment of itch and seasonal allergic rhinitis.
- Many of these drugs are available over the counter for the relief of the symptoms of hay fever. Note that they are less effective than topical corticosteroids.
- A sedative antihistamine is helpful for relief of itch associated with eczema. They are not a treatment for the eczema itself; consider a topical steroid for this.
- Give antihistamines orally for the relief of pruritus. Topical use is not recommended, as this route is not very effective and may induce contact sensitivity.

- Topical antihistamines can be useful for the relief of allergic conjunctivitis, but ensure that other diagnoses have been properly excluded first. Note that these drugs can be absorbed systemically when given by this route and so may cause sedation.

Anaphylaxis

- Antihistamines (e.g. chlorphenamine 10–20 mg slowly iv) are a useful adjunct to the treatment of anaphylaxis. Intramuscular adrenaline (0.5 mL adrenaline injection 1 in 1000) is the first-line treatment (see adrenoceptor agonists, p. 194).
- Continue treatment with an antihistamine for 24–48 hours after an episode of anaphylaxis.

Cough

- Antihistamines are common components of cough and cold remedies. The sedative effect is probably the most useful one in these cases. Advise patients in whom sputum retention would be harmful (e.g. those with chronic bronchitis, bronchiectasis) to avoid these proprietary remedies.
- Cough is a symptom, not a diagnosis; always consider the underlying cause.

Sedation

- Diphenhydramine is available over the counter as a short-term hypnotic. Note that it has a long duration of action ('hangover effect'). It is not recommended.

- Sedation may be the desired effect, but will interfere with skilled motor tasks, especially driving. Even the 'non-sedative' antihistamines can cause some sedation.
- In some patients, these drugs can cause paradoxical stimulation, confusion, and even convulsions.
- As well as being a treatment for hypersensitivity, they may cause hypersensitivity, especially when administered topically (avoid this route).
- The antimuscarinic actions of these drugs can cause problems (see caution above).

- The antihistamines potentiate the effects of other CNS depressants such as alcohol, benzodiazepines, and phenothiazines.
- Terfenadine has potentially serious interactions with grapefruit juice, ketoconazole, and erythromycin (see teaching point below). It should not be used.

Safety and efficacy

- These drugs are principally used for symptomatic relief; always ensure that you have a clear idea of the diagnosis that is responsible for the symptoms. Reconsider the diagnosis if the patient does not improve.

- Warn the patient about the sedative effects of these drugs (including those that are less sedative). Those with a long duration of action may have a considerable hangover effect.

Drugs and the long QT syndrome

- Some commonly used drugs prolong the QT interval.
- Prolongation of the QT interval predisposes to the potentially fatal dysrhythmia torsade de pointes.

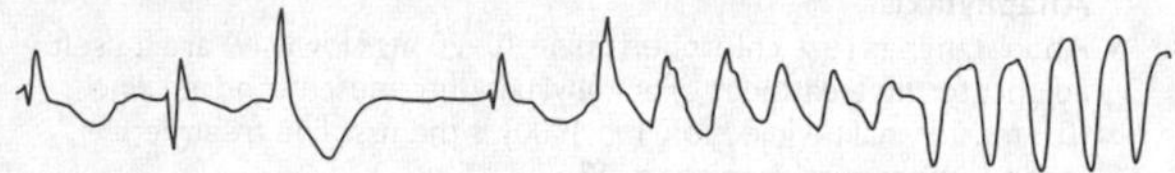

ECG showing the development of torsade des pointes. Source www.ecglibrary.com

- The mechanism is thought to involve inhibition of HERG-type potassium channels in the heart. Some individuals may be particularly susceptible, but the risk is greater when these drugs are present in high concentrations.
- Grapefruit contains a number of substances that inhibit cytochrome P450 enzymes. This can lead to marked rises in the plasma concentrations of drugs, and so put the patient at risk of dysrhythmias.
- Drugs such as erythromycin and ketoconazole also inhibit cytochrome P450 enzymes and produce the same effect.
- Antihistamines such as astemizole and terfenidine were some of the first drugs to be identified as causes of the long QT syndrome. Astemizole has now been withdrawn from the market, and terfenadine is not recommended.

Drugs capable of prolonging the QT interval

This list is not exhaustive but gives some of the most commonly prescribed drugs.

- Chlorpromazine, thioridazine, haloperidol, droperidol, risperidone.
- Cisapride (now withdrawn).
- Ondansetron and related compounds.
- Some SSRIs and related compounds (fluoxetine, paroxetine, sertraline, venlafaxine).
- Serotonin receptor agonists (drugs ending in -triptan).
- Quinolone antibiotics (drugs ending in -floxacin).
- Macrolide antibiotics (erythromycin and clarithromycin).
- Antiarrhythmic drugs that prolong the QT: amiodarone, sotalol, dofetilide, butilide, class 1a and 1c antiarrhythmic drugs.

Prescribing information: **Antihistamines**

Many drugs are available; the following are given as examples.

Chlorphenamine (chlorpheniramine)

- Treatment by mouth, 4 mg every 4–6 hours, maximum 24 mg daily.
- Adjunct to treatment of anaphylaxis (see adrenoceptor agonists, p. 194), by intravenous injection over 1 minute, 10–20 mg.

Promethazine

- Treatment by mouth, 25 mg at night, increased to 25 mg twice daily if necessary, or 10–20 mg 2 or 3 times daily.

Cetirizine (less sedative)

- Treatment by mouth, 10 mg daily or 5 mg twice daily.

Loratadine (less sedative)

- Treatment by mouth, 10 mg daily.

TEACHING POINT Treatment of itch

- Distinguish between generalized and localized symptoms.
- The pattern of local itching will often indicate the cause and direct treatment.
  - Insect bite itch is mediated by histamine and so responds well to H_1 histamine receptor antagonists.
  - Contact dermatitis from a deodorant. Change to an unperfumed deodorant.
  - Localized eczema. Treat with emollients and topical steroids.
- Generalized itch is more difficult to treat and can be a considerable cause of distress in palliative care.

Specific treatments

- These are uncommon, but can be important.
  - For example, reduction in the haematocrit will relieve itch in polycythemia, malathion for scabies, change of washing powder or toilet soap for generalized contact dermatitis.
- Do not forget that hypersensitivity to a medicine could be the cause.

Specific symptomatic treatments

- Opioid analgesics cause itch by causing histamine release; opioid antagonists will relieve the itch but reduce the anagesic effect. Ondansetron can also be effective for this type of itch (unlicensed indication).
- If the cause is cholestatic jaundice, a bile acid sequestrant can help, but only if the obstruction is not complete (see colestyramine, p. 46).
- Uraemia causes itch; narrow-band ultraviolet light can be effective. Thalidomide is sometimes made available on a named-patient basis (unlicensed drug; see 'off-licence' drugs, p. 4).

General symptomatic treatments

- Discourage scratching and cut nails to reduce damage to skin.
- Use emollients to soothe and hydrate the skin (e.g. aqueous cream, white soft paraffin).
- A sedative antihistamine can be helpful. The sedative action is probably the most important.
- Seek expert advice in difficult cases. SSRI drugs (e.g. paroxetine) have been used for treatment of paraneoplastic itch.

TEACHING POINT Treatment of seasonal allergic rhinitis ('hay fever')

- Try to identify the allergen; avoidance is an important part of the treatment.
- Identify whether nasal or eye symptoms are the most troublesome.
- Nasal symptoms are effectively treated by topical nasal corticosteroids (available over the counter). Steroids should not be applied to the eye for this indication as they cause cataracts.
- Systemic antihistamines are effective for nasal and eye symptoms. Less sedative ones are used most commonly but a sedative one can be useful if symptoms disturb sleep. Note that even the less sedative antihistamines can cause some drowsiness.
- Systemic nasal decongestants are of doubtful value and are not recommended.
- Treat acute attacks of asthma as usual (see p. 217).
- Systemic corticosteroid treatment should be reserved for the most severe cases and should be given for the shortest possible period.

Retinoids

Analogues of vitamin A (retinoic acid)

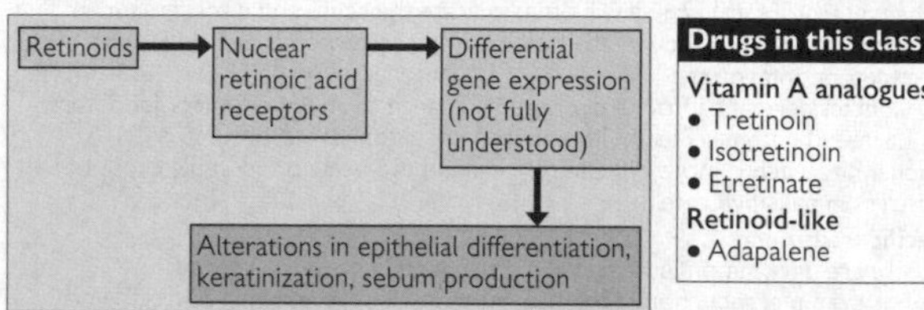

Drugs in this class

Vitamin A analogues
- Tretinoin
- Isotretinoin
- Etretinate

Retinoid-like
- Adapalene

- These drugs should only be used by specialists.
- The drugs are not equivalent; as a class they can used for:
  - Remission of acute promyelocytic leukaemia.
  - Treatment of acne.
    - Topical treatment for moderate to severe acne.
    - Oral treatment for severe, unresponsive, scarring acne. Limited to consultant dermatologists only.
  - Treatment of severe, unresponsive psoriasis. Limited to consultant dermatologists only.
  - Treatment of photodamaged skin. Limited to consultant dermatologists only.

- Do not give these drugs to women who are pregnant; they are teratogenic.
  - Ensure that women know not to become pregnant while taking these drugs.
  - Women should also avoid becoming pregnant for 1 month after stopping isotretinoin, and for 1 year after stopping etretinate.
  - Advise premenopausal women to use adequate contraception.
  - Perform a pregnancy test before starting these drugs.
  - This guidance applies to both topical and oral administration.
- Do not give these drugs to patients with a history of cutaneous epithelioma.
- Reduce the dose in hepatic insufficiency.
- Avoid these drugs in renal insufficiency.

- Treatment with retinoids should always be under the supervision of a specialist familiar with the condition and the role of the drugs in treatment.

Acne
- (Other uses are very specialized and are not discussed further here.)
- See tetracyclines (p. 339) for more information on the treatment of acne.

Topical treatment for moderate to severe acne
- Do not start treatment if the patient has peeling skin.
- Do not apply to large areas of skin and do not apply to mucous membranes.
- Avoid damaged skin and advise the patient to avoid ultraviolet radiation (direct sunlight, solariums).
- Do not use in combination with astringent or mechanical skin cleansers.

Systemic treatment for acne

- This is limited to consultant dermatologists. Those most likely to benefit are:
  - Those with severe, scarring acne.
  - Those unresponsive to systemic antibacterial drugs.
  - Women with late-onset acne (often unresponsive to antibiotics).
- Stop the treatment once no new lesions appear.
  - This usually takes 3 months.

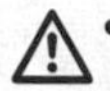

- The retinoids are effective drugs, but their use is limited by their considerable potential for toxicity.
- Topical effects.
  - Local burning and stinging. Drying of the skin and ulceration of mucous membranes. See note above.
- Treatment can initially worsen the acne.
- The first month of treatment is associated with an increased risk of thromboembolic disease.
- CNS effects.
  - Retinoids can cause benign intracranial hypertension ('pseudotumor cerebri'). The risk is greater in children.
  - They can cause headache (note above), visual disturbances, insomnia, and paraesthesia.
- These drugs can cause 'retinoic acid syndrome'. This is rare.
  - It is a severe capillary leakage syndrome characterized by fever, shortness of breath, pulmonary infiltrates, pleural effusions, and multi-organ failure.
- Retinoids can cause gastrointestinal disturbance and pancreatitis.
- They can raise plasma lipid concentrations.

- The risk of benign intracranial hypertension is greater if the patient is also taking tetracyclines or corticosteroids; avoid these combinations.
- Treatment with retinoids by mouth reduces the efficacy of the progestogen-only oral contraceptive.
- Take care if the patient is taking other cytotoxic drugs; the risk of toxicity is higher.
- Do not use with any topical treatments containing alcohol (methanol, perfumes, or other astringents).

Safety

- Measure a full blood count, clotting screen, liver function tests, calcium, and serum lipids before starting treatment.
- Make sure that adequate contraception is being used (see notes above). Perform a pregnancy test before starting these drugs.
- Repeat the blood tests listed above during treatment. Beware of liver toxicity. Plasma triglyceride concentrations can rise.

- Warn the patient that the skin may worsen before it improves. Stop the drug if peeling of the skin becomes severe.
- Make sure patients understand the importance of advice about contraception.
- Advise the patient to report symptoms such as headache or visual disturbance.
- Warn the patient about avoiding direct sunlight, and that they should not use a sunbed.

Prescribing information: **Retinoids**

- These drugs should only be prescribed systemically by specialists, usually consultant dermatologists.

Topical treatment for acne

Tretinoin

- Available as a cream, gel, and lotion. Usual concentration 0.025%. Apply thinly 1 or 2 times daily.

Isotretinoin

- Available as a gel 0.05%. Apply thinly 1 or 2 times daily.

Chapter 13

Poisoning

Contents

An approach to the poisoned patient

Poisoning by drugs is very common; it is said to be a factor in about 10% of UK hospital admissions. Poisoned patients present in several ways:

- The unconscious patient (deliberate or accidental overdose).
- The deliberate overdose. The patient may state what they have taken.
- Iatrogenic (commonly a consequence of polypharmacy, especially in elderly people).
- Accidental (especially children).

Assessment

Absolutely diagnostic features are rare. Always consider poisoning in your differential diagnosis of an unconscious patient. Look for clinical patterns.

- Coma, hypotension, flaccidity (benzodiazepines, barbiturates, ethanol, opiates).
- Coma, hyper-reflexia, tachycardia, dilated pupils (tricyclic antidepressants, anticholinergic drugs, phenothiazines).
- Behavioural disturbance (psychotropic drugs, organic solvents, anticholinergic drugs).
- Convulsions (tricyclic antidepressants, phenothiazines, carbon monoxide, MAOIs, mefenamic acid, theophylline, salicylates).
- Skin blisters (benzodiazepines, carbon monoxide, tricyclic antidepressants, opiates, barbiturates).

Use these to focus your initial investigations.

Management

- How can you reduce the absorption of the drug?
  - See activated charcoal (p. 620).
- Can you increase the elimination of the drug?
  - Is the drug excreted by the kidney or liver?
  - Elimination by the kidney can be increased by increasing urine flow (e.g. salicylate poisoning).
  - See activated charcoal (p. 620).
- What are the supportive treatments?
  - Begin with the ABC (airway, breathing, and circulation).
  - Hypoglycaemia and altered potassium handling are common in severe poisoning.
  - Cardiac monitoring may be required (e.g. poisoning by tricyclic antidepressants).
- Is there a specific antidote?
  - For example, acetylcysteine for paracetamol (see p. 622).
- What are the most likely complications and how can you treat them?
  - Respiratory depression and cardiac arrhythmias are the most likely to kill the patient in the short term.
- What can you do to reduce the risk of repeat overdose?
  - Psychiatric/psychological assessment of intent.
  - Is there a safer alternative drug (e.g. SSRIs are safer in overdose than tricyclic antidepressants).
  - Issue short-term prescriptions (1–2 weeks rather than 3 months).
- Seek advice from the National Poisons Information Service (0870-6006266; *www.spib.axl.co.uk*)

Activated charcoal

Activated charcoal

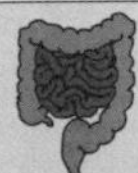

- Activated charcoal adsorbs (not absorbs) many drugs on to its surface.
- Because it has a very large surface area it reduces the amount of a drug that is available for absorption into the body from the gut lumen.
- Some drugs (see box for a list) undergo enterohepatic or enteroenteric recirculation. Some are excreted into the bile and so can be reabsorbed in the small bowel; others are secreted into the gut lumen by P glycoprotein, and can be reabsorbed. In these cases repeated doses of activated charcoal can interrupt this recirculation.

Drugs that undergo enteric recirculation

Consider repeated doses of activated charcoal if the patient has taken a life-threatening overdose of these drugs.

- Carbamazepine
- Cardiac glycosides
- Dapsone
- Phenobarbital
- Quinine
- Theophylline

- An adjunct to the treatment of poisoning.

- Do not give activated charcoal to patients who cannot swallow properly or do not have a secure airway.
- Some drugs are not adsorbed by activated charcoal.

Substances that are not adsorbed by charcoal

- Boric acid
- Cyanide
- Ethanol
- Ethylene glycol
- Iron
- Lithium
- Malathion
- Methanol
- Petroleum distillates
- Strong acids and alkalis

- Activated charcoal is widely used in the treatment of poisoning, but evidence for its effectiveness is limited.
  - In volunteer studies, the absorption of many drugs has been reduced by the administration of activated charcoal up to 1 hour after ingestion.
  - One study in patients poisoned with paracetamol supports the use of a single dose of activated charcoal in reducing drug absorption.
  - A large study in self-poisoning with yellow oleander seeds (commonly taken in Sri Lanka and South India) which contain cardiac glycosides, showed that repeated doses of activated charcoal reduced mortality.
- Detailed guidance is available from the National Poisons Information Service to NHS institutions via the TOXBASE website (*www.spib.axl.co.uk*, password required), and by 24-hour telephone service (NPIS UK telephone 0870 600 6266).
- Activated charcoal is most likely to be effective if given soon after the overdose.
  - Do not expose the patient to risk from the charcoal (see above) if they present late, unless multiple-dose charcoal therapy is indicated.
- A single dose of activated charcoal can be given by mouth or nasogastric tube.
  - If given by nasogastric tube, check for correct placement before administering the charcoal. The suspension of charcoal is thick and can easily block a narrow-bore tube. Only give charcoal via large-bore nasogastric tubes.

- A single dose of activated charcoal is unlikely to save the patient's life. Always consider other interventions; see the previous section on an approach to the poisoned patient.

Other methods of gut decontamination

- Gastric lavage is potentially hazardous. Evidence for its effectiveness is lacking. It should be considered only if a patient has ingested a life-threatening amount of a toxic substance within 1 hour.
  - Ensure that the airway is protected (e.g. by a cuffed endotracheal tube).
- There is no evidence that the administration of syrup of ipecacuanha to poisoned patients reduces drug absorption significantly. It has adverse effects that increase morbidity and make diagnosis more difficult. Charcoal adsorbs ipecacuanha and inactivates it.

- All formulations of activated charcoal are unpalatable and commonly cause nausea and vomiting.
- Charcoal can cause constipation.

- Activated charcoal will reduce the absorption of many drugs given by mouth, not just those taken in overdose.

Safety and efficacy

- The mainstay of the treatment of poisoning is supportive treatment. See individual drug articles for likely adverse effects and guidance on treatment of overdose.

- Explain that the activated charcoal is unpalatable.

Prescribing information: **Activated charcoal**

- To reduce drug absorption
  - By mouth, 50 g
  - Repeated oral doses, 50 g 4-hourly.

Acetylcysteine (Parvolex®)

An amino acid derivative

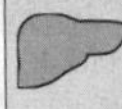

In toxic doses, the metabolism of paracetamol by cytochrome P450 enzymes in the liver produces the highly reactive intermediate NAPQI. Acetylcysteine acts as a scavenger to 'mop up' this reactive intermediate, thus protecting the liver from damage.

Alternative if acetylcysteine is not available
Methionine, given by mouth.

- Paracetamol (acetaminophen) overdose
  - Effective in acute poisoning, markedly reducing the risk of liver damage.
  - There is some evidence of benefit in established liver damage due to paracetamol, although the mechanism is unclear (seek advice from a liver unit). See below for a list of criteria for referral to a liver unit.

- Can cause bronchospasm; take care if the patient has asthma. This reaction is anaphylactoid (for explanation see box). Consider reducing the initial rate of infusion in those with asthma.
- The safety of acetylcysteine in pregnancy has not been formally assessed, but in most cases the risks of paracetamol poisoning outweigh the risks of the drug.
- Dosage adjustments are not usually required in hepatic or renal insufficiency.

Acute paracetamol poisoning

- Detailed guidance is available from the National Poisons Information Service to NHS institutions via the TOXBASE website (*www.spib.axl.co.uk*, password required) and 24-hour telephone advice service (see the 'Emergency Treatment of Poisoning' section in the BNF for contact details).
- Acetylcysteine provides a replacement for glutathione depleted by the production of the reactive paracetamol metabolite NAPQI.
- Used appropriately and early (within 8 hours) it is almost completely effective in averting significant liver damage in paracetamol poisoning. There is established benefit when it is given up to 24 hours after the overdose, but patients who present late (after 15 hours) are at much greater risk of liver damage.
- A nomogram for determining those who require acetylcysteine treatment is shown the box on p. 624.
- Paracetamol concentrations taken earlier than 4 hours after an overdose can mislead (they do not accurately reflect the peak tissue concentrations).
- Plasma paracetamol concentrations measured more than 24 hours after ingestion are meaningless, and should not be used to decide about treatment.
- The treatment regimen is based on an intravenous loading dose, followed by a continuous infusion (see prescribing information).
- If acetylcysteine is not available, consider oral methionine.
- If the patient is deteriorating, contact your liver unit for advice early. They may advise that the acetylcysteine infusion be continued, as there is some evidence for its use in established liver failure.

- Dose-related anaphylactoid reactions (see teaching point) are common, affecting up to 15% of patients during infusion.
  - Stopping the infusion is usually all that is required.
  - Give an antihistamine (e.g. chlorphenamine) if necessary.
  - Corticosteroids are only indicated if the reaction is severe.
  - Give nebulized salbutamol if bronchospasm is significant.
  - Once the reaction has settled restart the acetylcysteine infusion at an infusion rate of 50 mg/kg over 4 hours. Further reactions are almost unknown.

- There are no major drug interactions with acetylcysteine.

Safety

- Anaphylactoid reactions are most common during infusion of the loading dose; ensure close supervision and that resuscitation facilities are available.

Efficacy

- The prothrombin time (PT) is the best measure of liver damage. Transaminases can rise but are poor predictors of liver failure. Treat with acetylcysteine until the PT returns to normal, or for 24 hours, whichever is longer.
- The following features suggest that the patient has significant liver damage. Discuss the patient with a liver unit if any of the following are present:
  - Rapid development of encephalopathy.
  - PT >45 seconds at 48 hours or >50 seconds at 72 hours.
  - Increasing plasma creatinine.
  - An arterial pH <7.3 more than 24 hours after the overdose.

- Warn the patient that this drug can cause flushing and that they must report any difficulty with breathing.
- Ensure that the patient's suicidal intent has been assessed before deciding whether they are fit for discharge and that appropriate follow-up has been arranged.

Prescribing information: **Acetylcysteine**

- Only available as an intravenous infusion.
- Make up in 5% glucose solution.
  - **Bag 1**: 150 mg/kg in 200 mL infused over 15 minutes.
  - Followed immediately by **bag 2**: 50 mg/kg in 500 mL infused over 4 hours.
  - Followed immediately by **bag 3**: 100 mg/kg in 1000 mL infused over 16 hours.
- If the patient requires treatment beyond 24 hours, continue repeating the prescription as for bag 3 (do not give repeat loading doses).
- Take care when calculating and drawing up these doses.
  - Audits have shown that mistakes are very common when prescribing and administering acetylcysteine. This can lead to an increased incidence of severe adverse drug reactions.

Nomogram for acetylcysteine treatment in paracetamol poisoning

Use the high-risk treatment line for patients who:

- Are taking enzyme-inducing drugs (carbamazepine, phenobarbital, phenytoin, rifampicin).
- Are malnourished through chronic alcoholism, anorexia, or chronic disease (especially malignancy and AIDS).

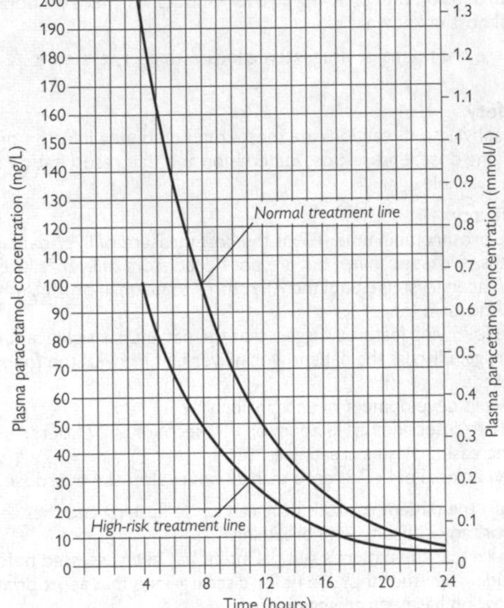

Reproduced with permission from the University of Wales College of Medicine, Therapeutics and Toxicology Centre.

TEACHING POINT Anaphylactoid drug reactions

- Anaphylactoid drug reactions have the same clinical features as anaphylactic reactions (bronchospasm, rash, etc), but the underlying mechanism is different (see adrenoceptor agonists, p. 194).
- In anaphylactoid reactions, the response is not mediated by IgE; rather the drug itself causes mast cells to degranulate.
- This is important, because the risk of the reaction does not increase with repeated exposure.
- Clinically, this means that it can be reasonable to restart treatment at a lower dose once the patient has recovered from the initial reaction.
- In settings such as the treatment of acute paracetamol poisoning, this can be life-saving.

Drugs that can cause anaphylactoid reactions

- Acetylcysteine.
- Colloid volume expanders and mannitol.
- Drugs that are formulated for intravenous use in the excipient known as Cremophor EL (polyethoxylated castor oil). These include ciclosporin, paclitaxel, and some vitamin K formulations.

Naloxone

Selective opioid μ receptor (OP_3 receptor) antagonist

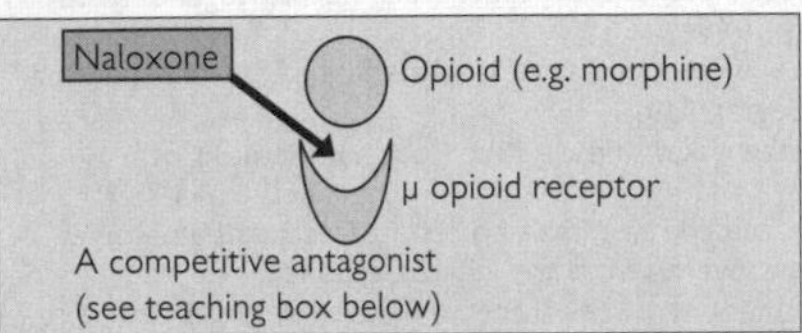

Examples of drugs reversed by naloxone

- Morphine
- Diamorphine (heroin)
- Fentanyl, alfentanil, remifentanil
- Codeine
- Methadone
- Tramadol
- Papaveretum
- Pethidine
- Dextropropoxyphene (e.g. in co-proxamol)

Buprenorphine is a partial opioid agonist and is less well reversed by naloxone than the other opiates. Consider treatment with glucagon or doxapram (see pp. 398 and 234).

- Treatment of overdose by opioids.
- Given postoperatively to reverse respiratory depression caused by opioids.

- Take care in patients who are dependent on opioids, in whom naloxone can cause an acute severe withdrawal reaction.
- Be careful if the patient is cardiovascularly unstable; naloxone can rarely cause ventricular arrhythmias postoperatively.
- No dosage change is usually required in renal or hepatic insufficiency.
- Naloxone can be used during pregnancy; hypoxia represents a greater risk to the fetus than naloxone.

- Available as intravenous, subcutaneous, and intramuscular formulations. Intravenous administration is preferred.
- Doses:
  - Opioid overdose: 400–2000 micrograms repeated every 2–3 minutes up to 10 mg.
    - May need continuous infusion (see below).
  - Respiratory depression: 100–200 micrograms every 2–3 minutes until the desired effect is achieved.
    - Note that naloxone does not work for other causes of respiratory depression; it is not a respiratory stimulant.

- The adverse effects of naloxone are usually those associated with acute opioid withdrawal: irritability, vomiting, sweating, hypertension, reversal of analgesia.
- Use repeated small doses to achieve the optimal effect.

- Naloxone is not usually subject to drug interactions.

Safety

- Most opioids have a longer duration of action than naloxone.
  - Repeat doses may be required.
  - Monitor the patient closely to ensure that they do not lapse into coma.
  - Consider a continuous infusion in severe overdose; 2 mg in 500 mL at a rate adjusted to the desired effect.

Efficacy

- Naloxone is very effective in opioid overdose.
  - If there is no effect reconsider the diagnosis.

- Naloxone is usually given in an emergency, when it is difficult to inform the patient; afterwards it may be important to explain to patients and their relatives what happened and why the naloxone was given, otherwise misunderstandings can occur.

Prescribing information: **Naloxone**

- *Intravenous injection* 0.4–2.0 mg repeated at intervals of 2–3 minutes to a maximum of 10 mg. If respiratory function does not improve, question the diagnosis.
- *Subcutaneous or intramuscular injection* As for intravenous injection, but only if the intravenous route is not feasible (onset of action slower).
- *Continuous intravenous infusion using an infusion pump* 2 mg diluted in 50 mL of intravenous infusion solution (5% glucose or 0.9% saline) at a rate adjusted according to the response.

TEACHING POINT Receptor antagonists

- Antagonists are drugs that bind to receptors and prevent their activation by agonists. Most antagonists are competitive. This means that they bind at the same site as agonists, and compete with the agonist for occupancy of the site. The overall effect will depend on which drug is present at higher concentration. Naloxone is a competitive antagonist at opioid receptors. When it is first given, its concentration usually exceeds that of the opioid, and so it antagonizes the effect of the opioid. Naloxone is metabolized more quickly (shorter half-life) than most opioids. With time, the naloxone concentration falls more rapidly than that of the opioid, causing the patient to lapse into coma again. For this reason, a continuous infusion of naloxone may be required.
- A non-competitive antagonist binds at an alterative site. There is no competition with the agonist (e.g. ketamine is a non-competitive NMDA receptor antagonist).
- Many drugs do not act on receptors but on other molecules such as enzymes (e.g. aspirin).

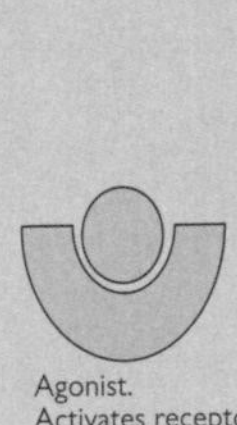

Agonist. Activates receptor. Can be a natural agonist or a drug.

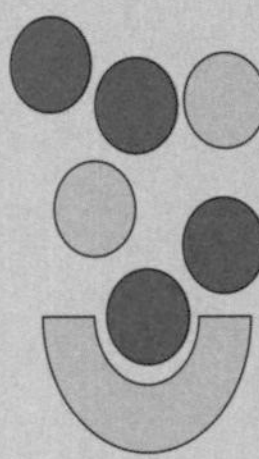

Competitive antagonist. If present at higher concentration than the agonist, will block the action of the agonist.

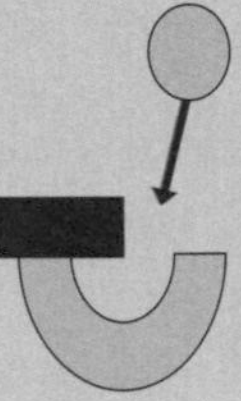

Non-competitive antagonist. Binds at another site, preventing binding by the agonist.

TEACHING POINT **Examples of agonists and antagonists**

Receptors	Subtypes	Sites in the body	Agonists	Antagonists
Cholino-ceptors	Muscarinic	Tissues innervated by parasympathetic nerves	Acetylcholine and analogues	Atropine and analogues Tricyclic antidepressants
	Nicotinic	Neuromuscular junction	Acetylcholine and analogues	Neuromuscular blocking drugs Aminoglycoside antibiotics
Histamine	H1	Smooth muscle	Histamine	Antihistamines
	H2	Stomach	Histamine	Ranitidine, etc.
Serotonin (5-HT)	Many subtypes	CNS, vascular smooth muscle, gastrointestinal tract	5-HT 5-HT1 agonists (triptans)	5-HT3 antagonists (ondansetron, etc.)
GABA	$GABA_A$	CNS	Benzodiazepines	Bicuculine
	$GABA_B$	CNS	GABA	Baclofen

Penicillamine

Chelating agent

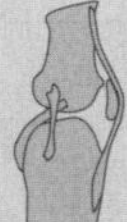

Penicillamine is a chelating agent. It is this action that is the basis of its action in the treatment of Wilson's disease, cystinuria, and heavy metal poisoning.

Penicillamine is also used as a disease modifying agent (DMARD) in the treatment of rheumatoid arthritis. The mechanism of action is not fully understood, but is thought to be similar to that of gold.

- As a DMARD in rheumatoid arthritis.
- As a chelating agent.
  - Wilson's disease.
  - Cystinuria.
  - Heavy metal poisoning (especially copper and lead).
- Also occasionally used for treatment of chronic active hepatitis once the disease has been controlled with corticosteroids (specialized use).

- Penicillamine is a derivative of penicillin; a small proportion of patients who are allergic to penicillin will also react to penicillamine. Avoid penicillamine if the patient is allergic to penicillin.
- Avoid penicillamine during pregnancy; it can cause rare, fatal abnormalities at all stages of pregnancy.
- Pencillamine is renally excreted; reduce the dose in mild renal insufficiency and avoid it in severe renal insufficiency. Penicillamine can also cause the nephrotic syndrome.
- Pencillamine can cause a lupus-like syndrome; do not give it to patients with systemic lupus erythematosus.

Rheumatoid arthritis

- The choice of a DMARD should be made by the supervising specialist.
- Sulfasalazine, methotrexate, gold salts, and penicillamine are of similar efficacy, but sulfasalazine and methotrexate tend to be used first, as they are better tolerated.
- Penicillamine should be stopped if there has been no response after treatment for 12 months.

Heavy metal poisoning

- See teaching point below.
- Seek advice from your local poisons information service (NPIS UK telephone 0870 600 6266)
- The laboratory reference blood lead concentration is 0.2–0.7 micromol/L for adults.
  - The reference range for pregnant women is much lower.
- Give penicillamine until the serum lead concentration falls into the reference range.

- Serious adverse effects from penicillamine are very common (30% of patients).
  - Serious adverse effects are more common if the patient is a slow sulfoxidizer, but this is not usually tested clinically.

Clinical features of lead poisoning

- Abdominal pain
- Fatigue
- Anaemia
- Heart failure
- Depression
- Gout
- Kidney failure
- High blood pressure
- Deficits in short-term memory
- Lead line (a blue/black line at the gingival–tooth border)

- Penicillamine commonly causes nausea; start with a low dose and give it with food.
- Penicillamine can cause loss of taste. This usually returns after 6 weeks treatment, whether or not the drug is stopped.
- Hypersensitivity phenomena are common and include the following syndromes: myasthenia-like, lupus-like, myositis, pemphigus (see below).
- Pencillamine can cause a rash.
  - Early rashes (1–6 months) are commonly morbilliform. They can resolve with continued therapy, especially if the dose is reduced.
  - Late rashes are commonly pemphigus-like; they do not resolve and usually require drug withdrawal.
- Penicillamine can cause an immune complex nephritis. This is common (30% of patients) and does not always require drug withdrawal. See monitoring section below for more guidance.
- Penicillamine causes thrombocytopenia in 4% of patients and leukopenia in 2%.
- High dosages reduce collagen synthesis, causing thinning of the skin.

- Do not give penicillamine with chloroquine, gold, or immunosuppressants; there is risk of severe exfoliative dermatitis.
- Do not take iron or zinc supplements within 2 hours of penicillamine; they will not be absorbed.
- Antacids reduce the absorption of penicillamine.

Safety and efficacy

- Perform the following investigations before treatment starts, every 2 weeks for the first 2 months of treatment, and then every 4 weeks. Perform an additional test 1 week after any dosage increases.
  - Full blood count. Stop the penicillamine if:
    - The platelet count falls below 120 x 10^9/L.
    - The white cell count falls below 2.5 x 10^9/L or falls on three successive measurements within the reference range.
  - Urine dipstick for protein. Proteinuria is common, but the treatment can continue if:
    - Renal function remains normal.
    - The patient has no oedema.
    - The 24-hour urinary protein excretion is below 2 g.
- If penicillamine is used for the treatment of lead poisoning, measure the urinary lead excretion rate.
- If penicillamine is used for rheumatoid arthritis, set clear targets against which the success of treatment can be judged. Ideally these should include functional outcomes.

- Explain that this drug affects the disease process but does not provide rapid pain relief.
- Advise the patient to report symptoms of bone marrow suppression immediately (e.g. easy bruising, bleeding).

Prescribing information: **Penicillamine**

Rheumatoid arthritis

- By mouth, initially 125–250 mg daily before food for 1 month.
- Increase by 125–250 mg at intervals of not less than 4 weeks to a usual maintenance dose of 500–750 mg daily.
- The maximum dose is 1.5 g daily.

Heavy metal poisoning

- By mouth, 1–2 g daily in divided doses before food. Give until the blood metal concentration falls below the toxic threshold.

TEACHING POINT Chelating agents

- Chelating drugs have an important role in the treatment of heavy metal poisoning, but their use is not straightforward.
- These drugs can cause redistribution of the heavy metal from soft tissues to the CNS, worsening the clinical features.
- Seek expert advice from your poisons centre.
- Drugs given for heavy metal poisoning:
  - Penicillamine (for lead poisoning).
  - Dimercaprol (largely superceded by DMSA).
  - Sodium calcium edetate (for lead poisoning).
  - Succimer (DMSA). This has been recommended in antimony, arsenic, bismuth, lead, and mercury poisoning (unlicensed indication). It has little effect on the urinary excretion of calcium, zinc, iron, and magnesium.
  - Unithiol (DMPS) (unlicensed indication for lead poisoning).

Diagnostic agents

- Diagnostic agents are not therapeutic drugs, but they are commonly given to patients.
- Fluorescein
  - Local administration to the eye to detect ulcers.
  - Systemic administration for retinal vessel angiography.
- Contrast agents
  - Imaging of the gastrointestinal tract:
    - Gastrograffin, oral contrast for computed tomography.
    - Barium.
  - Intravenous agents for angiography and computed tomography (iodine-containing).
    - High-osmolar ionic monomers: ditrizoate, iothalamate, metrizoate.
    - Low-osmolar ionic dimers: ioxaglate.
    - Low-osmolar non-ionic monomers: iopitridole, iohexol, iomepril, iopamidole, ioprolimide, ioversol.
    - Iso-osmolar non-ionic dimers: iodixonal, iotrolam.
- Gases
  - Radiolabelled xenon or krypton for ventilation scanning.
  - Pneumoventriculography.
  - Small gas bubbles used for contrast ultrasound (e.g. echocardiography).
- Radiochemicals.
  - Diagnostic (e.g. lung perfusion scan (^{99}Tc)).
    - ^{125}iodine thyroid scan.
    - ^{99}Tc for MUGA scan (cardiac).
  - Therapeutic ^{131}iodine for Graves' disease.
- Agents for magnetic resonance imaging.
  - Gadolinium (e.g. gadodiamide, gadobenate, dimeglumine).

- These agents should only be given by a specialist.
- Always consider whether there are any contraindications to ionizing radiation (e.g. pregnancy) or administration of contrast media before you request an investigation.
- The specialist (often a radiologist) is usually responsible for selection of the appropriate agent and dose calculation.
- Some contrast agents contain iodine; advise the radiologist if the patient has a history of hypersensitivity to iodine or has thyroid disease.

- The principal risk from these agents is hypersensitivity.
  - Always ask if the patient has reacted to contrast agents in the past.
  - Ensure that adequate resuscitation facilities are available whenever these agents are administered.
  - Make sure you know how to recognize and treat anaphylaxis (see adrenoceptor agonists, p. 194).
- Intravenous contrast agents can cause renal impairment; this is usually transient but can be severe. Ensure that the patient is well hydrated and that renal function is optimal. Avoid drugs (e.g. NSAIDs) that impair renal function.
  - Warn the radiologist if the patient has renal insufficiency.
- Take care to avoid unnecessary exposure to radiation from patients who have been given radioisotopes.

- Metformin is a biguanide drug used in the treatment of diabetes mellitus. There have been reports of metformin-induced lactic acidosis precipitated by contrast media.
- The Royal College of Radiologists advises that:
  - Metformin should be withheld on the day of investigation, and for 48 hours thereafter.
  - The referring doctor should inform the radiologist in advance and take steps to optimize the patient's renal function beforehand.
  - Provision is made for the adequate control of the patient's diabetes.
  - Renal function is measured before and 48 hours after the investigation.

Safety and efficacy

- Identify patients who are at risk of contrast-induced renal failure by measuring renal function in advance.
- Re-measure renal function after the procedure and adjust the dose of any renally excreted or nephrotoxic drugs accordingly.
- Take a careful history of any allergies before the procedure. If a reaction occurs, make sure it is documented clearly in the notes and that the patient's GP is informed.

- Many patients experience a sensation of warmth when they are given an intravenous contrast agent.
- Make sure the patient understands what the procedure involves, and its purpose.

Chapter 14

Immunological products and vaccines

Contents

Immunoglobulins

Human antibodies

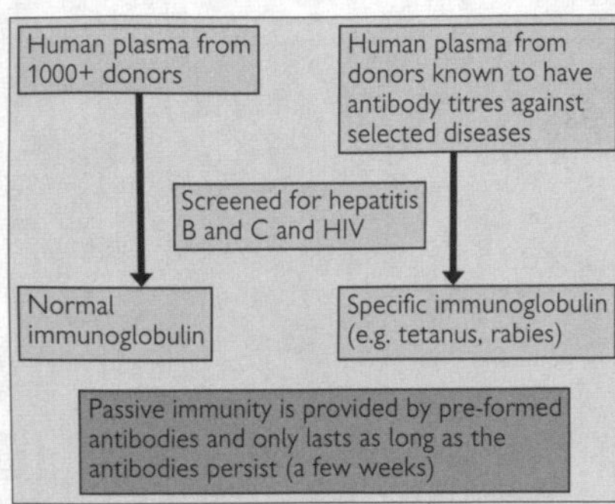

These are polyclonal blood products. Monoclonal antibodies have a number of other clinical uses, for example:

- Abciximab for acute coronary syndromes
- Anti-TNF antibodies for rheumatoid arthritis
- Infliximab for rheumatoid arthritis and ankylosing spondylitis
- Rituximab for advanced follicular lymphoma
- Trastuzumab for breast cancer

- Most of the uses of immunoglobulins are specialized.
- Normal immunoglobulin.
  - Intravenous immunoglobulin is given for:
    - Congenital agammaglobulinaemia, hypogammaglobulinaemia, and after bone marrow transplant.
    - Treatment of idiopathic thrombocytopenic purpura, Kawasaki's disease, Guillan–Barré syndrome.
  - Can be given to treat and prevent measles, mumps, rubella, and hepatitis A.
  - Sometimes given for severe myasthenia gravis with bulbar involvement, before more definitive treatment (unlicensed use).
- Specific immunoglobulin is used to treat:
  - Tetanus, rabies, hepatitis B, *Varicella zoster* infection (chickenpox), cytomegalovirus (CMV).
  - Anti-D immunoglobulin is given to prevent haemolytic disease of the newborn (see below).

- Do not give immunoglobulins to patients known to have class-specific antibodies to IgA.
- The protection that immunogloblins offer depends on pre-formed antibodies. Unlike active immunity, there can be no adaptive response.
- Prevention is more effective than treatment with immunoglobulins. When a vaccine is available this is recommended.
  - Do not give live viral vaccine for 3 weeks before and 3 weeks after an immunoglobulin has been given; it interferes with the immunological response. See vaccines (p. 646).

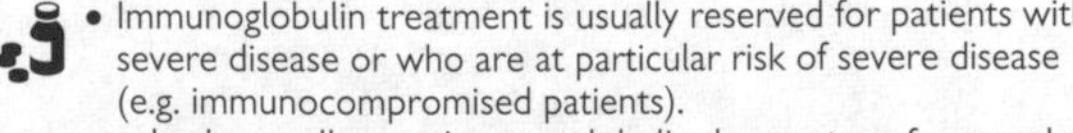

- Immunoglobulin treatment is usually reserved for patients with severe disease or who are at particular risk of severe disease (e.g. immunocompromised patients).
  - In almost all cases, immunoglobulin does not confer complete protection; prior active immunization is preferred.

- Seek expert advice. Detailed information is available in the UK Government publication *Immunization against infection* ('The Green Book') (*http://www.doh.gov.uk/greenbook*).

Chickenpox *(Varicella zoster)* and pregnancy

- Chickenpox during the first trimester can cause limb hypoplasia and loss of the fetus (1–2%). Maternal infection in the second or third trimester does not usually affect development of the baby. Maternal infection in the last week of pregnancy or first 28 days of life can cause infection in the baby; this can be severe and life-threatening.
- Passive immunization with *Varicella* immunoglobulin (VZIG) is recommended in the following circumstances (always seek expert advice as well):

For the mother

- Chickenpox in the first trimester or last 21 days of pregnancy.

For the baby

- If the mother develops chickenpox (or is exposed to chickenpox) in the last week of pregnancy.
- If the baby is exposed in the first 4 weeks of life.
- Despite this, over half the infants exposed will develop chickenpox. This should be managed by an expert.
- VZIG prophylaxis is not required if:
  - The baby is born more than 7 days after the start of the maternal infection.
  - If the mother develops zoster (shingles).

- Patients who are immunosuppressed (e.g. after transplantation), taking corticosteroids, have symptomatic HIV infection, or have immunoglobulin deficiency may also benefit from passive immunization if they are exposed to chickenpox. Seek expert guidance.

Prevention of rhesus disease

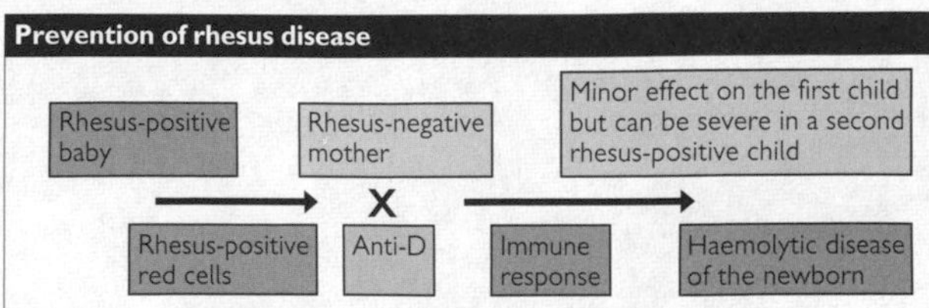

- Anti-D immunoglobulin should be given to the mother:
  - Within 72 hours of birth, abortion, or miscarriage.
  - Routine prophylaxis (at 24 and 34 weeks of gestation) in all rhesus-negative women. Also give postpartum.
- The dose is 500 units.
- Do not give measles, mumps, and rubella (MMR) vaccine within 3 months of giving anti-D immunoglobulin.

- Immunoglobulins can cause hypersensitivity reactions, most commonly fever and chills.
  - Anaphylaxis is rare.
- These products are screened for hepatitis B and C and HIV, but they cannot be guaranteed to be free from other, as yet unidentified, infections.

⇄

- Immunoglobulins are not usually subject to drug interactions.
- Note the advice above regarding live vaccines.

Efficacy

- The efficacy of immunoglobulins is measured in terms of the clinical response. They are rarely completely effective; other treatment will usually be required.

- Warn at-risk patients to avoid others with chickenpox and to report any inadvertent exposure immediately. See box for a list of those at risk and advice about pregnancy and newborn babies.

Prescribing information: **Immunoglobulins**

Seek expert advice. Consult *Immunization against infection* ('The Green Book') (*http://www.doh.gov.uk/greenbook*).

Interferons

Naturally occurring peptide cytokines

Interferons are naturally occurring peptide cytokines, most commonly produced in response to viral infections. They have several actions:
- Antiviral actions.
- Antiproliferative actions.
- Immunomodulatory actions.

For this reason, they have applications in several clinical settings, but are not very specific in their effects.

- All the uses of these drugs are specialized.
- Interferon alfa:
  - Treatment of chronic infection with hepatitis B or C virus in selected patients.
- Interferon beta:
  - Can be given to reduce the number of attacks in relapsing–remitting multiple sclerosis.
  - The use of interferon beta and glatiramer (see box) for this indication is not recommended by NICE.
- Interferon gamma is given for chronic granulomatous disease to reduce the frequency of serious infection.
- Interferons alfa and gamma are given as part of some specialized regimens for the treatment of cancer.

- Avoid interferons if the patient has severe or decompensated hepatic insufficiency.
- Avoid interferons during pregnancy, unless the indication is compelling.
- Avoid interferons if the patient has:
  - Poorly controlled epilepsy.
  - Suicidal ideation.
- The following are contraindications to the use of interferon alfa for the treatment of hepatitis B or C.
  - Intravenous drug use (high risk if reinfection).
  - Alcohol abuse with liver damage.

Drugs in this class

Interferon alfa
- Treatment of hepatitis B and C
- Hairy-cell leukaemia
- AIDS-related Kaposi's sarcoma

Interferon beta
- Relapsing–remitting multiple sclerosis

Interferon gamma
- Chronic granulomatous disease

Other drugs used in conjunction with interferons

Lamivudine (3TC)
- Nucleoside reverse transcriptase inhibitor.
- Licensed for use in chronic hepatitis B infection, in selected patients, and in combination with other drugs for the treatment of HIV infection. Principal use in chronic hepatitis B is for patients who require a transplant, or who have decompensated cirrhosis.

Ribavirin
- A nucleoside analogue.
- Licensed for use with interferon alfa for chronic hepatitis C, and for severe respiratory syncitial virus infection in children.
- Teratogenic; must exclude in pregnancy.
- Most important adverse effect is a haemolytic anaemia; monitor full blood count.

Glatiramer

Immunomodulating synthetic peptide. Reduces inflammation around nerves. Licensed for use in the treatment of multiple sclerosis. Similar efficacy to beta interferon. Not recommended by NICE.

- Interferons are given by subcutaneous injection.
- See guanosine analogues (p. 367) for advice on the approach to viral infections.

Treatment of hepatitis B or C (interferon alfa)

- The effectiveness is relatively low. Prevention is much more effective than treatment.
  - Immunization for hepatitis B.
  - Universal precautions for hepatitis B and C (e.g. protective gloves and eye wear).
- The response rate from interferon alfa given for chronic hepatitis B is less then 50%. Selecting the patients who are most likely to benefit is crucial. Seek expert advice.
  - It is recommended that treatment be stopped if there has been no response after 3 months.
  - Do not give if the patient is taking other immunosuppressant drugs.
  - Selected patients benefit from treatment with lamivudine (see box).
- Early treatment of hepatitis C infection with interferon alfa can reduce persistence, but this indication is unlicensed.
- Interferon alfa is usually given with ribavirin (see box) for the treatment of chronic hepatitis C. Initial treatment is for 6 months, but this may be extended to 12 months, depending on the viral genotype. The combination increases the response rate from 16% to 41% at 48 weeks.
  - NICE has recommended that the combination be offered to those patients who have not been treated with interferon before, or who have relapsed with interferon monotherapy.
- Pegylated interferon (peginterferon alfa) has a longer duration of action. It is slightly more effective than the standard formulation, but is more expensive. It is licensed for use in combination with ribavirin.

Treatment of multiple sclerosis (interferon beta)

- Relapsing–remitting multiple sclerosis is defined as at least two attacks of neurological dysfunction in the previous 2–3 years followed by complete or incomplete recovery.
- Interferon beta 1b is licensed for use in secondarily progressive multiple sclerosis.
- The results of clinical trials suggest that these drugs prevent one relapse per patient every 2.5 years. The natural history of relapsing–remitting multiple sclerosis is very variable, and this effect was not felt to be sufficient to allow NICE to recommend the use of these drugs in the NHS in the UK.
- Therapy for multiple sclerosis requires a multidisciplinary approach to address:
  - The symptoms that result from neurological impairment (e.g. speech therapy).
  - The emotional and social consequences of neurological disability.
  - Treatment of acute relapses with corticosteroids.
  - Consideration of treatment with disease-modifying drugs. However, at present, interferon beta and glatiramer are the only options.

- Adverse effects from these drugs are common.
  - The most common is a flu-like syndrome characterized by fever, chills, myalgia, headache, nausea, vomiting, and malaise.
  - Injection site reactions are also common.

- The following adverse effects are uncommon but serious:
  - Bone marrow depression.
  - Hepatotoxicity.
  - Hypersensitivity.
  - Psychiatric reactions, including suicidal ideation.
  - Thyroid dysfunction (interferon beta 1b).

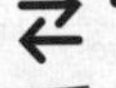

- The effectiveness of these drugs in, for example, chronic viral hepatitis, is increased by combination with another drug (see above).

Safety and efficacy

- Monitoring the action of interferon alfa in chronic viral hepatitis is complex and should be directed by a specialist. This includes assessment of liver function and viral DNA (hepatitis B) or RNA (hepatitis C). It may also include monitoring for the appearance of drug-resistant forms.
- The manufacturers of interferon beta recommend monitoring liver function tests in patients with multiple sclerosis.

- Warn patients that these drugs can cause a flu-like syndrome; some find it intolerable.
- Make sure that the patient understands that the effectiveness of these drugs is modest.

Prescribing information: **Interferons**

Dosage regimens are complex and should be directed by a specialist.

Vaccines

Stimulants of active immunity

- Immunization with vaccines is one of the most effective (and cost-effective) means of reducing the burden of human disease.
- Vaccines stimulate the immune system, producing active immunity; this is in contrast to short-lived passive immunity provided by immunoglobulins (see p. 638). Active immunity has a cellular component (mediated by T cells) and a humoral component (mediated by antibodies from B cells). Vaccines usually produce both, but the relative importance of each depends on the vaccine; for example, BCG immunization produces cell-mediated immunity, whereas measles vaccine produces a long-lasting antibody response. The immunogenicity of vaccines can be increased by the inclusion of molecules such as aluminium hydroxide; these are called adjuvants.
- Vaccines are of two broad types—those that are based on live (attenuated) organisms (e.g. rubella, pertussis), and those based on immunizing components of the organism (e.g. tetanus toxoid).
- Vaccines are usually given to prevent disease, and are especially important for the prevention of viral disease, for which treatments are often poor.

- Vaccines are given:
  - As part of a childhood preventive programme (e.g. MMR).
  - To prevent disease in healthy groups identified to be at special risk (e.g. hepatitis B vaccine for healthcare workers, rubella vaccine for non-immune pregnant women).
  - To prevent disease in patients with diseases that put them at increased risk (e.g. influenza vaccine for patients with chronic lung disease).
  - To prevent diseases in travellers (e.g. typhoid, Japanese B encephalitis).
- See below for the UK immunization schedule.

- Immunization should be postponed if the patient has an acute systemic illness; postponement is not necessary for focal or minor illnesses.
- Do not give a vaccine to a patient who has a definite history of a severe local or generalized reaction to previous vaccines. Seek specialist advice, so that a proper assessment of potential harms and benefits can be made.
- Some vaccines contain small amounts of polymixins or neomycin; avoid them if the patient is hypersensitive to these drugs.
- Patients with anaphylaxis to egg protein should not be given influenza or yellow fever vaccine.
- Live vaccines (e.g. polio) should not usually be given to women who are pregnant, because of a theoretical risk to the fetus. If, however, the risk of harm from the disease is great (e.g. yellow fever), immunization is justified.
- Live vaccines should not be given to:
  - Patients receiving cytotoxic chemotherapy or generalized radiotherapy.
  - Patients receiving immunosuppressive doses of corticosteroids (more than 40 mg/day prednisolone equivalents in adults).

  - Patients who have received a bone marrow transplant in the last 6 months.
  - Patients with inherited disorders of cell-mediated immunity; minor deficiencies of antibody formation are not a contraindication.
- Patients with acquired immunodeficiency due to HIV infection are a special case. They should be offered immunization against:
  - Measles, mumps, rubella, and polio (live vaccines).
  - Pertussis, diphtheria, tetanus, polio, typhoid (injection), cholera, hepatitis A, hepatitis B, and *Haemophilus influenzae* type b (Hib), meningococcus, pneumococcus, and rabies (inactivated vaccines).
  - They should not be given BCG vaccine or oral typhoid vaccine; in addition, there is insufficient evidence to recommend yellow fever vaccine.
- Do not give intramuscular injections to patients with a bleeding tendency.
- There is a theoretical risk of congenital malformation from live vaccines given during pregnancy, but the benefit/harm balance must be assessed on an individual basis.
- It is beyond our scope to include details of all vaccines. Detailed advice is available from the UK Department of Health at *http://www.dh.gov.uk*.
- You should obtain consent before giving any vaccine. This is especially important when giving vaccines to children; parents and guardians should be given an opportunity to make their wishes known.
- Most vaccines need to be stored in a refrigerator; care should be taken to confirm that they have been stored correctly. This has been one barrier to their widespread availability in developing countries.
- If you plan to give two vaccines at the same time, check that they are compatible, and record the sites of administration of each in case there is a local reaction.
- A few vaccines are given by mouth (e.g. oral polio vaccine), but most are injected. It is very important that they are injected into the correct site (usually the lateral thigh); check the packaging for detailed instructions.
- BCG is the most common vaccine given by intradermal injection. The needle (25 gauge) should be inserted at an angle almost parallel to the skin 2 mm into the dermis. Injection should be against considerable resistance and should raise a bleb.
- Almost all other vaccines are given by deep subcutaneous or intramuscular injection; a 23 gauge needle is used and the angle of injection is close to perpendicular to the skin.
  - In infants, the anterolateral aspect of the thigh (vastus lateralis muscle) is recommended. For immunization against hepatitis B and influenza in adults and older children, use the deltoid muscle; otherwise use the vastus lateralis.
- Tetnus toxoid immunization should be offered to all patients who present with a wound potentially contaminated by soil or manure, unless they have received a booster within the past 10 years. For treatment of tetanus see p. 355.
- For information on the treatment and prevention of influenza, see p. 366.
- Local reactions at sites of injection are common and can indicate a good antibody response. These reactions can be accompanied by local lymph node enlargement.

- Some vaccines can cause systemic fever, headache, and malaise; this usually lasts only a few days.
- Hypersensitivity to the constituents of some vaccines (e.g. egg albumin, neomycin) can occur and can be severe. See cautions above.
- Live vaccines can cause severe local reactions, or even systemic infections in patients with impaired immune responses. See the cautions above for groups that should not be given live vaccines.

Measles, mumps, and rubella vaccine (MMR)

- Controversy has surrounded the MMR vaccine since it was suggested that there was a link between exposure to the vaccine and the development of intestinal inflammation and autism.
- However, the evidence is overwhelming that there is no such link.
- Despite this, members of the public remain confused about the safety of MMR.
- There has been a suggestion that the vaccines should be given singly, but this is not recommended. Children remain susceptible to disease for longer if the vaccines are given singly, and several cases of disease in part-immunized children have been reported.
- This is an area that engenders strong emotions, and you should be prepared to discuss the issues with concerned parents.
- Immunization rates in the UK have now fallen to a level at which epidemics are expected.

- Live vaccines should not be given to patients who are receiving cytotoxic chemotherapy or immunosuppressive doses of corticosteroids; there is a risk of severe local reactions and systemic infection.

Efficacy

- The immune response to most vaccines is not measured routinely. However, the following are commonly assessed.

Hepatitis B (HBV)

- Measure the concentration of anti-HBs antibodies 2–4 months after a course of immunization.

Anti-HBs antibody concentration (miu/mL)	Recommended response	Comments
<10 ('non-responder')	Repeat course of immunization	Require HBIg if exposed to infection
10–100 ('poor response')	Give booster dose immediately and re-test	
>100 ('good response'/protective)	Booster usually recommended after 5 years	Duration of protection not fully characterized

Rubella

- Measure the anti-rubella antibody concentration and offer immunization to all women of childbearing age if they have not been immunized.
- Measure the anti-rubella antibody concentration in all women at antenatal screening, whether they have been immunized or not. If the result is negative, give rubella vaccine after delivery and before discharge from the antenatal unit. Warn women who do not have anti-rubella antibodies of the risks of rubella infection to the unborn child.

BCG

- The role of BCG immunization in the protection of the general population against TB is undergoing revaluation. You should perform a tuberculin skin test before giving BCG vaccine. If the test is positive, BCG should not be given; it is unnecessary and can cause severe reactions. Two tuberculin skin tests are recommended — the Heaf test and Mantoux test. The proper administration and interpretation of these tests requires training, and you should seek advice (e.g. from a specialist nurse) before undertaking them.

- Warn the patient about local reactions and the possibility of a systemic response.
- See box for specific advice about the MMR vaccine.

UK immunization schedule

This is offered as a general guide; it is correct at the time of going to press, but you should check the BNF and Government guidance documents regularly, as the schedule is frequently updated.

During the first year of life

- Adsorbed diphtheria, tetanus, and (whole-cell) pertussis vaccine (DTwP) *plus*
- *Haemophilus influenzae* type b vaccine (Hib) *plus*
- Meningococcal group C conjugate vaccine *plus*
- Poliomyelitis vaccine, live (oral)
  - Each 3 doses given at intervals of 4 weeks; give the first dose at 2 months of age.
- BCG vaccine (for neonates at risk only)

During the second year of life

- Measles, mumps, and rubella vaccine, live (MMR)
  - A single dose given at 12–15 months of age.
- *Haemophilus influenzae* type b vaccine (Hib) (if not previously immunized)
  - A single dose given at 13 months–4 years of age.

Before school or nursery school entry

- Give single booster doses of:
- Adsorbed diphtheria, tetanus, and pertussis (acellular component) vaccine (DTaP) *plus*
- Poliomyelitis vaccine, live (oral) *plus*
- Measles, mumps, and rubella vaccine, live (MMR)
  - MMR can be given at same session as DtaP vaccine, but use a separate syringe and needle, and use a different limb.

10–14 years of age

- BCG vaccine (for tuberculin-negative children)
  - A single dose.

Before leaving school or before employment or further education

- Adsorbed diphtheria (low dose) and tetanus vaccine for adults and adolescents *plus*
- Poliomyelitis vaccine, live (oral)
- **Note**: adsorbed diphtheria and tetanus vaccine (DT/Vac/Ads(Child)) is not to be used for children aged over 10 years and for adults.

During adult life

- Poliomyelitis vaccine, live (oral) (if not previously immunized)
  - 3 doses at intervals of 4 weeks.
  - No adult should remain unimmunized; booster doses for adults are not necessary unless they are at special risk, such as health-care workers in possible contact with poliomyelitis and travellers to areas where poliomyelitis is epidemic or endemic.
- Rubella vaccine (as MMR), live (for susceptible women of childbearing age)
  - A single dose. See monitoring notes above.
- Adsorbed diphtheria (low dose) and tetanus vaccine for adults and adolescents (if not previously immunized)
  - 3 doses at intervals of 4 weeks.

    - A booster dose given 10 years after primary course and again 10 years later maintains a satisfactory level of protection.
- **Note:** adsorbed diphtheria and tetanus vaccine (DT/Vac/Ads(Child)) is not to be used for children aged over 10 years and for adults.

TEACHING POINT Treatment of patients without a spleen

- Patients without a spleen, or who have functional hyposplenism, are at risk of bacterial infections, especially those caused by encapsulated organisms.
- Whenever possible patients should be offered immunization against the following at least 2 weeks before the removal of the spleen:
    - Pneumococcus. Measure the titre of all 23 pneumococcal antibodies 6 weeks after immunization. If the titres are low, seek expert advice.
    - *Haemophilus influenzae* type b
    - Influenza
    - Meningococcus types A and C
- If prior immunization is not possible, it should be given as soon as possible; asplenia is not a contraindication to immunization.
- In addition, patients should be warned about the risks of bacterial infection, should receive a patient information card, and should be given antibiotic prophylaxis before any dental or surgical procedures.
- Patients should take penicillin V 500 mg bd (or erythromycin 250 mg bd if there is penicillin allergy). A 3-day supply of amoxicillin should be issued, and the patient should be told to take 1 g at the first sign of infection and 500 mg tds thereafter; they should also be advised to seek medical attention immediately.

Chapter 15

The treatment of pain

Contents

Palliative care

- Many forms of care do not affect the underlying pathology of disease and could be considered palliative in the sense that they only relieve symptoms. However, the term 'palliative care' has traditionally been associated with terminal care of patients with cancer.
- One of the principles of palliative care is to focus on the problems that are of greatest concern to the patient, rather than those of most interest to healthcare professionals. This approach, developed in the care of patients with terminal cancer, is now applied to the care of patients with other terminal conditions, such as emphysema and heart failure.
- Relief of symptoms is an essential goal of many drug treatments, and guidance on this is threaded throughout this book. The following topics are commonly associated with palliative care:
  - Relief of pain p. 657
  - Starting oral morphine p. 672
  - Relief of itch p. 611
  - Pruritus p. 46
  - Vomiting p. 73

Use of syringe drivers

- In most cases, drugs used in palliative care can be given by mouth, but a parenteral route is sometimes required. Reasons for parental administration include severe nausea and vomiting or bowel obstruction.
- Syringe drivers deliver drugs by continuous subcutaneous infusion. There are two kinds: those that run at a fixed rate, and those that can run at variable rates. The wording of the prescription for each is different. Familiarize yourself with the machines that are used in your area, so that errors and confusion do not occur.
- Diamorphine is the drug that is most commonly given by a syringe driver. Diamorphine is preferred to morphine because it is more soluble. As a general guide, the equivalent dose of subcutaneous diamorphine over 24 hours is about one third to a half of the total daily dose of oral morphine (see p. 668).
- The following drugs can be mixed with diamorphine for subcutaneous infusion:
  - *Cyclizine* An antiemetic.
  - *Dexamethasone* A corticosteroid.
  - *Haloperidol* An antipsychotic drug that can be used to treat nausea and vomiting.
  - *Hyoscine hydrobromide** An antimuscarinic drug given to reduce excessive respiratory secretions.
  - *Hyoscine butylbromide** An antimuscarinic drug given to relieve bowel colic.
  - *Levomepromazine* An antipsychotic drug given for its sedative effect.
  - *Metoclopramide* An antiemetic.
  - *Midazolam* A benzodiazepine given for its sedative and antiepileptic actions.

  (*Take care — the dosages of these drugs are very different. See p. 196.)
- Solutions for subcutaneous administration are usually dissolved in sterile water for injection, because drugs are more soluble in water than isotonic saline.

Paracetamol (acetaminophen)

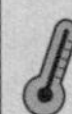

Paracetamol was introduced into clinical practice in 1893, but its mechanism of action remains unclear. It is probable that it involves inhibition of cyclo-oxygenase enzymes, but the site (brain or periphery) has not been fully established.

- Treatment of mild to moderate pain.
- Antipyretic.

- Paracetamol is metabolized by the liver and can cause hepatic toxicity. Avoid in patients with hepatic impairment, especially if acute.
- Paracetamol is not known to be harmful in pregnancy.
- No dosage adjustment is usually required in renal insufficiency.

Analgesia

- As with all analgesics, paracetamol is most effective when given regularly (see teaching point below).
- If additional breakthrough analgesia is required, add an opiate such as codeine or dihydrocodeine.
- Combination formulations are not recommended, since a regular opiate is not usually required. In addition, combination formulations are associated with increased mortality when taken in overdose.
- Paracetamol is available over the counter in blister packs containing up to 32 tablets. There is evidence that the introduction of limited size blister packs has reduced the frequency and severity of paracetamol overdose.

- Paracetamol is usually very well tolerated; at therapeutic dosages adverse effects are rare.
- In rare cases, paracetamol causes a rash or blood disorders.
- Long-term frequent use can cause analgesic nephropathy and analgesic-induced headache.

Overdose

- Paracetamol is the drug that is most commonly taken in deliberate overdose in the UK.
- Individuals vary up to 50-fold in their ability to metabolize paracetamol. Toxic dosages can vary enormously.
- Measure the plasma paracetamol concentration 4 hours after the overdose was taken or later. Concentrations measured before this time can be falsely reassuring, since not all of the drug may have been absorbed.
- Certain groups of patients are at increased risk of liver toxicity from paracetamol.
  - Patients in whom hepatic enzymes have been induced (e.g. those taking carbamazepine or phenytoin, chronic alcoholics).
  - Patients with poor antioxidant reserve: those who are poorly nourished or anorexic, and those with cancer or other chronic debilitating illnesses.
- For details on treatment of paracetamol toxicity, see acetylcysteine (p. 622).

- Regular paracetamol (e.g 1 g 4 times daily for 1 week) can increase the INR in patients taking warfarin. Measure the INR more frequently if the patient requires regular analgesia. Intermittent doses are unlikely to produce a measurable adverse effect.

Efficacy

- Ensure that your analgesia regimen is providing adequate relief from pain. Review the patient regularly.

- Remind the patient of the maximum daily dosage (4 g).

Prescribing information: **Paracetamol**

Analgesia

- By mouth 500–1000 mg every 4–6 hours up to a maximum of 4 g daily.

TEACHING POINT

The analgesic ladder for the treatment of postoperative pain

- Many medical procedures cause predictable pain. The table below has been developed for the treatment of postsurgical pain, but it can usefully be applied to other procedures.
- Regular analgesia is more effective than 'as-required' treatment. If pain is predictable, give analgesia early and regularly enough to control the pain. Pain is easier to prevent than to control once it has occurred.
- Individuals vary greatly in their analgesic requirements. Pain is what the patient says it is; treat it appropriately.
- The table is based on analgesic drugs, but do not forget to consider the cause of the pain. For example, glyceryl trinitrate is not an analgesic but is very effective for ischaemic cardiac pain because it treats the cause. If the patient has pain from a pressure sore, the most appropriate treatment is a pressure-relieving mattress, rather than large doses of analgesics.

Severity	Nature of procedure	Suggested treatment
Mild	Day case/in-patient on discharge	Regular paracetamol
Mild–moderate	Day case/in-patient on discharge	Regular paracetamol + as-required mild opioid (codeine, dihydrocodeine)
Moderate–severe	Day case/in-patient	Regular paracetamol + as-required mild opioid (codeine, dihydrocodeine) + NSAID
Severe	In-patient	Intravenous/intramuscular opioid (e.g. morphine) + NSAID
Very severe	In-patient (e.g. bowel resection)	Patient-controlled analgesia (PCA); usually morphine + NSAID
Excruciating	In-patient (e.g. oesophagectomy)	Epidural opioid + local anaesthetic

Non-steroidal anti-inflammatory drugs (NSAIDs)

Inhibitors of cyclo-oxygenase

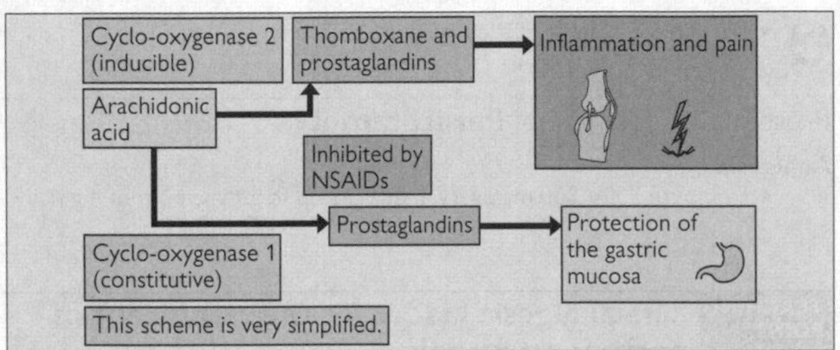

- Analgesic and anti-inflammatory drugs, especially:
  - In chronic inflammation.
    - Rheumatoid arthritis.
    - Severe osteoarthritis.
    - Chronic back pain.
  - In acute injury with inflammation.
  - Dysmenorrhoea.
  - Pain from lytic bone metastases.

- NSAIDs can cause gastrointestinal bleeding.
  - Do not give them to patients with active peptic ulceration.
  - Do not give them to patients with a history of gastrointestinal bleeding.
  - Elderly patients are at greater risk. Consider very carefully before giving them any NSAID.
  - Renal or hepatic insufficiency increases the risk (see also below).
  - Acute severe illness increases the risk.
- Because these drugs can cause gastrointestinal bleeding, they should not be given with anticoagulant drugs unless accompanied by a proton pump inhibitor (see p. 26).
- NSAIDs can cause asthma and worsen the control of intrinsic asthma.
- NSAIDs can worsen renal function; avoid them in renal insufficiency.
  - They can cause fluid retention, which will worsen hepatic or cardiac failure.
- Pregnant women.
  - Avoid NSAIDs if possible.
  - Risk of intrauterine bleeding and closure of ductus arteriosus in utero.
  - Can delay the onset and increase the duration of labour (occasionally used to delay labour; specialized use).

NSAIDs

- Non-selective
  - Aceclofenac
  - Acemetacin
  - Azapropazone
  - Dexketoprofen
  - Diclofenac
  - Etodolac
  - Fenbrufen
  - Fenoprofen
  - Flurbiprofen
  - Ibuprofen
  - Indometacin
  - Ketoprofen
  - Ketorolac
  - Lornoxicam
  - Nabumetone
  - Naproxen
  - Phenylbutazone
  - Piroxicam
  - Sulindac
  - Tenoxicam
  - Tiaprofenic acid
- Relatively COX-2 selective ('coxibs')
  - Celecoxib
  - Rofecoxib
  - Parecoxib
  - Etoricoxib
  - Meloxicam
- Note that aspirin is an NSAID at high dosages.
- Mefenamic acid
  - Has only minor anti-inflammatory properties.

- When given in single doses these drugs are only as effective as paracetamol, which is safer and is the drug of choice for intermittent mild pain.
- See box below for selection guidance.
- To achieve an anti-inflammatory effect these drugs need to be given regularly.
  - A full analgesic effect is usually achieved within 1 week.
  - The full anti-inflammatory effect can take 3 weeks to develop.
- The principal problem with these drugs is their propensity to cause gastrointestinal bleeding; avoid them in patients who are at high risk (see cautions above). If the patient is of intermediate risk consider the following factors:
  - Use a drug that is effective but has the lowest risk of bleeding.
  - Give the drug for the shortest possible time.
  - Many patients require long-term treatment. Consider gastroprotection with:
    - Misoprostol.
    - A proton pump inhibitor.
- Drugs that are selective inhibitors of COX-2 have a lower risk of gastrointestinal haemorrhage. See below for a fuller discussion.
- Enteric-coated tablets may reduce the incidence of dyspeptic symptoms, but do not reduce the risk of gastrointestinal bleeding.
- NSAIDs are widely used as an adjunct to anaesthesia. See paracetamol (p. 657) for their place in the analgesic ladder.
- Some NSAIDs are available as topical over-the-counter formulations for acute muscle injury. The evidence for their effectiveness is slight.
- These drugs can have a small antiplatelet action, but they should not be used as antiplatelet drugs (see aspirin, p. 116).

Drug selection guidance for non-selective NSAIDs

If an NSAID is appropriate, choose a drug that carries the lowest risk of gastrointestinal haemorrhage while offering the desired anti-inflammatory activity. The anti-inflammatory potency of these drugs is roughly proportional to the risk of causing gastrointestinal haemorrhage. The differences between the drugs in the intermediate categories are small.

Risk of bleeding/anti-inflammatory potency

	Low	Low–intermediate	Intermediate	Intermediate–high	High
'Benchmark' drug	Ibuprofen	Diclofenac	Indometacin	Piroxicam	Azapropazone
Other options		Fenbufen, flurbiprofen, nabumetone, naproxen, tenoxicam			

- In addition to the risk of gastrointestinal haemorrhage, NSAIDs commonly cause nausea and dyspeptic symptoms.
- NSAIDs can cause a rash.
  - This can be severe, including toxic epidermal necrolysis or Stevens–Johnson syndrome.
  - The risk of rash is greatest with fenbufen and azapropazone.
- NSAIDs can cause bronchospasm. Some patients with asthma can tolerate them, but they are contraindicated.
  - Do not give NSAIDs to patients with aspirin allergy.
- NSAIDs can be nephrotoxic and can cause an interstitial nephritis. Stop them if the patient has or develops renal insufficiency, or if they suffer an acute illness that may transiently worsen renal function.
- NSAIDs can cause an aseptic meningitis; this is very rare, but the risk is greater in patients with systemic vasculitis (e.g. systemic lupus erythematosus).
- Phenylbutazone can cause an acute pulmonary syndrome associated with fever and dyspnoea, and the risk of neutropenia and aplastic anaemia is high. Its use is now limited to in-patient treatment of ankylosing spondylitis under the direction of a specialist.
- Tiaprofenic acid can cause cystitis.
- Mefenamic acid is effective for the treatment of dysmenorrhoea and menorrhagia, but has few anti-inflammatory properties. It can cause a haemolytic anaemia and severe diarrhoea. In overdose it can cause convulsions (treat these with diazepam).
  - Other NSAIDs are also licensed for the treatment of dysmenorrhoea.

Risk factors for NSAID-induced gastric ulceration

- Linear increase in risk with increasing age (especially >65 years).
- History of peptic ulceration.
- Debilitated patients.
- Long-term treatment with maximal doses of NSAIDs.
- Concomitant treatment with drugs that can cause bleeding.

- Take care when giving NSAIDs to patients taking drugs that increase their risk of bleeding: warfarin, antiplatelet drugs (e.g. aspirin), and corticosteroids.
  - In some cases this increased risk will be justified, but ensure that you have considered it before prescribing the drug.
- Avoid giving NSAIDs to patients taking drugs that can cause renal impairment (e.g. ciclosporin, tacrolimus).
- NSAIDs can cause liver toxicity, characterized by increased transaminases.
- NSAIDs antagonize the action of diuretics and can cause fluid retention; withdrawal can improve control of heart failure.
- NSAIDs block the actions of ACE inhibitors and increase the risk of hyperkalaemia.
- NSAIDs reduce the excretion of methotrexate and lithium, increasing the risk of toxicity.

Safety and efficacy

- Routine monitoring is not usually required for low dosages, but the key to successful treatment with NSAIDs is appropriate patient selection.
- Measure renal function if regular treatment is required. Stop the drug if renal function deteriorates.
- Manufacturers of these drugs suggest regular measurement of liver function tests, but the predictive benefit of this has not been established.
- Blood loss due to NSAIDs can be occult and chronic. Have a low threshold for measuring a full blood count. Chronic diseases are often associated with anaemia, but ensure that it is not due to iron deficiency through blood loss.

- Advise the patient to stop the drug if they suffer severe abdominal pain. Advise them to seek immediate medical attention if they have blood in the stool or dark, tarry stools.
- Advise patients with asthma not to take NSAIDs or aspirin if they think it makes their asthma worse. Patients with nasal polyps are most at risk.

Prescribing information: **NSAIDs**

The box shows how many drugs are available; the following are given as examples.

Ibuprofen

- By mouth, anti-inflammatory dose 400 mg tds or qds. Maximum daily dose 2.4 g.

Naproxen

- By mouth, anti-inflammatory dose 0.5–1.0 g in 1 or 2 divided doses.

Diclofenac

- By mouth, anti-inflammatory dose 75–150 mg daily in 2 or 3 divided doses.
- By rectum (suppositories), 75–150 mg daily in divided doses.
- By deep intramuscular injection into the gluteal muscle, 75 mg. May be given twice daily, for a maximum of 2 days in severe pain.
  - Do not give by this route for prolonged periods; there is a risk of sterile abscess formation and rarely the Nicolau syndrome.

Indometacin

- By mouth, anti-inflammatory dose 50–200 mg daily in divided doses.

Selective cyclo-oxygenase 2 inhibitors (COX-2 inhibitors)

Selective COX-2 inhibitors
- Celecoxib
- Rofecoxib*
- Parecoxib
- Etoricoxib
- Meloxicam

* Withdrawn

Most of the properties of these drugs are the same as the other NSAIDs, but there are some important differences; these are outlined here.

Indications

NICE has given the following guidance:
- These drugs should not be used in the routine management of rheumatoid arthritis or osteoarthritis.
- COX-2 inhibitors can be used for patients who have a previous history of gastrointestinal haemorrhage or who are at high risk (see inset).
- Patients with cardiovasular disease, in whom aspirin is indicated, should not be given COX-2 inhibitors, they offer us additional benefits in these patients.
- There is no evidence to suggest that adding a gastroprotective drug (misoprostol or a proton pump inhibitor) to treatment with these drugs reduces the risk of bleeding any further.

Practical use
- These drugs have a similar efficacy to naproxen or diclofenac. They are therefore not suitable for patients who require a more potent NSAID.
- To achieve an anti-inflammatory effect theses drugs need to be given regularly.
  - A full analgesic effect is usually achieved within 1 week.
  - The full anti-inflammatory effect may take 3 weeks to develop.
- Note that meloxicam is only licensed for short-term use.
- There is no evidence that these drugs provide any protection from ischaemic heart disease. They should not be given as antiplatelet drugs. If aspirin is indicated, they are unsuitable (see above).

Adverse effects
- The risk of gastrointestinal haemorrhage is lower with these drugs, but is not zero. They may also cause nausea and dyspeptic symptoms.
- Clinical experience with these drugs is considerably more limited than for the NSAIDs. There may be adverse effects that are not fully recognized yet (see carbimazole, p. 419). Apart from the risk of gastrointestinal haemorrhage, the adverse effect profile of these drugs is very similar to conventional NSAIDs. However, rofecoxib is associated with an increased risk of cardiovascular disease; it is not yet known whether this is a class effect.

Prescribing information

The following is given as an example.
- *Celecoxib*
  - Osteoarthritis, by mouth, 200 mg daily in 1 or 2 divided doses. May be increased to 200 mg bd.
  - Rheumatoid arthritis, by mouth, 200–400 mg daily in 2 divided doses.

Codeine phosphate and dihydrocodeine

Agonists at μ opioid receptors (OP_3 receptors)

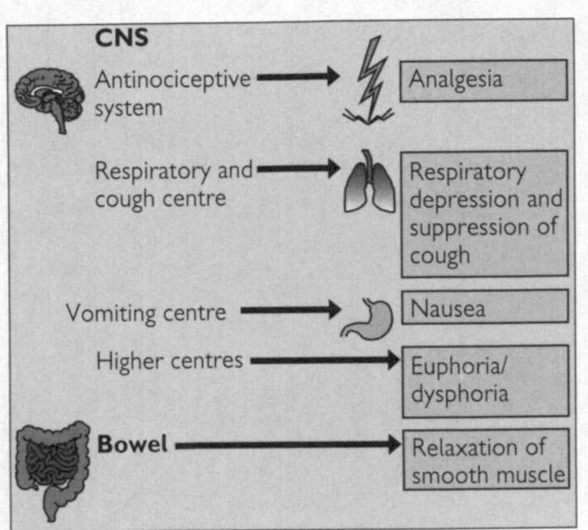

Alternative antimotility drugs

- Morphine
- Co-phenotrope
- Loperamide
- Bile salt sequestrants (e.g. colestyramine or aluminium hydroxide) for patients who have had an ileal resection or who have ileal disease.

- Relief of mild to moderate pain.
- Codeine is also used:
  - As an adjunct to rehydration in acute diarrhoea.
  - In some forms of chronic diarrhoea.
  - As a cough suppressant.
- See also opioids (p. 668).

- Avoid these drugs when there is a suspicion of acute infective diarrhoea.
- Contraindicated in active ulcerative colitis and antibiotic-associated colitis.
  - Risk of toxic dilatation of the colon.
- Can cause sputum retention; avoid in patients with bronchiectasis and chronic bronchitis.
- Avoid opioid drugs in patient with severe hepatic insufficiency; they can precipitate coma.
- These drugs have a prolonged duration of action in patients with moderate to severe renal insufficiency; reduce the dose.
- These drugs have been used during pregnancy and labour, but they depress neonatal respiration. In addition, they cause gastric stasis and so increase the risk of inhalation of stomach contents.

Analgesia

- Used alone these drugs are relatively poor analgesics. They are of greatest use when used as required in addition to regular paracetamol. See teaching point in paracetamol (p. 657).
- Codeine and dyhydrocodeine are of similar efficacy.
- These drugs are not suitable for long-term use as they are very constipating.

Diarrhoea

- See below for general advice.
- Acute diarrhoea is usually a symptom of another disease. Do not use antimotility drugs when there is any suspicion that the cause may be an infection.

- Do not use instead of rehydration.
- Codeine may be of use in chronic diarrhoea when the cause is known, but cannot be treated directly. Titrate the dose to the optimal effect; higher doses can cause nausea.

Antitussive (cough suppressant)

- Cough is usually a symptom of another disease. Do not use in patients in whom the drug might cause sputum retention.

- Excessive use can lead to bowel obstruction (both mechanical and paralytic).
  - Warn the patient to stop if bloating or distension develop.
- In overdose, may see other opioid effects (e.g. drowsiness, respiratory depression) (see p. 668).
  - These can be treated with intravenous naloxone.

- These drugs potentiate the actions of the drugs that depress the CNS (e.g. antipsychotic drugs)
- They antagonize the gastric emptying actions of domperidone and metoclopramide.

Efficacy

- Review patients' analgesia requirements regularly; titrate the dose up and down as the problem changes.
- Review patients with acute diarrhoea after a few days to ensure that the episode has resolved; if it has not resolved, review the diagnosis.

- Codeine is not a controlled drug in the UK, but it is an opioid; travellers who carry it with them may require an explanatory letter for authorities in other countries.

Prescribing information: **Codeine phosphate and dihydrocodeine**

Codeine

- Pain relief
  - By mouth or intramuscular injection, 30–60 mg every 4 hours.
  - Maximum of 240 mg daily.
- Diarrhoea
  - By mouth, 30 mg 3 or 4 times daily.
- Cough suppressant
  - By mouth as linctus (15 mg/5 mL), 5–10 mL 3 or 4 times daily.

Dihydrocodeine

- Pain relief
  - By mouth or intramuscular injection, 30 mg every 4–6 hours.
  - Increasing the dose to 60 mg may provide additional benefit, but the risk of nausea is greater.

- Codeine is available in combination with a number of other drugs, some of which are available over the counter.
    - Kaolin.
    - Ibuprofen.
    - Paracetamol.
    - Buclizine (an antihistamine).
    - Dicycloverine/dicyclomine; atropine-like antimuscarinic drug.
- Remember that these other drugs have their own therapeutic and adverse effects.

TEACHING POINT Drugs and diarrhoea

- Diarrhoea is defined as the passage of more than 300 mL of liquid faeces daily. Drugs can be used to treat diarrhoea, but they can also contribute to it.
- Identify whether the diarrhoea is acute or chronic:
    - An acute history suggests an infective cause. Widespread use of broad-spectrum antibiotics promotes the development of antibiotic-associated diarrhoea (see cephalosporins, p. 331).
    - A chronic history may represent irritable bowel syndrome, but can also be a symptom of antacid misuse.
- Is the history suggestive of a large bowel cause (typically watery, with mucus or blood) or small bowel cause (typically a pale bulky stool)?
    - For example, somatostatin analogues can be used to treat secretory diarrhoea associated with the carcinoid syndrome, but they can cause fat malabsorption, resulting in steatorrhoea.
- 'Overflow' diarrhoea can result from drugs that slow gut transit (e.g. opioid analgesics).
- In most cases, the treatment of diarrhoea is of the underlying cause. Treatment with drugs that slow gut transit is only indicated in chronic diarrhoea when the underlying cause cannot be treated. If symptomatic treatment is required consider:
    - Loperamide
    - Codeine
    - Co-phenotrope (diphenoxylate + atropine)

Opiates and non-opiate narcotic analgesics

Opiates and non-opiate narcotic analgesics

Agonists at μ opioid receptors (OP_3 receptors)

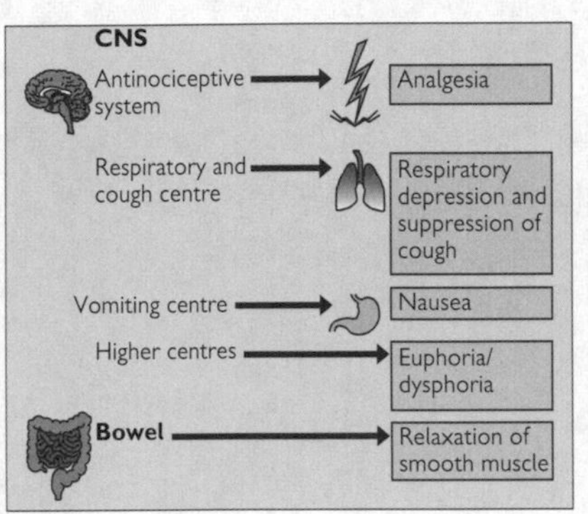

Drugs in this group

Opioids
- Morphine and diamorphine (heroin)*
- Papaveretum*
- Buprenorphine*
- Codeine and dihydrocodeine (see p. 664)

Non-opiate opioids
- Fentanyl, alfentanil, remifentanil*
- Methadone*
- Pethidine*
- Dextropropoxyphene
- Tramadol

Less commonly used
- Meptazinol
- Nalbuphine
- Oxycodone*
- Dextromoramide*
- Diphenoxylate
- Dipipanone*

*Controlled drugs

- Relief of pain.
- Particularly effective for:
  - Ischaemic pain (e.g. myocardial infarction).
  - Visceral pain (postoperative).
  - Palliative care.
- Symptomatic treatment of diarrhoea (see codeine, p. 664).

- These drugs cause respiratory depression.
  - Avoid them if the patient has acute respiratory insufficiency.
  - Avoid them if the patient has raised intracranial pressure; respiratory depression will worsen this.
  - Can cause sputum retention and thus harm in patients with bronchiectasis and chronic bronchitis.
  - Respiratory depression is not usually a problem when these drugs are used for relief of pain and the dose is titrated carefully.
- Avoid opioids in patients with severe hepatic insufficiency; they can precipitate encephalopathy.
- Opioids are contraindicated in active ulcerative colitis and antibiotic-associated colitis. There is a risk of toxic dilatation of the colon.
- Opioids have a prolonged duration of action in patients with moderate to severe renal insufficiency; reduce the dose.
- Do not give these drugs to patients with phaeochromocytoma; they can precipitate a hypertensive crisis by causing histamine release.
- Opioids can cause confusion; this is more common in elderly patients.
- Opioids are used during pregnancy and labour, but they depress neonatal respiration. In addition, they cause gastric stasis and so increase the risk of inhalation of stomach contents.

- **Opiate**—a drug that is structurally related to morphine.
- **Opioid**—any drug, opiate or non-opiate, that acts on opioid receptors.

- Most of these drugs are controlled drugs. See teaching point below for guidance on writing an out-patient or 'to-take-home' prescription.
  - In hospital you do not need to write a special prescription, but the drugs are kept in a special locked cupboard.
  - Controlled drugs must be drawn up and signed for by two authorized members of staff (usually two nurses, or a nurse and a doctor).
  - Once drawn up, the drug must be given immediately. If any drug is not used it must be disposed of immediately. Record on the drug chart the amount given to the patient.

Analgesia

- Acute severe pain.
  - Morphine is the drug of choice. Draw up 10 mg in 10 mL of water for injection. Inject slowly intravenously, 1 mg every 2 minutes, until the pain is controlled. In this way, pain is relieved rapidly without overdose.
  - Avoid giving large single doses; patients vary greatly in their requirements.
- Opioids are the mainstay of the management of postoperative pain. See paracetamol (p. 657) for the 'ladder' of analgesia. Analgesia is most effective when given early and regularly, before severe pain develops.
- Intermittent intramuscular or intravenous opioids will control pain well, but logistic issues (requires two members of staff) often delay administration of the drug. Patient-controlled analgesia (PCA) is increasingly popular, as it allows the patient a degree of control.

PCA pumps

- A PCA pump consists of a locked syringe containing (usually) 50 mg of morphine in 50 mL of isotonic (0.9%) saline, connected to a patient-activated switch.
- When the patient presses the button the pump delivers a pre-determined amount (volume) of morphine intravenously.
- The PCA pump also has a lock–out time, during which no more morphine is delivered, even if the button is pressed.
- The volume delivered by each button press and the lock–out time can be tailored to the patient's requirements. The PCA unit is locked with a key and you will need this to alter the bolus volume or lock–out time.
- Many hospitals have an acute pain team that provides advice and management, but you should familiarize yourself with the operation of these pumps in case the dose delivered is either inadequate or excessive.

- Opioids are commonly given by epidural infusion, usually in combination with local anaesthetic drugs (an unlicensed route of delivery). This is a specialized use, but you should be able to assess the adequacy of analgesia and manage adverse effects (see below).

Long-term use *(e.g. palliative care)*

- See box at end of topic.

Notes on addicts

- A special licence, issued by the Home Secretary, is required in the UK to prescribe diamorphine, dipipanone, and cocaine in the treatment of drug addiction.
- A licence is not required if an addict requires any of these drugs for clinical reasons. They may require higher doses.
- Doctors are expected to report cases of drug misuse to the National Drugs Treatment Monitoring System.

Notes on combination formulations (e.g. paracetamol plus dextropropoxyphene, co-proxamol)

- These drugs are not usually recommended, as the combination provides less flexible analgesia (see paracetamol (p. 657) for analgesic ladder), although co-codamol is widely used and is effective for postoperative pain.
- In addition, these formulations are associated with a higher incidence of fatal outcome in overdose, owing to respiratory depression from the opioid component.
- Only use a combination formulation if the patient requires both drugs regularly.

Notes on specific drugs

- Diamorphine is more soluble than morphine. This makes it easier to give in small volumes for subcutaneous administration in palliative care. However, its pharmacological properties are the same as those of morphine. The equivalent dose is about one-third to a half of that of morphine.
- Fentanyl, alfentanil, and remifentanil are used during anaesthesia. They have a rapid onset and offset of action. They have relatively few cardiovascular effects and so are commonly used for cardiac anaesthesia. Their short duration of action makes them less suitable for postoperative analgesia. Fentanyl is available as a transdermal patch for long-term analgesia.
- Methadone is used for treatment of opioid addiction. It causes less respiratory depression than other opioids, but this is dose-related; patients on opioid maintenance schemes should be monitored.
- Buprenophine is a partial agonist at opioid receptors. This means that in overdose its actions are only partially reversed by naloxone (see naloxone, p. 626).
- Dextropropoxyphene (see notes above) is less potent than codeine. It is also more likely to cause confusion in elderly people.
- Tramadol is not as effective as other opioids for severe pain.

⚠

- Opioids commonly cause nausea and vomiting. This can be reduced by giving them with an antiemetic (e.g. metoclopramide). In acute myocardial infarction the beneficial effects of morphine are partly due to the release of histamine; so do not use an antihistamine or phenothiazine drug as an antiemetic.
- Opioid effects on the bowel can lead to constipation.
  - Excessive use can lead to bowel obstruction (both mechanical and paralytic).
  - Advise the patient to take plenty of water and eat a high-fibre diet.
- Opioids can cause drowsiness and respiratory depression.
  - These can be treated with intravenous naloxone (see naloxone, p. 626).
- Opioids commonly cause itch, due to release of histamine.
- Pethidine is metabolized to norpethidine. This can accumulate in renal insufficiency and cause seizures.
- Long-term use can cause dependency, but there is no evidence that opioids cause dependency when used appropriately to control pain in palliative care.

- Opioids potentiate the actions of drugs that depress the CNS (e.g. antipsychotic drugs, alcohol).
- Opioids antagonize the gastric emptying actions of domperidone and metoclopramide.

- Pethidine can cause effects on the CNS; the risk of toxicity is increased if it is given with an SSRI or MAOI; avoid these combinations.
- Tramadol inhibits neuronal reuptake of noradrenaline and enhances serotonin release; it can interact with tricyclic antidepressant drugs and SSRIs; avoid these combinations.

Safety and efficacy

- Review patients' analgesia regularly; titrate the dose up and down as the problem changes.
  - Monitor the respiratory rate and oxygen saturation when these drugs are given acutely.
- Make sure the patient is not becoming constipated.

- Patients are often worried that they will become dependent on opioids. There is no evidence that this occurs when they are used appropriately for pain relief. Reassurance may be required.
- Advise the patient how to avoid constipation if they are taking long-term opioids
  - Avoid becoming dehydrated.
  - Include plenty of fibre in the diet.

Prescribing information: **Opioids**

There are many opioid drugs and formulations; morphine is given as an example. Suggested dosages are given in the text.

Morphine

- Oral solution
  - Oramorph® by mouth, 10 mg/5 mL (also available in other concentrations).
- Immediate-release tablets
  - Sevredol®. Tablet sizes 10 mg, 20 mg, 50 mg.
- Modified-release capsules
  - Zomorph®. Tablet sizes 10 mg, 20 mg, 30 mg, 60 mg, 100 mg, 200 mg.
  - Capsules can be opened and the drug suspended in fruit juice or yoghurt, but do not chew the granules.
- Injection
  - By intravenous or intramuscular injection: note that the dose is not the same.
  - Ampoules contain varying amounts of morphine (10–60 mg/ampoule); check carefully before drawing up.

Guidelines for starting oral morphine (e.g. in palliative care)

- The starting dose of morphine is calculated to give a greater analgesic effect than the medication already in use; for example, a dose of 5–10 mg is enough to replace a weaker analgesic (such as paracetamol or co-codamol), but 10–30 mg or more is required to replace a stronger one (e.g. morphine given by injection).
- Continue non-opioid analgesics (e.g. NSAIDs).
- Morphine should be given in the form of the oral solution or standard formulation tablets (immediate-release).
  - If the first dose of morphine is no more effective than the previous analgesic, increase the next dose by 30–50%; the aim is to choose the lowest dose that prevents pain.
  - Give the dose of morphine every 4 hours by the clock. A double dose at bedtime obviates the need to wake the patient for a dose during the night.
  - If pain occurs between regular doses of morphine ('breakthrough pain'), give additional doses of an equal amount ('rescue dose'), as required.
  - Increase the regular dose by 30–50% every 2 or 3 days until there is adequate relief throughout each 4-hour period.
- If the response is unsatisfactory, it may be necessary to add in, or substitute, an adjuvant analgesic (antidepressants or anticonvulsant drugs). Seek advice from a specialist in palliative care.
- When the pain is controlled and the patient's 24-hour morphine requirement is established, give the daily dose as two 12-hourly doses in the form of modified-release capsules (e.g. Zomorph®). Give the first dose of the modified-release morphine 4 hours after the last dose of the standard formulation.
  - Prescribe standard formulation morphine (oral solution or tablets) for breakthrough pain. A suggested dose is one-sixth of the total daily dose of modified-release morphine.

Guidelines for prescribing controlled drugs for out-patients or for patients who are going home from hospital

- To comply with legal requirements, prescriptions ordering controlled drugs must be written legibly in **INK** and **ENTIRELY** in the prescriber's own handwriting.
- The prescription must have all the following details:
  1. The name and address of the patient (written by hand, not a sticky label).
  2. The name of the formulation and strength when more than one strength is available.
  3. The type of formulation, (e.g. modified-release capsules, oral liquid, suppositories).
  4. The dose and frequency, (e.g. 10 mg bd).
  5. The total quantity to be supplied, in **words** and **figures**. This can be stated either as the number of dosage units or the total amount of controlled drug to be supplied in milligrams.
  6. The date and usual signature of the prescriber.
- For an example of a prescription for a controlled drug in the UK, see the *British National Formulary.*

Gabapentin

Neuropathic pain

Gabapentin

Structural analogue of gamma-aminobutyric acid (GABA)

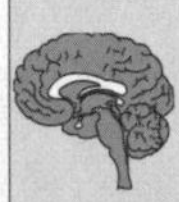

Gamma-aminobutyric acid (GABA) is an inhibitory neurotransmitter. It is likely that gabapentin exerts an anticonvulsant action by affecting GABA. However, the exact mechanism is not known. For example, it also has inhibitory effects on the neuronal transmembrane transport of amino acids and on sodium-dependent action potentials.

These actions are presumably also responsible for gabapentin's actions in the treatment of neuropathic pain.

Drugs used for neuropathic pain

This is often a very difficult condition to treat. Drug treatment should be part of a multidisciplinary approach involving physiotherapy and psychological support.

First-line
- Paracetamol (with or without an NSAID)

Second-line
- Tricyclic antidepressant drugs (e.g. amitriptyline, nortriptyline); drugs of choice but not licensed for this indication
- Gabapentin (licensed indication)
- Carbamazepine (unlicensed indication)
- Capsaicin

Third-line
- Opioids—the response is often poor; the most effective include dextropropoxyphene, tramadol, and methadone

Specialist use
- Sodium valproate
- Ketamine

- Adjunctive treatment of epilepsy.
  - For partial seizures, with or without secondary generalization unsatisfactorily controlled with other antiepileptic drugs.
- Treatment of neuropathic pain.

- Pregnancy.
  - Experience with gabapentin is limited.
  - In general, good control of epilepsy outweighs the risks from the drug.
  - Counsel women about this; seek specialist advice in women considering pregnancy.
- Gabapentin is not metabolized; there is no need to adjust the dose in patients with hepatic insufficiency.
- Gabapentin is excreted in the urine; as creatinine clearance deteriorates, so the plasma gabapentin concentration increases proportionally. Reduce the dose accordingly.

Epilepsy

- Gabapentin is given orally for the long-term control of seizures. It is not licensed for monotherapy.
  - It is not used for control of acute seizures; see benzodiazepines (p. 269) for guidance on this.
- Titration to an effective dose can progress rapidly; see prescribing section below.
- Only 10% of patients require two or more drugs to control their epilepsy.
- Avoid abrupt withdrawal of gabapentin; there is a risk of rebound seizures.
  - If the drug needs to be withdrawn, taper the dose over a period of weeks under cover of another antiepileptic drug.

Neuropathic pain

- Neuropathic pain is complex in its aetiology. Patients with troublesome neuropathic pain should be assessed by a specialist.

- The different treatment options for neuropathic pain are very different in their modes of action. Careful consideration should be given as to which may be the best for the individual patient.
- Drug treatment should form part of a multidisciplinary approach.

- Adverse effects are less common than with other antiepileptic drugs.
- CNS adverse effects include drowsiness, dizziness, sleepiness, tremor, and ataxia.
- Uncommon adverse effects include pharyngitis, weight gain, and myalgia.

- Gabapentin is not subject to many drug interactions.
  - In particular, gabapentin does not interact with other antiepileptic drugs or oral contraceptives.
- The tricyclic antidepressant drugs and mefloquine antagonize the anticonvulsant action of gabapentin; avoid these combinations.
- Antacid drugs reduce the absorption of gabapentin.

Efficacy

- Plasma concentration measurement is not used.
- Efficacy must be judged on the basis of seizure frequency and adverse effects.

Safety

- No specific monitoring is required.
- Note that gabapentin can cause a false-positive reaction with some urinary protein tests.

- Always ensure that the patient is aware of the law regarding seizures and driving (see lamotrigine, p. 261).
- Advise women of childbearing age to seek an expert opinion before trying to become pregnant.
- No treatment for neuropathic pain is 100% effective; make sure that the patient does not have unrealistic expectations of the treatment.

Prescribing information: **Gabapentin**

Adjunctive treatment of epilepsy

- Give 300 mg once on day 1.
- 300 mg twice on day 2.
- 300 mg thrice on day 3.
- Thereafter the dose can be increased, in increments of 300 mg per day (given in 3 equally divided doses).
- The maximum daily dose is 2400 mg.

Treatment of neuropathic pain

- Regimen as above, except that the maximum daily dose is 1800 mg.

Capsaicin

Counter irritant

- Capsaicin is the ingredient of peppers that makes them taste hot.
- Its exact mechanism is not fully understood, but it probably acts by depleting the neurotransmitter substance P within tissues.

Drugs used for painful neuropathies

See gabapentin, p. 674.

- Used topically for:
  - Treatment of postherpetic neuralgia (only after lesions have healed).
  - Painful neuropathy due to diabetes mellitus.
  - Osteoarthritis.

- Capsaicin can cause intense burning during initial use (especially in those with diabetic neuropathy).
- Capsaicin is only used topically; no dosage reduction is required in renal or hepatic insufficiency.
- Capsaicin is unlikely to have any systemic effect during pregnancy.
- Capsaicin is not a conventional analgesic and should not be used in place of analgesia.

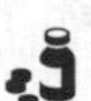

- The treatment of chronic pain is difficult. There are several treatment options. Patients with severe or persistent symptoms should be assessed by a specialist.
- Capsaicin should be applied sparingly to the affected area.
- Do not apply to broken or damaged skin.
- It must be used regularly (3 or 4 times daily) to prevent a burning sensation with every application.

- The major adverse effect of capsaicin is an intense burning sensation. This can be intolerable, but it abates during repeated administration.
- Capsaicin should not cause systemic adverse effects.

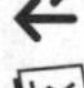

- No systemic drug interactions have been identified.

Efficacy

- Review the patient regularly. Capsaicin will usually form part of a wider strategy for the treatment of chronic pain.

- Warn the patient that this drug will initially cause a burning sensation but that this should subside with continued use.

Prescribing information: **Capsaicin**

- Capsaicin cream 0.025% or 0.075% for topical application. Apply sparingly to the affected area 3 or 4 times daily.

Lidocaine (lignocaine)

[illegible]

Local anaesthesia

[illegible]

Lidocaine (lignocaine)

Antiarrhythmic drug and local anaesthetic

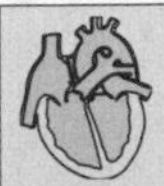

- In the Vaughan–Williams classification, lidocaine is a class Ib antiarrhythmic drug. All of these drugs have complex actions on the electrophysiology of cardiac tissue. At the simplest level, lidocaine inhibits the fast depolarizing sodium channels. The effect is to reduce the rate of depolarization, but lidocaine has less effect on the conduction velocity. The duration of the action potential is reduced, but the refractory period is reduced to a lesser extent. Overall, this increases the proportion of time the tissue is refractory.
- In the heart, the principal effect of lidocaine is on Purkinje fibres and the ventricle.
- As with all antiarrhythmic drugs, it can be difficult to correlate the electrophysiological actions with the clinical effects.
- Lidocaine is a local anaesthetic; its effect is greater on sensory rather than motor fibres.

Class I antiarrhythmic drugs

- Ia. Drugs that prolong the action potential: *quinidine, procainamide, disopyramide, propafenone*
- Ib. Drugs that shorten the action potential: *lidocaine, mexiletine, tocainide*
- Ic. Drugs that leave the action potential duration unchanged: *flecainide*

- Lidocaine is a first-line drug treatment for ventricular tachycardia, but cardioversion may be preferred.
- Lidocaine is used widely as a local anaesthetic.
- Lidocaine is occasionally used intravenously for the treatment of neuropathic pain (unlicensed, specialist use).

- The kinetics of lidocaine are altered in patients with heart failure; reduce the dose.
- Hypokalaemia (a common adverse effect of diuretics) reduces the efficacy of lidocaine and predisposes to cardiac arrhythmias. Correct hypokalaemia as a matter of urgency in patients at risk of arrhythmias.
- Avoid using lidocaine in patients with 2nd or 3rd degree heart block or sinus node disease.
- Avoid lidocaine in pregnancy. It can cause neonatal bradycardia and, after large doses, respiratory and CNS depression.
- Lidocaine penetrates the CNS; take care in patients with epilepsy.
- Reduce the dose or avoid in severe hepatic insufficiency; lidocaine is metabolized by the liver.

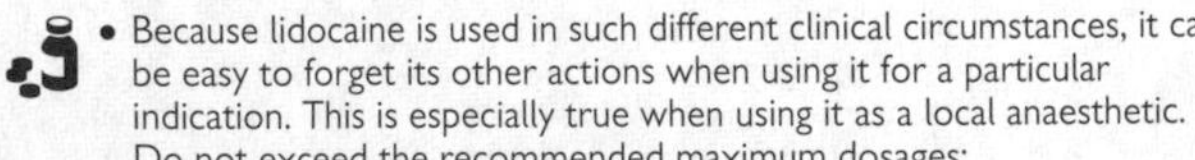

- Because lidocaine is used in such different clinical circumstances, it can be easy to forget its other actions when using it for a particular indication. This is especially true when using it as a local anaesthetic. Do not exceed the recommended maximum dosages:
  - Plain lidocaine 200 mg.
  - Lidocaine plus adrenaline (see below) 500 mg.

Local anaesthesia

- Lidocaine is available as an injection, a topical cream, a gel for urethral instillation, eye drops, and a mouth spray.
- Reduce the risk of cardiac adverse effects by reducing systemic exposure:
  - Do not inject lidocaine into inflamed or traumatized tissue.

  - Take particular care to avoid intravascular injection. Draw back on the needle before injecting.
  - Do not apply topical lidocaine to raw or inflamed skin.
  - Do not use the instillation gel if the urethra is inflamed.
- Maximal systemic concentrations are reached 30 minutes after injecting lidocaine into tissues. Make sure the patient is monitored during this period.
- Lidocaine can be used with adrenaline (which causes local vasoconstriction) to prolong its duration of action.
  - This increases the duration of lidocaine to 90 minutes.
  - The maximum dose of adrenaline that can be used is 500 micrograms.
  - Use a very dilute solution (1:200 000) of adrenaline.
  - Do not use lidocaine with adrenaline on appendages and fingers; it can cause ischaemic necrosis.
- Lidocaine is available with fluorescein as eye drops.
  - This is to provide anaesthesia during tonometry and other ocular investigations.
  - It should not be used for the relief of ocular symptoms.

Bupivacaine

- Lidocaine is limited in its usefulness, particularly after surgery, on account of its short duration of action. Bupivacaine has a longer duration of action, but takes 30 minutes to act. It is widely used in spinal and epidural anaesthesia, when this can be taken into account. Bupivacaine is available in a 'heavy' formulation for spinal anaesthesia.
- Bupivacaine has similar pharmacological effects to lidocaine, but its slow onset of action makes it an inappropriate choice as an antiarrhythmic drug.

Treatment of ventricular tachycardia

- Lidocaine is a first-line drug treatment for ventricular tachycardia. It is given initially by bolus injection of 50–100 mg.
  - This may be repeated after 10 minutes if required.
- Lidocaine has a short half-life, so its duration of action is only about 15–20 minutes. An intravenous infusion is required for a sustained action.
- Prophylactic use of lidocaine is not useful in patients with myocardial infarction (see also results of the CAST study in flecainide, p. 89).
- The rapid metabolism of lidocaine in the liver means that it does not reach the systemic circulation when given by mouth; it is not an option for long-term treatment.
- Long-term prophylaxis and treatment of ventricular arrhythmias is complex; seek specialist advice.
- The development of ventricular arrhythmias may indicate new ischaemia or other complications. Reassess the patient once the arrhythmia has been controlled.

- All drugs that block fast sodium channels can interfere with neuronal conduction in the CNS. This can cause toxicity, which occurs in up to 6% of patients given lidocaine systemically.
  - This is characterized by initial lightheadedness, followed by sedation and twitching. If severe, it can progress to seizures and coma.
- Cardiac adverse effects of lidocaine include hypotension, conduction defects, and asystole.

- Avoid using lidocaine in patients given quinupristin/dalfopristin; there is an increased risk of ventricular tachycardia.
- Take care in patients taking diuretics; hypokalaemia increases the risk of cardiac arrhythmias.

Safety and efficacy

- The patient should have continuous cardiac monitoring when lidocaine is given systemically.
- Close monitoring is also good practice when lidocaine or bupivacaine are given for spinal or epidural anaesthesia.
- Remember that hypokalaemia predisposes to cardiac arrhythmias; measure the plasma potassium concentration and correct it urgently if low.

- When using lidocaine for minor procedures, ensure that you have achieved adequate anaesthesia before you begin.
- Check with the patient that the skin is anaesthetized.

Prescribing information: **Lidocaine**

Treatment of ventricular arrhythmias

- By intravenous injection, 100 mg as a bolus over a few minutes.
- Reduce the dose to 50 mg in lighter patients or those whose circulation is severely impaired.
- Follow this with an infusion of 4 mg/minute for 30 minutes, 2 mg/minute for 2 hours, then 1 mg/minute.
- Reduce the concentration further if the infusion is continued beyond 24 hours.

Local anaesthesia

- Infiltration anaesthesia by injection according to the patient's weight and the nature of procedure.
- The maximum dose is 200 mg.
- This can be increased to 500 mg if given in solutions containing adrenaline (see notes above).

Spinal and epidural anaesthesia

- Specialist use only.

TEACHING POINT Surface anaesthesia with lidocaine for minor procedures

- Ensure that you have all the equipment you need (including specimen pots) before starting. Do not begin a procedure unless you have adequate experience.
- Decide whether plain lidocaine or lidocaine with adrenaline is appropriate. Calculate how much lidocaine you expect to use for the procedure. Take note of the maximum dosages.
- Check that you have the correct strength of lidocaine; this can range from 1% to 4%, and the vials look very similar.
- Maintain aseptic technique throughout.
- Having cleaned the skin, raise a small bleb of lidocaine under the skin to anaesthetize a small area. Use a small-gauge needle (usually orange), and warn the patient that this will sting.
- Lidocaine works quickly but not instantly; wait a minute before proceeding. Check with the patient that the area is anaesthetic.
- Use this small area as your entry point to anaesthetize the required area of skin and underlying tissues. A 21-gauge (green) needle is usually used for this; never use a needle of a larger gauge as this will traumatize the tissues.
- Insert the needle a single time and move it back and forth to deliver the lidocaine. Be systematic to ensure even and complete anaesthesia. Before injecting an area, pull back on the syringe gently to ensure that you have not entered a blood vessel. Do not keep pulling the needle in and out of the skin, as this will damage it.
- Plan to keep a small amount of lidocaine in reserve in case you discover an area that has inadequate anaesthesia.
- Again, wait a minute or two to allow the lidocaine to act before proceeding.
- Lidocaine has a limited duration of action (about 30 minutes), but this is usually more than adequate to complete a minor procedure. Do not hurry and become careless, thinking that the anaesthesia will wear off.

Drug index

Subject index

NOTE: Entries in bold indicate *medical emergencies.*